# Principles and Labs for Fitness and Wellness

**Tenth Edition**

**Werner W.K. Hoeger**
*Boise State University*

**Sharon A. Hoeger**
*Fitness & Wellness, Inc.*

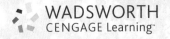

WADSWORTH
CENGAGE Learning™

Australia • Brazil • Japan • Korea • Mexico • Singapore • Spain • United Kingdom • United States

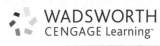
WADSWORTH
CENGAGE Learning

**Principles and Labs for Fitness and Wellness,
Tenth Edition**
Werner W.K. Hoeger, Sharon A. Hoeger

Publisher: Yolanda Cossio

Development Editor: Anna Lustig

Assistant Editor: Elesha Feldman

Editorial Assistant: Jenny Hoang

Technology Project Manager: Lauren Tarson

Marketing Manager: Tom Ziolkowski

Marketing Assistant: Elizabeth Wong

Marketing Communications Manager: Belinda Krohmer

Project Manager, Editorial Production: Trudy Brown

Creative Director: Rob Hugel

Art Director: John Walker

Print Buyer: Karen Hunt

Permissions Editor: Bob Kauser

Production Service: Graphic World Inc.

Text Designer: Riezebos Holzbaur Design Group

Photo Researcher: Pre-PressPMG

Copy Editor: Graphic World Inc.

Illustrator: Graphic World Inc.

Cover Designer: Riezebos Holzbaur Design Group

Cover Image: Jupiterimages

Compositor: Graphic World Inc.

# Brief Contents

# Contents

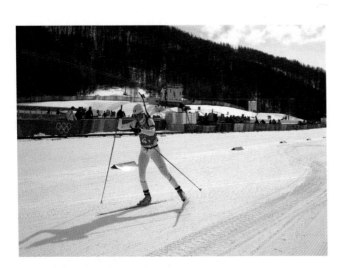

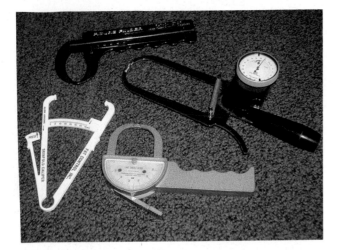

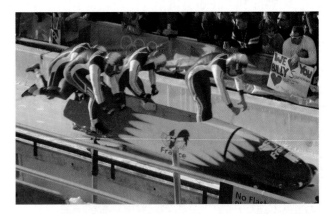

## Chapter 11

# Preventing Cardiovascular Disease 391

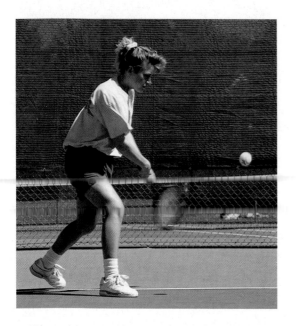

## Chapter 12

# Cancer Prevention 423

## Chapter 13

# Addictive Behavior 453

## Chapter 14

# Preventing Sexually Transmitted Infections 485

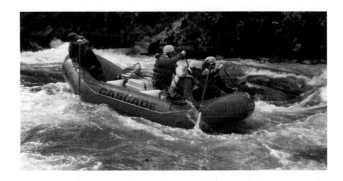

## Chapter 15
## Lifetime Fitness and Wellness 503

# Preface

The current American way of life does not provide the human with sufficient physical activity to maintain good health and improve quality of life. Actually our way of life is such a serious threat to our health that it increases the deterioration rate of the human body and leads to premature illness and mortality.

Approximately one half of the adults in the United States do not achieve the minimum recommended amount of daily physical activity, and 16 percent are not physically active at all. Yet, most people in the United States say they believe that physical activity and positive lifestyle habits promote better health, but many do not reap benefits because they simply do not know how to implement a sound fitness and wellness program that will yield the desired results.

The U.S. Surgeon General has determined that lack of physical activity is detrimental to good health. As a result, the importance of sound fitness and wellness programs has assumed an entirely new dimension. The Office of the Surgeon General has identified physical fitness as a top health priority by stating that: "The nation's top health goals as we begin the new millennium are: exercise, increased consumption of fruits and vegetables, smoking cessation, and the practice of safe sex." All four of these fundamental healthy lifestyle factors are thoroughly addressed in this book.

Furthermore, the science of behavioral therapy has established that many of the behaviors we adopt are a product of our environment. Unfortunately, we live in a "toxic" health/fitness environment. Becoming aware of how the environment affects our health is vital if we wish to achieve and maintain wellness. Yet, we are so habituated to this modern-day environment that we miss the subtle ways it influences our behaviors, personal lifestyle, and health each day.

Along with the most updated health, fitness, and nutrition guidelines, the information in this book provides extensive behavior modification strategies to help you abandon negative habits and adopt and maintain healthy behaviors. As you study and assess physical fitness and wellness parameters, you will need to take a critical look at your behaviors and lifestyle and most likely make selected permanent changes to promote overall health and wellness.

*Principles and Labs for Fitness and Wellness* contains 15 chapters and 42 laboratories (labs) that serve as a guide to implement a complete lifetime fitness and wellness program. The book contents point out the need to go beyond the basic components of fitness to achieve total well-being.

In addition to a thorough discussion on physical fitness, including all health- and skill-related components, extensive and up-to-date information is provided on behavior modification, nutrition, weight management, stress management, cardiovascular and cancer risk reduction, exercise and aging, prevention of sexually transmitted infections, and substance abuse control (including tobacco, alcohol, and other psychoactive drugs). The information has been written to provide you with the necessary tools and guidelines for an active lifestyle and a wellness way of life.

Scientific evidence has clearly shown that improving the quality—and most likely the longevity—of our lives is a matter of personal choice. As you work through the various chapters and laboratories in the book, you will be able to develop and regularly update your own healthy lifestyle program to improve physical fitness and personal wellness. The emphasis throughout the book is on teaching you how to take control of your own health and lifestyle habits so that you can make a constant and deliberate effort to stay healthy and achieve the highest potential for well-being.

## New in the Tenth Edition

The chapters in this tenth edition of *Principles and Labs for Fitness and Wellness* have been revised and updated to conform to recent advances and recommendations in the field and include new information reported in literature and at professional health and fitness, sports medicine, and physical education meetings.

Significant changes in this tenth edition include a new "FAQ" section at the start of each chapter, new study cards to help students learn key fitness and wellness concepts, and additional Behavior Modification Planning boxes in several chapters. New photography is also included throughout the textbook.

## Chapter Updates

In Chapter 1, "Physical Fitness and Wellness," all statistics related to the leading causes of death in the United States have been brought up to date according to the latest publications from the U.S. Centers for Disease Control and Prevention (CDC).

New information is also included in the 2007 guidelines of the American College of Sports Medicine (ACSM)/American Heart Association (AHA) and the 2008 federal guidelines on physical activity and public health recommendations. An update on environmental wellness and the benefits of vigorous-intensity exercise versus moderate-intensity physical activity is also provided. Basic principles to improve personal finance that will lead to "financial fitness," a typically neglected topic among college students, are also included in this opening chapter. Further guidelines on the number of steps that people take per mile, based on the most recent research available, are provided to help students determine additional walking or jogging distances required, beyond normal activities of daily living, to achieve the national recommended standard of accumulating 10,000 steps on most days of the week.

In Chapter 2, "Behavior Modification," the concept of self-efficacy, sources of self-efficacy, and the role of core values and emotions in triggering the process of behavioral change have been added to the chapter.

"Nutrition for Wellness," Chapter 3, includes extensive new information on the benefits of omega-3 fatty acids, an expanded discussion on the benefits of vitamin D, probiotics, fiber, and nutrient supplementation. A new Behavior Modification Planning box on minimizing the risk of food contamination and pesticide residues is also provided. Frequently asked questions include information on the controversy between conventional foods and organic foods, mercury in fish, the glycemic index, and the difference between antioxidants and phytonutrients.

Due to several requests, the tables to assess percent body fat according to girth measurements are again included in Chapter 4, "Body Composition." This technique is very useful to individuals who are unable to assess percent body fat through other body composition techniques.

The topic of Chapter 5, "Weight Management," includes an update on popular diet plans, information on the new diet drug Alli, a section on emotional eating, an expanded discussion on the role of strength training on resting metabolism, and activity guidelines for weight gain prevention and weight loss maintenance.

In Chapter 6, "Cardiorespiratory Endurance," a clear distinction on the benefits and differences between moderate-intensity and vigorous-intensity exercise have been updated. Although moderate-intensity exercise provides substantial health benefits, the most recent research indicates that vigorous exercise provides even greater health and fitness benefits to the participant. With this knowledge, students can decide the best approach to aerobic fitness training. A new Physical Activity Perceived Exertion (H-PAPE) scale is also introduced in this chapter. Unlike the previous scale that used phrases difficult to differentiate by participants (e.g., "very, very light" vs. "very light" vs. "fairly light"), the new scale includes intensity phrases based on common

physical activity and exercise prescription terminology (low, moderate, somewhat hard, vigorous).

An expanded discussion on strength-training principles involving number of sets, repetition maximum (RM) training zone, and rest intervals between sets is provided in Chapter 7, "Muscular Strength and Endurance." An introduction to Elastic-Band Resistive Exercise is also new to this chapter.

In Chapter 8, "Muscular Flexibility," a revision on the best time to stretch and the relationship between stretching time and injuries are addressed in the chapter.

In Chapter 9, "Skill Fitness and Fitness Programming," updated information is provided on nutrition guidelines for optimal performance and recovery following exercise. Updates were also made to several of the questions related to specific exercise considerations, and in particular the exercise guidelines for diabetics. The section on "Preparing for Sports Participation" has been expanded in this edition. A new Activity for students to update and demonstrate their competence in writing their personal comprehensive fitness program is included in the chapter.

New Behavior Modification Planning boxes and additional stress coping techniques are included in Chapter 10, "Stress Assessment and Management Techniques."

Data on the incidence and prevalence of cardiovascular diseases have been brought up to date in Chapter 11, "Preventing Cardiovascular Disease." New Behavior Modification Planning boxes have also been included to emphasize lifestyle changes students can implement to decrease their personal risk and prevent diseases of the cardiovascular system.

As with cardiovascular disease, all cancer statistics were brought up to date in Chapter 12, "Cancer Prevention." A comprehensive revision of the cancer risk questionnaire has been included in this edition. The risk factors for several cancer sites have been updated, along with healthy lifestyle recommendations to prevent cancer. New information is also included on the role of sugar in cancer risk, as well as updates on the effects of vitamin D, phytonutrients, tea, soy, and excessive body weight on cancer risk. Increased emphasis is placed on the roles of physical activity and diet in cancer prevention, the benefits of "safe sun" exposure, and additional strategies for skin cancer prevention. A new Behavior Modification Planning box on lifestyle factors that decrease cancer risk is now also provided in this chapter.

As with previous editions, a complete update on the most current trends in drug abuse according to the National Survey on Drug Use and Health (NSDUH) by the U.S. Department of Health and Human Services is included in Chapter 13, "Addictive Behavior." Trends in cigarette smoking have been brought up to date using the latest available information. Additionally, new information on the nonmedical use of prescription drugs, social consequences of alcohol abuse, and sobering statistics on the repercussions of alcohol abuse on college campuses were added to this chapter.

The most recent figures available from the Centers for Disease Control and Prevention on the prevalence of sexually transmitted infections (STIs) are included in Chapter 14, "Preventing Sexually Transmitted Infections." The guidelines for the prevention of STIs were also updated, along with current information on the health consequences of HIV infection and a revision of Lab 14A, the Self-Quiz on HIV and AIDS.

The final chapter, Chapter 15, "Lifetime Fitness and Wellness," includes updates on reliable sources of health, fitness, nutrition, wellness information, and reliable health Web sites. A new lab, Fitness and Wellness Community Resources, is also included to help students identify resources available for them to continue on the path toward lifetime fitness and wellness.

## ANCILLARIES

- **CengageNOW 1-Semester Instant Access Code**
  Get instant access to CengageNOW! This exciting online resource is a powerful new learning companion that helps students gauge their unique study needs—and provides them with a Personalized Change Plan that enhances their problem-solving skills and conceptual understanding. A click of the mouse allows students to enter and explore the system whenever they choose, with no instructor set-up necessary. The Personalized Change Plan section guides students through a behavior change process tailored specifically to their needs and personal motivation. An excellent tool to give as a project, this plan is easy to assign, track, and grade, even for large sections.

- **CengageNOW Printed Access Code** This exciting online resource is a powerful new learning companion that helps students gauge their unique study needs—and provides them with a Personalized Change Plan that enhances their problem-solving skills and conceptual understanding. A click of the mouse allows students to enter and explore the system whenever they choose, with no instructor set-up necessary. The Personalized Change Plan section guides students through a behavior change process tailored specifically to their needs and personal motivation. An excellent tool to give as a project, this plan is easy to assign, track, and grade, even for large sections.

- **Online Instructor's Manual and Test Bank** The Instructor's Manual helps instructors plan and coordinate lectures by providing detailed chapter outlines, student assignments, and ideas for incorporating the material into classroom activities and discussions. The newly expanded Test Bank includes more than 70 questions per chapter, correlated to the chapter learning objectives to ease item selection. The Instructor's Manual can be downloaded from the instructor companion website; contact your Cengage Learning representative to receive the Test Bank questions.

- **PowerLecture DVD-ROM** This teaching tool contains lecture presentations, art for PowerPoint, video clips, and resources such as the Instructor's Manual with Test Bank, all on one convenient DVD-ROM. The PowerLecture also includes JoinIn on TurningPoint content for use with Personal Response Systems. JoinIn content allows you to pose book-specific questions in class and display students' answers seamlessly within the PowerPoint slides of your lecture, in conjunction with the "clicker" hardware of your choice.

- **ExamView® Computerized Testing** Create, deliver, and customize tests and study guides (both print and online) in minutes with this easy-to-use assessment and tutorial system. ExamView offers a Quick Test Wizard that guides you step by step through the process of creating tests, while allowing you to see the test you are creating on the screen exactly as it will print or display online. You can build tests of up to 250 questions and, using ExamView's word processing capabilities, you can enter an unlimited number of questions and can edit existing questions.

- **Transparency Acetates and Correlation Chart** There are approximately 100 color transparency acetates available of charts, tables, and illustrations from the text. The correlation chart shows how the acetates are correlated with the new edition of the book.

- **Personal Daily Log** This log contains an exercise pyramid, ethnic food pyramid, time-management strategies, goal-setting worksheets, cardiorespiratory endurance and strength training forms, and much more.

- **Behavior Change Workbook** This workbook includes a brief discussion of current theories about making positive lifestyle changes, plus exercises to help students make changes in everyday life.

- **Diet Analysis Plus 9.0** Diet Analysis Plus, the market-leading online diet assessment program used by colleges and universities, allows students to create personal profiles and determine the nutritional value of the diet. The program calculates nutrition intakes, goal percentages, and actual percentages of nutrients, vitamins, and minerals, customized to the student's profile. Students can use this tool to gain an understanding of the way nutrition relates to personal health goals.

- **Testwell** This online assessment tool allows students to complete a 100-question wellness inventory related to the dimensions of wellness. Students can evaluate their nutrition, emotional health, spirituality, sexuality, physical health, self-care, safety, environmental health, occupational health, and intellectual health.

- **Careers in Health, Physical Education, and Sport** This essential manual for majors who are interested in pursuing a position in their chosen field guides them through the complicated process of picking the type of career they want to pursue. The manual also provides suggestions on how to prepare for the working world and offers information about different career paths, education requirements, and reasonable salary expectations. The supplement also describes the differences in credentials found in the field and testing requirements for certain professions.

- **Health and Wellness Resource Center at http://www.gale.com/HealthRC/index.htm** Gale's Health and Wellness Resource Center is a new, comprehensive website that provides easy-to-find answers to health questions

- **Walk4life® Elite Model Pedometer** This pedometer tracks steps, elapsed time, distance, and calories burned. Whether used as a class activity or simply to encourage students to track their steps and walk toward better fitness, this is a valuable item for everyone.

- **Web site (http://www.cengage.com/health/ hoeger/plfw10e)** When you adopt *Principles and Labs for Fitness and Wellness*, tenth edition, you and your students will have access to a rich array of teaching and learning resources that you won't find anywhere else. Resources include a downloadable study guide for students, web links, flash cards, and more.

## BRIEF AUTHOR BIOGRAPHIES

**Werner W.K. Hoeger** is the most successful fitness and wellness college textbook author. Dr. Hoeger is a full professor and director of the Human Performance Laboratory at Boise State University. He completed his undergraduate and master's degrees in physical education at the age of 20 and received his doctorate degree with an emphasis in exercise physiology at the age of 24. Dr. Werner Hoeger is a fellow of the American College of Sports Medicine. In 2002, he was recognized as the Outstanding Alumnus from the College of Health and Human Performance at Brigham Young University. He is the recipient of the 2004 Presidential Award for Research and Scholarship in the College of Education at Boise State University. In 2008, he was asked to be the keynote speaker at the VII Iberoamerican Congress of Sports Medicine and Applied Sciences in Mérida, Venezuela, and was presented with the Distinguished Guest of the City recognition.

Dr. Hoeger uses his knowledge and personal experiences to write engaging, informative books that thoroughly address today's fitness and wellness issues in a format accessible to students. He has written several textbooks for Wadsworth, Cengage Learning, including *Lifetime Physical Fitness and Wellness*, tenth edition; *Fitness and Wellness*, seventh edition; *Principles and Labs for Physical Fitness*, seventh edition; *Wellness: Guidelines for a Healthy Lifestyle*, fourth edition; and *Water Aerobics for Fitness and Wellness*, third edition (with Terry-Ann Spitzer Gibson).

He was the first author to write a college fitness textbook that incorporated the "wellness" concept. In 1986, with the release of the first edition of *Lifetime Physical Fitness and Wellness*, he introduced the principle that to truly improve fitness, health, quality of life, and achieve wellness, a person needed to go beyond the basic health-related components of physical fitness. His work was so well received that almost every fitness author immediately followed his lead in the field.

As an innovator in the field, Dr. Hoeger has developed many fitness and wellness assessment tools, including fitness tests such as the Modified Sit-and-Reach, Total Body Rotation, Shoulder Rotation, Muscular Endurance, Muscular Strength and Endurance, and Soda Pop Coordination Tests. Proving that he "practices what he preaches," at 48, he was the oldest male competitor in the 2002 Winter Olympics in Salt Lake City, Utah. He raced in the sport of luge along with his then 17-year-old son Christopher. It was the first time in Winter Olympics history that father and son competed in the same event. In 2006, at the age of 52, he was the oldest competitor at the Winter Olympics in Turin, Italy.

**Sharon A. Hoeger** is vice-president of Fitness & Wellness, Inc., of Boise, Idaho. Sharon received her degree in computer science from Brigham Young University. She is extensively involved in the research process used in retrieving the most current scientific information that goes into the revision of each textbook. She is also the author of the software that accompanies all of the fitness and wellness textbooks. Her innovations in this area since the publication of the first edition of *Lifetime Physical Fitness and Wellness* set the standard for fitness and wellness computer software used in this market today.

Sharon is a co-author in five of the seven fitness and wellness titles. Husband and wife have been jogging and strength training together for more than 31 years. They are the proud parents of five children, all of whom are involved in sports and lifetime fitness activities. Their motto: "Families that exercise together, stay together." She also served as chef de mission (head of delegation) for the Venezuelan Olympic team at the 2006 Winter Olympics in Turin, Italy.

## Acknowledgments

The authors would like to thank the reviewers of the ninth edition for their valuable contribution and suggestions to this new edition. In particular, we express gratitude to the following colleagues:

Kym Y. Atwood, *University of West Florida*

Joan C. Barch, *Lansing Community College*

Michelle Cook, *University of Northern Iowa*

Amy Howton, *Kennesaw State University*

Wayne Jacobs, *LeTourneau University*

Joe L. Jones, *Cameron University*

Connie Kunda, *Muhlenberg College*

Toni LaSala, *William Paterson University*

Karen E. McConnell, *Pacific Lutheran University*

Paul A. Smith, *McMurry University*

Deborah Varland, *Spring Arbor University*

Catherine Zubrod, *University of Northern Iowa*

We also wish to thank the following individuals for their kind help with new photography in this edition: Jonathan and Cherie Hoeger, Jorge Kleiss, Erica Gonzalez, David Gonzalez, Heather Perry, Tori Markus, Megan Perner, and Angela Hoeger.

# Physical Fitness and Wellness

1

## Objectives

- Understand the health and fitness consequences of physical inactivity
- Identify the major health problems in the United States
- Learn how to monitor daily physical activity
- Define wellness and list its dimensions
- Define physical fitness and list health-related, skill-related, and physiologic components
- State the differences between physical fitness, health promotion, and wellness
- Distinguish between health fitness standards and physical fitness standards
- Understand the benefits and significance of participating in a comprehensive wellness program
- List key national health objectives for 2010
- Identify risk factors that may interfere with safe participation in exercise
- Learn to assess resting heart rate and blood pressure

Chronicle your daily activities using the exercise log. Determine the safety of exercise participation using the health history questionnaire. Check your understanding of the chapter contents by logging on to CengageNOW and accessing the pre-test, personalized learning plan, and post-test for this chapter.

# FAQ

**Why should I take a fitness and wellness course?**

Most people go to college to learn how to make a living, but a fitness and wellness course will teach you how to *live*—how to truly live life to its fullest potential. Some people seem to think that success is measured by how much money they make. Making a good living will not help you unless you live a wellness lifestyle that will allow you to enjoy what you earn. You may want to ask yourself: Of what value is a nice income, a beautiful home, and a solid retirement portfolio if at age 45 I suffer a massive heart attack that will seriously limit my physical capacity or end life itself?

**Will the attainment of good physical fitness be sufficient to ensure good health?**

Regular participation in a sound physical fitness program will provide substantial health benefits and significantly decrease the risk of many chronic diseases. And while good fitness often motivates toward adoption of additional positive lifestyle behaviors, to maximize the benefits for a healthier, more productive, happier, and longer life we have to pay attention to all seven dimensions of wellness: physical, social, mental, emotional, occupational, environmental, and spiritual. These dimensions are interrelated, and one frequently affects the other. A wellness way of life requires a constant and deliberate effort to stay healthy and achieve the highest potential for well-being within all dimensions of wellness.

**If a person is going to do only one thing to improve health, what would it be?**

This is a common question. It is a mistake to think, though, that you can modify just one factor and enjoy wellness. Wellness requires a constant and deliberate effort to change unhealthy behaviors and reinforce healthy behaviors. While it is difficult to work on many lifestyle changes all at once, being involved in a regular physical activity program and proper nutrition are two behaviors I would work on first. Others should follow, depending on your lifestyle.

Movement and physical activity are basic functions that the human organism evolved to perform with vigor and proficiency. Modern-day technology, however, has almost completely eliminated the necessity for physical exertion in daily life. Physical activity is no longer a natural part of our existence. We live in an automated society, where most of the activities that used to require strenuous exertion can be accomplished by machines with the simple pull of a handle or push of a button.

Research findings in the last three decades have clearly shown that physical inactivity and a negative lifestyle seriously threaten health and hasten the deterioration rate of the human body. Most of the world's industrialized nations are experiencing an epidemic of physical inactivity. In the United States, physical inactivity is the second greatest threat to public health and has been termed **Sedentary Death Syndrome** or **SeDS** (the number-one threat is tobacco use—the largest cause of preventable deaths).

Widespread interest in **health** and preventive medicine in recent years, nonetheless, is motivating people to participate in organized fitness and wellness programs. The growing number of participants is attributed primarily to scientific evidence linking regular physical activity and positive lifestyle habits to better health, longevity, quality of life, and overall well-being.

At the beginning of the 20th century, **life expectancy** for a child born in the United States was only 47 years. The most common health problems in the Western world were infectious diseases, such as tuberculosis, diphtheria, influenza, kidney disease, polio, and other diseases of infancy. Progress in the medical field largely eliminated these diseases. Then, as more people started to enjoy the "good life" (sedentary living, alcohol, fatty foods, excessive sweets, tobacco, drugs), we saw a parallel increase in the incidence of **chronic diseases** such as cardiovascular disease, cancer, diabetes, and chronic respiratory diseases (see Figure 1.1). According to the World Health Organization (WHO), chronic diseases account for 60 percent of all deaths worldwide.[1]

As the incidence of chronic diseases climbed, we recognized that prevention was the best medicine. Consequently, a fitness and wellness movement developed gradually in the 1980s. People began to realize that good health was mostly self-controlled and that the leading causes of premature death and illness could be prevented by adhering to positive lifestyle habits. We all desire to live a long life, and wellness programs seek to enhance the overall quality of life—for as long as we live.

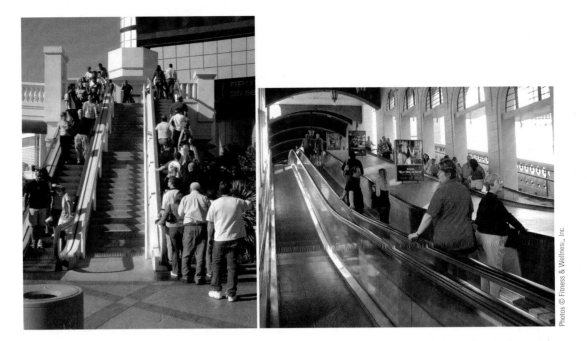
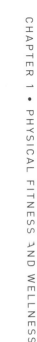

Modern-day conveniences lull people into a sedentary lifestyle.

**FIGURE 1.1 Causes of deaths in the United States for selected years.**

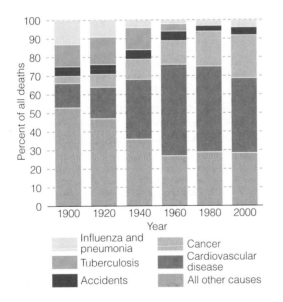

*Source:* National Center for Health Statistics, Division of Vital Statistics.

**FIGURE 1.2 Factors that determine our health and longevity.**

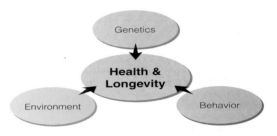

# Life Expectancy Versus Healthy Life Expectancy

Based on 2008 government data, the average life expectancy in the United States is 75.4 years for men and 80.7 years for women. The WHO, however, has calculated

There are three basic factors that determine our health and longevity: genetics, the environment, and our behavior (see Figure 1.2). Although we cannot change our genetic pool, we can exert control over the environment and our health behaviors so that we may reach our full physical potential based on our own genetic code. How we accomplish this goal will be thoroughly discussed through the chapters of this book.

**Sedentary Death Syndrome (SeDS)** Cause of deaths attributed to a lack of regular physical activity.

**Health** A state of complete well-being—not just the absence of disease or infirmity.

**Life expectancy** Number of years a person is expected to live based on the person's birth year.

**Chronic diseases** Illnesses that develop as a result of an unhealthy lifestyle and last a long time.

**healthy life expectancy (HLE)** estimates for 191 nations. HLE is obtained by subtracting the years of ill health from total life expectancy. The United States ranked 24th in this report, with an HLE of 70 years; Japan was first with an HLE of 74.5 years (see Figure 1.3). This finding was a major surprise, given the status of the United States as a developed country with one of the best medical care systems in the world. The rating indicates that Americans die earlier and spend more time disabled than people in most other advanced countries. The WHO points to several factors that may account for this unexpected finding:

1. The extremely poor health of some groups, such as Native Americans, rural African Americans, and the inner-city poor. Their health status is more characteristic of a poor developing nation than a rich industrialized country.

2. The epidemic of human immunodeficiency virus (HIV), which causes more deaths and disability in the United States than in other developed nations

3. The high incidence of tobacco use

4. The high incidence of coronary heart disease

5. Fairly high levels of violence, notably homicides, compared with other developed countries

Although life expectancy in the United States gradually increased by 30 years over the last century, scientists from the National Institute of Aging believe that in the coming decades the average lifespan may decrease by as much as 5 years. This decrease in life expectancy will be related primarily to the growing epidemic of obesity. According to estimates from the Centers for Disease Control and Prevention, more than 34 percent of the adult population in the United States is obese. Additional information on the obesity epidemic and its detrimental health consequences is given in Chapter 5.

# Leading Health Problems in the United States

The leading causes of death in the United States today are largely lifestyle related (see Figure 1.4). The U.S. Surgeon General stated that in 2008, 7 of 10 Americans died of preventable chronic diseases such as heart disease, many forms of cancer, and diabetes.[2] Specifically, about 60 percent of all deaths in the United States are caused by cardiovascular disease and cancer.[3] Almost 80 percent of the latter deaths could be prevented through a healthy lifestyle program. The third and fourth leading causes of death, respectively, are chronic lower respiratory disease (CLRD) and accidents.

The most prevalent degenerative diseases in the United States are those of the cardiovascular system. Thirty-five percent of all deaths in this country are attributed to diseases of the heart and blood vessels. According to the American Heart Association (AHA), 80.7 million people in the United States are afflicted with diseases of the cardiovascular system, including 73 million with hypertension

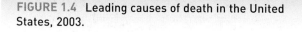

**FIGURE 1.3** Healthy life expectancy for selected countries.

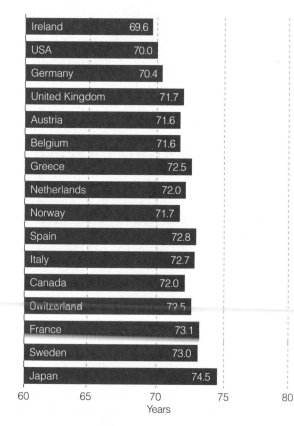

| Country | Years |
|---|---|
| Ireland | 69.6 |
| USA | 70.0 |
| Germany | 70.4 |
| United Kingdom | 71.7 |
| Austria | 71.6 |
| Belgium | 71.6 |
| Greece | 72.5 |
| Netherlands | 72.0 |
| Norway | 71.7 |
| Spain | 72.8 |
| Italy | 72.7 |
| Canada | 72.0 |
| Switzerland | 72.5 |
| France | 73.1 |
| Sweden | 73.0 |
| Japan | 74.5 |

*Source:* World Health Organization, http://www.who.int/inf-pr-2000/en/pr2000-life.html. Retrieved June 4, 2000.

**FIGURE 1.4** Leading causes of death in the United States, 2003.

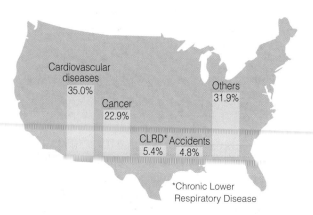

Cardiovascular diseases 35.0%
Cancer 22.9%
Others 31.9%
CLRD* 5.4%
Accidents 4.8%
*Chronic Lower Respiratory Disease

*Source:* U.S. Department of Health and Human Services, Centers for Disease Control and Prevention, National Center for Health Statistics, National Vital Statistics reports, *Deaths: Preliminary Data for 2003,* 56:10 (April 24, 2008).

(high blood pressure) and 16 million with coronary heart disease. (Many of these people have more than one type of cardiovascular disease.) About 1.2 million people have heart attacks each year, and nearly 500,000 of them die as a result. The estimated cost of heart and blood vessel disease in 2008 exceeded $448 billion.[4] A complete cardiovascular disease prevention program is outlined in Chapter 11.

The second leading cause of death in the United States is cancer. Even though cancer is not the number-one killer, it is the number-one health fear of the American people. Almost 23 percent of all deaths in the United States are attributable to cancer. More than 565,650 people died from this disease in 2008, and an estimated 1,437,180 new cases were reported the same year.[5] The major contributor to the increase in the incidence of cancer during the last five decades is lung cancer, of which 87 percent is caused by tobacco use. Furthermore, smoking accounts for more than 30 percent of all deaths from cancer. Another 33 percent of deaths are related to nutrition, physical inactivity, excessive body weight, and other faulty lifestyle habits.

The American Cancer Society maintains that the most influential factor in fighting cancer today is prevention through health education programs. Evidence indicates that as much as 80 percent of all human cancer can be prevented through positive lifestyle behaviors. A comprehensive cancer-prevention program is presented in Chapter 12.

The third leading cause of death, CLRD, is a general category that includes chronic obstructive pulmonary disease, emphysema, and chronic bronchitis (all diseases of the respiratory system). Although CLRD is related mostly to tobacco use (see Chapter 13 for discussion on how to stop smoking), lifetime nonsmokers also can develop CLRD. Precautions to prevent CLRD include:[6]

1. Consuming a low-fat, low-sodium, nutrient-dense diet (similar to a cardio- and cancer-protective diet)
2. Staying physically active
3. Not smoking and staying clear of cigarette smoke
4. Avoiding swimming pools, for individuals sensitive to chlorine vapor
5. Getting a pneumonia vaccine if over age 50 and a current or ex-smoker

Accidents are the fourth leading cause of death. Even though not all accidents are preventable, many are. Fatal accidents are often related to abusing drugs and not wearing seat belts.

Most people do not perceive accidents as a health problem. Even so, accidents affect the total well-being of millions of Americans each year. Accident prevention and personal safety are part of a health enhancement program aimed at achieving a better quality of life. Proper nutrition, exercise, stress management, and abstinence from cigarette smoking are of little help if the person is involved in a disabling or fatal accident as a result of distraction, a single reckless decision, or not wearing seat belts properly.

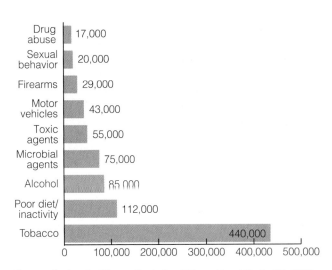

**FIGURE 1.5** Underlying causes of death in the United States, 2000.

*Source:* Centers for Disease Control and Prevention, Atlanta, GA, 2005.

Accidents do not just happen. We cause accidents, and we are victims of accidents. Although some factors in life, such as earthquakes, tornadoes, and airplane accidents, are completely beyond our control, more often than not, personal safety and accident prevention are a matter of common sense. Most accidents stem from poor judgment and confused mental states, which occur when people are upset, are not paying attention to the task at hand, or are abusing alcohol or other drugs.

Alcohol abuse is the number-one cause of all accidents. About half of accidental deaths and suicides in the United States are alcohol related. Further, alcohol intoxication is the leading cause of fatal automobile accidents. Other commonly abused drugs alter feelings and perceptions, generate mental confusion, and impair judgment and coordination, greatly enhancing the risk for accidental **morbidity** and mortality (see Chapter 13).

The underlying causes of death in the United States (see Figure 1.5) indicate that eight of the nine causes are related to lifestyle and lack of common sense. Of the approximately 2.4 million yearly deaths in the United States, the "big three"—tobacco use, poor diet and inactivity, and alcohol abuse—are responsible for about 637,000 deaths each year.

**Lifestyle as a Health Problem** As the incidence of chronic diseases rose, it became obvious that prevention was—and remains—the best medicine. Accord-

**Healthy life expectancy (HLE)** Number of years a person is expected to live in good health; this number is obtained by subtracting ill-health years from the overall life expectancy.

**Morbidity** A condition related to or caused by illness or disease.

**FIGURE 1.6** Factors that affect health and well-being.

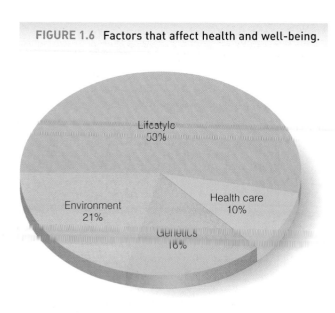

Lifestyle
53%

Environment
21%

Health care
10%

Genetics
16%

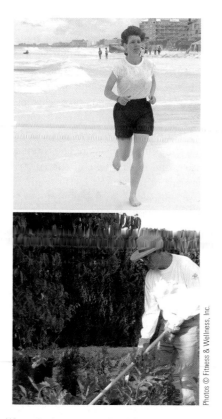

An active lifestyle increases health, quality of life, and longevity.

ing to Dr. David Satcher, former U.S. Surgeon General, more than half of the people who die in this country each year die because of what they do. Based on estimates, more than half of disease is lifestyle related, a fifth is attributed to the environment, and a tenth is influenced by the health care that the individual receives. Only 16 percent is related to genetic factors (see Figure 1.6). Thus, the individual controls as much as 84 percent of his or her vulnerability to disease—and thus quality of life. The same data indicate that 83 percent of deaths before age 65 are preventable. In essence, most people in the United States are threatened by the very lives they lead today.

Because of the unhealthy lifestyles that many young adults lead, their bodies may be middle-aged or older! Many physical education programs do not emphasize the skills necessary for youth to maintain a high level of fitness and health throughout life. The intent of this book is to provide those skills and help to prepare you for a lifetime of physical fitness and wellness. A healthy lifestyle is self-controlled, and you can learn how to be responsible for your own health and fitness. Healthy choices made today influence health for decades.

# Physical Activity and Exercise Defined

Abundant scientific research over the past three decades has established a distinction between physical activity and exercise. **Physical activity** is bodily movement produced by skeletal muscles. It requires energy expenditure and produces progressive health benefits. Physical activity typically requires only a low to moderate intensity of effort. Examples of physical activity include walking to and from work, taking the stairs instead of elevators and escalators, gardening, doing household chores, dancing, and washing the car by hand. Physical inactivity, by contrast, implies a level of activity that is lower than that required to maintain good health.

**Exercise** is a type of physical activity that requires planned, structured, and repetitive bodily movement to improve or maintain one or more components of physical fitness. Examples of exercise are walking, running, cycling, aerobics, swimming, and strength training. Exercise is usually viewed as an activity that requires a high-intensity effort.

## 2007 ACSM/AHA Physical Activity and Public Health Recommendations
In August 2007, the American College of Sports Medicine (ACSM) and the AHA released a joint statement on physical activity recommendations for healthy adults.[7] These recommendations were issued to update and clarify the previous recommendations issued in 1995 and to help clarify the 1996 landmark report by the U.S. Surgeon General on physical activity and health.[8]

The updated recommendations by the ACSM and AHA indicate that to promote and maintain good health, all healthy adults between 18 and 65 years of age need:

1. Moderate-intensity aerobic physical activity for a minimum of 30 minutes five days a week or vigorous-intensity aerobic physical activity for a minimum of 20 minutes three days a week. The 30 minutes of moderate-intensity activity can be achieved by accumulating aerobic bouts of activity that last at least 10 minutes each. The aerobic activity recommendation is

in addition to light-intensity routine activities of daily living such as casual walking, self-care, shopping, or those lasting less than 10 minutes in duration.

2. Activities that maintain or increase muscular strength and endurance a minimum of two days per week on nonconsecutive days. Eight to 10 exercises should be performed that include a resistance (weight) that will be heavy enough to provide substantial fatigue after 8 to 12 repetitions of each exercise.

The ACSM/AHA report further states that a greater amount of physical activity, to exceed the minimum recommendations given, will provide even greater benefits and is recommended for individuals who wish to further improve personal fitness, reduce the risk for chronic disease and disabilities, prevent premature mortality, or prevent unhealthy weight gain.

A combination of moderate- and vigorous-intensity activities can be used to meet the aerobic activity recommendation. That is, a person could participate in moderate-intensity activity twice a week for 30 minutes and vigorous-intensity activity for 20 minutes on another two days. Moderate intensity activity is defined as the equivalent of a brisk walk that noticeably increases the heart rate. Vigorous-intensity activity is described as an activity similar to jogging that causes rapid breathing and a substantial increase in heart rate.

The report also states that only 49.1 percent of the U.S. adult population meets the recommendations. College graduates are more likely to adhere to the recommendations (about 53 percent of them), followed by individuals with some college education, then high school graduates; and the least likely to meet the recommendations are those with less than a high school diploma (37.8 percent).

In conjunction with the report, the ACSM and the American Medical Association (AMA) have launched a new nationwide *Exercise Is Medicine* program.[9] The goal of this initiative is to help improve the health and wellness of the nation through exercise prescriptions from physicians and health-care providers: "Exercise is medicine and it's free." All physicians should be prescribing exercise to all patients and participate in exercise themselves. Exercise is considered to be the much needed vaccine of our time to prevent chronic diseases. Physical activity and exercise are powerful tools for both the treatment and the prevention of chronic diseases and premature death.

## 2008 Federal Guidelines for Physical Activity

Because of the importance of physical activity to our health, in October 2008, the U.S. Department of Health and Human Services issued federal *Physical Activity Guidelines for Americans* for the first time. These guidelines complement the *Dietary Guidelines for Americans* published in 2005 (see Chapter 3, pages 108–110) and further substantiate the ACSM/AHA recommendations. These documents provide science-based guidance on the importance of being physically active and eating a healthy diet to promote health and reduce the risk of chronic diseases. The guidelines were developed by an advisory committee appointed by the secretary of Health and Human Services. This advisory committee conducted an extensive analysis of the scientific information on physical activity and health and issued the following recommendations:[10]

Adults between 18 and 64 years of age
- Adults should do 2 hours and 30 minutes a week of moderate-intensity aerobic (cardiorespiratory) physical activity, 1 hour and 15 minutes (75 minutes) a week of vigorous-intensity aerobic physical activity, or an equivalent combination of moderate- and vigorous-intensity aerobic physical activity (also see Chapter 6). Aerobic activity should be performed in episodes of at least 10 minutes, preferably spread throughout the week.
- Additional health benefits are provided by increasing to 5 hours (300 minutes) a week of moderate-intensity aerobic physical activity, 2 hours and 30 minutes a week of vigorous-intensity physical activity, or an equivalent combination of both.
- Adults should also do muscle-strengthening activities that involve all major muscle groups, performed on 2 or more days per week.

Older adults (ages 65 and older)
- Older adults should follow the adult guidelines. If this is not possible due to limiting chronic conditions, older adults should be as physically active as their abilities allow. They should avoid inactivity. Older adults should do exercises that maintain or improve balance if they are at risk of falling.

Children 6 years of age and older and adolescents
- Children and adolescents should do 1 hour (60 minutes) or more of physical activity every day.
- Most of the 1 hour or more a day should be either moderate- or vigorous-intensity aerobic physical activity.
- As part of their daily physical activity, children and adolescents should do vigorous-intensity activity on at least 3 days per week. They also should do muscle-strengthening and bone-strengthening activities on at least 3 days per week.

Pregnant and postpartum women
- Healthy women who are not already doing vigorous-intensity physical activity should get at least 2 hours and 30 minutes (150 minutes) of moderate-intensity aerobic activity a week. Preferably, this activity should be spread throughout the week. Women who regularly

Physical activity Bodily movement produced by skeletal muscles; requires expenditure of energy and produces progressive health benefits. Examples include walking, taking the stairs, dancing, gardening, yard work, house cleaning, snow shoveling, washing the car, and all forms of structured exercise.

Exercise A type of physical activity that requires planned, structured, and repetitive bodily movement with the intent of improving or maintaining one or more components of physical fitness.

**TABLE 1.1** Physical Activity Guidelines

| Benefits | Duration | Intensity | Frequency per Week | Weekly Time |
|---|---|---|---|---|
| Health | 30 min | MI* | ≥5 times | ≥150 min |
| Health and fitness | ≥20 min | VI* | ≥3 times | ≥ 75 min |
| Health, fitness, and weight gain prevention | 60 min | MI/VI† | 5–7 times | >300 min |
| Health, fitness, and weight regain prevention | 60–90 min | MI/VI | 5–7 times | ≥450 min |

*MI = moderate intensity, VI = vigorous intensity
†MI/VI = You may use MI or VI or a combination of the two

## Health Benefits of Physical Activity: A Review of the Strength of the Scientific Evidence

### For adults and older adults

There is strong evidence that physical activity:

Lowers the risk of

- early death
- heart disease
- stroke
- type 2 diabetes
- high blood pressure
- adverse blood lipid profile
- metabolic syndrome
- colon and breast cancers

Helps

- prevent weight gain
- with weight loss when combined with diet
- improve cardiorespiratory and muscular fitness
- prevent falls
- reduce depression
- improve cognitive function in older adults

There is moderate to strong evidence that physical activity:

Improves functional health in older adults

Reduces abdominal obesity

Helps maintain weight after weight loss

Lowers the risk of hip fracture

Increases bone density

Improves sleep quality

Lowers the risk of lung and endometrial cancers

***Source:*** U.S. Department of Health and Human Services, *2008 Physical Activity Guidelines for Americans. www.health.gov/ paguidelines.* Downloaded October 15, 2008.

engage in vigorous-intensity aerobic activity or high amounts of activity can continue their activity provided that their condition remains unchanged and they talk to their health-care provider about their activity level throughout their pregnancy.

## Importance of Increased Physical Activity

The U.S. Surgeon General has stated that poor health as a result of lack of physical activity is a serious public health problem that must be met head-on at once. Regular **moderate physical activity** provides substantial benefits in health and well-being for the vast majority of people who are not physically active. For those who are already moderately active, even greater health benefits can be achieved by increasing the level of physical activity.

Among the benefits of regular physical activity and exercise are significantly reduced risks for developing or dying from heart disease, stroke, type 2 diabetes, colon and breast cancers, high blood pressure, and osteoporotic fractures.[11] Regular physical activity also is important for the health of muscles, bones, and joints, and it seems to reduce symptoms of depression and anxiety, improve mood, and enhance one's ability to perform daily tasks throughout life. It also can help control health-care costs and maintain a high quality of life into old age.

Moderate physical activity has been defined as any activity that requires an energy expenditure of 150 calories per day, or 1,000 calories per week. The general health recommendation is that people strive to accumulate at least 30 minutes of physical activity a minimum of five days per week (see Table 1.1). Whereas 30 minutes of continuous activity is preferred, on days when time is limited, three activity sessions of at least 10 minutes each provide about half the aerobic benefits. Examples of moderate physical activity are walking, cycling, playing basketball or volleyball, swimming, doing water aerobics, dancing fast, pushing a stroller, raking leaves, shoveling snow, washing or waxing a car, washing windows or floors, and even gardening.

Because of the ever growing epidemic of obesity in the United States, a 2002 guideline by American and Canadian scientists from the Institute of Medicine of the National Academy of Sciences increased the recommendation to 60 minutes of moderate-intensity physical activity every day.[12] This recommendation was based on evidence indicating that people who maintain healthy weight typically accumulate one hour of daily physical activity.

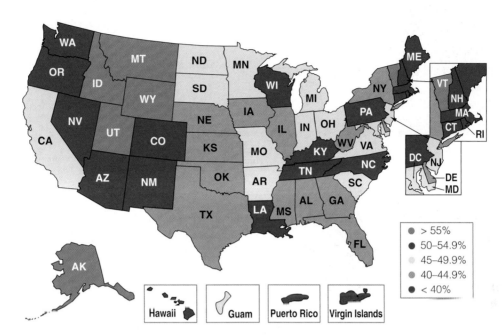

**FIGURE 1.7** Prevalence of recommended physical activity in the United States, 2003.

Legend:
- > 55%
- 50–54.9%
- 45–49.9%
- 40–44.9%
- < 40%

*Note:* Recommended physical activity is moderate-intensity physical activity at least 5 days a week for 30 minutes a day, or vigorous-intensity physical activity 3 days a week for 20 minutes a day.
*Source:* Centers for Disease Control and Prevention, Atlanta, 2005.

Subsequently, the 2005 Dietary Guidelines for Americans released by the U.S. Department of Health and Human Services and the Department of Agriculture recommend that up to 60 minutes of moderate- to vigorous-intensity physical activity per day may be necessary to prevent weight gain, and between 60 and 90 minutes of moderate-intensity physical activity daily is recommended to sustain weight loss for previously significantly overweight people.[13]

In sum, although health benefits are derived with 30 minutes per day, people with a tendency to gain weight need to be physically active daily for an hour to an hour and a half to prevent weight gain. And 60 to 90 minutes of activity per day provides additional health benefits, including a lower risk for cardiovascular disease and diabetes.

## Critical Thinking

Do you consciously incorporate physical activity into your daily lifestyle? Can you provide examples? Do you think you get sufficient daily physical activity to maintain good health?

**Monitoring Daily Physical Activity** According to the Centers for Disease Control and Prevention, the majority of U.S. adults are not sufficiently physically active to promote good health. The data indicate that only

49 percent of adults meet the minimal recommendation of 30 minutes of moderate physical activity at least five days per week, 25 percent report no leisure physical activity at all, and 16 percent are completely inactive (less than 10 minutes per week of moderate- or vigorous-intensity physical activity). The prevalence of physical activity by state in the United States is displayed in Figure 1.7.

Other than carefully monitoring actual time engaged in activity, an excellent tool to monitor daily physical activity is a **pedometer.** A pedometer is a small mechanical device that senses vertical body motion and counts footsteps. Wearing a pedometer throughout the day allows you to determine the total steps you take that day. Some pedometers also record distance, calories burned, speeds, and actual time of activity each day. A pedometer is a great motivational tool to help increase, maintain, and monitor daily physical activity that involves lower-body motion (walking, jogging, running). The use of pedometers most likely will increase in the next few years to help promote and quantify daily physical activity.

Before purchasing a pedometer, be sure to verify its accuracy. Many of the free and low-cost pedometers provided

**Moderate physical activity** Activity that uses 150 calories of energy per day, or 1,000 calories per week.

**Pedometer** An electronic device that senses body motion and counts footsteps. Some pedometers also record distance, calories burned, speeds, "aerobic steps," and time spent being physically active.

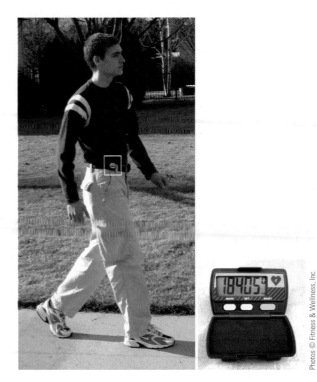

Photos © Fitness & Wellness, Inc.

Pedometers are used to monitor daily physical activity; the recommendation is a minimum of 10,000 steps per day.

by corporations for promotion and advertisement purposes are inaccurate, so their use is discouraged. Pedometers also tend to lose accuracy at a very slow walking speed (slower than 30 minutes per mile) because the vertical movement of the hip is too small to trigger the spring-mounted lever arm inside the pedometer to properly record the steps taken.

You can obtain a good pedometer for about $25, and ratings are available online. The most accurate pedometer brands are Walk4Life, Yamax, Kenz, and New Lifestyles. To test the accuracy of a pedometer, follow these steps: Clip the pedometer on the waist directly above the kneecap, reset the pedometer to zero, carefully close the pedometer, walk exactly 50 steps at your normal pace, carefully open the pedometer, and look at the number of steps recorded. A reading within 10 percent of the actual steps taken (45 to 55 steps) is acceptable.

In the United States, men typically take about 6,000 steps per day, in comparison with women, who take about 5,300 steps. The general recommendation for adults is 10,000 steps per day. Table 1.2 provides specific activity categories based on the number of daily steps taken.

All daily steps count, but some of your steps should come in bouts of at least 10 minutes, so as to meet the national physical activity recommendation of accumulating 30 minutes of moderate-intensity physical activity in at least three 10-minute sessions five days per week. A 10-minute brisk walk (a distance of about 1,200 yards at a pace of 15 minutes per mile) is approximately 1,300 steps. A 15-minute-mile walk (1,770 yards) is about 1,900 steps.[14] Thus, new pedometer brands have an "aero-

## TABLE 1.2 Adult Activity Levels Based on Total Number of Steps Taken per Day

| Steps per Day | Category |
|---|---|
| <5,000 | Sedentary Lifestyle |
| 5,000–7,499 | Low Active |
| 7,500–9,999 | Somewhat Active |
| 10,000–12,499 | Active |
| ≥12,500 | Highly Active |

*Source:* C. Tudor-Locke and D. R. Basset, "How many steps/day are enough? Preliminary pedometer indices for public health," *Sports Medicine* 34 (2004): 1–8.

bic steps" function that records steps taken in excess of 60 steps per minute over a 10-minute period of time.

If you do not accumulate the recommended 10,000 daily steps, you can refer to Table 1.3 to determine the additional walking or jogging distance required to reach your goal. For example, if you are 5'8" tall and male and you typically accumulate 5,200 steps per day, you would need an additional 4,800 daily steps to reach your 10,000-steps goal. You can do so by jogging 3 miles at a 10-minute-per-mile pace (1,602 steps × 3 miles = 4,806 steps) on some days, and you can walk 2.5 miles at a 15-minute-per-mile pace (1,908 steps × 2.5 miles = 4,770 steps) on other days. If you do not find a particular speed (pace) that you typically walk or jog at in Table 1.3, you can estimate the number of steps at that speed using the prediction equations at the bottom of the table.

The first practical application that you can undertake in this course is to determine your current level of daily activity. The log provided in Lab 1A will help you do this. Keep a four-day log of all physical activities you do daily. Record the time of day, type and duration of the exercise/activity, and, if possible, steps taken while engaged in the activity. The results will indicate how active you are and serve as a basis to monitor changes in the next few months and years.

# Wellness

Most people recognize that participating in fitness programs improves their quality of life. At the end of the 20th century, however, we came to realize that physical fitness alone was not always sufficient to lower the risk for disease and ensure better health. For example, individuals who run three miles (about 5 km) a day, lift weights regularly, participate in stretching exercises, and watch their body weight might be easily classified as having good or excellent fitness. Offsetting these good habits, however, might be **risk factors,** including high blood pressure, smoking, excessive stress, drinking too much alcohol, and eating too many foods high in saturated fat. These factors place people at risk for cardiovascular disease and other chronic diseases of which they may not be aware.

**TABLE 1.3** Estimated Number of Steps to Walk or Jog a Mile Based on Gender, Height, and Pace

| | Pace (min/mile) | | | | | | | |
|---|---|---|---|---|---|---|---|---|
| | Walking | | | | Jogging | | | |
| Height | 20 | 18 | 16 | 15 | 12 | 10 | 8 | 6 |
| **Women** | | | | | | | | |
| 5'0" | 2,371 | 2,244 | 2,117 | 2,054 | 1,997 | 1,710 | 1,423 | 1,136 |
| 5'2" | 2,343 | 2,216 | 2,089 | 2,026 | 1,970 | 1,683 | 1,396 | 1,109 |
| 5'4" | 2,315 | 2,188 | 2,061 | 1,998 | 1,943 | 1,656 | 1,369 | 1,082 |
| 5'6" | 2,286 | 2,160 | 2,033 | 1,969 | 1,916 | 1,629 | 1,342 | 1,055 |
| 5'8" | 2,258 | 2,131 | 2,005 | 1,941 | 1,889 | 1,602 | 1,315 | 1,028 |
| 5'10" | 2,230 | 2,103 | 1,976 | 1,913 | 1,862 | 1,575 | 1,288 | 1,001 |
| 6'0" | 2,202 | 2,075 | 1,948 | 1,885 | 1,835 | 1,548 | 1,261 | 974 |
| 6'2" | 2,174 | 2,047 | 1,920 | 1,857 | 1,808 | 1,521 | 1,234 | 947 |
| **Men** | | | | | | | | |
| 5'2" | 2,310 | 2,183 | 2,056 | 1,993 | 1,970 | 1,683 | 1,396 | 1,109 |
| 5'4" | 2,282 | 2,155 | 2,028 | 1,965 | 1,943 | 1,656 | 1,369 | 1,082 |
| 5'6" | 2,253 | 2,127 | 2,000 | 1,937 | 1,916 | 1,629 | 1,342 | 1,055 |
| 5'8" | 2,225 | 2,098 | 1,872 | 1,908 | 1,889 | 1,602 | 1,315 | 1,028 |
| 5'10" | 2,197 | 2,070 | 1,943 | 1,880 | 1,862 | 1,575 | 1,288 | 1,001 |
| 6'0" | 2,169 | 2,042 | 1,915 | 1,852 | 1,835 | 1,548 | 1,261 | 974 |
| 6'2" | 2,141 | 2,014 | 1,887 | 1,824 | 1,808 | 1,521 | 1,234 | 947 |
| 6'4" | 2,112 | 1,986 | 1,859 | 1,795 | 1,781 | 1,494 | 1,207 | 920 |

Prediction Equations (pace in min/mile and height in inches):
Walking
Women: Steps/mile = 1,949 + [(63.4 × pace) − (14.1 × height)]
Men: Steps/mile = 1,916 + [(63.4 × pace) − (14.1 × height)]
Running
Women and Men: Steps/mile = 1,084 + [(143.6 × pace) − (13.5 × height)]
**Source:** Werner W. K. Hoeger et al., "One- mile step count at walking and running speeds." *ACSM's Health & Fitness Journal,* Vol 12(1):14–19, 2008.

Even though most people are aware of their unhealthy behaviors, they seem satisfied with life as long as they are free from symptoms of disease or illness. They do not contemplate change until they incur a major health problem. Nevertheless, present lifestyle habits dictate the health and well-being of tomorrow.

Good health no longer is viewed as simply the absence of illness. The notion of good health has evolved considerably in the last few years and continues to change as scientists learn more about lifestyle factors that bring on illness and affect wellness. Furthermore, once the idea took hold that fitness by itself would not always decrease the risk for disease and ensure better health, **health promotion** programs and the **wellness** concept followed.

Wellness implies a constant and deliberate effort to stay healthy and achieve the highest potential for well-being. Wellness requires implementing positive lifestyle habits to change behavior and thereby improve health and quality of life, prolong life, and achieve total well-being. Living a wellness way of life is a personal choice,

but you may need additional support to achieve wellness goals. Thus, health promotion programs have been developed to educate people regarding healthy lifestyles and provide the necessary support to achieve wellness.

For example, you may be prepared to initiate an aerobic exercise program, but if you are not familiar with exercise prescription guidelines or places to exercise safely, or if you lack peer support or flexible scheduling to do so,

**Risk factors** Lifestyle and genetic variables that may lead to disease.

**Health promotion** The science and art of enabling people to increase control over their lifestyles to move toward a state of wellness.

**Wellness** The constant and deliberate effort to stay healthy and achieve the highest potential for well-being. It encompasses seven dimensions—physical, emotional, mental, social, environmental, occupational, and spiritual—and integrates them all into a quality life.

**FIGURE 1.8** Dimensions of wellness.

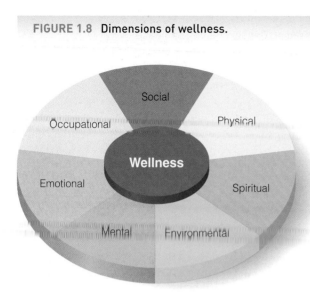

you may have difficulty accomplishing your goal. Similarly, if you want to quit smoking but do not know how to do it and everyone else around you smokes, the chances for success are limited. To some extent, the environment limits your choices. Hence, the availability of a health promotion program would provide the much-needed support to get started and implement a wellness way of life.

**The Seven Dimensions of Wellness** Wellness has seven dimensions: physical, emotional, mental, social, environmental, occupational, and spiritual (see Figure 1.8). These dimensions are interrelated: One frequently affects the others. For example, a person who is emotionally "down" often has no desire to exercise, study, socialize with friends, or attend church, and he or she may be more susceptible to illness and disease.

The seven dimensions of wellness show how the concept clearly goes beyond the absence of disease. Wellness incorporates factors such as adequate fitness, proper nutrition, stress management, disease prevention, spirituality, not smoking or abusing drugs, personal safety, regular physical examinations, health education, and environmental support.

For a wellness way of life, individuals must be physically fit and manifest no signs of disease, and they also must be free of risk factors for disease (such as hyperten-

sion, hyperlipidemia, cigarette smoking, negative stress, faulty nutrition, careless sex). The relationship between adequate fitness and wellness is illustrated in the continuum in Figure 1.9. Even though an individual tested in a fitness center may demonstrate adequate or even excellent fitness, indulging in unhealthy lifestyle behaviors will still increase the risk for chronic diseases and diminish the person's well-being.

**Physical Wellness** **Physical wellness** is the dimension most commonly associated with being healthy. It entails confidence and optimism about one's ability to protect physical health and take care of health problems.

Physically well individuals are physically active, exercise regularly, eat a well balanced diet, maintain recommended body weight, get sufficient sleep, practice safe sex, minimize exposure to environmental contaminants, avoid harmful drugs (including tobacco and excessive alcohol), and seek medical care and exams as needed. Physically well people also exhibit good cardiorespiratory endurance, adequate muscular strength and flexibility, proper body composition, and the ability to carry out ordinary and unusual demands of daily life safely and effectively.

**Emotional Wellness** **Emotional wellness** involves the ability to understand your own feelings, accept your limitations, and achieve emotional stability. Furthermore, it implies the ability to express emotions appropriately, adjust to change, cope with stress in a healthy way, and enjoy life despite its occasional disappointments and frustrations.

Emotional wellness brings with it a certain stability, an ability to look both success and failure squarely in the face and keep moving along a predetermined course. When success is evident, the emotionally well person radiates the expected joy and confidence. When failure seems evident, the emotionally well person responds by making the best of circumstances and moving beyond the failure. Wellness enables you to move ahead with optimism and energy instead of spending time and talent worrying about failure. You learn from it, identify ways to avoid it in the future, and then go on with the business at hand.

Emotional wellness also involves happiness—an emotional anchor that gives meaning and joy to life. Happiness is a long-term state of mind that permeates the various facets of life and influences our outlook. Although there is no simple recipe for creating happiness, research-

**FIGURE 1.9** Wellness continuum.

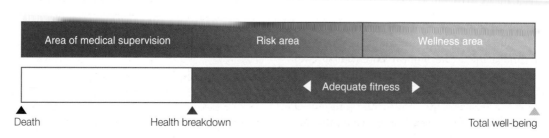

| Area of medical supervision | Risk area | Wellness area |
| --- | --- | --- |

◀ Adequate fitness ▶

Death  Health breakdown  Total well-being

ers agree that happy people are usually participants in some category of a supportive family unit where they feel loved. Healthy, happy people enjoy friends, work hard at something fulfilling, get plenty of exercise, and enjoy play and leisure time. They know how to laugh, and they laugh often. They give of themselves freely to others and seem to have found deep meaning in life.

An attitude of true happiness signals freedom from the tension and depression that many people endure. Emotionally well people are obviously subject to the same kinds of depression and unhappiness that occasionally plague us all, but the difference lies in the ability to bounce back. Well people take minor setbacks in stride and have the ability to enjoy life despite it all. They don't waste energy or time recounting the situation, wondering how they could have changed it, or dwelling on the past.

## Mental Wellness

**Mental wellness**, also referred to as intellectual wellness, implies that you can apply the things you have learned, create opportunities to learn more, and engage your mind in lively interaction with the world around you. When you are mentally well, you are not intimidated by facts and figures with which you are unfamiliar, but you embrace the chance to learn something new. Your confidence and enthusiasm enable you to approach any learning situation with eagerness that leads to success.

Mental wellness brings with it vision and promise. More than anything else, mentally well people are open-minded and accepting of others. Instead of being threatened by people who are different from themselves, they show respect and curiosity without feeling they have to conform. They are faithful to their own ideas and philosophies and allow others the same privilege. Their self-confidence guarantees that they can take their place among others in the world without having to give up part of themselves and without requiring others to do the same.

## Social Wellness

**Social wellness,** with its accompanying positive self-image, endows you with the ease and confidence to be outgoing, friendly, and affectionate toward others. Social wellness involves a concern for oneself and also an interest in humanity and the environment as a whole.

One of the hallmarks of social wellness is the ability to relate to others and to reach out to other people, both within one's family and outside it. Similar to emotional wellness, it involves being comfortable with your emotions and thus helps you understand and accept the emotions of others. Your own balance and sense of self allow you to extend respect and tolerance to others. Healthy people are honest and loyal. This dimension of wellness leads to the ability to maintain close relationships with other people.

## Environmental Wellness

**Environmental wellness** refers to the effect that our surroundings have on our well-being. Our planet is a delicate **ecosystem,** and its health depends on the continuous recycling of its elements. Environmental wellness implies a lifestyle that maximizes harmony with the earth and takes action to protect the world around us.

Environmental threats include air pollution, chemicals, ultraviolet radiation in the sunlight, water and food contamination, secondhand smoke, noise, inadequate shelter, unsatisfactory work conditions, lack of personal safety, and unhealthy relationships. Health is affected negatively when we live in a polluted, toxic, unkind, and unsafe environment.

Unfortunately, a national survey of first-year college students showed that less than 20 percent were concerned about the health of the environment.[15] To enjoy environmental wellness, we are responsible for educating and protecting ourselves against environmental hazards and also protecting the environment so that we, our children, and future generations can enjoy a safe and clean environment.

Steps that you can take to live an environmentally conscious life include conserving energy (walk to your destination or ride on public transportation, do not drive unless absolutely necessary, turn off lights and computers when not in use); not littering and politely asking others not to do it either; recycling as much as possible (paper, glass, cans, plastics, cardboard); conserving paper and water (take shorter showers, don't let the water run while brushing your teeth); not polluting the air, water, or earth if you can avoid doing so; not smoking; planting trees and keeping plants and shrubs alive; evaluating purchases and conveniences based on their environmental impact; donating old clothes to Goodwill, veterans' groups, or other charities; and enjoying, appreciating, and spending time outdoors in natural settings.

## Occupational Wellness

**Occupational wellness** is not tied to high salary, prestigious position, or extravagant working conditions. Any job can bring occupational wellness if it provides rewards that are important to the individual. To one person, salary might be the most important factor, whereas another might place much greater value on creativity. Those who are occupationally well have their own "ideal" job, which allows them to thrive.

---

**Physical wellness** Good physical fitness and confidence in your personal ability to take care of health problems.

**Emotional wellness** The ability to understand your own feelings, accept your limitations, and achieve emotional stability.

**Mental wellness** A state in which your mind is engaged in lively interaction with the world around you.

**Social wellness** The ability to relate well to others, both within and outside the family unit.

**Environmental wellness** The capability to live in a clean and safe environment that is not detrimental to health.

**Ecosystem** A community of organisms interacting with each other in an environment.

**Occupational wellness** The ability to perform your job skillfully and effectively under conditions that provide personal and team satisfaction and adequately reward each individual.

People with occupational wellness face demands on the job, but they also have some say over demands placed on them. Any job has routine demands, but in occupational wellness, routine demands are mixed with new, unpredictable challenges that keep a job exciting. Occupationally well people are able to maximize their existing skills and have the opportunity to broaden them or gain new ones. Their occupation offers the opportunity for advancement and recognition for achievement. Occupational wellness encourages collaboration and interaction among co-workers, which fosters a sense of teamwork and support.

## Spiritual Wellness

**Spiritual wellness** provides a unifying power that integrates all dimensions of wellness. Basic characteristics of spiritual people include a sense of meaning and direction in life and a relationship to a higher being. Pursuing these avenues may lead to personal freedom, including prayer, faith, love, closeness to others, peace, joy, fulfillment, and altruism.

Several studies have reported positive relationships among spiritual well-being, emotional well-being, and satisfaction with life. People who attend church and regularly participate in religious organizations enjoy better health, have a lower incidence of chronic diseases, handle stress more effectively, and apparently live longer.[16]

**Prayer** is a signpost of our spirituality, at the core of most spiritual experiences. It is communication with a higher power. At least 200 studies have been conducted on the effects of prayer on health. About two-thirds of these studies have linked prayer to positive health outcomes—as long as these prayers are offered with sincerity, humility, love, empathy, and compassion. Some studies have shown faster healing time and fewer complications in patients who didn't even know they were being prayed for, compared with patients who were not prayed for.[17]

**Altruism,** a key attribute of spiritual people, seems to enhance health and longevity. Studies indicate that people who regularly volunteer live longer. Research has found that health benefits of altruism are so powerful that doing good for others is good for oneself, especially for the immune system.

The relationship between spirituality and wellness is meaningful in our quest for a better quality of life. As with the other dimensions, development of the spiritual dimension to its fullest potential contributes to wellness. Wellness requires a balance among all of its seven dimensions.

## Critical Thinking

Now that you understand the seven dimensions of wellness, rank them in order of importance to you and explain your rationale in doing so.

# Wellness, Fitness, and Longevity

During the second half of the 20th century, scientists began to realize the importance of good fitness and improved lifestyle in the fight against chronic diseases, particularly those of the cardiovascular system. Because of more participation in wellness programs, cardiovascular mortality rates dropped. The decline began in about 1963, and between 1960 and 2000 the incidence of cardiovascular disease dropped by 26 percent, according to national vital statistics from the Centers for Disease Control and Prevention. This decrease is credited to higher levels of wellness and better health care in the United States. More than half of the decline is attributed specifically to improved diet and reduction in smoking.

Furthermore, several studies showed an inverse relationship between physical activity and premature mortality rates. The first major study in this area was conducted among 16,936 Harvard alumni linking physical activity habits and mortality rates.[18] As the amount of weekly physical activity increased, the risk of cardiovascular deaths decreased. The largest decrease in cardiovascular deaths was observed among alumni who used more than 2,000 calories per week through physical activity.

A landmark study subsequently conducted at the Aerobics Research Institute in Dallas upheld the findings of the Harvard alumni study.[19] Based on data from 13,344 people followed over an average of eight years, the study revealed a graded and consistent inverse relationship between physical activity levels and mortality, regardless of age and other risk factors. As illustrated in Figure 1.10, the higher the level of physical activity, the longer the lifespan. The death rate during the eight-year study from all causes for the least-fit men was 3.4 times higher than that of the most-fit men. For the least-fit women, the death rate was 4.6 times higher than that of most-fit women.

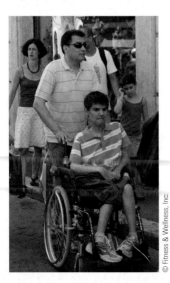

Altruism enhances health and well-being.

© Fitness & Wellness, Inc.

FIGURE 1.10 Death rates by physical fitness groups.

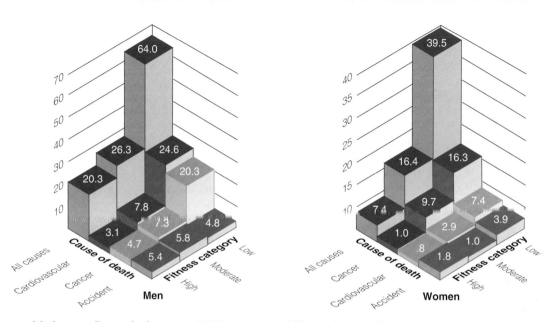

Numbers on top of the bats are all-cause death rates per 10,000 person-years of follow up for each cell, 1 person-year indicates one person who was followed up one year later.
***Source:*** Based on data from S. N. Blair, H. W. Kohl III, R. S. Paffenbarger, Jr., D. G. Clark, K. H. Cooper, and L. W. Gibbons, "Physical fitness and all-cause mortality: a prospective study of healthy men and women," *Journal of the American Medical Association* 262 (1989): 2395–2401.

This study also reported a greatly reduced rate of premature death, even at moderate fitness levels that most adults can achieve easily. The participants attained more protection by combining higher fitness levels with reduction in other risk factors such as hypertension, serum cholesterol, cigarette smoking, and excessive body fat.

A subsequent five-year follow-up study at this institute on fitness and mortality found a substantial (44 percent) reduction in mortality risk when people abandoned a **sedentary** lifestyle and became moderately fit.[20] The lowest death rate was found in people who were fit at the start of the study and remained fit; the highest death rate was found in men who were unfit at the beginning of the study and remained unfit. The results of these studies indicate that fitness improves wellness, quality of life, and longevity.

While it is clear that moderate-intensity exercise does provide substantial health benefits, research data also show a dose-response relationship between physical activity and health. That is, greater health and fitness benefits occur at higher duration and/or intensity of physical activity. **Vigorous activity** and longer duration are preferable to the extent of one's capabilities because they are most clearly associated with better health and longer life.

Vigorous-intensity exercise seems to provide the best benefits.[21] As compared with prolonged moderate-intensity activity, vigorous intensity has been shown to provide the best improvements in aerobic capacity, coronary heart disease risk reduction, and overall cardiovascular health.[22]

A recent comprehensive review of research studies found a lower rate of heart disease in vigorous-intensity exercisers compared with those who exercised at moderate intensity.[23] While no differences were found in weight loss between the two groups, greater improvements are seen in cardiovascular risk factors in the vigorous-intensity groups, including aerobic fitness, blood pressure, and blood glucose control.

A word of caution, however, is in order. Vigorous exercise should be reserved for healthy individuals who have been cleared to do so (see Lab 1C) and who have been participating regularly in at least moderate-intensity activities.

Since the release of the aforementioned landmark studies, scientific research continues on the benefits of regular physical activity and exercise. Almost universally,

**Spiritual wellness** The sense that life is meaningful, that life has purpose, and that some power brings all humanity together; the ethics, values, and morals that guide you and give meaning and direction to life.

**Prayer** Sincere and humble communication with a higher power.

**Altruism** Unselfish concern for the welfare of others.

**Sedentary** Description of a person who is relatively inactive and whose lifestyle is characterized by a lot of sitting.

**Vigorous activity** Any exercise that requires a MET level equal to or greater than 6 METs (21 mL/kg/min). 1 MET is the energy expenditure at rest, 3.5 mL/kg/min, and METs are defined as multiples of this resting metabolic rate (examples of activities that require a 6-MET level include aerobics, walking uphill at 3.5 mph, cycling at 10 to 12 mph, playing doubles in tennis, and vigorous strength training).

the results confirm the benefits of physical activity and exercise on health, longevity, and quality of life. The benefits are so impressive that researchers and sports medicine leaders state that if the benefits of exercise could be packaged in a pill, it would be the most widely prescribed medication throughout the world today.

# Types of Physical Fitness

As the fitness concept grew at the end of the last century, it became clear that several specific components contribute to an individual's overall level of fitness. **Physical fitness** is classified into health-related, skill-related, and physiologic fitness.

1. **Health-related fitness** is the ability to perform activities of daily living without undue fatigue and is conducive to a low risk for premature **hypokinetic diseases.**[24] Health-related fitness components are cardiorespiratory (aerobic) endurance, muscular strength and endurance, muscular flexibility, and body composition (see Figure 1.11).

2. **Skill-related fitness** components consist of agility, balance, coordination, reaction time, speed, and power (see Figure 1.12). These components are related primarily to successful sports and motor skill performance and may not be as crucial to better health.

3. **Physiologic fitness** is a term used primarily in the field of medicine in reference to biological systems that are affected by physical activity and the role the latter plays in preventing disease. The components of physiologic fitness are **metabolic fitness, morphologic fitness,** and **bone integrity** (see Figure 1.13).[25]

Critical Thinking

What role do the four health-related components of physical fitness play in your life? Rank them in order of importance to you and explain the rationale you used.

**FIGURE 1.11 Health-related components of physical fitness.**

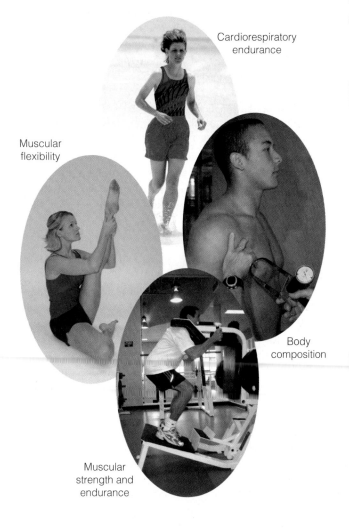

Cardiorespiratory endurance

Muscular flexibility

Body composition

Muscular strength and endurance

**Fitness Standards: Health Versus Physical Fitness** A meaningful debate regarding age- and gender-related fitness standards has resulted in two stan-

**FIGURE 1.12 Motor skill–related components of physical fitness.**

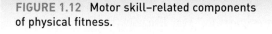

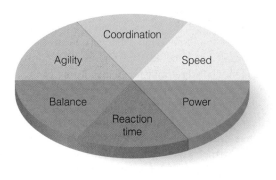

Coordination

Agility

Speed

Balance

Power

Reaction time

**FIGURE 1.13 Components of physiologic fitness.**

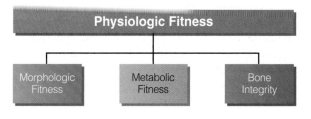

Physiologic Fitness

Morphologic Fitness

Metabolic Fitness

Bone Integrity

FIGURE 1.14  Health and fitness benefits based on the type of lifestyle and physical activity program.

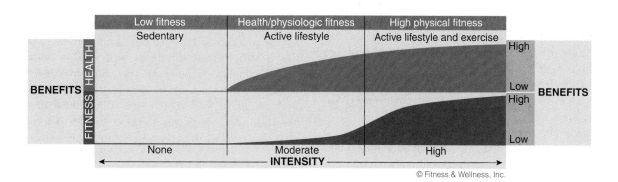

© Fitness & Wellness, Inc.

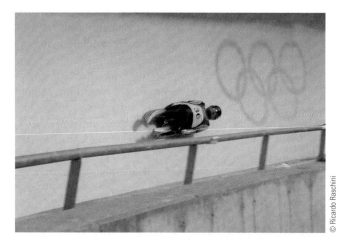

Good health-fitness and skill-related fitness are required to participate in highly skilled activities.

© Ricardo Raschini

dards: health fitness (also referred to as *criterion referenced*) and physical fitness. Following are definitions of both. The assessment of health-related fitness is presented in Chapters 4, 6, 7, and 8; where appropriate, physical fitness standards are included for comparison.

## Health Fitness Standards
The **health fitness standards** proposed here are based on data linking minimum fitness values to disease prevention and health. Attaining the health fitness standard requires only moderate physical activity. For example, a 2-mile walk in less than 30 minutes, five or six times a week, seems to be sufficient to achieve the health-fitness standard for cardiorespiratory endurance.

As illustrated in Figure 1.14, significant health benefits can be reaped with such a program, although fitness improvements, expressed in terms of maximum oxygen uptake, or $VO_{2max}$ (explained next and in Chapter 6), are not as notable. Nevertheless, health improvements are quite striking. These benefits include reduction in blood lipids, lower blood pressure, weight loss, stress release, less risk for diabetes, and lower risk for disease and premature mortality.

More specifically, improvements in the **metabolic profile** (measured by insulin sensitivity, glucose tolerance, and improved cholesterol levels) can be notable despite little or no weight loss or improvement in aerobic capacity. Physiologic and metabolic fitness can be attained through an active lifestyle and moderate-intensity physical activity.

An assessment of health-related fitness uses **cardiorespiratory endurance**, measured in terms of the

**Physical fitness** The ability to meet the ordinary as well as the unusual demands of daily life safely and effectively without being overly fatigued and still have energy left for leisure and recreational activities.

**Health-related fitness** Fitness programs that are prescribed to improve the individual's overall health.

**Hypokinetic diseases** "Hypo" denotes "lack of"; "kinetic" denotes "motion"; therefore, illnesses related to lack of physical activity.

**Skill-related fitness** Fitness components important for success in skillful activities and athletic events; encompasses agility, balance, coordination, power, reaction time, and speed.

**Physiologic fitness** A term used primarily in the field of medicine in reference to biological systems affected by physical activity and the role of activity in preventing disease.

**Metabolic fitness** A component of physiologic fitness that denotes reduction in the risk for diabetes and cardiovascular disease through a moderate-intensity exercise program in spite of little or no improvement in cardiorespiratory fitness.

**Morphologic fitness** A component of physiologic fitness used in reference to body composition factors such as percent body fat, body fat distribution, and body circumference.

**Bone integrity** A component of physiologic fitness used to determine risk for osteoporosis based on bone mineral density.

**Health fitness standards** The lowest fitness requirements for maintaining good health, decreasing the risk for chronic diseases, and lowering the incidence of muscular-skeletal injuries.

**Metabolic profile** A measurement of plasma insulin, glucose, lipid, and lipoprotein levels to assess risk for diabetes and cardiovascular disease.

**Cardiorespiratory endurance** The ability of the lungs, heart, and blood vessels to deliver adequate amounts of oxygen to the cells to meet the demands of prolonged physical activity.

maximal amount of oxygen the body is able to utilize per minute of physical activity ($VO_{2max}$)—essentially, a measure of how efficiently the heart, lungs, and muscles can operate during aerobic exercise (see Chapter 6). $VO_{2max}$ is commonly expressed in milliliters (mL) of oxygen (volume of oxygen) per kilogram (kg) of body weight per minute (mL/kg/min). Individual values can range from about 10 mL/kg/min in cardiac patients to more than 80 mL/kg/min in world-class runners, cyclists, and cross-country skiers.

Research data from the study presented in Figure 1.10 reported that achieving $VO_{2max}$ values of 35 and 32.5 mL/kg/min for men and women, respectively, may be sufficient to lower the risk for all-cause mortality significantly. Although greater improvements in fitness yield a lower risk for premature death, the largest drop is seen between the least fit and the moderately fit. Therefore, the 35 and 32.5 mL/kg/min values could be selected as the health fitness standards.

## Physical Fitness Standards

**Physical fitness standards** are set higher than health fitness standards and require a more intense exercise program. Physically fit people of all ages have the freedom to enjoy most of life's daily and recreational activities to their fullest potentials. Current health fitness standards may not be enough to achieve these objectives.

Sound physical fitness gives the individual a degree of independence throughout life that many people in the United States no longer enjoy. Most adults should be able to carry out activities similar to those they conducted in their youth, though not with the same intensity. These standards do not require being a championship athlete, but activities such as changing a tire, chopping wood, climbing several flights of stairs, playing basketball, mountain biking, playing soccer with children or grandchildren, walking several miles around a lake, and hiking through a national park do require more than the current "average fitness" level in the United States.

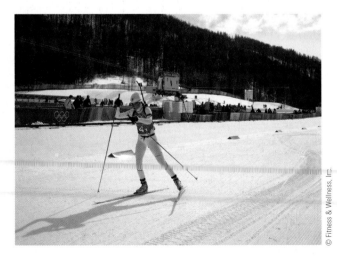

© Fitness & Wellness, Inc.

Individuals who wish to participate in vigorous fitness activities should train to achieve the high physical fitness standard.

# Which Program Is Best?

Your own personal objectives will determine the fitness program you decide to use. If the main objective of your fitness program is to lower the risk for disease, attaining the health fitness standards will provide substantial health benefits. If, however, you want to participate in vigorous fitness activities, achieving a high physical fitness standard is recommended. This book gives both health fitness and physical fitness standards for each fitness test so you can personalize your approach.

## Benefits of a Comprehensive Wellness Program

An inspiring story illustrating what fitness can do for a person's health and well-being is that of George Snell from Sandy, Utah. At age 45, Snell weighed approximately 400 pounds, his blood pressure was 220/180, he was blind because of undiagnosed diabetes, and his blood glucose level was 487.

Snell had determined to do something about his physical and medical condition, so he started a walking/jogging program. After about 8 months of conditioning, he had lost almost 200 pounds, his eyesight had returned, his glucose level was down to 67, and he was taken off medication. Just 2 months later—less than 10 months after beginning his personal exercise program—he completed a marathon, a running course of 26.2 miles!

## Health Benefits

Most people exercise because it improves their personal appearance and makes them feel good about themselves. Although many benefits accrue from participating in a regular fitness and wellness program, and active people generally live longer, the greatest benefit of all is that physically fit individuals enjoy a better quality of life. These people live life to its fullest, with fewer health problems than inactive individuals (who also may indulge in other negative lifestyle behaviors). Although compiling an all-inclusive list of the benefits reaped from participating in a fitness and wellness program is difficult, the following list summarizes many of them. A fitness and wellness program:

- Improves and strengthens the cardiorespiratory system
- Maintains better muscle tone, muscular strength, and endurance
- Improves muscular flexibility
- Enhances athletic performance
- Helps maintain recommended body weight
- Helps preserve lean body tissue
- Increases resting metabolic rate
- Improves the body's ability to use fat during physical activity
- Improves posture and physical appearance
- Improves functioning of the immune system
- Lowers the risk for chronic diseases and illness (such as cardiovascular diseases and cancer)
- Decreases the mortality rate from chronic diseases

- Thins the blood so it doesn't clot as readily (thereby decreasing the risk for coronary heart disease and strokes)
- Helps the body manage cholesterol levels more effectively
- Prevents or delays the development of high blood pressure and lowers blood pressure in people with hypertension
- Helps prevent and control diabetes
- Helps achieve peak bone mass in young adults and maintain bone mass later in life, thereby decreasing the risk for osteoporosis
- Helps people sleep better
- Helps prevent chronic back pain
- Relieves tension and helps in coping with life stresses
- Raises levels of energy and job productivity
- Extends longevity and slows the aging process
- Promotes psychological well-being, including higher morale, self-image, and self-esteem
- Reduces feelings of depression and anxiety
- Encourages positive lifestyle changes (improving nutrition, quitting smoking, controlling alcohol and drug use)
- Speeds recovery time following physical exertion
- Speeds recovery following injury or disease
- Regulates and improves overall body functions
- Improves physical stamina and counteracts chronic fatigue
- Helps to maintain independent living, especially in older adults
- Enhances quality of life: People feel better and live a healthier and happier life.

**Economic Benefits** Sedentary living can have a strong impact on a nation's economy. As the need for physical exertion in Western countries decreased steadily during the last century, health-care expenditures increased dramatically. Health-care costs in the United States rose from $12 billion in 1950 to more than $2 trillion in 2006 (see Figure 1.15), or about 16 percent of the gross domestic product (GDP). In 1980, health-care costs represented 8.8 percent of the GDP and are projected to reach about 20 percent by 2015.

In terms of yearly health-care costs per person, U.S. citizens spend more than any other industrialized nation. In 2006, U.S. health-care costs per capita were about $7,026; they are expected to reach almost $9,000 in 2010. Yet, overall, the U.S. health-care system ranks only 37th in the world.

One of the reasons for the low overall ranking is the overemphasis on state-of-the-art cures instead of prevention programs. The United States is the best place in the world to treat people once they are sick, but the system does a poor job of keeping people healthy in the first place. Ninety-five percent of our health-care dollars are spent on treatment strategies, and less than 5 percent is spent on prevention. Another factor is that the United States fails to provide good health care for

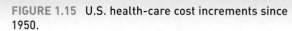

**FIGURE 1.15 U.S. health-care cost increments since 1950.**

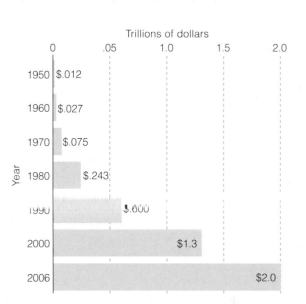

all: More than 44 million residents do not have health insurance.

Unhealthy behaviors also contribute to the staggering U.S. health-care costs. Risk factors for disease such as obesity and smoking carry a heavy price tag. An estimated 1 percent of the people account for 30 percent of health-care costs.[26] Half of the people use up about 97 percent of health-care dollars. Furthermore, the average health-care cost per person in the United States is almost twice as high as that in most other industrialized nations.

Scientific evidence now links participation in fitness and wellness programs to better health and also to lower medical costs and higher job productivity. As a result of the staggering rise in medical costs, many organizations offer health-promotion programs, because keeping employees healthy costs less than treating them once they are sick.

Another reason some organizations are offering health promotion programs to their employees—overlooked by many because they do not seem to affect the bottom line directly—is simply top management's concern for the employees' well-being. Whether the program lowers medical costs is not the main issue; more important is that wellness helps individuals feel better about themselves and improve their quality of life.

**Physical fitness standards** A fitness level that allows a person to sustain moderate-to-vigorous physical activity without undue fatigue and the ability to closely maintain this level throughout life.

# Behavior Modification Planning

## FINANCIAL FITNESS PRESCRIPTION

Although not one of the components of physical fitness, taking control of your personal finances is critical for your success and well-being. The sooner you start working on a lifetime personal financial plan, the more successful you will be in becoming financially secure and being able to retire early, in comfort, if you choose to do so. Most likely, you have not been taught basic principles to improve personal finance and enjoy "financial fitness." Thus, start today using the following strategies:

**I PLAN TO**
**I DID IT**

1. *Develop a personal financial plan.* Set short-term and long-term financial goals for yourself. If you do not have financial goals, you cannot develop a plan or work toward that end.

2. *Subscribe to a personal finance magazine or newsletter.* In the same way that you should regularly read reputable fitness/wellness journals or newsletters, you should regularly peruse a "financial fitness" magazine. If you don't enjoy reading financial materials, then find a periodical that is quick and to the point; there are many available. You don't have to force yourself to read the *Wall Street Journal* to become financially knowledgeable. Many periodicals have resources to help you develop a financial plan. Educate yourself and stay current on personal finances and investment matters.

3. *Set up a realistic budget and live on less than you make.* Pay your bills on time and keep track of *all* expenses. Then develop your budget so that you spend less than you earn. Your budget may require that you either cut back on expenses and services or figure out a way to increase your income. Balance your checkbook regularly and do not overdraft your checking account.

4. *Learn to differentiate between wants and needs.* It is fine to reward yourself for goals that you have achieved (see Chapter 2), but limit your spending to items that you truly need. Avoid simple impulse spending because "it's a bargain" or something you just want to have.

5. *Pay yourself first; save 10 percent of your income each month.* Before you take any money out of your paycheck, put 10 percent of your income into a retirement or investment account. If possible, ask for an automatic withdrawal at your bank from your paycheck to avoid the temptation to spend this money. This strategy may allow you to have a solid retirement fund or even provide for an early retirement. If you start putting away $100 a month at age 20, and earn an average 6 percent interest rate, at age 65 you will have more than $275,000.

6. *Set up an emergency savings fund.* Whether you ultimately work for yourself or for someone else, there may be uncontrollable financial setbacks or even financial disasters in the future. So, as you are able, start an emergency fund equal to three to six months of normal monthly earnings. Additionally, start a second savings account for expensive purchases such as a car, a down payment on a home, or a vacation.

7. *Use credit, gas, and retail cards responsibly and sparingly.* As soon as you receive new cards, sign them promptly and store them securely. Due to the prevalence of identity theft (someone stealing your creditworthiness), cardholders should even consider a secure post office box, rather than a regular mailbox, for all high-risk mail. Pay off all credit card debt monthly and do not purchase on credit unless you have the cash to pay it off when the monthly statement arrives.

Develop a plan at this very moment to pay off your debt if you have such. Credit card balances, high interest rates, and frequent credit purchases lead to financial disaster. Credit card debt is the worst enemy to your personal finances!

☐ ☐ 8. *Understand the terms of your student loans.* Do not borrow more money than you absolutely need for actual educational expenses. Student loans are not for wants but needs (see item 4). Remember, loans must be repaid, with interest, once you leave college. Be informed regarding the repayment process and do not ever default on your loan. If you do, the entire balance (principal, interest, and collection fees) is due immediately and serious financial and credit consequences will follow.

☐ ☐ 9. *Eat out infrequently.* Besides saving money that you can then pay to yourself, you will eat healthier and consume fewer calories.

☐ ☐ 10. *Make the best of tax "motivated" savings and investing opportunities available to you.* For example, once employed, your company may match your voluntary 401(k) contributions (or other retirement plan), so contribute at least up to the match (you may use the 10 percent you "pay yourself first"—see item 5—or part of it). Also, under current tax law, maximize your Roth IRA contribution personally. Always pay attention to current tax rules that provide tax incentives for investing in retirement plans. If at all possible, *never* cash out a retirement account early. You may pay penalties in addition to tax, in most situations. As you are able, employ a tax professional or financial planner to avoid serious missteps in your tax planning.

☐ ☐ 11. *Stay involved in your financial accumulations.* You may seek professional advice, but you stay in control. Ultimately, no one will look after your interests as well as you.

☐ ☐ 12. *Protect your assets.* As you start to accumulate assets, get proper insurance coverage (yes, even renter's insurance) in case of an accident or disaster. You have disciplined yourself and worked hard to obtain those assets, now make sure they are protected.

☐ ☐ 13. *Review your credit report.* The best way to ensure that your credit "identity" is not stolen and ruined is to regularly review your credit report, at least once a year, for accuracy.

☐ ☐ 14. *Contribute to charity and the needy.* Altruism (doing good for others) is good for heart health and emotional well-being. Remember the less fortunate and donate regularly to some of your favorite charitable organizations and volunteer time to worthy causes.

### THE POWER OF INVESTING EARLY

Jon and Jim are both 20 years old. Jon begins investing $100 a month starting on his 20th birthday. He stops investing on his 30th birthday (he has set aside a total of $12,000). Jim does not start investing until he's 30. He chooses to invest $100 a month as Jon had done, but he does so for the next 30 years (Jim invests a total of $36,000). Although Jon stopped investing at age 30, assuming an 8 percent annual rate of return in a tax-deferred account, by the time both Jon and Jim are 60, Jon will have accumulated $199,035, whereas Jim will have $150,029. At a 6 percent rate of return, they would both accumulate about $100,000, but Jim invested three times as much as Jon did.

## Try It

Post these principles of financial fitness in a visible place at home where you can review them often. Start implementing these strategies as soon as you can and watch your financial fitness level increase over the years.

© David Johnson, CPA and Fitness & Wellness, Inc.

## Behavior Modification Planning

### HEALTHY LIFESTYLE HABITS

Research indicates that adhering to the following 12 lifestyle habits will significantly improve health and extend life.

I PLAN TO

I DID IT

❑ ❑ 1. *Participate in a lifetime physical activity program.* Exercise regularly at least 3 times per week and try to accumulate a minimum of 60 minutes of moderate-intensity physical activity each day of your life. The 60 minutes should include 20 to 30 minutes of aerobic exercise at least 3 times per week, along with strengthening and stretching exercises 2 to 3 times per week.

❑ ❑ 2. *Do not smoke cigarettes.* Cigarette smoking is the largest preventable cause of illness and premature death in the United States. If we include all related deaths, smoking is responsible for more than 440,000 unnecessary deaths each year.

❑ ❑ 3. *Eat right.* Eat a good breakfast and two additional well-balanced meals every day. Avoid eating too many calories, processed foods, and foods with a lot of sugar, fat, and salt. Increase your daily consumption of fruits, vegetables, and whole-grain products.

❑ ❑ 4. *Avoid snacking.* Some researchers recommend refraining from frequent between-meal snacks. Every time a person eats, insulin is released to remove sugar from the blood. Such frequent spikes in insulin may contribute to the development of heart disease. Less-frequent increases of insulin are more conducive to good health.

❑ ❑ 5. *Maintain recommended body weight through adequate nutrition and exercise.* This is important in preventing chronic diseases and in developing a higher level of fitness.

❑ ❑ 6. *Get enough rest.* Sleep 7 to 8 hours each night.

❑ ❑ 7. *Lower your stress levels.* Reduce your vulnerability to stress and practice stress management techniques as needed.

# The Wellness Challenge for Our Day

Because a better and healthier life is something every person should strive for, our biggest challenge in the new century is to teach people how to take control of their personal health habits and adhere to a positive lifestyle. A wealth of information on the benefits of fitness and wellness programs indicates that improving the quality and possible length of our lives is a matter of personal choice.

Even though people in the United States believe that a positive lifestyle has a great impact on health and longevity, most people do not reap the benefits because they simply do not know how to implement a safe and effective fitness and wellness program. Others are exercising incorrectly and, therefore, are not reaping the full benefits of

their program. How, then, can we meet the health challenges of the 21st century? That is the focus of this book—to provide the necessary tools that will enable you to write, implement, and regularly update your personal lifetime fitness and wellness program.

## Critical Thinking

What are your thoughts about lifestyle habits that enhance health and longevity? How important are they to you? What obstacles keep you from adhering to these habits or incorporating new habits into your life?

☐ ☐ 8. *Be wary of alcohol.* Drink alcohol moderately or not at all. Alcohol abuse leads to mental, emotional, physical, and social problems.

☐ ☐ 9. *Surround yourself with healthy friendships.* Unhealthy friendships contribute to destructive behaviors and low self-esteem. Associating with people who strive to maintain good fitness and health reinforces a positive outlook in life and encourages positive behaviors. Constructive social interactions enhance well-being. Researchers have also found that mortality rates are much higher among people who are socially isolated. People who aren't socially integrated are more likely to "give up when seriously ill"—which accelerates dying.

☐ ☐ 10. *Be informed about the environment.* Seek clean air, clean water, and a clean environment. Be aware of pollutants and occupational hazards: asbestos fibers, nickel dust, chromate, uranium dust, and so on. Take precautions when using pesticides and insecticides.

☐ ☐ 11. *Increase education.* Data indicate that people who are more educated live longer. The theory is that as education increases, so do the number of connections between nerve cells. The increased number of connections in turn helps the individual make better survival (healthy lifestyle) choices.

☐ ☐ 12. *Take personal safety measures.* Although not all accidents are preventable, many are. Taking simple precautionary measures—such as using seat belts and keeping electrical appliances away from water—lessens the risk for avoidable accidents.

## Try It

Look at the list above and indicate which habits are already a part of your lifestyle. What changes could you make to incorporate some additional healthy habits into your daily life?

# National Health Objectives for 2010

Every 10 years, the U.S. Department of Health and Human Services releases a list of objectives for preventing disease and promoting health. Since its initiation in 1980, this 10-year plan has helped instill a new sense of purpose and focus for public health and preventive medicine. These national health objectives are intended to be realistic goals to improve the health of all Americans. Two unique goals of the 2010 objectives (a) emphasize increased quality and years of healthy life and (b) seek to eliminate health disparities among all groups of people. The objectives address three important points:[27]

1. *Personal responsibility for health behavior.* Individuals need to become ever more health conscious. Responsible and informed behaviors are the keys to good health.

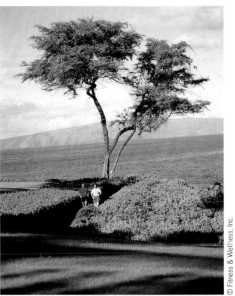

No current drug or medication provides as many health benefits as a regular physical activity program.

2. *Health benefits for all people and all communities.* Lower socioeconomic conditions and poor health often are interrelated. Extending the benefits of good health to all people is crucial to the health of the nation.

3. *Health promotion and disease prevention.* A shift from treatment to preventive techniques will drastically cut health-care costs and help all Americans achieve a better quality of life.

Developing these health objectives involves more than 10,000 people representing 300 national organizations, including the Institute of Medicine of the National Academy of Sciences, all state health departments, and the federal Office of Disease Prevention and Health Promotion. Figure 1.16 summarizes the key 2010 objectives. Unfortunately, none of the goals to increase participation in physical activity and fitness are being met. Living the fitness and wellness principles provided in this book will enhance the quality of your life and also will allow you to be an active participant in achieving the Healthy People 2010 Objectives.

# Wellness Education: Using This Book

Although everyone would like to enjoy good health and wellness, most people don't know how to reach this objective. Lifestyle is the most important factor affecting personal well-being. Granted, some people live long because of genetic factors, but quality of life during middle age and the "golden years" is more often related to wise choices initiated during youth and continued throughout life. In a few short years, lack of wellness can lead to a loss of vitality and gusto for life, as well as premature morbidity and mortality.

**A Personalized Approach** Because fitness and wellness needs vary significantly from one individual to another, all exercise and wellness prescriptions must be personalized to obtain best results. The Wellness Lifestyle Questionnaire in Lab 1B will provide an initial rating of your current efforts to stay healthy and well. Subsequent chapters of this book and their respective labs discuss the components of a wellness lifestyle and set forth the necessary guidelines that will allow you to develop a personal lifetime program to improve fitness and promote your own preventive health care and personal wellness.

The labs in this book have been prepared on tear-out sheets so they can be turned in to class instructors. As you study this book and complete the worksheets, you will learn to:

- Implement motivational and behavior modification techniques to help you adhere to a lifetime fitness and wellness program
- Determine whether medical clearance is needed for your safe participation in exercise
- Conduct nutritional analyses and follow the recommendations for adequate nutrition
- Write sound diet and weight-control programs
- Assess the health-related components of fitness (cardiorespiratory endurance, muscular strength and endurance, muscular flexibility, and body composition)

**FIGURE 1.16** Selected health objectives for 2010.

1. Increase quality and years of healthy life.
2. Eliminate health disparities.
3. Improve the health, fitness, and quality of life of all Americans through the adoption and maintenance of regular, daily physical activity.
4. Promote health and reduce chronic disease risk, disease progression, debilitation, and premature death associated with dietary factors and nutritional status among all people in the United States.
5. Reduce disease, disability, and death related to tobacco use and exposure to secondhand smoke.
6. Increase the quality, availability, and effectiveness of educational and community-based programs designed to prevent disease and improve the health and quality of life of the American people.
7. Promote health for all people through a healthy environment.
8. Reduce the incidence and severity of injuries from unintentional causes, as well as violence and abuse.
9. Promote worker health and safety through prevention.
10. Improve access to comprehensive, high-quality health care.
11. Ensure that every pregnancy in the United States is intended.
12. Improve maternal and pregnancy outcomes and reduce rates of disability in infants.
13. Improve the quality of health-related decisions through effective communication.
14. Decrease the incidence of functional limitations due to arthritis, osteoporosis, and chronic back conditions.
15. Decrease cancer incidence, morbidity, and mortality.
16. Promote health and prevent secondary conditions among persons with disabilities.
17. Enhance the cardiovascular health and quality of life of all Americans through prevention and control of risk factors and promotion of healthy lifestyle behaviors.
18. Prevent HIV transmission and associated morbidity and mortality.
19. Improve the mental health of all Americans.
20. Raise the public's awareness of the signs and symptoms of lung disease.
21. Increase awareness of healthy sexual relationships and prevent all forms of sexually transmitted diseases.
22. Reduce the incidence of substance abuse by all people, especially children.

- Write exercise prescriptions for cardiorespiratory endurance, muscular strength and endurance, and muscular flexibility
- Understand the relationship between fitness and aging
- Determine your levels of tension and stress, lessen your vulnerability to stress, and implement a stress management program if necessary
- Determine your potential risk for cardiovascular disease and implement a risk-reduction program
- Follow a cancer risk-reduction program
- Implement a smoking cessation program, if applicable
- Avoid chemical dependency and know where to find assistance if needed
- Learn the health consequences of sexually transmitted infections (STIs), including HIV/acquired immune deficiency syndrome (AIDS), and guidelines for preventing STIs
- Write goals and objectives to improve your fitness and wellness and learn how to chart a wellness program for the future
- Differentiate myths from facts about exercise and health-related concepts

# Exercise Safety

Even though testing and participation in exercise are relatively safe for most apparently healthy individuals under age 45, the reaction of the cardiovascular system to higher levels of physical activity cannot be totally predicted.[28] Consequently, a small but real risk exists for exercise-induced abnormalities in people with a history of cardiovascular problems and those who are at higher risk for disease. These factors include abnormal blood pressure, irregular heart rhythm, fainting, and, in rare instances, a heart attack or cardiac arrest.

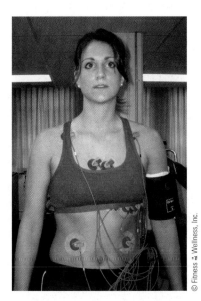

© Fitness & Wellness, Inc.

An exercise tolerance test with 12-lead electrocardiographic monitoring (stress ECG test) may be required of some individuals prior to initiating an exercise program.

**TABLE 1.4  Resting Heart Rate Ratings**

| Heart Rate (beats/minute) | Rating |
|---|---|
| ≤59 | Excellent |
| 60–69 | Good |
| 70–79 | Average |
| 80–89 | Fair |
| ≥90 | Poor |

Before you engage in an exercise program or participate in any exercise testing, you should fill out the questionnaire in Lab 1C. If your answer to any of the questions is yes, you should see a physician before participating in a fitness program. Exercise testing and participation are not wise under some of the conditions listed in Lab 1C and may require a medical evaluation, including a stress electrocardiogram (ECG) test. If you have any questions regarding your current health status, consult your doctor before initiating, continuing, or increasing your level of physical activity.

# Assessment of Resting Heart Rate and Blood Pressure

Heart rate can be obtained by counting your pulse either on the wrist over the radial artery or over the carotid artery in the neck (see Chapter 6, pages 201–206). In Lab 1D you will learn how to determine your heart rate and blood pressure and calculate the extra heart rate life years an increase in exercise may produce.

You may count your pulse for 30 seconds and multiply by 2 or take it for a full minute. The heart rate usually is at its lowest point (resting heart rate) late in the evening after you have been sitting quietly for about half an hour watching a relaxing TV show or reading in bed, or early in the morning just before you get out of bed.

Unless you have a pathological condition, a lower resting heart rate indicates a stronger heart. To adapt to cardiorespiratory or aerobic exercise, blood volume increases, the heart enlarges, and the muscle gets stronger. A stronger heart can pump more blood with fewer strokes.

Resting heart rate categories are given in Table 1.4. Although resting heart rate decreases with training, the extent of **bradycardia** depends not only on the amount of training but also on genetic factors. Although most

---

**Bradycardia** Slower heart rate than normal.

highly trained athletes have a resting heart rate of around 40 beats per minute, occasionally one of these athletes has a resting heart rate in the 60s or 70s even during peak training months of the season. For most individuals, however, the resting heart rate decreases as the level of cardiorespiratory endurance increases.

Blood pressure is assessed using a **sphygmomanometer** and a stethoscope. Use a cuff of the appropriate size to get accurate readings. Size is determined by the width of the inflatable bladder, which should be about 80 percent of the circumference of the midpoint of the arm.

Blood pressure usually is measured while the person is in the sitting position, with the forearm and the manometer at the same level as the heart. The arm should be flexed slightly and placed on a flat surface. At first, the pressure is recorded from each arm, and after that from the arm with the highest reading.

The cuff should be applied approximately an inch above the antecubital space (natural crease of the elbow), with the center of the bladder directly over the medial (inner) surface of the arm. The stethoscope head should be applied firmly, but with little pressure, over the brachial artery in the antecubital space.

To determine how high the cuff should be inflated, the person recording the blood pressure monitors the subject's radial pulse with one hand and, with the other hand, inflates the manometer's bladder to about 30 to 40 mm Hg above the point at which the feeling of the pulse in the wrist disappears. Next, the pressure is released, followed by a wait of about one minute, then the bladder is inflated to the predetermined level to take the blood pressure reading. The cuff should not be overinflated, as this may cause blood vessel spasm, resulting in higher blood pressure readings. The pressure should be released at a rate of 2 to 4 mm Hg per second.

As the pressure is released, **systolic blood pressure** (SBP) is recorded as the point where the sound of the pulse becomes audible. The **diastolic blood pressure** (DBP) is the point where the sound disappears. The recordings should be expressed as systolic over diastolic pressure—for example, 124/80.

If you take more than one reading, be sure the bladder is completely deflated between readings and allow at least a full minute before making the next recording. The person measuring the pressure also should note whether the

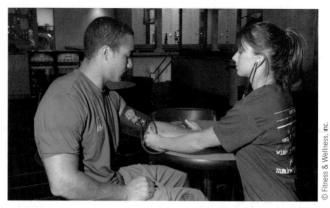

Assessment of resting blood pressure with an aneroid manometer.

pressure was recorded from the left or the right arm. Resting blood pressure ratings are given in Table 1.5.

In some cases the pulse sounds become less intense (point of muffling sounds) but still can be heard at a lower pressure (50 or 40 mm Hg) or even all the way down to zero. In this situation DBP is recorded at the point of a clear, definite change in the loudness of the sound (also referred to as fourth phase) and at complete disappearance of the sound (fifth phase) (for example, 120/78/60 or 120/82/0).

**Mean Blood Pressure** During a normal resting contraction/relaxation cycle of the heart, the heart spends more time in the relaxation (diastolic) phase than in the contraction (systolic) phase. Accordingly, mean blood pressure (MBP) cannot be computed by taking an average of SBP and DBP. The equations used to determine MBP are shown in Lab 1D.

When measuring blood pressure, be aware that a single reading may not be an accurate value because of the various factors (rest, stress, physical activity, food) that can affect blood pressure. Thus, if you are able, ask different people to take several readings at different times of the day, to establish the real values. You can record the results of your resting heart rate and your SBP, DBP, and MBP assessments in Lab 1D. You can also calculate the effects of aerobic activity on resting heart rate in this lab.

**Sphygmomanometer** Inflatable bladder contained within a cuff and a mercury gravity manometer (or aneroid manometer) from which blood pressure is read.

**Systolic blood pressure** Pressure exerted by blood against walls of arteries during forceful contraction (systole) of the heart.

**Diastolic blood pressure** Pressure exerted by the blood against the walls of the arteries during the relaxation phase (diastole) of the heart.

**TABLE 1.5  Resting Blood Pressure Guidelines (in mm Hg)**

| Rating | Systolic | Diastolic |
|---|---|---|
| Normal | ≤120 | ≤80 |
| Prehypertension | 120–139 | 80–89 |
| Hypertension | ≥140 | ≥90 |

*Source:* National Heart, Lung and Blood Institute.

# ASSESS YOUR BEHAVIOR

 Log on to http://www.cengage.com/sso/ and take a wellness inventory to assess the behaviors that might benefit most from healthy change.

1. Are you aware of your family health history and life-style factors that may negatively impact your health?

2. Do you accumulate at least 30 minutes of moderate-intensity physical activity five days per week?

3. Do you make a constant and deliberate effort to stay healthy and achieve the highest potential for well-being?

# ASSESS YOUR KNOWLEDGE

 Log on to http://www.cengage.com/sso/ to assess your understanding of this chapter's topics by taking the Student Practice Test and exploring the modules recommended in your Personalized Study Plan.

1. Advances in modern technology
   a. help people achieve higher fitness levels
   b. have led to a decrease in chronic diseases
   c. have almost completely eliminated the necessity for physical exertion in daily life
   d. help fight hypokinetic disease
   e. make it easier to achieve good aerobic fitness

2. Most activities of daily living in the United States help people
   a. get adequate physical activity on a regular basis
   b. meet health-related fitness standards
   c. achieve good levels of skill-related activities
   d. Choices a, b, and c are correct.
   e. None of the choices is correct.

3. The leading cause of death in the United States is
   a. cancer
   b. accidents
   c. CLRD
   d. diseases of the cardiovascular system
   e. drug abuse

4. Bodily movement produced by skeletal muscles is called
   a. physical activity
   b. kinesiology
   c. exercise
   d. aerobic exercise
   e. muscle strength

5. Among the benefits of regular physical activity and exercise are significantly reduced risks for developing or dying from
   a. heart disease
   b. type 2 diabetes
   c. colon and breast cancers
   d. osteoporotic fractures
   e. All are correct choices.

6. To be ranked in the "active" category, an adult has to take between
   a. 3,500 and 4,999 steps per day
   b. 5,000 and 7,499 steps per day
   c. 7,500 and 9,999 steps per day
   d. 10,000 and 12,499 steps per day
   e. 12,500 and 15,000 steps per day

7. The constant and deliberate effort to stay healthy and achieve the highest potential for well-being is defined as
   a. health
   b. physical fitness
   c. wellness
   d. health-related fitness
   e. physiologic fitness

8. Research on the effects of fitness on mortality indicates that the largest drop in premature mortality is seen between
   a. the average and excellent fitness groups
   b. the low and moderate fitness groups
   c. the high and excellent fitness groups
   d. the moderate and good fitness groups
   e. The drop is similar among all fitness groups.

9. Metabolic fitness can be achieved through
   a. a moderate-intensity exercise program
   b. a high-intensity speed-training program
   c. an increased basal metabolic rate
   d. anaerobic training
   e. an increase in lean body mass

10. What is the greatest benefit of being physically fit?
   a. absence of disease
   b. a higher quality of life
   c. improved sports performance
   d. better personal appearance
   e. maintenance of ideal body weight

Correct answers can be found at the back of the book.

# MEDIA MENU

You can find the links below at the book companion site: www.cengage.com/health/hoeger/plfw10e

- Chronicle your daily activities using the exercise log.

- Determine the safety of exercise participation.

- Check how well you understand the chapter's concepts.

## Internet Connections

- Healthy People 2010. Healthy People, a national health promotion and disease prevention initiative, lists national goals for improving the health of all Americans by 2010. *http://www.health.gov/healthypeople*

- The National Association for Health and Fitness (NAHF). This nonprofit organization promotes physical fitness, sports, and healthy lifestyles; it fosters and supports governors' and states' councils on physical fitness and sports in every state and U.S. territory. NAHF is also the national sponsor of the largest U.S. worksite health and fitness event, "Let's Get Physical" (the national fitness challenge) and "Make Your Move!" (an incentive-based health promotion campaign). *http://www.physicalfitness.org*

- Lifescan Health Risk Appraisal. This site was created by Bill Hettler, M.D., of the National Wellness Institute and features questions to help you identify the specific lifestyle factors that can impair your health and longevity. *http://wellness.uwsp.edu/other/lifescan*

- My Family Health Portrait. This helpful profile was developed by Ralph Carmona, Surgeon General of the United States, and is available on the U.S. Department of Health and Human Services Web site. It allows you to create a family medical history that identifies possible health risks you might face. *http://www.hhs.gov/familyhistory*

# NOTES

1. World Health Organization, *Global Strategy on Diet, Physical Activity, and Health*, http://who.int/dietphysicalactivity/en; downloaded July 2, 2008.

2. U.S. Department of Health and Human Services, Office of the Surgeon General, *Disease Prevention*, http://surgeongeneral.gov/publichealthpriorities.html#disease; downloaded July 2, 2008.

3. U.S. Department of Health and Human Services, Centers for Disease Control and Prevention, National Center for Health Statistics, *National Vital Statistics Reports: Deaths Final Data for 2005*, 56, no. 10 (April 24, 2008).

4. American Heart Association, *Heart Disease and Stroke Statistics—2008 Update* (Dallas: American Heart Association, 2008).

5. American Cancer Society, *2006 Cancer Facts and Figures* (New York: ACS, 2006).

6. N. Schachter, "Lung Disease Can Affect All Adults," *Bottom Line/Health* 17 (May 2003): 13–14.

7. W. L. Haskell, "Physical Activity and Public Health: Updated Recommendations for Adults from the American College of Sports Medicine and the American Heart Association," *Medicine and Science in Sports and Exercise* 39 (2007): 1423–1434.

8. U.S. Department of Health and Human Services, *Physical Activity and Health: A Report of the Surgeon General* (Atlanta: Centers for Disease Control and Prevention, National Center for Chronic Disease Prevention and Health Promotion, 1996).

9. American College of Sports Medicine and American Medical Association, *Exercise Is Medicine*, http://www.exercise is medicine.org/physicians.htm; downloaded July 2, 2008.

10. U.S. Department of Health and Human Services, *2008 Physical Activity Guidelines for Americans*. www.health.gov/paguidelines. Downloaded October 15, 2008.

11. American College of Sports Medicine, *ACSM's Guidelines for Exercise Testing and Prescription* (Baltimore: Williams & Wilkins, 2006).

12. National Academy of Sciences, Institute of Medicine, *Dietary Reference Intakes for Energy, Carbohydrates, Fiber, Fat, Protein and Amino Acids (Macronutrients)* (Washington, DC: National Academy Press, 2002).

13. U.S. Department of Health and Human Services and Department of Agriculture, *Dietary Guidelines for Americans, 2005* (Washington, DC: DHHS, 2005).

14. W. W. K. Hoeger et al., "One-Mile Step Count at Walking and Running Speeds," *ACSM's Health & Fitness Journal* 11, no. 1 (2008):14–19.

15. L. Sax et al., *The American Freshman: National Norms for Fall 2000* (Los Angeles: UCLA, Higher Education Research Institute, 2000).

16. H. G. Koenig, "The Healing Power of Faith," *Bottom Line/Health* 18 (May 2004): 3–4.

17. L. Dossey, "Can Spirituality Improve Your Health?" *Bottom Line/Health* 15 (July 2001): 11–13.

18. R. S. Paffenbarger, Jr., R. T. Hyde, A. L. Wing, and C. H. Steinmetz, "A Natural History of Athleticism and Cardiovascular Health," *Journal of the American Medical Association* 252 (1984): 491–495.

19. S. N. Blair, H. W. Kohl III, R. S. Paffenbarger, Jr., D. G. Clark, K. H. Cooper, and L. W. Gibbons, "Physical Fitness and All-Cause Mortality: A Prospective Study of Healthy Men and Women," *Journal of the American Medical Association* 262 (1989): 2395–2401.

20. S. N. Blair, H. W. Kohl III, C. E. Barlow, R. S. Paffenbarger, Jr., L. W. Gibbons, and C. A. Macera, "Changes in Physical Fitness and All-Cause Mortality: A Prospective Study of Healthy and Unhealthy Men," *Journal of the American Medical Association* 273 (1995): 1193–1198.

21. D. P. Swain, "Moderate- or Vigorous-Intensity Exercise: What Should We Prescribe?" *ACSM's Health & Fitness Journal* 10, no. 5 (2007): 7–11.

22. P. T. Williams, "Physical Fitness and Activity as Separate Heart Disease Risk Factors: A Meta-analysis," *Medicine & Science in Sports & Exercise* 33 (2001): 754–761.

23. D. P. Swain and B. A. Franklin, "Comparative Cardioprotective Benefits of Vigorous vs. Moderate Intensity Aerobic Exercise," *American Journal of Cardiology* 97 (2006): 141–147.

24. See ACSM, note 10.

25. Ibid.

26. "Wellness Facts," *University of California at Berkeley Wellness Letter* (Palm Coast, FL: The Editors, April 1995).

27. U.S. Department of Health and Human Services, *Healthy People 2010* (Washington, DC: U.S. Government Printing Office, November 2000).

28. See ACSM, note 10.

# SUGGESTED READINGS

American College of Sports Medicine. ACSM Fit Society Page, http://acsm.org/health1fitness/fit_ society.htm.

Blair, S. N., et al. "Influences of Cardiorespiratory Fitness and Other Precursors on Cardiovascular Disease and All-Cause Mortality in Men and Women." *Journal of the American Medical Association* 276 (1996): 205–210.

Booth, F. W., and B. S. Tseng. "America Needs to Exercise for Health." *Medicine and Science in Sports and Exercise* 27 (1995): 462–465.

Bouchard, C., S. N. Blair, and W. Haskell. *Physical Activity and Health.* Champaign, IL: Human Kinetics, 2007.

Haskell, W. L., et al., "Physical Activity and Public Health: Updated Recommendations for Adults from the American College of Sports Medicine and the American Heart Association," *Medicine and Science in Sports and Exercise* 39 (2007): 1423–1434.

Hoeger, W. W. K., L. W. Turner, and B. Q. Hafen. *Wellness: Guidelines for a Healthy Lifestyle.* Belmont, CA: Wadsworth/ Thomson Learning, 2007.

National Academy of Sciences, Institute of Medicine. *Dietary Reference Intakes for Energy, Carbohydrates, Fiber, Fat, Protein and Amino Acids (Macronutrients).* Washington, DC: National Academy Press, 2002.

Pate, R., et al. "Physical Activity and Public Health: A Recommendation from the Centers for Disease Control and Prevention and the American College of Sports Medicine." *Journal of the American Medical Association* 273 (1995): 402–407.

U.S. Department of Health and Human Services. *Physical Activity and Health: A Report of the Surgeon General.* Atlanta: Centers for Disease Control and Prevention, National Center for Chronic Disease Prevention and Health Promotion, 1996.

U.S. Department of Health and Human Services, Public Health Service. *Healthy People 2010: Conference Edition,* http:// www.health.gov/healthypeople/ Document/ tableofcontents.htm.

# LAB 1A: Daily Physical Activity Log

Name _____    Date _____    Grade/Age _____

Instructor _____    Course _____    Section _____

**Necessary Lab Equipment**
None.

**Objective**
To indicate how active you are and serve as a basis to monitor future changes.

**Instructions**
Record the time of day, type and duration of the exercise/activity, and if possible, steps taken while engaged in the activity.

Date: [ ]    Day of the Week: [ ]

| Time of Day | Exercise/Activity | Duration | Number of Steps | Comments |
|---|---|---|---|---|
| | | | | |
| | | | | |
| | | | | |
| | | | | |
| | | | | |
| | | | | |
| | | | | |

Totals: [ ] [ ]

Activity category based on steps per day (use Table 1.2, page 10): [ ]

Date: [ ]    Day of the Week: [ ]

| Time of Day | Exercise/Activity | Duration | Number of Steps | Comments |
|---|---|---|---|---|
| | | | | |
| | | | | |
| | | | | |
| | | | | |
| | | | | |
| | | | | |
| | | | | |

Totals: [ ] [ ]

Activity category based on steps per day (use Table 1.2, page 10): [ ]

Date: _____  Day of the Week: _____

| Time of Day | Exercise/Activity | Duration | Number of Steps | Comments |
|---|---|---|---|---|
| | | | | |
| | | | | |
| | | | | |
| | | | | |
| | | | | |
| | | | | |
| | | | | |

Totals: _____  _____  🏃

Activity category based on steps per day (use Table 1.2, page 10): _____

Date: _____  Day of the Week: _____

| Time of Day | Exercise/Activity | Duration | Number of Steps | Comments |
|---|---|---|---|---|
| | | | | |
| | | | | |
| | | | | |
| | | | | |
| | | | | |
| | | | | |
| | | | | |

Totals: _____  _____  🏃

Activity category based on steps per day (use Table 1.2, page 10): _____

Briefly evaluate your current activity patterns, discuss your feelings about the results, and provide a goal for the weeks ahead.

_____

_____

_____

_____

_____

# LAB 1B: Wellness Lifestyle Questionnaire

Name _____  Date _____  Grade/Age _____

Instructor _____  Course _____  Section _____

The purpose of this questionnaire is to analyze current lifestyle habits and help determine changes necessary for future health and wellness. Check the appropriate answer to each question and obtain a final score according to the guidelines provided at the end of the questionnaire.

| | ALWAYS | NEARLY ALWAYS | OFTEN | SELDOM | NEVER |
|---|---|---|---|---|---|
| 1. I participate in vigorous aerobic activity for 20 minutes on three or more days per week, and I accumulate at least 30 minutes of moderate-intensity (or vigorous-intensity) physical activity a minimum of five days per week. | 5 | 4 | ③ | 2 | 1 |
| 2. I participate in strength-training exercises, using a minimum of eight different exercises, two or more nonconsecutive days per week. | 5 | 4 | 3 | 2 | 1 |
| 3. I perform flexibility exercises two or more days per week. | 5 | 4 | 3 | 2 | 1 |
| 4. I maintain recommended body weight (includes avoidance of excessive body fat, excessive thinness, or frequent fluctuations in body weight). | 5 | 4 | 3 | 2 | 1 |
| 5. Every day, I eat three regular meals that include a wide variety of foods. | 5 | 4 | 3 | 2 | 1 |
| 6. I limit the amount of saturated fat and trans fats in my diet on most days of the week. | 5 | 4 | 3 | 2 | 1 |
| 7. I eat a minimum of five servings of fruits and vegetables and six servings from grain products daily. | 5 | 4 | 3 | 2 | 1 |
| 8. I regularly avoid snacks, especially those that are high in calories and fat and low in nutrients and fiber. | 5 | 4 | 3 | 2 | 1 |
| 9. I avoid cigarettes or tobacco in any other form. | 5 | 4 | 3 | 2 | 1 |
| 10. I avoid alcoholic beverages. If I drink, I do so in moderation (one daily drink for women and two for men), and I do not combine alcohol with other drugs. | 5 | 4 | 3 | 2 | 1 |
| 11. I avoid addictive drugs and needles that have been used by others. | 5 | 4 | 3 | 2 | 1 |
| 12. I use prescription drugs and over-the-counter drugs sparingly, only when needed, and I follow all directions for their proper use. | 5 | 4 | 3 | 2 | 1 |
| 13. I readily recognize when I am under excessive tension and stress (distress). | 5 | 4 | 3 | 2 | 1 |
| 14. I am able to perform effective stress-management techniques. | 5 | 4 | 3 | 2 | 1 |
| 15. I have close friends and relatives with whom I can discuss personal problems and approach for help when needed, and with whom I can express my feelings freely. | 5 | 4 | 3 | 2 | 1 |
| 16. I spend most of my daily leisure time in wholesome recreational activities. | 5 | 4 | 3 | 2 | 1 |
| 17. I sleep 7 to 8 hours each night. | 5 | 4 | 3 | 2 | 1 |
| 18. I floss my teeth every day and brush them at least twice daily. | 5 | 4 | 3 | 2 | 1 |
| 19. I avoid overexposure to the sun, and I use sunscreen and appropriate clothing when I am out in the sun for an extended time. | 5 | 4 | 3 | 2 | 1 |
| 20. I avoid using products that have not been shown by science to be safe and effective. (This includes anabolic steroids and unproven nutrient and weight loss supplements). | 5 | 4 | 3 | 2 | 1 |
| 21. I stay current with the warning signs for heart attack, stroke, and cancer. | 5 | 4 | 3 | 2 | 1 |
| 22. I practice monthly breast/testicle self-exams, get recommended screening tests (blood lipids, blood pressure, Pap tests), and seek a medical evaluation when I am not well or disease symptoms arise. | 5 | 4 | 3 | 2 | 1 |
| 23. I have a dental checkup at least once a year, and I get regular medical exams according to age recommendations. | 5 | 4 | 3 | 2 | 1 |
| 24. I am not sexually active / I practice safe sex. | 5 | 4 | 3 | 2 | 1 |
| 25. I can deal effectively with disappointments and temporary feelings of sadness, loneliness, and depression. If I am unable to deal with these feelings, I seek professional help. | 5 | 4 | 3 | 2 | 1 |
| 26. I can work out emotional problems without turning to alcohol or other drugs. | 5 | 4 | 3 | 2 | 1 |

| | ALWAYS | NEARLY ALWAYS | OFTEN | SELDOM | NEVER |
|---|---|---|---|---|---|
| 27. I associate with people who have a positive attitude about life. | 5 | 4 | 3 | 2 | 1 |
| 28. I respond to temporary setbacks by making the best of the circumstances and by moving ahead with optimism and energy. I do not spend time and talent worrying about failures. | 5 | 4 | 3 | 2 | 1 |
| 29. I wear a seat belt whenever I am in a car, I ask others in my vehicle to do the same, and I make sure that children are in an infant seat or wear a shoulder harness. | 5 | 4 | 3 | 2 | 1 |
| 30. I do not drive under the influence of alcohol or other drugs, and I make an effort to keep others from doing the same. | 5 | 4 | 3 | 2 | 1 |
| 31. I avoid being alone in public places, especially after dark; I seek escorts when I visit or exercise in unfamiliar places. | 5 | 4 | 3 | 2 | 1 |
| 32. I seek to make my living quarters accident-free, and I keep doors and windows locked, especially when I am home alone. | 5 | 4 | 3 | 2 | 1 |
| 33. I try to minimize environmental pollutants, and I support community efforts to minimize pollution. | 5 | 4 | 3 | 2 | 1 |
| 34. I use energy conservation strategies and encourage others to do the same. | 5 | 4 | 3 | 2 | 1 |
| 35. I study and/or work in a clean environment (including avoidance of secondhand smoke). | 5 | 4 | 3 | 2 | 1 |
| 36. I participate in recycling programs for paper, cardboard, glass, plastic, and aluminum. | 5 | 4 | 3 | 2 | 1 |

## How to Score

Enter the score you have circled for each question in the spaces provided below. Next, total the score for each specific wellness lifestyle category and obtain a rating for each category according to the criteria provided below.

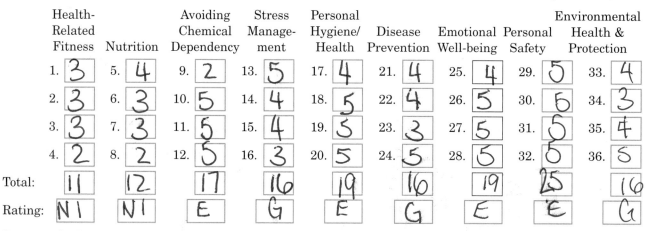

| | Health-Related Fitness | Nutrition | Avoiding Chemical Dependency | Stress Management | Personal Hygiene/Health | Disease Prevention | Emotional Well-being | Personal Safety | Environmental Health & Protection |
|---|---|---|---|---|---|---|---|---|---|
| | 1. 3 | 5. 4 | 9. 2 | 13. 5 | 17. 4 | 21. 4 | 25. 4 | 29. 5 | 33. 4 |
| | 2. 3 | 6. 3 | 10. 5 | 14. 4 | 18. 5 | 22. 4 | 26. 5 | 30. 5 | 34. 3 |
| | 3. 3 | 7. 3 | 11. 5 | 15. 4 | 19. 5 | 23. 3 | 27. 5 | 31. 5 | 35. 4 |
| | 4. 2 | 8. 2 | 12. 5 | 16. 3 | 20. 5 | 24. 5 | 28. 5 | 32. 5 | 36. 5 |
| Total: | 11 | 12 | 17 | 16 | 19 | 16 | 19 | 25 | 16 |
| Rating: | NI | NI | E | G | E | G | E | E | G |

## Category Rating

Excellent (E) = ≥17 Your answers show that you are aware of the importance of this category to your health and wellness. You are putting your knowledge to work for you by practicing good habits. As long as you continue to do so, this category should not pose a health risk. You are also setting a good example for family and friends to follow. Because you got a very high test score on this part of the test, you may want to consider other categories in which your score indicates room for improvement.

Good (G) = 13–16 Your health practices in this area are good, but you have room for improvement. Look again at the items you answered with a 4 or lower and identify changes that you can make to improve your lifestyle. Even small changes often can help you achieve better health.

Needs Improvement (NI) = ≤12 Your health risks are showing. You may be taking serious and unnecessary risks with your health. Perhaps you are not aware of the risks and what to do about them. Most likely you need additional information and help in deciding how to successfully make the changes you desire. You can easily get the information that you need to improve, if you wish. The next step is up to you.

Please note that no final overall rating is provided for the entire questionnaire because it may not be indicative of your overall wellness. For example, an excellent rating in most categories will not offset the immediate health risks and life-threatening consequences of using addictive drugs or not wearing a seat belt.

# LAB 1C: Health History Questionnaire

Name _____    Date _____    Grade _____

Instructor _____    Course _____    Section _____

### Necessary Lab Equipment
None.

### Objective
To determine the safety of exercise participation.

### Introduction
Although exercise testing and exercise participation are relatively safe for most apparently healthy individuals under the age of 45, the reaction of the cardiovascular system to increased levels of physical activity cannot always be totally predicted. Consequently, there is a small but real risk of certain changes occurring during exercise testing and participation. Some of these changes may be abnormal blood pressure, irregular heart rhythm, fainting, and in rare instances a heart attack or cardiac arrest. Therefore, you must provide honest answers to this questionnaire. Exercise may be contraindicated under some of the conditions listed below; others may simply require special consideration. **If any of the conditions apply, consult your physician before you participate in an exercise program.** Also, promptly report to your instructor any exercise-related abnormalities that you may experience during the course of the semester.

**A.** Have you ever had or do you now have any of the following conditions?

- [ ] 1. A myocardial infarction
- [ ] 2. Coronary artery disease
- [ ] 3. Congestive heart failure
- [ ] 4. Elevated blood lipids (cholesterol and triglycerides)
- [ ] 5. Chest pain at rest or during exertion
- [ ] 6. Shortness of breath
- [ ] 7. An abnormal resting or stress electrocardiogram
- [ ] 8. Uneven, irregular, or skipped heartbeats (including a racing or fluttering heart)
- [ ] 9. A blood embolism
- [ ] 10. Thrombophlebitis
- [ ] 11. Rheumatic heart fever
- [ ] 12. Elevated blood pressure
- [ ] 13. A stroke
- [ ] 14. Diabetes
- [ ] 15. A family history of coronary heart disease, syncope, or sudden death before age 60
- [ ] 16. Any other heart problem that makes exercise unsafe

**B.** Do you have any of the following conditions?

- [ ] 1. Arthritis, rheumatism, or gout
- [ ] 2. Chronic low-back pain
- [ ] 3. Any other joint, bone, or muscle problems
- [ ] 4. Any respiratory problems
- [ ] 5. Obesity (more than 30 percent overweight)
- [ ] 6. Anorexia
- [ ] 7. Bulimia
- [ ] 8. Mononucleosis
- [ ] 9. Any physical disability that could interfere with safe participation in exercise

**C.** Do any of the following conditions apply?

- [ ] 1. Do you smoke cigarettes?
- [ ] 2. Are you taking any prescription drugs?
- [ ] 3. Are you 45 years or older?

**D.** Do you have any other concern regarding your ability to safely participate in an exercise program? If so, explain:

_____

_____

Student's Signature: _____    Date: _____

Personal Challenge

In your own words, indicate what the Wellness Lifestyle Questionnaire in Lab 1B tells you about your current state of wellness. Also, identify categories where you can personally make changes in the next few months and indicate what may help you accomplish your goals.

Lab 1B suggests that _____

_____

_____

_____

I can make these changes in the next few months: _____

_____

_____

_____

The following could help me accomplish my goals: _____

_____

_____

_____

_____

Do you feel that it is safe for you to proceed with an exercise program? Explain any concerns or limitations that you may have regarding your safe participation in a comprehensive exercise program that will target cardiorespiratory endurance, muscular strength, muscular flexibility, and weight management.

I believe it ☐ is ☐ is not safe for me to exercise. I have the following concerns or limitations: _____

_____

_____

_____

_____

_____

# LAB 1D: Resting Heart Rate and Blood Pressure

Name _____   Date _____   Grade _____

Instructor _____   Course _____   Section _____

### Necessary Lab Equipment
Stopwatches, stethoscopes, and blood pressure sphygmomanometers.

### Objective
To determine resting heart rate and blood pressure.

### Preparation
The instructions to determine heart rate and blood pressure are given on pages 25–26. Many factors can affect heart rate and blood pressure. Factors such as excite-

ment, nervousness, stress, food, smoking, pain, temperature, and physical exertion all can alter heart rate and blood pressure significantly. Therefore, whenever possible, readings should be taken in a quiet, comfortable room following a few minutes of rest in the recording position. Avoid any form of exercise several hours prior to the assessment. Wear exercise clothing, including a shirt with short or loose-fitting sleeves to allow for placement of the blood pressure cuff around the upper arm.

### I. Resting Heart Rate and Blood Pressure
Determine your resting heart rate and blood pressure in the right and left arms while sitting comfortably in a chair.

Resting Heart Rate: [        ] bpm    Rating (see Table 1.4, page 25): [        ]

| **Blood Pressure:** | **Right Arm** | **Rating (from Table 1.5, page 26)** | **Left Arm** | **Rating (from Table 1.5, page 26)** |
|---|---|---|---|---|
| Systolic | [    ] | [        ] | [    ] | [        ] |
| Diastolic | [    ] | [        ] | [    ] | [        ] |

### II. Standing, Walking, Jogging Heart Rate and Blood Pressure
Have one individual measure your heart rate and another individual your blood pressure immediately after standing for one minute, after walking for one minute, and after jogging in place for one minute. For blood pressure assessment use the arm that showed the highest reading in the sitting position (in Part I, above).

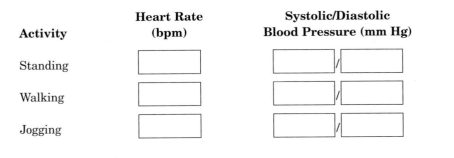

| Activity | **Heart Rate (bpm)** | **Systolic/Diastolic Blood Pressure (mm Hg)** | |
|---|---|---|---|
| Standing | [    ] | [    ] / | [    ] |
| Walking | [    ] | [    ] / | [    ] |
| Jogging | [    ] | [    ] / | [    ] |

## III. Effects of Aerobic Activity on Resting Heart Rate

Using your actual resting heart rate (RHR) from Part I of this lab, compute the total number of times your heart beats each day and each year:

A.  Beats per day = _____ (RHR bpm) × 60 (min per hour) × 24 (hours per day) = _____ beats per day

B.  Beats per year = _____ (heart rate in beats per day, use item A) × 365 = _____ beats per year

If your RHR dropped 20 bpm through an aerobic exercise program, determine the number of beats that your heart would save each year at that lower RHR:

C.  Beats per day = _____ (your current RHR − 20) × 60 × 24 = _____ beats per day

D.  Beats per year = _____ (heart rate in beats per day, use item C) × 365 = _____ beats per year

E.  Number of beats saved per year (B − D) _____ − _____ = _____ beats saved per year

Assuming that you will reach the average US life expectancy of 80 years for women or 75 for men, determine the additional number of "heart rate life years" available to you if your RHR were 20 bpm lower:

F.  Years of life ahead = _____ (use 80 for women and 75 for men) − _____ (current age) = _____ years

G.  Number of beats saved = _____ (use item E) × _____ (use item F) = _____ beats saved

H.  Number of heart rate life years based on the lower RHR = _____ (use item G) ÷ _____ (use item D) = _____ years

## IV. Mean Blood Pressure Computation

During a normal resting contraction/relaxation cycle of the heart, the heart spends more time in the relaxation (diastolic) phase than in the contraction (systolic) phase. Accordingly, mean blood pressure (MBP) cannot be computed by taking an average of the systolic (SBP) and diastolic (DBP) blood pressures. The following equations are, therefore, used to determine MBP:

$MBP = DBP + \frac{1}{3} PP$     Where PP = pulse pressure or the difference between the systolic and diastolic pressures.

A.  Compute your MBP using your own blood pressure results:

PP = _____ (systolic) − _____ (diastolic) = _____ mm Hg

MBP = _____ (DBP) + $\dfrac{\text{_____(PP)}}{3}$ = _____ mm Hg

B.  Determine the MBP for a person with a BP of 130/80 and a second person with a BP of 120/90.

_____

_____

_____

_____

Which subject has the lower MBP? _____

## V. What I Learned

Draw conclusions based on your observed resting and activity heart rates and blood pressures. Discuss the importance of a lower resting heart rate to your health and comment on the effects of a higher systolic versus diastolic blood pressure on the mean arterial blood pressure.

_____

_____

_____

_____

_____

# Behavior Modification

# 2

Jim Cummins/Getty Images

## Objectives

- Learn the effects of environment on human behavior
- Understand obstacles that hinder the ability to change behavior
- Explain the concepts of motivation and locus of control
- Identify the stages of change
- Describe the processes of change
- Explain techniques that will facilitate the process of change
- Describe the role of SMART goal setting in the process of change
- Be able to write specific objectives for behavioral change

Prepare for a healthy change in lifestyle. Check your understanding of the chapter contents by logging on to CengageNOW and accessing the pre-test, personalized learning plan, and post-test for this chapter.

# FAQ

### Why is it so hard to change?

Change is incredibly difficult for most people. Our behaviors are based on our core values. Whether we are trying to increase physical activity, quit smoking, change unhealthy eating habits, or reverse heart disease, it is human nature to resist change even when we know that change will provide substantial benefits. Furthermore, Dr. Richard Earle, managing director of the Canadian Institute of Stress and the Hans Selye Foundation, explains that people have a tendency toward pessimism. In every spoken language, there is a ratio of three pessimistic adjectives to one positive adjective. Thus, linguistically, psychologically, and emotionally, we focus on what can go wrong and we lose motivation before we even start. "That's why we have the saying, 'The only person who truly welcomes a change is a baby with a full diaper.'"

### What triggers the desire to change?

Motivation comes from within. In most instances, no amount of pressure, reasoning, or fear will inspire people to take action. Change in behavior is most likely to occur by speaking to people's feelings. Most people start contemplating change when there is a change in core values that will make them feel uncomfortable with the present behavior(s) or lack thereof. Core values change when feelings are addressed. The challenge is to find ways that will help people understand the problems and solutions in a manner that will influence emotions and not just the thought process. Once the problem behavior is understood and "felt," the person may become uncomfortable with the situation and will be more inclined to address the problem behavior or adoption of a healthy behavior.

Dr. Jan Hill, a Toronto-based life skills specialist, stated that discomfort is a great motivator. People tolerate any situation until it becomes too uncomfortable for them: "Then they have to take steps to make changes in their lives." It is at this point that the skills presented in this chapter will help you implement a successful plan for change. Keep in mind that as you make lifestyle changes, your relationships and friendships also need to be addressed. You need to distance yourself from those individuals who share your bad habits (smoking, drinking, sedentary lifestyle) and associate with people who practice healthy habits. Are you prepared to do so?

The benefits of regular physical activity and living a healthy lifestyle to achieve wellness are well documented. Nearly all Americans accept that exercise is beneficial to health and see a need to incorporate it into their lives. Seventy percent of new and returning exercisers, however, are at risk for early dropout.[1] As the scientific evidence continues to mount each day, most people still are not adhering to a healthy lifestyle program.

Let's look at an all-too-common occurrence on college campuses. Most students understand that they should be exercising, and they contemplate enrolling in a fitness course. The motivating factor might be improved physical appearance, health benefits, or simply fulfillment of a college requirement. They sign up for the course, participate for a few months, finish the course—and stop exercising! They offer a wide array of excuses: too busy, no one to exercise with, already have the grade, inconvenient open-gym hours, job conflicts, and so on. A few months later they realize once again that exercise is vital, and they repeat the cycle (see Figure 2.1).

The information in this book will be of little value to you if you are unable to abandon your negative habits and adopt and maintain healthy behaviors. Before looking at any physical fitness and wellness guidelines, you will need

**FIGURE 2.1** Exercise/exercise-dropout cycle.

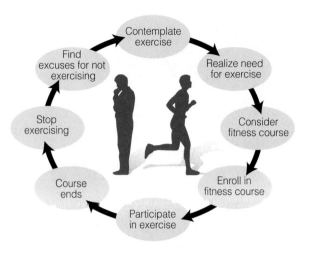

to take a critical look at your behaviors and lifestyle—and most likely make some permanent changes to promote your overall health and wellness.

# Living in a Toxic Health and Fitness Environment

Most of the behaviors we adopt are a product of our environment—the forces of social influences we encounter and the thought processes we go through (also see self-efficacy on pages 46–47). This environment includes our families, friends, peers, homes, schools, workplaces, television, radio, and movies, as well as our communities, country, and culture in general.

Unfortunately, when it comes to fitness and wellness, we live in a "toxic" environment. Becoming aware of how the environment affects us is vital if we wish to achieve and maintain wellness. Yet, we are so habituated to the environment that we miss the subtle ways it influences our behaviors, personal lifestyle, and health each day.

From a young age, we observe, we learn, we emulate, and without realizing it, we incorporate into our own lifestyle the behaviors of people around us. We are transported by parents, relatives, and friends who drive us nearly anyplace we need to go. We watch them drive short distances to run errands. We see them take escalators and elevators and ride moving sidewalks at malls and airports. We notice that the adults around us use remote controls, pagers, and cell phones. We observe them stop at fast-food restaurants and pick up supersized, calorie-dense, high-fat meals. They watch television and surf the 'Net for hours at a time. Some smoke, some drink heavily, and some have hard-drug addictions. Others engage in risky behaviors by not wearing seat belts, by drinking and driving, and by having unprotected sex. All of these un-

healthy habits can be passed along, unquestioned, to the next generation.

# Environmental Influences on Physical Activity

Among the leading underlying causes of death in the United States are physical inactivity and poor diet. This is partially because most activities of daily living, which a few decades ago required movement or physical activity, now require almost no effort and negatively impact health, fitness, and body weight. Small movements that have been streamlined out of daily life quickly add up, especially when we consider these over 7 days a week and 52 weeks a year.

We can examine the decrease in the required daily energy (caloric) expenditure as a result of modern-day conveniences that lull us into physical inactivity. For example, short automobile trips that replace walking or riding a bike decrease energy expenditure by 50 to 300 calories per day; automatic car window and door openers represent about 1 calorie at each use; automatic garage door openers, 5 calories; drive-through windows at banks, fast-food restaurants, dry cleaners, and pharmacies add up to about 5 to 10 calories each time; elevators and escalators, 3 to 10 calories per trip; food processors, 5 to 10 calories; riding lawnmowers, about 100 calories; automatic car washes, 100 calories; hours of computer use to e-mail, surf the 'Net, and conduct Internet transactions represent another 50 to 300 calories; and excessive television viewing can add up to 200 or more calories. Little wonder that we have such a difficult time maintaining a healthy body weight.

Health experts recommend that to be considered active, a person accumulate the equivalent of five to six miles of walking per day. This level of activity equates to about 10,000 to 12,000 daily steps. If you have never clipped on a pedometer, try to do so. When you look at the total number of steps it displays at the end of the day, you may be shocked by how few steps you took.

With the advent of now-ubiquitous cell phones, people are moving even less. Family members call each other on the phone even within the walls of their own home. Some people don't get out of the car anymore to ring a doorbell. Instead, they wait in front and send a text message to have the person come out.

Even modern-day architecture reinforces unhealthy behaviors. Elevators and escalators are often of the finest workmanship and are located conveniently. Many of our newest, showiest shopping centers and convention centers don't provide accessible stairwells, so people are all but forced to ride escalators. If they want to walk up the escalator, they can't because the people in front of them obstruct the way. Entrances to buildings provide electric

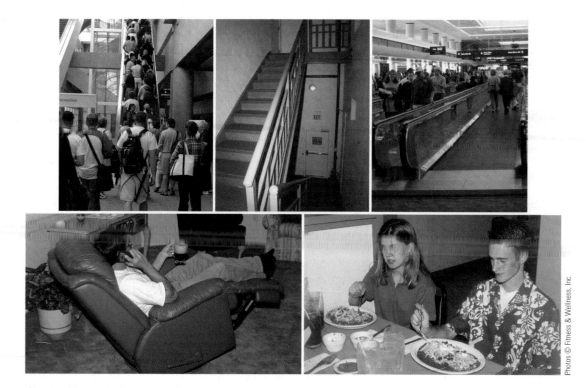

Photos © Fitness & Wellness, Inc.

Our environment is not conducive to a healthy, physically active lifestyle.

sensors and automatic door openers. Without a second thought, people walk through automatic doors instead of taking the time to push a door open.

At work, most people have jobs that require them to sit most of the day. We don't even get up and walk a short distance to talk to co-workers. Instead, we use intercoms and telephones.

Leisure time is no better. When people arrive home after work, they surf the 'Net, play computer games, or watch television for hours at a time. The first thing people consider when setting up a family room is where to put the television. This little (or big-screen) box has truly lulled us into inactivity. Excessive TV viewing is directly linked to obesity, and the amount of time people choose to spend watching television programs and DVDs is climbing. The average household watches close to 8 hours of programming each day—up one hour from 1982 and two from 1970.[2]

Television viewing is more than just a sedentary activity. Think about people's habits before they sit down to watch a favorite show. They turn on the television, then stop by the kitchen for a box of crackers and processed cheese. They return to watch the show, start snacking, and are bombarded with commercials about soft drinks, beer, and unhealthy foods. Viewers are enticed to purchase and eat unhealthy, calorie-dense foods in an unnecessary and mindless "snacking setting." Television viewing has been shown to reduce the number of fruits and vegetables some people consume, most likely because people are eating the unhealthy foods advertised on television.[3]

Our communities aren't much help either. Walking, jogging, and bicycle trails are too sparse in most cities, further discouraging physical activity. Places for safe exercise

are hard to find in many metropolitan areas, motivating many people to remain indoors during leisure hours for fear of endangering their personal safety and well-being.

In addition to sitting most of the day at work and at home, we also sit in our cars. We are transported or drive everywhere we have to go. Safety concerns also keep people in cars instead of on sidewalks and in parks. And communities are designed around the automobile. City streets make driving convenient and walking or cycling difficult, impossible, or dangerous. Streets typically are rated by traffic engineers according to their "level of service"—that is, based on how well they facilitate motorized traffic. A wide, straight street with few barriers to slow motorized traffic gets a high score. According to these guidelines, pedestrians are "obstructions." Only recently have a few local governments and communities started to devise standards to determine how useful streets are for pedestrians and bicyclists.

For each car in the United States, there are seven parking spaces.[4] Drivers can almost always find a parking spot, but walkers often run out of sidewalks and crosswalks in modern streets. Sidewalks have not been a priority in city, suburban, or commercial development. Whereas British street design manuals recommend sidewalks on both sides of the street, American manuals recommend sidewalks on one side of the street only.

One measure that encourages activity is the use of "traffic-calming" strategies: intentionally slowing traffic to make the pedestrian's role easier. These strategies were developed and are widely used in Europe. Examples include narrow streets, rough pavement (cobblestone), pedestrian islands, and raised crosswalks.

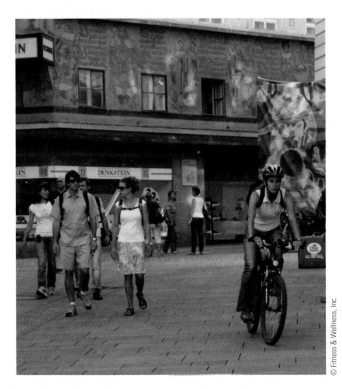

Walking and cycling are priority activities in many European communities.

Many European communities place a high priority on walking and cycling, which makes up 40 to 54 percent of all daily trips taken by people in Austria, the Netherlands, Denmark, Italy, and Sweden. By contrast, in the United States, walking and biking account for 10 percent of daily trips, whereas the automobile accounts for 84 percent (although these figures may change in the near future due to the high cost of fuel).[5]

Granted, many people drive because the distances to cover are on a vast scale. We live in bedroom communities and commute to work. When people live near frequently visited destinations, they are more likely to walk or bike for transportation. Neighborhoods that mix commercial and residential uses of land encourage walking over driving because of the short distances between home, shopping, and work.

Children also walk or cycle to school today less frequently than in the past. The reasons? Distance, traffic, weather, perceived crime, and school policy. Distance is a significant barrier because the trend during the last few decades has been to build larger schools on the outskirts of communities instead of small schools within neighborhoods.

# Environmental Influence on Diet and Nutrition

The present obesity epidemic in the United States and other developed countries has been getting worse every year. We are becoming a nation of overweight and obese people. You may ask why. Let's examine the evidence.

According to the U.S. Department of Agriculture's Center for Nutrition Policy and Promotion, the amount of daily food supply available in the United States is about 3,900 calories per person, before wastage. This figure represents a 700-calorie rise over the early 1980s,[6] which means that we have taken the amount of food available to us and tossed in a Cinnabon for every person in the country.

The overabundance of food increases pressure on food suppliers to advertise and try to convince consumers to buy their products. The food industry spends more than $33 billion each year on advertising and promotion, and most of this money goes toward highly processed foods. The few ads and campaigns promoting healthy foods and healthful eating simply cannot compete. Most of us would be hard-pressed to recall a jingle for brown rice or kale. The money spent advertising a single food product across the United States is often 10 to 50 times more than the money the federal government spends promoting MyPyramid or encouraging us to eat fruits and vegetables.[7]

Coupled with our sedentary lifestyle, many activities of daily living in today's culture are associated with eating. We seem to be eating all the time. We eat during coffee breaks, when we socialize, when we play, when we watch sports, at the movies, during television viewing, and when the clock tells us it's time for a meal. Our lives seem to be centered on food, a nonstop string of occasions to eat and overeat. And much of the overeating is done without a second thought. For instance, when people rent a video, they usually end up in line with the video and also with popcorn, candy, and soft drinks. Do we really have to eat while watching a movie?

As a nation, we eat out more often than in the past, portion sizes are larger, and we have an endless variety of foods to choose from. We also snack more than ever before. Unhealthy food is relatively inexpensive and is sold in places where it was not available in the past.

Increasingly, people have decided that they no longer require special occasions to eat out. Mother's Day, a birthday, or someone's graduation are no longer reasons to eat at a restaurant. Eating out is part of today's lifestyle. In the late 1970s, food eaten away from home represented about 18 percent of our energy intake. In the mid-1990s, this figure rose to 32 percent. Almost half of the money Americans spend on food today is on meals away from home.[8]

Eating out would not be such a problem if portion sizes were reasonable or if restaurant food were similar to food prepared at home. Compared with home-cooked meals, restaurant and fast-food meals are higher in fat and calories and lower in essential nutrients and fiber.

Food portions in restaurants have increased substantially in size. Patrons consume huge amounts of food, almost as if this were the last meal they would ever have. They drink entire pitchers of soda pop or beer instead of the traditional 8-ounce-cup size. Some restaurant menus may include selections that are called "healthy choices," but these items may not provide nutritional information, including calories. In all likelihood, the menu has many other choices that look delicious but provide larger serving sizes with more fat and calories and fewer fruits and vegetables. Making a healthy selection is difficult, because people tend to choose food for its taste, convenience, and cost instead of nutrition.

Restaurant food is often less healthy than we think. Trained dietitians were asked to estimate nutrition information for five restaurant meals. The results showed that the dietitians underestimated the number of calories and amount of fat by 37 percent and 49 percent, respectively.[9] Findings such as these do not offer much hope for the average consumer who tries to make healthy choices when eating out.

We can also notice that most restaurants are pleasurable places to be: colorful, well lit, and thoughtfully decorated. These intentional features are designed to enhance comfort, appetite, and length of stay, with the intent to entice more eating. Employees are formally trained in techniques that urge patrons to eat more and spend more. Servers are prepared to approach the table and suggest specific drinks, with at least one from the bar. When the drink is served, they recommend selected appetizers. Drink refills are often free while dining out. Following dinner, the server offers desserts and coffee. A person could literally get a full day's worth of calories in one meal without ever ordering an entree.

Fast-food restaurants do not lag far behind. Popular menu items frequently are introduced at one size and, over time, are increased two to five times.[10] Large portion sizes are a major problem because people tend to eat what they are served. A study by the American Institute for Cancer Research found that with bigger portion sizes, 67 percent of Americans ate the larger amount of food they were served.[11] The tendency of most patrons is to clean their plates.

Individuals seem to have the same disregard for hunger cues when snacking. Participants in one study were randomly given an afternoon snack of potato chips in different bag sizes. They received bags from 1 to 20 ounces for five days. The results showed that the larger the bag, the more the person ate. Men ate 37 percent more chips from the largest than the smallest bag. Women ate 18 percent more. Of significant interest, the size of the snack did not change the amount of food the person ate during the next meal.[12] Another study found no major difference in reported hunger or fullness after participants ate different sizes of sandwiches that were served to them, even though they ate more when they were given larger sandwiches.[13]

Other researchers set out to see if the size of the package—not just the amount of food—affected how much people ate. Study participants received two different sized packages with the same number of spaghetti strands. The larger package was twice the size of the smaller package. When participants were asked to take out enough spaghetti to prepare a meal for two adults, they took out an average of 234 strands from the small package versus 302 strands from the larger package.[14] In our own kitch-

ens, and in restaurants, we seem to have taken away from our internal cues the decision of how much to eat. Instead we have turned that choice over to businesses that profit from our overindulgence.

Also working against our hunger cues is our sense of thrift. Many of us consider cost ahead of nutrition when we choose foods. Restaurants and groceries often appeal to this sense of thrift by using "value marketing," meaning that they offer us a larger portion for only a small price increase. Customers think they are getting a bargain, and the food providers turn a better profit because the cost of additional food is small compared with the cost of marketing, production, and labor.

The National Alliance for Nutrition has further shown that a little more money buys a lot more calories. Ice cream upsizing from a kid's scoop to a double scoop, for example, adds an extra 390 calories for only an extra $1.62. A medium-size movie theater popcorn (unbuttered) provides 500 additional calories over a small-size popcorn for just an extra 71 cents. Equally, king-size candy bars provide about 230 additional calories for just another 33 cents over the standard size.[15] We often eat more simply because we get more for our money, without taking into consideration the detrimental consequences to our health and waistlines.

Another example of financial but not nutritional sense is free soft-drink refills. When people choose a high-calorie drink over diet soda or water, the person does not compensate by eating less food later that day.[16] Liquid calories seem to be difficult for people to account for. A 20-ounce bottle of regular soda contains the equivalent of one-third cup of sugar. One extra can of soda (160 calories) per day represents an extra 16.5 pounds of fat per year (160 calories $\times$ 365 days = 3,500 calories). Even people who regularly drink diet sodas tend to gain weight. In their minds, they may rationalize that a calorie-free drink allows them to consume more food.

A larger variety of food also entices overeating. Think about your own experiences at parties that have a buffet of snacks. Do you eat more when everyone brings something to contribute to the snack table? When unhealthy choices outnumber healthy choices, people are less likely to follow their natural cues to choose healthy food.

The previously mentioned environmental factors influence our thought processes and hinder our ability to determine what constitutes an appropriate meal based on actual needs. The result: On average, American women consume 335 more daily calories than they did 20 years ago, and men an additional 170 calories.[17]

Now you can analyze and identify the environmental influences on your behaviors. Lab 2A provides you with the opportunity to determine whether you control your environment or the environment controls you.

Living in the 21st century, we have all the modern-day conveniences that lull us into overconsumption and sedentary living. By living in America, we adopt behaviors that put our health at risk. And though we understand that lifestyle choices affect our health and well-being, we still have an extremely difficult time making changes.

Let's look at weight gain. Most people do not start life with a weight problem. By age 20, a man may weigh 160 pounds. A few years later, the weight starts to climb and may reach 170 pounds. He now adapts and accepts 170 pounds as his weight. He may go on a diet but not make the necessary lifestyle changes. Gradually his weight climbs to 180, 190, 200 pounds. Although he may not like it and would like to weigh less, once again he adapts and accepts 200 pounds as his stable weight.

The time comes, usually around middle age, when values change and people want to make changes in their lives but find this difficult to accomplish, illustrating the adage that "old habits die hard." Acquiring positive behaviors that will lead to better health and well-being is a long-term process and requires continual effort. Understanding why so many people are unsuccessful at changing their behaviors and are unable to live a healthy lifestyle may increase your readiness and motivation for change. Next we will examine barriers to change, what motivates people to change, behavior change theories, the transtheoretical or stages-of-change model, the process of change, techniques for change, and actions required to make permanent changes in behavior.

# Barriers to Change

In spite of the best intentions, people make unhealthy choices daily. The most common reasons are:

1. **Lack of core values.** Most people recognize the benefits of a healthy lifestyle but are unwilling or unable to trade convenience (sedentary lifestyle, unhealthy eating, substance abuse) for health or other benefits.

   *Tip to initiate change.* Educate yourself regarding the benefits of a healthy lifestyle and subscribe to several reputable health, fitness, and wellness newsletters (see Chapter 15). The more you read about, understand, and then start living a wellness lifestyle, the more your core values will change. At this time you should also break relationships with individuals who are unwilling to change with you.

2. **Procrastination.** People seem to think that tomorrow, next week, or after the holiday is the best time to start change.

   *Tip to initiate change.* Ask yourself: Why wait until tomorrow when you can start changing today? Lack of motivation is a key factor in procrastination (motivation is discussed later in this chapter).

3. **Preconditioned cultural beliefs.** If we accept the idea that we are a product of our environment, our cultural beliefs and our physical surroundings pose significant barriers to change. In Salzburg, Austria, people of both genders and all ages use bicycles as a primary mode of transportation. In the United States, few people other than children ride bicycles.

   *Tip to initiate change.* Find a like-minded partner. In the pre-Columbian era, people thought the world was flat. Few dared to sail long distances for fear that they would fall off the edge. If your health and fitness are at stake, preconditioned cultural beliefs shouldn't keep you from making changes. Finding people who are willing to "sail" with you will help overcome this barrier.

4. **Gratification.** People prefer instant gratification to long-term benefits. Therefore, they will overeat (instant pleasure) instead of using self-restraint to eat moderately to prevent weight gain (long-term satisfaction). We like tanning (instant gratification) and avoid paying much attention to skin cancer (long-term consequence).

   *Tip to initiate change.* Think ahead and ask yourself: How did I feel the last time I engaged in this behavior? How did it affect me? Did I really feel good about myself or about the results? In retrospect, was it worth it?

5. **Risk complacency.** Consequences of unhealthy behaviors often don't manifest themselves until years later. People tell themselves, "If I get heart disease, I'll deal with it then. For now, let me eat, drink, and be merry."

   *Tip to initiate change.* Ask yourself: How long do I want to live? How do I want to live the rest of my life and what type of health do I want to have? What do I want to be able to do when I am 60, 70, or 80 years old?

6. **Complexity.** People think the world is too complicated, with too much to think about. If you are living the typical lifestyle, you may feel overwhelmed by everything that seems to be required to lead a healthy lifestyle, for example:
   • Getting exercise
   • Decreasing intake of saturated and trans fats
   • Eating high-fiber meals and cutting total calories
   • Controlling use of substances
   • Managing stress
   • Wearing seat belts
   • Practicing safe sex
   • Getting annual physicals, including blood tests, Pap smears, and so on
   • Fostering spiritual, social, and emotional wellness

   *Tip to initiate change.* Take it one step at a time. Work on only one or two behaviors at a time so the task won't seem insurmountable.

7. **Indifference and helplessness.** A defeatist thought process often takes over, and we may believe that the way we live won't really affect our health, that we have no control over our health, or that our destiny is all in our genes (also see discussion of locus of control, pages 47–48).

   *Tip to initiate change.* As much as 84 percent of the leading causes of death in the United States are preventable. Realize that only you can take control of your personal health and lifestyle habits and affect the qual-

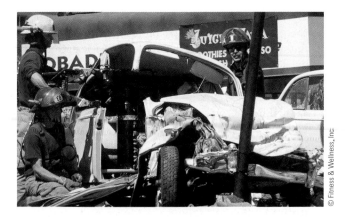

Feelings of invincibility are a strong barrier to change that can bring about life-threatening consequences.

ity of your life. Implementing many of the behavioral modification strategies and programs outlined in this book will get you started on a wellness way of life.

8. **Rationalization.** Even though people are not practicing healthy behaviors, they often tell themselves that they do get sufficient exercise, that their diet is fine, that they have good, solid relationships, or that they don't smoke/drink/get high enough to affect their health.

*Tip to initiate change.* Learn to recognize when you're glossing over or minimizing a problem. You'll need to face the fact that you have a problem before you can commit to change. Your health and your life are at stake. Monitoring lifestyle habits through daily logs and then analyzing the results can help you change self-defeating behaviors.

9. **Illusions of invincibility.** At times people believe that unhealthy behaviors will not harm them. Young adults often have the attitude that "I can smoke now, and in a few years I'll quit before it causes any damage." Unfortunately, nicotine is one of the most addictive drugs known to us, so quitting smoking is not an easy task. Health problems may arise before you quit, and the risk of lung cancer lingers for years after you quit. Another example is drinking and driving. The feeling of "I'm in control" or "I can handle it" while under the influence of alcohol is a deadly combination. Others perceive low risk when engaging in negative behaviors with people they like (for example, sex with someone you've recently met and feel attracted to) but perceive themselves at risk just by being in the same classroom with an HIV-infected person.

*Tip to initiate change.* No one is immune to sickness, disease, and tragedy. The younger you are when you implement a healthy lifestyle, the better are your odds to attain a long and healthy life. Thus, initiating change right now will help you enjoy the best possible quality of life for as long as you live.

When health and appearance begin to deteriorate—usually around middle age—people seek out health care professionals in search of a "magic pill" to reverse and cure the many ills they have accumulated during years of abuse and overindulgence. The sooner we implement a healthy lifestyle program, the greater will be the health benefits and quality of life that lie ahead.

# Self-Efficacy

At the heart of behavior modification is the concept of **self-efficacy,** or the belief in one's own ability to perform a given task. Self-efficacy exerts a powerful influence on people's behaviors and touches virtually every aspect of their lives. It determines how you feel, think, behave, motivate yourself, make choices, set goals, and pursue courses of action, as well as the effort you put into all of your tasks or activities. It also influences your vulnerability to stress and depression. Furthermore, your confidence in your coping skills determines how resilient you are in the face of adversity. Possessing high self-efficacy enhances wellness in countless ways, including your desire to learn, be productive, be fit, and be healthy.

The knowledge and skills you possess and further develop determine your goals and what you do and choose not to do. Mahatma Gandhi once stated: "If I have the belief that I can do it, I shall surely acquire the capacity to do it even if I may not have it at the beginning." Likewise, Teilhard de Chardin, a French paleontologist and philosopher, stated: "It is our duty as human beings to proceed as though the limits of our capabilities do not exist." With this type of attitude, how can you not strive to be the best that you can possibly be?

As you have already learned in this chapter, the environment has a tremendous effect on our behaviors. We can therefore increase self-efficacy by the type of environment we choose. Experts agree that four different sources affect self-efficacy (discussed next). If you understand these sources and learn from them, you can use them to improve your degree of efficacy. Subsequently, you can apply the concepts for change provided in this chapter to increase confidence in your abilities to master challenging tasks and succeed at implementing change.

Sources of Self-Efficacy The best contributors to self-efficacy are mastery experiences, or personal experiences that one has had with successes and failures. Successful past performances greatly enhance self-efficacy: "Nothing succeeds like success." Failures, on the other hand, undermine confidence, in particular if they occur before a sense of efficacy is established.

You should structure your activities in such ways that they will bring success. Don't set your goals too high or make them too difficult to achieve. Your success at a particular activity increases your confidence in being able to repeat that activity. Once strong self-efficacy is developed through successful mastery experiences, an occasional setback does not have a significant effect on one's beliefs.

Vicarious experiences provided by role models or those one admires also influence personal efficacy. This involves the thought process of your belief that you can also do it. When you observe a peer of similar capabilities master a task, you are more likely to develop a belief that you too can perform that task—"If he can do it, so can I." Here you imitate the model's skill or you follow the same approach demonstrated by your model to complete the task. You may also visualize success. Visual imagery of successful personal performance, that is, watching yourself perform the skill in your mind, also increases personal efficacy.

Although not as effective as past performances and vicarious experiences, verbal persuasion of one's capabilities to perform a task also contributes to self-efficacy. When you are verbally persuaded that you possess the capabilities, you will be more likely to try the task and believe that you can get it done. The opposite is also true. Negative verbal persuasion has a far greater effect in lowering efficacy than positive messages do to enhance it. If you are verbally persuaded that you lack the skills to master a task, you will tend to avoid the activity and will be more likely to give up without giving yourself a fair chance to succeed.

The least significant source of self-efficacy beliefs are physiological cues that people experience when facing a challenge. These cues in turn affect performance. For example, feeling calm, relaxed, and self-confident enhances self-efficacy. Anxiety, nervousness, perspiration, dryness of the mouth, and a rapid heart rate are cues that may adversely affect performance. You may question your competence to successfully complete the task.

# Motivation and Locus of Control

The explanation given for why some people succeed and others do not is often **motivation.** Although motivation comes from within, external factors trigger the inner desire to accomplish a given task. These external factors, then, control behavior.

When studying motivation, understanding locus of control is helpful. People who believe that they have control over events in their lives are said to have an internal **locus of control.** People with an external locus of control believe that what happens to them is a result of chance or the environment and is unrelated to their behavior. People with an internal locus of control generally are healthier and have an easier time initiating and adhering to a wellness program than those who perceive that they have no control and think of themselves as powerless and vulnerable. The latter people also are at greater risk for illness. When illness does strike a person, establishing a sense of control is vital to recovery.

Few people have either a completely external or a completely internal locus of control. They fall somewhere along a continuum. The more external one's locus of control is, the greater is the challenge to change and adhere to exercise and other healthy lifestyle behaviors. Fortunately, people can develop a more internal locus of control. Understanding that most events in life are not determined genetically or environmentally helps people pursue goals and gain control over their lives. Three impediments, however, can keep people from taking action: lack of competence, lack of confidence, and lack of motivation.[18]

1. *Problems of competence.* Lacking the skills to get a given task done leads to reduced competence. If your friends play basketball regularly but you don't know how to play, you might be inclined not to participate. The solution to this problem of competence is to master the skills required to participate. Most people are not born with all-inclusive natural abilities, including playing sports.

   Another alternative is to select an activity in which you are skilled. It may not be basketball, but it well could be aerobics. Don't be afraid to try new activities. Similarly, if your body weight is a problem, you could learn to cook healthy, low-calorie meals. Try different recipes until you find foods that you like.

2. *Problems of confidence.* Problems of confidence arise when you have the skill but don't believe you can get it done. Fear and feelings of inadequacy often interfere with the ability to perform the task. You shouldn't talk yourself out of something until you have given it a fair try. If you have the skills, the sky is the limit. Initially, try to visualize yourself doing the task and getting it done. Repeat this several times, then actually try it. You will surprise yourself.

   Sometimes, lack of confidence arises when the task seems insurmountable. In these situations, dividing a goal into smaller, more realistic objectives helps to accomplish the task. You might know how to swim but may need to train for several weeks to swim a continu-

---

**Self-efficacy** One's belief in the ability to perform a given task.

**Motivation** The desire and will to do something.

**Locus of control** A concept examining the extent to which a person believes he or she can influence the external environment.

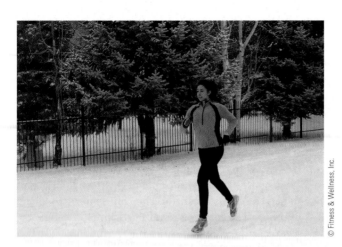

© Fitness & Wellness, Inc.

The higher quality of life experienced by people who are physically fit is hard to explain to someone who has never achieved good fitness.

ous mile. Set up your training program so you swim a little farther each day until you are able to swim the entire mile. If you don't meet your objective on a given day, try it again, reevaluate, cut back a little, and, most important, don't give up.

3. *Problems of motivation.* With problems of motivation, both the competence and the confidence are there but individuals are unwilling to change because the reasons to change are not important to them. For example, people begin contemplating a smoking-cessation program only when the reasons for quitting outweigh the reasons for smoking. The primary causes of unwillingness to change are lack of knowledge and lack of goals. Knowledge often determines goals, and goals determine motivation. How badly you want something dictates how hard you'll work at it.

Many people are unaware of the magnitude of benefits of a wellness program. When it comes to a healthy lifestyle, however, you may not get a second chance. A stroke, a heart attack, or cancer can have irreparable or fatal consequences. Greater understanding of what leads to disease can help initiate change. Joy, however, is a greater motivator than fear. Even fear of dying often doesn't instigate change.

Two years following coronary bypass surgery (for heart disease), most patients' denial returns, and surveys show that they have not done much to alter their unhealthy lifestyle. The motivating factor for the few who do change is the "joy of living." Rather than dwelling on the "fear of dying" and causing patients to live in emotional pain, point out the fact that change will help them feel better. They will be able to enhance their quality of life by carrying out activities of daily living without concern for a heart attack, go for a walk without chest pain, play with children, and even resume an intimate relationship.

Also, feeling physically fit is difficult to explain to people unless they have experienced it themselves. Feelings of fitness, self-esteem, confidence, health, and better quality of life cannot be conveyed to someone who is constrained by sedentary living. In a way, wellness is like reaching the top of a mountain. The quiet, the clean air, the lush vegetation, the flowing water in the river, the wildlife, and the majestic valley below are difficult to explain to someone who has spent a lifetime within city limits.

# Changing Behavior

The first step in addressing behavioral change is to recognize that you indeed have a problem. The five general categories of behaviors addressed in the process of willful change are:

1. Stopping a negative behavior
2. Preventing relapse of a negative behavior
3. Developing a positive behavior
4. Strengthening a positive behavior
5. Maintaining a positive behavior

People do not change all at once. Thus, psychotherapy has been used successfully to help people change their behavior. But most people do not seek professional help. They usually attempt to change by themselves with limited or no knowledge of how to achieve change. In essence, the process of change moves along a continuum from not willing to change, to recognizing the need for change, to taking action and implementing change.

The simplest model of change is the two-stage model of unhealthy behavior and healthy behavior. This model states that either you do it or you don't. Most people who use this model attempt self-change but end up asking themselves why they're unsuccessful. They just can't do it (exercise, perhaps, or quit smoking). Their intent to change may be good, but to accomplish it, they need knowledge about how to achieve change.

## Behavior Change Theories
For most people, changing chronic/unhealthy behaviors to stable, healthy behaviors is challenging. The "do it or don't do it" approach seldom works when attempting to implement lifestyle changes. Thus, several theories or models have been developed over the years. Among the most accepted are learning theories, the problem-solving model, social cognitive theory, the relapse prevention model, and the transtheoretical model.

**Learning Theories** **Learning theories** maintain that most behaviors are learned and maintained under complex schedules of reinforcement and anticipated outcomes. The process involved in learning a new behavior requires modifying many small behaviors that shape the new pattern behavior. For example, a previously inactive individual who wishes to accumulate 10,000 steps per day may have to gradually increase the number of steps daily, park farther away from the office and stores, decrease television and Internet use, take stairs instead of elevators and escalators, and avoid the car and telephone when running errands that are only short distances away. The outcomes are better health and body weight management and feelings of well-being.

**FIGURE 2.2** Stages of change model: Behavior modification accomplished through progressive stages.

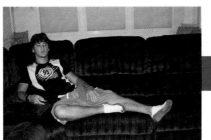

**Precontemplation**
Do not wish to change

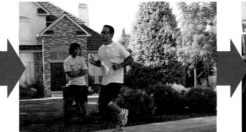

**Contemplation**
Contemplating change
over next 6 months

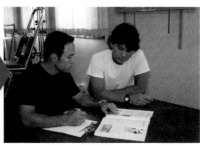

**Preparation**
Looking to change in the next month

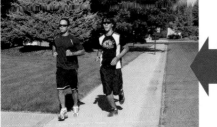

**Termination/Adoption**
Change has been maintained
for more than 5 years

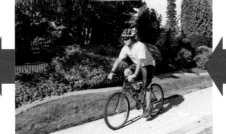

**Maintenance**
Maintaining change for 5 years

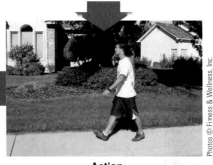

**Action**
Implementing change for 6 months

Photos © Fitness & Wellness, Inc.

**Problem-Solving Model** The **problem-solving model** proposes that many behaviors are the result of making decisions as we seek to change the problem behavior. The process of change requires conscious attention, the setting of goals, and a design for a specific plan of action. For instance, to quit smoking cigarettes, one has to understand the reasons for smoking, know under what conditions each cigarette is smoked, decide that one will quit, select a date to do so, and then draw up a plan of action to reach the goal (a complete smoking-cessation program is outlined in Chapter 13).

**Social Cognitive Theory** In **social cognitive theory**, behavior change is influenced by the environment, self-efficacy, and characteristics of the behavior itself. You can increase self-efficacy by educating yourself about the behavior, developing the skills to master the behavior, performing smaller mastery experiences successfully, and receiving verbal reinforcement and vicarious experiences. If you desire to lose weight, for example, you need to learn the principles of proper weight management, associate with people who are also losing weight or who have lost weight, eat less, shop and cook wisely, be more active, set small weight loss goals of 1 to 2 pounds per week, praise yourself for your accomplishments, and visualize losing the weight as others you admire have done.

**Relapse Prevention Model** In **relapse prevention,** people are taught to anticipate high-risk situations and develop action plans to prevent **lapses** and **relapses.** Examples of factors that disrupt behavior change include negative physiological or psychological states (stress, ill-ness), social pressure, lack of support, limited coping skills, change in work conditions, and lack of motivation. For example, if the weather turns bad for your evening walk, you can choose to walk around an indoor track (or at the mall), do water aerobics, swim, or play racquetball.

**Transtheoretical Model** The **transtheoretical model,** developed by psychologists James Prochaska, John Norcross, and Carlo DiClemente, is based on the theory that change

**Learning theories** Behavioral modification perspective stating that most behaviors are learned and maintained under complex schedules of reinforcement and anticipated outcomes.

**Problem-solving model** Behavioral modification model proposing that many behaviors are the result of making decisions as the individual seeks to solve the problem behavior.

**Social cognitive theory** Behavioral modification model holding that behavior change is influenced by the environment, self-efficacy, and characteristics of the behavior itself.

**Relapse prevention model** Behavioral modification model based on the principle that high-risk situations can be anticipated through the development of strategies to prevent lapses and relapses.

**Lapse** (v.) To slip or fall back temporarily into unhealthy behavior(s); (n.) short-term failure to maintain healthy behaviors.

**Relapse** (v.) To slip or fall back into unhealthy behavior(s) over a longer time; (n.) longer-term failure to maintain healthy behaviors.

**Transtheoretical model** Behavioral modification model proposing that change is accomplished through a series of progressive stages in keeping with a person's readiness to change.

is a gradual process that involves several stages.[19] The model is used most frequently to change health-related behaviors such as physical inactivity, smoking, poor nutrition, weight problems, stress, and alcohol abuse.

An individual goes through five stages in the process of willful change. The stages describe underlying processes that people go through to change problem behaviors and replace them with healthy behaviors. A sixth stage (termination/adoption) was subsequently added to this model. The six stages of change are precontemplation, contemplation, preparation, action, maintenance, and termination/adoption.

After years of study, researchers indicate that applying specific behavioral-change processes during each stage of the model increases the success rate for change (the specific processes for each stage are shown in Table 2.1). Understanding each stage of this model will help you determine where you are in relation to your personal healthy-lifestyle behaviors. It also will help you identify processes to make successful changes. The discussion in the remainder of the chapter focuses on the transtheoretical model, with the other models integrated as applicable with each stage of change.

1. Precontemplation

Individuals in the **precontemplation stage** are not considering change or do not want to change a given behavior. They typically deny having a problem and have no intention of changing in the immediate future. These people are usually unaware or underaware of the problem. Other people around them, including family, friends, health care practitioners, and co-workers, however, identify the problem clearly. Precontemplators do not care about the problem behavior and may even avoid information and materials that address the issue. They tend to avoid free screenings and workshops that might help identify and change the problem, even if they receive financial compensation for attending. Often they actively resist change and seem resigned to accepting the unhealthy behavior as their "fate."

Precontemplators are the most difficult people to inspire toward behavioral change. Many think that change isn't even a possibility. At this stage, knowledge is power. Educating them about the problem behavior is critical to help them start contemplating the process of change. The challenge is to find ways to help them realize that they are ultimately responsible for the consequences of their behavior. Typically, they initiate change only when people they respect or job requirements pressure them to do so.

2. Contemplation

In the **contemplation stage,** individuals acknowledge that they have a problem and begin to think seriously about overcoming it. Although they are not quite ready for change, they are weighing the pros and cons of changing. Core values are starting to change. Even

**TABLE 2.1** Applicable Processes of Change During Each Stage of Change

| Precontemplation | Contemplation | Preparation | Action | Maintenance | Termination/ Adoption |
|---|---|---|---|---|---|
| Consciousness-raising | Consciousness-raising | Consciousness-raising | | | |
| Social liberation | Social liberation | Social liberation | Social liberation | | |
| | Self-analysis | Self-analysis | | | |
| | Emotional arousal | Emotional arousal | | | |
| | Positive outlook | Positive outlook | Positive outlook | | |
| | | Commitment | Commitment | Commitment | Commitment |
| | | Behavior analysis | Behavior analysis | | |
| | | Goal setting | Goal setting | Goal setting | |
| | | Self-reevaluation | Self-reevaluation | Self-reevaluation | |
| | | | Countering | Countering | |
| | | | Monitoring | Monitoring | Monitoring |
| | | | Environment control | Environment control | Environment control |
| | | | Helping relationships | Helping relationships | Helping relationships |
| | | | Rewards | Rewards | Rewards |

**Source:** *Adapted from J. O. Prochaska, J. C. Norcross, and C. C. DiClemente, Changing for Good (New York: William Morrow, 1994); and W. W. K. Hoeger and S. A. Hoeger, Lifetime Physical Fitness & Wellness (Belmont, CA: Wadsworth / Cengage, 2009).*

though they may remain in this stage for years, in their minds they are planning to take some action within the next six months. Education and peer support remain valuable during this stage.

3. Preparation

In the **preparation stage,** individuals are seriously considering change and planning to change a behavior within the next month. They are taking initial steps for change and may even try the new behavior for a short while, such as stopping smoking for a day or exercising a few times during the month. During this stage, people define a general goal for behavioral change (for example, to quit smoking by the last day of the month) and write specific objectives (or strategies) to accomplish this goal. The discussion on goal setting later in this chapter will help you write SMART goals and specific objectives to reach your goal. Continued peer and environmental support is helpful during the preparation stage.

A key concept to keep in mind during the preparation stage is that in addition to being prepared to address the behavioral change or goal you are attempting to reach, you must prepare to address the specific objectives (supportive behaviors) required to reach that goal (see Figure 2.3). For example, you may be willing to give weight loss a try, but are you prepared to start eating less, eating out less often, eating less calorie-dense foods, shopping and cooking wisely, exercising more, watching television less, and becoming much more active? Achieving goals generally requires changing these supportive behaviors, and you must be prepared to do so.

4. Action

The **action stage** requires the greatest commitment of time and energy. Here, the individual is actively doing things to change or modify the problem behavior or to adopt a new, healthy behavior. The action stage requires that the person follow the specific guidelines set forth for that behavior. For example, a person has actually stopped smoking completely, is exercising aerobically three times a week according to exercise prescription guidelines, or is maintaining a healthy diet.

Relapse is common during this stage, and the individual may regress to a previous stage. If unsuccessful, a person should reevaluate his or her readiness to change supportive behaviors as required to reach the overall goal. Problem solving that includes identifying barriers to change and specific strategies (objectives) to overcome supportive behaviors is useful during relapse. Once people are able to maintain the action stage for six consecutive months, they move into the maintenance stage.

5. Maintenance

During the **maintenance stage,** the person continues the new behavior for up to five years. This stage requires the person to continue to adhere to the specific guidelines that govern the behavior (such as complete smoking cessation, exercising aerobically three times a week, or practicing proper stress management techniques). At this time, the person works to reinforce the gains made through the various stages of change and strives to prevent **lapses** and **relapses.**

6. Termination/Adoption

Once a person has maintained a behavior for more than five years, he or she is said to be in the **termination/ adoption stage** and exits from the cycle of change without fear of relapse. In the case of negative behaviors that are terminated, the stage of change is referred to as termination. If a positive behavior has been adopted successfully for more than five years, this stage is designated as adoption.

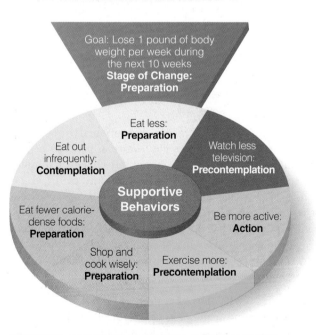

FIGURE 2.3 **Goal setting and supportive behaviors**

Goal: Lose 1 pound of body weight per week during the next 10 weeks
**Stage of Change: Preparation**

Eat less:
**Preparation**

Eat out infrequently:
**Contemplation**

Watch less television:
**Precontemplation**

**Supportive Behaviors**

Eat fewer calorie-dense foods:
**Preparation**

Be more active:
**Action**

Shop and cook wisely:
**Preparation**

Exercise more:
**Precontemplation**

**NOTE: This example may not lead to goal achievement. All supportive behaviors should be in the preparation stage to enhance success in the action stage.**

**Precontemplation stage** Stage of change in the transtheoretical model in which an individual is unwilling to change behavior.

**Contemplation stage** Stage of change in the transtheoretical model in which the individual is considering changing behavior within the next 6 months.

**Preparation stage** Stage of change in the transtheoretical model in which the individual is getting ready to make a change within the next month.

**Action stage** Stage of change in the transtheoretical model in which the individual is actively changing a negative behavior or adopting a new, healthy behavior.

**Maintenance stage** Stage of change in the transtheoretical model in which the individual maintains behavioral change for up to 5 years.

**Termination/adoption stage** Stage of change in the transtheoretical model in which the individual has eliminated an undesirable behavior or maintained a positive behavior for more than 5 years.

FIGURE 2.4  Model of progression and relapse.

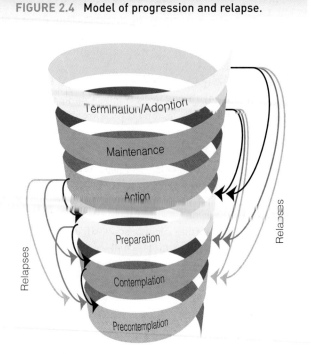

FIGURE 2.4  Model of progression and relapse.

Terminal/Adoption

Maintenance

Action

Preparation

Contemplation

Precontemplation

Relapses

Relapses

Relapses

Many experts believe that once an individual enters the termination/adoption stage, former addictions, problems, or lack of compliance with healthy behaviors no longer presents an obstacle in the quest for wellness. The change has become part of one's lifestyle. This phase is the ultimate goal for all people searching for a healthier lifestyle.

For addictive behaviors such as alcoholism and hard-drug use, however, some health-care practitioners believe that the individual never enters the termination stage. Chemical dependency is so strong that most former alcoholics and hard-drug users must make a lifetime effort to prevent relapse. Similarly, some behavioral scientists suggest that the adoption stage might not be applicable to health behaviors such as exercise and weight control because the likelihood of relapse is always high.

Use the guidelines provided in Lab 2B to determine where you stand in respect to behaviors you want to change or new ones you wish to adopt. As you follow the guidelines, you will realize that you might be at different stages for different behaviors. For instance, you might be in the preparation stage for aerobic exercise and smoking cessation, in the action stage for strength training, but only in the contemplation stage for a healthy diet. Realizing where you are with respect to different behaviors will help you design a better action plan for a healthy lifestyle.

## Relapse

After the precontemplation stage, relapse may occur at any level of the model. Even individuals in the maintenance and termination/adoption stages may regress to any of the

first three stages of the model (see Figure 2.4). Relapse, however, does not mean failure. Failure comes only to those who give up and don't use prior experiences as building blocks for future success. The chances of moving back up to a higher stage of the model are far better for someone who has previously made it into one of those stages.

# The Process of Change

Using the same plan for everyone who wishes to change a behavior will not work. With exercise, for instance, we provide different prescriptions to people of varying fitness levels (see Chapter 6). The same prescription would not provide optimal results for a person who has been inactive for 20 years, compared with one who already walks regularly three times each week. This principle also holds true for individuals who are attempting to change their behaviors.

Timing is also important in the process of willful change. People respond more effectively to selected **processes of change** in keeping with the stage of change they have reached at any given time. Thus, applying appropriate processes at each stage of change enhances the likelihood of changing behavior permanently. The following description of 14 of the most common processes of change will help you develop a personal plan for change. The respective stages of change in which each process works best are summarized in Table 2.1.

### Consciousness-Raising  The first step in a **behavior modification** program is consciousness-raising. This step involves obtaining information about the problem so you can make a better decision about the problem behavior. For example, the problem could be physical inactivity. Learning about the benefits of exercise or the difference in benefits between physical activity and exercise (see Chapter 1) can help you decide the type of fitness program (health or high fitness) that you want to pursue. Possibly, you don't even know that a certain behavior is a problem, such as being unaware of saturated and total fat content in many fast-food items. Consciousness-raising may continue from the precontemplation stage through the preparation stage.

### Social Liberation  Social liberation stresses external alternatives that make you aware of problem behaviors and make you begin to contemplate change. Examples of social liberation include pedestrian-only traffic areas, nonsmoking areas, health-oriented cafeterias and restaurants, advocacy groups, civic organizations, policy interventions, and self-help groups. Social liberation often provides opportunities to get involved, stir up emotions, and enhance self-esteem—helping you gain confidence in your ability to change.

### Self-Analysis  The next process in modifying behavior is developing a decisive desire to do so, called self-analysis. If you have no interest in changing a behavior, you won't do it. You will remain a precontemplator or a contemplator. A person who has no intention of quitting

smoking will not quit, regardless of what anyone may say or how strong the evidence in favor of quitting may be. In your self-analysis, you may want to prepare a list of reasons for continuing or discontinuing the behavior. When the reasons for changing outweigh the reasons for not changing, you are ready for the next stage—either the contemplation stage or the preparation stage.

### Emotional Arousal

In emotional arousal, a person experiences and expresses feelings about the problem and its solutions. Also referred to as "dramatic release," this process often involves deep emotional experiences. Watching a loved one die from lung cancer caused by cigarette smoking may be all that is needed to make a person quit smoking. As in other examples, emotional arousal might be prompted by a dramatization of the consequences of drug use and abuse, a film about a person undergoing open-heart surgery, or a book illustrating damage to body systems as a result of unhealthy behaviors.

### Positive Outlook

Having a positive outlook means taking an optimistic approach from the beginning and believing in yourself. Following the guidelines in this chapter will help you design a plan so you can work toward change and remain enthused about your progress. Also, you may become motivated by looking at the outcome—how much healthier you will be, how much better you will look, or how far you will be able to jog.

### Commitment

Upon making a decision to change, you accept the responsibility to change and believe in your ability to do so. During the commitment process, you engage in preparation and may draw up a specific plan of action. Write down your goals and, preferably, share them with others. In essence, you are signing a behavioral contract for change. You will be more likely to adhere to your program if others know you are committed to change.

### Behavior Analysis

How you determine the frequency, circumstances, and consequences of the behavior to be altered or implemented is known as behavior analysis. If the desired outcome is to consume less trans and saturated fats, you first must find out what foods in your diet are high in these fats, when you eat them, and when you don't eat them—all part of the preparation stage. Knowing when you don't eat them points to circumstances under which you exert control over your diet and will help as you set goals.

### Goals

Goals motivate change in behavior. The stronger the goal or desire, the more motivated you'll be either to change unwanted behaviors or to implement new, healthy

---

**Processes of change** Actions that help you achieve change in behavior.

**Behavior modification** The process of permanently changing negative behaviors to positive behaviors that will lead to better health and well-being.

## Behavior Modification Planning

### STEPS FOR SUCCESSFUL BEHAVIOR MODIFICATION

I PLAN TO / I DID IT

- ☐ ☐ 1. Acknowledge that you have a problem.
- ☐ ☐ 2. Describe the behavior to change (increase physical activity, stop overeating, quit smoking).
- ☐ ☐ 3. List advantages and disadvantages of changing the specified behavior.
- ☐ ☐ 4. Decide positively that you will change.
- ☐ ☐ 5. Identify your stage of change.
- ☐ ☐ 6. Set a realistic goal (SMART goal), completion date, and sign a behavioral contract.
- ☐ ☐ 7. Define your behavioral change plan: List processes of change, techniques of change, and objectives that will help you reach your goal.
- ☐ ☐ 8. Implement the behavior change plan.
- ☐ ☐ 9. Monitor your progress toward the desired goal.
- ☐ ☐ 10. Periodically evaluate and reassess your goal.
- ☐ ☐ 11. Reward yourself when you achieve your goal.
- ☐ ☐ 12. Maintain the successful change for good.

### Try It

In your Online Journal or class notebook, record your answers to the following questions:

Have you consciously attempted to incorporate a healthy behavior into or eliminate a negative behavior from your lifestyle? If so, what steps did you follow, and what helped you achieve your goal?

behaviors. The discussion on goal setting (beginning on page 55) will help you write goals and prepare an action plan to achieve them. This will aid with behavior modification.

**Self-Reevaluation** During the process of self-reevaluation, individuals analyze their feelings about a problem behavior. The pros and cons or advantages and disadvantages of a certain behavior can be reevaluated at this time. For example, you may decide that strength training will help you get stronger and tone up, but implementing this change will require you to stop watching an hour of TV three times per week. If you presently have a weight problem and are unable to lift certain objects around the house, you may feel good about weight loss and enhanced physical capacity as a result of a strength-training program. You also might visualize what it would be like if you were successful at changing.

**Countering** The process whereby you substitute healthy behaviors for a problem behavior, known as countering, is critical in changing behaviors as part of the action and maintenance stages. You need to replace unhealthy behaviors with new, healthy ones. You can use exercise to combat sedentary living, smoking, stress, or overeating. Or you may use exercise, diet, yard work, volunteer work, or reading to prevent overeating and achieve recommended body weight.

**Monitoring** During the action and maintenance stages, continuous behavior monitoring increases awareness of the desired outcome. Sometimes this process of monitoring is sufficient in itself to cause change. For ex-

ample, keeping track of daily food intake reveals sources of excessive fat in the diet. This can help you gradually cut down or completely eliminate high-fat foods. If the goal is to increase daily intake of fruit and vegetables, keeping track of the number of servings consumed each day raises awareness and may help increase intake.

**Environment Control** In environment control, the person restructures the physical surroundings to avoid problem behaviors and decrease temptations. If you don't buy alcohol, you can't drink any. If you shop on a full stomach, you can reduce impulse-buying of junk food.

Similarly, you can create an environment in which exceptions become the norm, and then the norm can flourish. Instead of bringing home cookies for snacks, bring fruit. Place notes to yourself on the refrigerator and pantry to avoid unnecessary snacking. Put baby carrots or sugarless gum where you used to put cigarettes. Post notes around the house to remind you of your exercise time. Leave exercise shoes and clothing by the door so they are visible as you walk into your home. Put an electric timer on the TV so it will shut off automatically at 7:00 p.m. All of these tactics will be helpful throughout the action, maintenance, and termination/adoption stages.

**Helping Relationships** Surrounding yourself with people who will work toward a common goal with you or those who care about you and will encourage you along the way—helping relationships—will be supportive during the action, maintenance, and termination/adoption stages.

Attempting to quit smoking, for instance, is easier when a person is around others who are trying to quit as well. The person also could get help from friends who have quit smoking already. Losing weight is difficult if meal planning and cooking are shared with roommates who enjoy foods that are high in fat and sugar. This situation can be even worse if a roommate also has a weight problem but does not desire to lose weight.

Peer support is a strong incentive for behavioral change, so the individual should avoid people who will not be supportive. Friends who have no desire to quit smoking or to lose weight, or whatever behavior a person is trying to change, may tempt one to smoke or overeat and encourage relapse into unwanted behaviors. People who have achieved the same goal already may not be supportive either. For instance, someone may say, "I can jog six consecutive miles." Your response should be, "I'm proud that I can jog three consecutive miles."

**Rewards** People tend to repeat behaviors that are rewarded and to disregard those that are not rewarded or are punished. Rewarding oneself or being rewarded by others is a powerful tool during the process of change in all stages. If you have successfully cut down your caloric intake during the week, reward yourself by going to a movie or buying a new pair of shoes. Do not reinforce yourself with destructive behaviors such as eating a high-fat/calorie-dense dinner. If you fail to change a desired behavior (or to implement a new one), you may want to put off

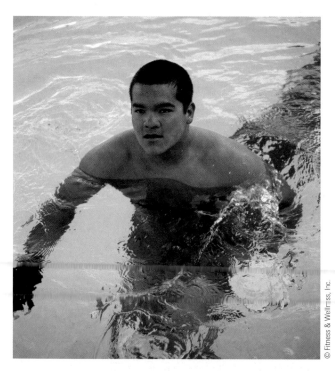

Countering: Substituting healthy behaviors for problem behaviors facilitates change.

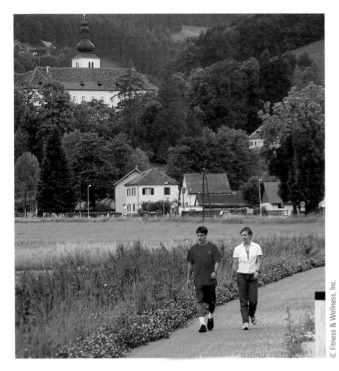

Rewarding oneself when a goal is achieved, such as scheduling a weekend getaway, is a powerful tool during the process of change.

© Fitness & Wellness, Inc.

buying those new shoes you had planned for that week. When a positive behavior becomes habitual, give yourself an even better reward. Treat yourself to a weekend away from home or buy a new bicycle.

## Critical Thinking

Your friend John is a 20-year-old student who is not physically active. Exercise has never been a part of his life, and it has not been a priority in his family. He has decided to start a jogging and strength-training course in two weeks. Can you identify his current stage of change and list processes and techniques of change that will help him maintain a regular exercise behavior?

## Techniques of Change

Not to be confused with the processes of change, you can apply any number of **techniques of change** within each process to help you through it (see Table 2.2). For example, following dinner, people with a weight problem often can't resist continuous snacking during the rest of the evening until it is time to retire for the night. In the process of countering, for example, you can use various techniques to avoid unnecessary snacking. Examples include going for a walk, flossing and brushing your teeth immediately after dinner, going for a drive, playing the piano, going to a show, or going to bed earlier.

As you develop a behavior modification plan, you need to identify specific techniques that may work for you within each process of change. A list of techniques for each process is provided in Table 2.2. This is only a sample list; dozens of other techniques could be used as well. For example, a discussion of behavior modification and adhering to a weight management program starts on page 175; getting started and adhering to a lifetime exercise program is presented on page 218; stress management techniques are provided in Chapter 12; and tips to help stop smoking are on pages 471–476. Some of these techniques also can be used with more than one process. Visualization, for example, is helpful in emotional arousal and self-reevaluation.

Now that you are familiar with the stages of change in the process of behavior modification, use Figure 2.5 and Lab 2B to identify two problem behaviors in your life. In the lab, you will be asked to determine your stage of change for two behaviors according to six standard statements. Based on your selection, determine the stage of change classification according to the ratings provided in Table 2.3. Next, develop a behavior modification plan according to the processes and techniques for change that you have learned in this chapter. (Similar exercises to identify stages of change for other fitness and wellness behaviors are provided in labs for subsequent chapters.)

## Goal Setting and Evaluation

To initiate change, **goals** are essential, as goals motivate behavioral change. Whatever you decide to accomplish, setting goals will provide the road map to help make your dreams a reality. Setting goals, however, is not as simple as it looks. Setting goals is more than just deciding what you want to do. A vague statement such as "I will lose weight" is not sufficient to help you achieve this goal.

SMART Goals   Only a well-conceived action plan will help you attain goals. Determining what you want to accomplish is the starting point, but to achieve ultimate success you need to write **SMART goals.** These goals are *s*pecific, *m*easurable, *a*cceptable, *r*ealistic, and *t*ime spe-

---

**Techniques of change** Methods or procedures used during each process of change.

**Goals** The ultimate aims toward which effort is directed.

**SMART** An acronym used in reference to specific, measurable, attainable, realistic, and time-specific goals.

**TABLE 2.2** Sample Techniques for Use with Processes of Change

| Process | Techniques |
|---|---|
| Consciousness-Raising | Become aware that there is a problem, read educational materials about the problem behavior or about people who have overcome this same problem, find out about the benefits of changing the behavior, watch an instructional program on television, visit a therapist, talk and listen to others, ask questions, take a class. |
| Social Liberation | Seek out advocacy groups (Overeaters Anonymous, Alcoholics Anonymous), join a health club, buy a bike, join a neighborhood walking group, work in non-smoking areas. |
| Self-Analysis | Become aware that there is a problem, question yourself on the problem behavior, express your feelings about it, analyze your values, list advantages and disadvantages of continuing (smoking) or not implementing a behavior (exercise), take a fitness test, do a nutrient analysis. |
| Emotional Arousal | Practice mental imagery of yourself going through the process of change, visualize yourself overcoming the problem behavior, do some role-playing in overcoming the behavior or practicing a new one, watch dramatizations (a movie) of the consequences or benefits of your actions, visit an auto salvage yard or a drug rehabilitation center. |
| Positive Outlook | Believe in yourself, know that you are capable, know that you are special, draw from previous personal successes. |
| Commitment | Just do it, set New Year's resolutions, sign a behavioral contract, set start and completion dates, tell others about your goals, work on your action plan. |
| Behavior Analysis | Prepare logs of circumstances that trigger or prevent a given behavior and look for patterns that prompt the behavior or cause you to relapse. |
| Goal Setting | Write goals and objectives; design a specific action plan. |
| Self-Reevaluation | Determine accomplishments and evaluate progress, rewrite goals and objectives, list pros and cons, weigh sacrifices (can't eat out with others) versus benefits (weight loss), visualize continued change, think before you act, learn from mistakes, and prepare new action plans accordingly. |
| Countering | Seek out alternatives: Stay busy, walk (don't drive), read a book (instead of snacking), attend alcohol-free socials, carry your own groceries, mow your yard, dance (don't eat), go to a movie (instead of smoking), practice stress management. |
| Monitoring | Use exercise logs (days exercised, sets and resistance used in strength training), keep journals, conduct nutrient analyses, count grams of fat, count number of consecutive days without smoking, list days and type of relaxation technique(s) used. |
| Environment Control | Rearrange your home (no TVs, ashtrays, large-sized cups), get rid of unhealthy items (cigarettes, junk food, alcohol), then avoid unhealthy places (bars, happy hour), avoid relationships that encourage problem behaviors, use reminders to control problem behaviors or encourage positive ones (post notes indicating "don't snack after dinner" or "lift weights at 8 pm"). Frequent healthy environments (a clean park, a health club, restaurants with low-fat/low-calorie/nutrient-dense menus, friends with goals similar to yours). |
| Helping Relationships | Associate with people who have and want to overcome the same problem, form or join self-help groups, join community programs specifically designed to deal with your problem. |
| Rewards | Go to a movie, buy a new outfit or shoes, buy a new bike, go on a weekend get-away, reassess your fitness level, use positive self-talk ("good job," "that felt good," "I did it," "I know I'd make it," "I'm good at this"). |

**FIGURE 2.5  Stage of change identification.**

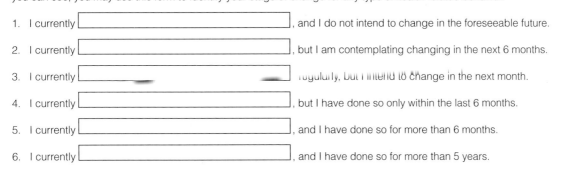

Please indicate which response most accurately describes your current [          ] behavior (in the blank space identify the behavior: smoking, physical activity, stress, nutrition, weight control). Next, select the statement below (select only one) that best represents your current behavior pattern. To select the most appropriate statement, fill in the blank for one of the first three statements if your current behavior is a problem behavior. (For example, you may say, "I currently smoke, and I do *not* intend to change in the foreseeable future," or "I currently *do not* exercise, but I am contemplating changing in the next 6 months.") If you have already started to make changes, fill in the blank in one of the last three statements. (In this case, you may say: "I currently *eat a low-fat diet*, but I have only done so within the last 6 months," or "I currently *practice adequate stress management techniques*, and I have done so for over 6 months.") As you can see, you may use this form to identify your stage of change for any type of health-related behavior.

1.  I currently [                          ], and I do not intend to change in the foreseeable future.

2.  I currently [                          ], but I am contemplating changing in the next 6 months.

3.  I currently [                          ] regularly, but I intend to change in the next month.

4.  I currently [                          ], but I have done so only within the last 6 months.

5.  I currently [                          ], and I have done so for more than 6 months.

6.  I currently [                          ], and I have done so for more than 5 years.

**TABLE 2.3  Stage of Change Classification**

| Selected Statements (see Figure 2.5 and Lab 2B) | Classification |
|:---:|:---:|
| 1 | Precontemplation |
| 2 | Contemplation |
| 3 | Preparation |
| 4 | Action |
| 5 | Maintenance |
| 6 | Termination/Adoption |

cific. In Lab 2C, you have an opportunity to set SMART goals for two behaviors that you wish to change or adopt.

1. *Specific.* When writing goals, state exactly and in a positive manner what you would like to accomplish. For example, if you are overweight at 150 pounds and at 27 percent body fat, to simply state, "I will lose weight" is not a specific goal. Instead, rewrite your goal to state, "I will reduce my body fat to 20 percent body fat (137 pounds) in 12 weeks."

Write them down. An unwritten goal is simply a wish. A written goal, in essence, becomes a contract with yourself. Show this goal to a friend or an instructor, and have him or her witness the contract you have made with yourself by signing alongside your signature.

Once you have identified and written down a specific goal, write the specific **objectives** that will help you reach it. These objectives are necessary steps. For example, a goal might be to achieve recommended body weight. Several specific objectives could be to:

a. lose an average of one pound (or one fat percentage point) per week

b. monitor body weight before breakfast every morning

c. assess body composition at three-week intervals

d. limit fat intake to less than 25 percent of total daily caloric intake

e. eliminate all pastries from the diet during this time

f. walk/jog in the proper target zone for 60 minutes, six times a week

2. *Measurable.* Whenever possible, goals and objectives should be measurable. For example, "I will lose weight" is not measurable, but "to reduce body fat to 20 percent" is measurable. Also note that all of the sample-specific objectives (a.) through (f.) under "Specific" above are measurable. For instance, you can figure out easily whether you are losing a pound or a percentage point per week; you can conduct a nutrient analysis to assess your average fat intake; or you can monitor your weekly exercise sessions to make sure you are meeting this specific objective.

3. *Acceptable.* Goals that you set for yourself are more motivational than goals that someone else sets for you. These goals will motivate and challenge you and should be consistent with your other goals. As you set an acceptable goal, ask yourself: Do I have the time, commitment, and necessary skills to accomplish this goal? If not, you need to restate your goal so that it is acceptable to you.

**Objectives** Steps required to reach a goal.

When successful completion of a goal involves others, such as an athletic team or an organization, an acceptable goal must be compatible with those of the other people involved. If a team's practice schedule is set Monday through Friday from 4:00 to 6:00 p.m., it is unacceptable for you to train only three times per week or at a different time of tho day.

Acceptable goals also embrace positive thoughts. Visualize and believe in your success. As difficult as some tasks may seem, where there's a will, there's a way. A plan of action, prepared according to the guidelines in this chapter, will help you achieve your goals.

4. **Realistic.** Goals should be within reach. On the one hand, if you currently weigh 190 pounds and your target weight is 140 pounds, setting a goal to lose 50 pounds in a month would be unsound, if not impossible. Such a goal does not allow you to implement adequate behavior modification techniques or ensure weight maintenance at the target weight. Unattainable goals only set you up for failure, discouragement, and loss of interest. On the other hand, do not write goals that are too easy to achieve and do not challenge you. If a goal is too easy, you may lose interest and stop working toward it.

You can write both short-term and long-term goals. If the long-term goal is to attain recommended body weight and you are 53 pounds overweight, you might set a short-term goal of losing 10 pounds and write specific objectives to accomplish this goal. Then the immediate task will not seem as overwhelming and will be easier.

At times, problems arise even with realistic goals. Try to anticipate potential difficulties as much as possible, and plan for ways to deal with them. If your goal is to jog for 30 minutes on six consecutive days, what are the alternatives if the weather turns bad? Possible solutions are to jog in the rain, find an indoor track, jog at a different time of day when the weather is better, or participate in a different aerobic activity such as stationary cycling, swimming, or step aerobics.

Monitoring your progress as you move toward a goal also reinforces behavior. Keeping an exercise log or doing a body composition assessment periodically enables you to determine your progress at any given time.

5. **Time specific.** A goal should always have a specific date set for completion. The above example to reach 20 percent body fat in 12 weeks is time specific. The chosen date should be realistic but not too distant in the future. Allow yourself enough time to achieve the goal, but not too much time, as this could affect your performance. With a deadline, a task is much easier to work toward.

**Goal Evaluation** In addition to the SMART guidelines provided, you should conduct periodic evaluations of your goals. Reevaluations are vital to success. You may find that after you have fully committed and put all your effort into a goal, that goal may be unreachable. If so, reassess the goal.

Recognize that you will face obstacles and you will not always meet your goals. Use your setbacks and learn from them. Rewrite your goal and create a plan that will help you get around self-defeating behaviors in the future. Once you achieve a goal, set a new one to improve upon or maintain what you have achieved. Goals keep you motivated.

# ASSESS YOUR BEHAVIOR

 Log on to http://www.cengage.com/sso/ to create a behavior change contract.

1. What are your feelings about the science of behavior modification and how its principles may help you on your journey to health and wellness?

2. Can you accept the fact that for various healthy lifestyle factors (for example, regular exercise, healthy eating, not smoking, stress management, prevention of sexually transmitted infections) you are in either the precontemplation or the contemplation stage of change? As such, are you willing to learn what is required to change and actually eliminate unhealthy behaviors and adopt healthy lifestyle behaviors?

3. Are you now in the action phase (or above) for exercise and healthy eating? If not, what barriers keep you from being in that phase?

# ASSESS YOUR KNOWLEDGE

 Log on to http://www.cengage.com/sso/ to assess your understanding of this chapter's topics by taking the Student Practice Test and exploring the modules recommended in your Personalized Study Plan.

1. Most of the behaviors that people adopt in life are
   a. a product of their environment
   b. learned early in childhood
   c. learned from parents
   d. genetically determined
   e. the result of peer pressure

2. Instant gratification is
   a. a barrier to change
   b. a factor that motivates change
   c. one of the six stages of change
   d. the end result of successful change
   e. a technique in the process of change

3. The desire and will to do something is referred to as
   a. invincibility
   b. confidence
   c. competence
   d. external locus of control
   e. motivation

4. People who believe they have control over events in their lives
   a. tend to rationalize their negative actions
   b. exhibit problems of competence
   c. often feel helpless over illness and disease
   d. have an internal locus of control
   e. often engage in risky lifestyle behaviors

5. A person who is unwilling to change a negative behavior because the reasons for change are not important enough is said to have problems of
   a. competence
   b. conduct
   c. motivation
   d. confidence
   e. risk complacency

6. Which of the following is a stage of change in the transtheoretical model?
   a. recognition
   b. motivation
   c. relapse
   d. preparation
   e. goal setting

7. A precontemplator is a person who
   a. has no desire to change a behavior
   b. is looking to make a change in the next six months
   c. is preparing for change in the next 30 days
   d. willingly adopts healthy behaviors
   e. is talking to a therapist to overcome a problem behavior

8. An individual who is trying to stop smoking and has not smoked for three months is in the
   a. maintenance stage
   b. action stage
   c. termination stage
   d. adoption stage
   e. evaluation stage

9. The process of change in which an individual obtains information to make a better decision about a problem behavior is known as
   a. behavior analysis
   b. self-reevaluation
   c. commitment
   d. positive outlook
   e. consciousness-raising

10. A goal is effective when it is
    a. specific
    b. measurable
    c. realistic
    d. time-specific
    e. all of the above

Correct answers can be found at the back of the book.

# MEDIA MENU

You can find the links below at the book companion site: www.cengage.com/health/hoeger/plfw10e

- Prepare for a healthy change in lifestyle.
- Check how well you understand the chapter's concepts.

## Internet Connections

- Transtheoretical Model—Cancer Prevention Research Center. This site describes the transtheoretical model, including effective interventions to promote change in health behavior, focusing on the individual's decision-making strategies. *http://www.uri.edu/research/cprc/TTM/detailedoverview.htm*

- Behavior Change Theories. This comprehensive site, by the Department of Health Promotion at California Polytechnic University at Pomona, describes all of the theories of behavioral change, including learning theories, the transtheoretical model, the health belief model, the relapse prevention model, reasoned action and planned behavior, social learning/social cognitive theory, and social support. *http://www.csupomona.edu/~jvgrizzell*

- How to Fit Exercise into Your Daily Routine. Offered by the Mayo Clinic, this site describes how you can incorporate simple exercises into your daily schedule—whether you're at home, at work, or traveling. Make time to exercise! *http://www.mayoclinic.com/health/fitness/HQ01217_D*

# NOTES

1. J. Annesi, "Using Emotions to Empower Members for Long-Term Exercise Success," *Fitness Management* 17 (2001): 54–58.

2. Television Bureau of Advertising Web site, "Time Spent Viewing Per TV Home: Per Day Annual Averages," available at http://www.tvb.org/nav/build_frameset.asp?url=/rcentral/index.asp; accessed March 26, 2005.

3. R. Boynton-Jarret, T. N. Thomas, K. E. Peterson, J. Wiecha, A. M. Sobol, and S. L. Gortmaker, "Impact of Television Viewing Patterns on Fruit and Vegetable Consumption among Adolescents," *Pediatrics* 113 (2003): 1321–1322.

4. League of California Cities Planners Institute, Pasadena Conference Center (April 13–15, 2005).

5. J. Pucher and C. Lefevre, *The Urban Transport Crisis in Europe and North America* (London: Macmillan Press Ltd., 1996).

6. S. Gerrior, L. Bente, and H. Hiza, "Nutrient Content of the U.S. Food Supply, 1909–2000," *Home Economics Research Report No. 56* (U.S. Department of Agriculture, Center for Nutrition Policy and Promotion, 2004): 74 (available online at http://www.usda.gov/cnpp/nutrient_content.html; accessed April 18, 2005).

7. Marion Nestle, *Food Politics* (Berkeley and Los Angeles: University of California Press, 2002), 1, 8, 22.

8. "Food Prepared Away from Home Is Increasing and Found to Be Less Nutritious," *Nutrition Research Newsletter* 21, no. 8 (August 2002): 10(2); A. Clauson, "Shares of Food Spending for Eating Reaches 47 Percent," *Food Review* 22 (1999): 20–22.

9. "A Diner's Guide to Health and Nutrition Claims in Restaurant Menus" (Center for Science in the Public Interest, 1997), available at http://www.cspinet.org/reports/dinersgu.html; accessed March 25, 2005.

10. Lisa R. Young and Marion Nestle, "Expanding Portion Sizes in the U.S. Marketplace: Implications for Nutrition Counseling," *Journal of the American Dietetic Association* 103, no. 2 (February 2003): 231.

11. American Institute for Cancer Research, "As Restaurant Portions Grow, Vast Majority of Americans Still Belong to 'Clean Plate Club,' New Survey Finds" (Washington, DC: AICR News Release, January 15, 2001).

12. T. V. E. Kral, L. S. Roe, J. S. Meengs, and D. E. Wall, "Increasing the Portion Size of a Packaged Snack Increases Energy Intake," *Appetite* 39 (2002): 86.

13. J. A. Ello-Martin, L. S. Roe, J. S. Meengs, D. E. Wall, and B. J. Rolls, "Increasing the Portion Size of a Unit Food Increases Energy Intake" *Appetite* 30 (2002): 74

14. B. Wansink, "Can Package Size Accelerate Usage Volume?" *Journal of Marketing* 60 (1996): 1–14.

15. National Alliance for Nutrition and Activity (NANA), "From Wallet to Waistline: The Hidden Costs of Super Sizing" (Washington, DC: NANA, 2002), available online at http://www.preventioninstitute.org/portion-sizerept.html

16. S. H. A. Holt, N. Sandona, and J. C. Brand-Miller, "The Effects of Sugar-Free vs. Sugar-Rich Beverages on Feelings of Fullness and Subsequent Food Intake," *International Journal of Food Sciences and Nutrition* 51, no. 1 (January 2000): 59.

17. "Wellness Facts," *University of California at Berkeley Wellness Letter* (Palm Coast, FL: The Editors, May 2004).

18. G. S. Howard, D. W. Nance, and P. Myers, *Adaptive Counseling and Therapy* (San Francisco: Jossey-Bass, 1987).

19. J. O. Prochaska, J. C. Norcross, and C. C. DiClemente, *Changing for Good* (New York: William Morrow, 1994).

# SUGGESTED READINGS

Bouchard, C., et al. *Physical Activity, Fitness, and Health.* Champaign, IL: Human Kinetics, 1994.

Blair, S. N., et al. *Active Living Every Day.* Champaign, IL: Human Kinetics, 2001.

Brehm, B. *Successful Fitness Motivation Strategies.* Champaign, IL: Human Kinetics, 2004.

Burgand, M., and K. Gallagher. "Self Monitoring: Influencing Effective Behavior Change in Your Clients." *ACSM's Health & Fitness Journal* 10, no 1 (2006): 14–19.

Dishman, R. *Advances in Exercise Adherence.* Champaign, IL: Human Kinetics, 1994.

Marcus, B., and L. Forsyth. *Motivating People to Be Physically Active.* Champaign, IL: Human Kinetics, 2003.

Prochaska, J. O., J. C. Norcross, and C. C. DiClemente. *Changing for Good.* New York: William Morrow, 1994.

Samuelson, M. "Stages of Change: From Theory to Practice." *The Art of Health Promotion* 2 (1998): 1–7.

# LAB 2A: Exercising Control over Your Physical Activity and Nutrition Environment

Name _____ Date _____ Gender/Age _____

Instructor _____ Course _____ Section _____

### Objective
To aid in the identification of environmental factors that have an effect on your physical activity and nutrition habits.

### Instructions
Select the appropriate answer to each question and obtain a final score for each section. Then rate yourself according to the guidelines at the end of the lab.

## I. Physical Activity
*Note:* Based on the definitions of *physical activity* and *exercise* (see page 7), as you take this questionnaire, keep in mind that you can be physically active without exercising, but you cannot exercise without being physically active.

| | NEARLY ALWAYS | OFTEN | SELDOM | NEVER |
|---|---|---|---|---|
| 1. Do you identify daily time slots to be *physically active?* | 4 | 3 | 2 | 1 |
| 2. Do you seek additional opportunities to be active each day (walk, cycle, park farther away, do yard work/gardening)? | 4 | 3 | 2 | 1 |
| 3. Do you avoid labor-saving devices/activities (escalators, elevators, self-propelled lawn mowers, snow blowers, drive-through windows)? | 4 | 3 | 2 | 1 |
| 4. Does physical activity improve your health and well-being? | 4 | 3 | 2 | 1 |
| 5. Does physical activity increase your energy level? | 4 | 3 | 2 | 1 |
| 6. Do you seek professional and/or medical (if necessary) advice prior to starting an exercise program or when increasing the intensity, duration, and frequency of exercise? | 4 | 3 | 2 | 1 |
| 7. Do you identify time slots to *exercise* most days of the week? | 4 | 3 | 2 | 1 |
| 8. Do you schedule exercise during times of the day when you feel most energetic? | 4 | 3 | 2 | 1 |
| 9. Do you have an alternative plan to be active or exercise during adverse weather conditions (walk at the mall, swim at the health club, climb stairs, skip rope, dance)? | 4 | 3 | 2 | 1 |
| 10. Do you cross-train (participate in a variety of activities)? | 4 | 3 | 2 | 1 |
| 11. Do you surround yourself with people who support your physical activity/exercise goals? | 4 | 3 | 2 | 1 |
| 12. Do you let family and friends know of your physical activity/exercise interests? | 4 | 3 | 2 | 1 |
| 13. Do you invite family and friends to exercise with you? | 4 | 3 | 2 | 1 |
| 14. Do you seek new friendships with people who are physically active? | 4 | 3 | 2 | 1 |
| 15. Do you select friendships with people whose fitness and skill levels are similar to yours? | 4 | 3 | 2 | 1 |
| 16. Do you plan social activities that involve physical activity? | 4 | 3 | 2 | 1 |
| 17. Do you plan activity/exercise when you are away from home (during business and vacation trips)? | 4 | 3 | 2 | 1 |
| 18. When you have a desire to do so, do you take classes to learn new activity/sport skills? | 4 | 3 | 2 | 1 |
| 19. Do you limit daily television viewing and Internet and computer game time? | 4 | 3 | 2 | 1 |
| 20. Do you spend leisure hours being physically active? | 4 | 3 | 2 | 1 |

Physical Activity Score: _____

Total number of daily steps: [ ]

## II. Nutrition

|   |   | NEARLY ALWAYS | OFTEN | SELDOM | NEVER |
|---|---|---|---|---|---|
| 1. | Do you prepare a shopping list prior to going to the store? | 4 | 3 | 2 | 1 |
| 2. | Do you select food items primarily from the perimeter of the store (site of most fresh/unprocessed foods)? | 4 | 3 | 2 | 1 |
| 3. | Do you limit the unhealthy snacks you bring into the home and the workplace? | 4 | 3 | 2 | 1 |
| 4. | Do you plan your meals and is your pantry well stocked so you can easily prepare a meal without a quick trip to the store? | 4 | 3 | 2 | 1 |
| 5. | Do you help cook your meals? | 4 | 3 | 2 | 1 |
| 6. | Do you pay attention to how hungry you are before and during a meal? | 4 | 3 | 2 | 1 |
| 7. | When reaching for food, do you remind yourself that you have a choice about what and how much you eat? | 4 | 3 | 2 | 1 |
| 8. | Do you eat your meals at home? | 4 | 3 | 2 | 1 |
| 9. | Do you eat your meals at the table only? | 4 | 3 | 2 | 1 |
| 10. | Do you include whole-grain products in your diet each day (whole-grain bread/cereal/crackers/rice/pasta)? | 4 | 3 | 2 | 1 |
| 11. | Do you make a deliberate effort to include a variety of fruits and vegetables in your diet each day? | 4 | 3 | 2 | 1 |
| 12. | Do you limit your daily saturated fat and trans fat intake (red meat, whole milk, cheese, butter, hard margarines, luncheon meats, baked goods, processed foods)? | 4 | 3 | 2 | 1 |
| 13. | Do you avoid unnecessary/unhealthy snacking (at work or play, during TV viewing, at the movies or socials)? | 4 | 3 | 2 | 1 |
| 14. | Do you plan caloric allowances prior to attending social gatherings that include food and eating? | 4 | 3 | 2 | 1 |
| 15. | Do you limit alcohol consumption to two drinks a day if you are a man or one drink a day if you are a woman? | 4 | 3 | 2 | 1 |
| 16. | Are you aware of strategies to decrease caloric intake when dining out (resist the server's offerings for drinks and appetizers, select a low-calorie/nutrient-dense item, drink water, resist cleaning your plate, ask for a doggie bag, share meals, request whole-wheat substitutes, get dressings on the side, avoid cream sauces, skip desserts)? | 4 | 3 | 2 | 1 |
| 17. | Do you avoid ordering larger meal sizes because you get more food for your money? | 4 | 3 | 2 | 1 |
| 18. | Do you avoid buying food when you hadn't planned to do so (gas stations, convenience stores, video rental stores)? | 4 | 3 | 2 | 1 |
| 19. | Do you fill your time with activities that will keep you away from places where you typically consume food (kitchen, coffee room, dining room)? | 4 | 3 | 2 | 1 |
| 20. | Do you know what situations trigger your desire for unnecessary snacking and overeating (vending machines, TV viewing, food ads, cookbooks, fast-food restaurants, buffet restaurants)? | 4 | 3 | 2 | 1 |

Nutrition Score: _____

## Ratings (Check the appropriate box.)

|   |   | Physical Activity | Nutrition |
|---|---|---|---|
| ≥71 | You have good control over your environment | ☐ | ☐ |
| 51–70 | There is room for improvement | ☐ | ☐ |
| 31–50 | Your environmental control is poor | ☐ | ☐ |
| ≤30 | You are controlled by your environment | ☐ | ☐ |

# LAB 2B: Behavior Modification Plan

Name _____ Date _____ Grade _____

Instructor _____ Course _____ Section _____

Necessary Lab Equipment

None.

Instructions

Chapter 2 must be read prior to this lab.

## Objective

To help you identify the stage of change for two problem behaviors and the processes and techniques for change.

## I. Stages of Change Instructions

Please indicate which response most accurately describes your current _____ behavior (in the blank space identify the behavior: smoking, physical activity, stress, nutrition, weight control). Next, select the statement below (select only one) that best represents your current behavior pattern. To select the most appropriate statement, fill in the blank for one of the first three statements if your current behavior is a problem behavior. For example, you may say:

"I currently smoke, and I do not intend to change in the foreseeable future" or

"I currently do not exercise, but I am contemplating changing in the next 6 months."

If you have already started to make changes, fill in the blank in one of the last three statements. In this case you may say:

"I currently eat a low-fat diet, but I have only done so within the last 6 months" or

"I currently practice adequate stress management techniques, and I have done so for over 6 months."

You may use this form to identify your stage of change for any health-related behavior. After identifying two problem behaviors, look up your stage of change for each one using Table 2.3 (on page 57).

Behavior #1. Fill in only one blank.

☐ 1. I currently _____, and do not intend to change in the foreseeable future.

☐ 2. I currently _____, but I am contemplating changing in the next 6 months.

☐ 3. I currently _____ regularly, but I intend to change in the next month.

☐ 4. I currently _____, but I have only done so within the last 6 months.

☐ 5. I currently _____, and I have done so for over 6 months.

☐ 6. I currently _____, and I have done so for over 5 years.

Stage of change: _____ (see Table 2.3 on page 57).

Behavior #2. Fill in only one blank.

☐ 1. I currently _____, and do not intend to change in the foreseeable future.

☐ 2. I currently _____, but I am contemplating changing in the next 6 months.

☐ 3. I currently _____ regularly, but I intend to change in the next month.

☐ 4. I currently _____, but I have only done so within the last 6 months.

☐ 5. I currently _____, and I have done so for over 6 months.

☐ 6. I currently _____, and I have done so for over 5 years.

Stage of change: _____ (see Table 2.3 on page 57).

## II. Processes of Change

According to your stage of change for the two behaviors you have identified, list the processes of change that apply to each behavior (see Table 2.1 on page 50).

Behavior #1: _____

_____

Behavior #2: _____

_____

## III. Techniques for Change

List a minimum of three techniques that you will use with each process of change (see Table 2.2 on page 56)

Behavior #1:  1. _____

2. _____

3. _____

Behavior #2:  1. _____

2. _____

3. _____

Will you continue to use techniques as a process of behavior modification in the future? Briefly, discuss the techniques that were most beneficial to you.

_____

_____

_____

_____

_____

_____

_____

_____

_____

_____

_____

_____

Today's date: _____    Completion Date: _____    Signature: _____

# LAB 2C: Setting SMART Goals

Name _____    Date _____    Grade _____

Instructor _____    Course _____    Section _____

Objective
To learn to write SMART goals.

**Objective**
To learn to write SMART goals.

**Instructions**
In Lab 2B you identified two behaviors that you wish to change. Using SMART goal guidelines, write goals and objectives that will provide a road map for behavioral change. In the spaces provided in this lab, indicate how your stated goals meet each one of the SMART goal guidelines.

## I. SMART Goals

Goal 1:
_____
_____

Indicate what makes your goal specific.
_____

How is your goal measurable?
_____
_____

Why is this an acceptable goal?
_____
_____

State why you consider this goal realistic?
_____
_____

How is this goal time-specific?
_____
_____

Goal 2:

_____

_____

Indicate what makes your goal specific.

_____

How is your goal measurable?

_____

_____

Why is this an acceptable goal?

_____

_____

State why you consider this goal realistic?

_____

_____

How is this goal time-specific?

_____

_____

## II. Specific Objectives

Write a minimum of five specific objectives that will help you reach your two SMART goals.

Goal 1: _____

Objectives:

1. _____

2. _____

3. _____

4. _____

5. _____

Goal 2: _____

Objectives:

1. _____

2. _____

3. _____

4. _____

5. _____

# Nutrition for Wellness

**3**

## Objectives

- Define nutrition and describe its relationship to health and well-being
- Learn to use the USDA MyPyramid guidelines for healthier eating
- Describe the functions of the nutrients—carbohydrates, fiber, fats, proteins, vitamins, minerals, and water—in the human body
- Define the various energy production mechanisms of the human body
- Be able to conduct a comprehensive nutrient analysis and implement changes to meet the Dietary Reference Intakes (DRIs)
- Identify myths and fallacies regarding nutrition
- Become aware of guidelines for nutrient supplementation
- Learn the 2005 Dietary Guidelines for Americans
- Analyze your diet and plan for a healthy change.

Ian O'Leary/Dorling Kindersley/Getty Images

Check your understanding of the chapter contents by logging on to CengageNOW and accessing the pre-test, personalized learning plan, and post-test for this chapter.

# FAQ

## Are organic foods better than conventional foods?

Concerns over food safety have led many people to turn to organic foods. Currently, less than 2 percent of imported food products is inspected by the FDA, and domestic food is seldom inspected at all. According to health officials, more than 76 million Americans each year get sick from food, resulting in 325,000 hospitalizations and 5,000 deaths. Health risks from pesticide exposure from foods are relatively small for healthy adults. The health benefits of produce far outweigh the risks. Children, older adults, pregnant and lactating women, and people with weak immune systems, however, may be vulnerable to some types of pesticides.

Organic foods, including crops, meat, poultry, eggs, and dairy products, are produced under strict government regulations. Organic crops have to be grown without the use of conventional pesticides, artificial fertilizers, human waste, or sewage sludge, and have been processed without ionizing radiation or food additives. Harmful microbes in manure must also be destroyed prior to use, and genetically modified organisms may not be used. Limited data suggest that organic crops may have more phytochemicals and a higher nutritional value. Organic livestock is raised under certain grazing conditions, using organic feed, and without the use of antibiotics and growth hormones.

While pesticide residues in organic foods are substantially lower than conventionally grown foods, organic foods can just as easily be contaminated with bacteria, pathogens, and heavy metals that pose major health risks. The soil itself may be- come contaminated, or if the produce comes in contact with feces of grazing cattle, wild animals/birds, farm workers, or any other source, potentially harmful microorganisms can contaminate the produce. The *Escherichia coli* California spinach contamination of 2006 had been grown in a field that was in transition from conventional crops to an organic field. The best safeguard to protect yourself is to follow the food safety guidelines provided on page 110.

## Fish is known to be heart healthy, but should we worry about mercury toxicity concerns?

Fish and shellfish contain high-quality protein, omega-3 fatty acids, and other essential nutrients. Fish is lower in saturated fat and cholesterol than meat or poultry. Data indicate that eating as little as 6 ounces of fatty fish per week can reduce the risk of premature death from heart disease by one-third and overall death rates by about one-sixth. Fish also appears to have anti-inflammatory properties that can help treat chronic inflammatory kidney disease, osteoarthritis, rheumatoid arthritis, Crohn's disease, and autoimmune disorders like asthma and lupus. Thus, fish is one of the healthiest foods we can consume.

Potential contaminants in fish, in particular mercury, have created concerns among some people. Mercury, a naturally occurring trace mineral, can be released into the air from industrial pollution. As mercury falls into streams and oceans, it accumulates in the aquatic food chain. Larger fish accumulate larger amounts of mercury because they eat medium and small fish. Of particular concern are shark, swordfish, king mackerel, pike, bass, and tilefish that have higher levels. Farm-raised

Good **nutrition** is essential to overall health and wellness. Proper nutrition means that a person's diet supplies all the essential nutrients for healthy body functioning, including normal tissue growth, repair, and maintenance. The diet should also provide enough **substrates** to produce the energy necessary for work, physical activity, and relaxation.

**Nutrients** should be obtained from a wide variety of sources. Figure 3.1 shows MyPyramid nutrition guidelines and recommended daily food amounts according to various caloric requirements. To lower the risk for chronic disease, an effective wellness program must incorporate healthy eating guidelines. These guidelines will be discussed throughout this chapter and in later chapters.

salmon also have slightly higher levels of polychlorinated biphenyls (PCBs), which the Environmental Protection Agency (EPA) lists as a "probable human carcinogen."

The American Heart Association recommends consuming fish twice a week. The risk of adverse effects from eating fish is extremely low and primarily theoretical in nature. For most people, eating two servings (up to 6 ounces) of fish per week poses no health threat. Pregnant and nursing women and young children, however, should avoid mercury in fish. The best recommendation is to balance the risks against the benefits. If you are still concerned, consume no more than 12 ounces per week of a variety of fish and shellfish that are lower in mercury, including canned light tuna, wild salmon, shrimp, pollock, catfish, and scallops. And check local advisories about the safety of fish caught by family and friends in local streams, rivers, lakes, and coastal areas. Dr. Dariush Mozaffarian, a physician who published a review of over 200 studies on the effects of fish consumption on health, has stated that the benefits of fish consumption exceed the potential risks and, "Seafood is likely the single most important food one can consume for good health."*

### What do the terms "glycemic index" and "glycemic load" mean?

The glycemic index is used to measure how rapidly a particular food increases blood sugar after eating it as compared with the same amount of carbohydrate in white bread. Foods high in glycemic index cause a rapid rise in blood sugar. Frequent consumption of high-glycemic foods by themselves can increase the risk for cardiovascular disease, especially in people with diabetes. The glycemic load is calculated by multiplying the glycemic index of a particular food by its carbohydrate content in grams and dividing by 100. The usefulness of the glycemic load is based on the theory that a high-glycemic-index food eaten in small quantities provides a similar effect in blood sugar rise as a consumption of a larger quantity of a low-glycemic food.

### What is the difference between antioxidants and phytonutrients?

Antioxidants, comprising vitamins, minerals, and phytonutrients, help prevent damage to cells from highly reactive and unstable molecules known as oxygen free radicals (see page 95). Antioxidants are found both in plant and animal foods, whereas phytonutrients are found in plant foods only, including fruits, vegetables, beans, nuts, and seeds. The actions of phytonutrients, however, go beyond those of most antioxidants. In particular, they appear to have powerful anticancer properties. For example, at almost every stage of cancer, phytonutrients can block, disrupt, slow, or even reverse the process. In terms of heart disease, they may reduce inflammation, inhibit blood clots, or prevent the oxidation of LDL cholesterol. People should consume ample amounts of plant-based foods to obtain a healthy supply of antioxidants, including a wide array of phytonutrients.

*D. Mozaffarian and E. B. Rimm, "Fish Intake, Contaminants, and Human Health," *Journal of the American Medical Association* 296 (2006): 1885–1899; "Eating Fish: Rewards Outweigh Risks," *Tufts University Health & Nutrition Letter* (January 2007).

Too much or too little of any nutrient can precipitate serious health problems. The typical U.S. diet is too high in calories, sugar, saturated fat, trans fat, and sodium, and not high enough in whole grains, fruits, and vegetables—factors that undermine good health. On a given day, nearly half of the people in the United States eat no fruit and almost one-fourth eat no vegetables.

**Nutrition** Science that studies the relationship of foods to optimal health and performance.

**Substrates** Substances acted upon by an enzyme (examples: carbohydrates, fats).

**Nutrients** Substances found in food that provide energy, regulate metabolism, and help with growth and repair of body tissues.

**FIGURE 3.1  MyPyramid: Steps to a healthier you.**

The colors of the pyramid illustrate variety: each color represents one of the five food groups, plus one for oils. Different band widths suggest the proportional contribution of each food group to a healthy diet.

A person climbing steps reminds consumers to be physically active.

The narrow slivers of color at the top imply moderation in foods rich in solid fats and added sugars.

The broad bases at the bottom represent nutrient-dense foods that should make up the bulk of the diet.

Greater intakes of grains, vegetables, fruit, and milk are encouraged by the broad bases of orange, green, red.

SOURCE: USDA, 2005.

**MyPyramid**
STEPS TO A HEALTHIER YOU
MyPyramid.gov

GRAINS  VEGETABLES  FRUITS  OIL  MILK  MEAT & BEANS

**GRAINS**

In general: 1 slice of bread, 1 cup of ready-to-eat cereal, ½ cup of cooked rice, cooked pasta, or cooked cereal can be considered as 1 oz equivalent of grains. Look for "whole" before the grain name on the list of ingredients and make at least half your grains whole.

**VEGETABLES**

In general: 1 cup of raw or cooked vegetables or vegetable juice, or 2 cups of raw leafy greens can be considered as 1 cup from the vegetable group. Try to eat more dark green and orange veggies, as well as dry beans and peas.

**FRUITS**

In general: 1 cup of fruit or 100% fruit juice, or ½ cup of dried fruit can be considered as 1 cup from the fruit group. Eat a variety of fruit, including fresh, frozen, canned, or dried fruit. Go easy on fruit juices.

**OILS**

Measured in teaspoons of either oils or solid fats. Most sources should come from fish, nuts, and vegetable oils. Limit solid fats such as butter, stick margarine, shortening, and lard.

**MILK**

In general: 1 cup of milk or yogurt, 1½ oz of natural cheese, or 2 oz of processed cheese can be considered as 1 cup from the milk group. Go low-fat or fat free. If you can't consume milk, choose lactose-free products or other calcium sources.

**MEATS & BEANS**

In general: 1 oz of meat, poultry, or fish, ¼ cup cooked dry beans, 1 egg, 1 tbsp of peanut butter, or ½ oz of nuts or seeds can be considered as 1 oz equivalent from the Meats & Beans group.

**Recommended Daily Amounts from Each Food Group**

| FOOD GROUP | 1600 cal | 1800 cal | 2000 cal | 2200 cal | 2400 cal | 2600 cal | 2800 cal | 3000 cal |
|---|---|---|---|---|---|---|---|---|
| Fruits | 1½ c | 1½ c | 2 c | 2 c | 2 c | 2 c | 2½ c | 2½ c |
| Vegetables | 2 c | 2½ c | 2½ c | 3 c | 3 c | 3½ c | 3½ c | 4 c |
| Grains | 5 oz | 6 oz | 6 oz | 7 oz | 8 oz | 9 oz | 10 oz | 10 oz |
| Meat and legumes | 5 oz | 5 oz | 5½ oz | 6 oz | 6½ oz | 6½ oz | 7 oz | 7 oz |
| Milk | 3 c | 3 c | 3 c | 3 c | 3 c | 3 c | 3 c | 3 c |
| Oils | 5 tsp | 5 tsp | 6 tsp | 6 tsp | 7 tsp | 8 tsp | 8 tsp | 10 tsp |
| Discretionary calorie allowance* | 132 cal | 195 cal | 267 cal | 290 cal | 362 cal | 410 cal | 426 cal | 512 cal |

*Discretionary calorie allowance: At each calorie level, people who consistently choose nutrient-dense foods may be able to meet their nutrient needs without consuming their full allotment of calories. The difference between the calories needed to supply nutrients and those needed for energy is known as the *discretionary calorie allowance*.

***Source:*** http://mypyramid.gov/. Additional information on MyPyramid can be obtained at this site, including an online individualized MyPyramid eating plan based on your age, gender, and activity level.

Food availability is not a problem. The problem is over-consumption of the wrong foods. Diseases of dietary excess and imbalance are among the leading causes of death in many developed countries throughout the world, including the United States.

Diet and nutrition often play a crucial role in the development and progression of chronic diseases. A diet high in saturated fat and cholesterol increases the risk for diseases of the cardiovascular system, including atherosclerosis, coronary heart disease (CHD), and strokes. In sodium-sensitive individuals, high salt intake has been linked to high blood pressure. Up to 50 percent of all cancers may be diet related. Obesity, diabetes, and osteoporosis also have been associated with faulty nutrition.

# Nutrients

The essential nutrients the human body requires are carbohydrates, fat, protein, vitamins, minerals, and water. The first three are called fuel nutrients because they are the only substances the body uses to supply the energy (commonly measured in calories) needed for work and normal body functions. The three others—vitamins, minerals, and water—are regulatory nutrients. They have no caloric value but are still necessary for a person to function normally and maintain good health. Many nutritionists add to this list a seventh nutrient: fiber. This nutrient is vital for good health. Recommended amounts seem to provide protection against several diseases, including cardiovascular disease and some cancers.

Carbohydrates, fats, proteins, and water are termed *macronutrients* because we need them in proportionately large amounts daily. Vitamins and minerals are required in only small amounts—grams, milligrams, and micrograms instead of, say, ounces—and nutritionists refer to them as micronutrients.

Depending on the amount of nutrients and calories they contain, foods can be classified by their **nutrient density.** Foods that contain few or a moderate number of calories but are packed with nutrients are said to have high nutrient density. Foods that have a lot of calories but few nutrients are of low nutrient density and are commonly called "junk food."

A **calorie** is the unit of measure indicating the energy value of food to the person who consumes it. It also is used to express the amount of energy a person expends in physical activity. Technically, a kilocalorie (kcal), or large calorie, is the amount of heat necessary to raise the temperature of 1 kilogram of water 1 degree centigrade. For simplicity, people call it a calorie rather than a kcal. For example, if the caloric value of a food is 100 calories (that is, 100 kcal), the energy in this food would raise the temperature of 100 kilograms of water 1 degree centigrade. Similarly, walking 1 mile would burn about 100 calories (again, 100 kcal).

## Carbohydrates  **Carbohydrates** constitute the major source of calories the body uses to provide energy for

FIGURE 3.2  Major types of carbohydrates.

**Simple carbohydrates**

| Monosaccharides | Disaccharides |
| --- | --- |
| Glucose | Sucrose (glucose+fructose) |
| Fructose | Lactose (glucose+galactose) |
| Galactose | Maltose (glucose+glucose) |

**Complex carbohydrates**

| Polysaccharides | Fiber |
| --- | --- |
| Starches | Cellulose |
| Dextrins | Hemicellulose |
| Glycogen | Pectins |
| | Gums |
| | Mucilages |

work and to maintain cells and generate heat. They also help regulate fat and metabolize protein. Each gram of carbohydrates provides the human body with 4 calories. The major sources of carbohydrates are breads, cereals, fruits, vegetables, and milk/dairy products. Carbohydrates are classified into **simple carbohydrates** and complex carbohydrates (see Figure 3.2).

**Simple Carbohydrates** Often called "sugars," simple carbohydrates have little nutritive value. Examples are candy, soda, and cakes. Simple carbohydrates are divided into monosaccharides and disaccharides. These carbohydrates—whose names end in "ose"—often take the place of more nutritive foods in the diet.

***Monosaccharides.*** The simplest sugars are **monosaccharides.** The three most common monosaccharides are glucose, fructose, and galactose.

---

**Nutrient density**  A measure of the amount of nutrients and calories in various foods.

**Calorie**  The amount of heat necessary to raise the temperature of 1 gram of water 1 degree Centigrade; used to measure the energy value of food and cost (energy expenditure) of physical activity.

**Carbohydrates**  A classification of a dietary nutrient containing carbon, hydrogen, and oxygen; the major source of energy for the human body

**Simple carbohydrates**  Formed by simple or double sugar units with little nutritive value; divided into monosaccharides and disaccharides.

**Monosaccharides**  The simplest carbohydrates (sugars), formed by five- or six-carbon skeletons. The three most common monosaccharides are glucose, fructose, and galactose.

1. Glucose is a natural sugar found in food and also produced in the body from other simple and complex carbohydrates. It is used as a source of energy, or it may be stored in the muscles and liver in the form of glycogen (a long chain of glucose molecules hooked together). Excess glucose in the blood is converted to fat and stored in **adipose tissue.**

2. Fructose, or fruit sugar, occurs naturally in fruits and honey and is converted to glucose in the body.

3. Galactose is produced from milk sugar in the mammary glands of lactating animals and is converted to glucose in the body.

**Disaccharides** The three major **disaccharides** are:

1. Sucrose, or table sugar (glucose + fructose)

2. Lactose (glucose + galactose)

3. Maltose (glucose + glucose)

These disaccharides are broken down in the body, and the resulting simple sugars (monosaccharides) are used as indicated above.

**Complex Carbohydrates** **Complex carbohydrates** are also called *polysaccharides.* Anywhere from about ten to thousands of monosaccharide molecules can unite to form a single polysaccharide. Examples of complex carbohydrates are starches, dextrins, and **glycogen.**

1. Starch is the storage form of glucose in plants that is needed to promote their earliest growth. Starch is commonly found in grains, seeds, corn, nuts, roots, potatoes, and legumes. In a healthful diet, grains, the richest source of starch, should supply most of the energy. Once eaten, starch is converted to glucose for the body's own energy use.

2. Dextrins are formed from the breakdown of large starch molecules exposed to dry heat, such as in baking bread or producing cold cereals. These complex carbohydrates of plant origin provide many valuable nutrients and can be an excellent source of fiber.

3. Glycogen is the animal polysaccharide synthesized from glucose and is found only in tiny amounts in meats. In essence, we manufacture it; we don't consume it. Glycogen constitutes the body's reservoir of glucose. Thousands of glucose molecules are linked, to be stored as glycogen in the liver and muscle. When a surge of energy is needed, enzymes in the muscle and the liver break down glycogen and thereby make glucose readily available for energy transformation. (This process is discussed under "Nutrition for Athletes," starting on page 102.)

*Fiber.* Fiber is a form of complex carbohydrate. A high-fiber diet gives a person a feeling of fullness without adding too many calories to the diet. **Dietary fiber** is present mainly in plant leaves, skins, roots, and seeds. Processing and refining foods removes almost all of their natural fi-

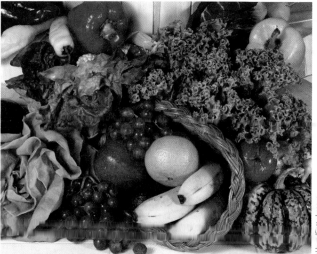

High-fiber foods are essential in a healthy diet.

ber. In our diet, the main sources of fiber are whole-grain cereals and breads, fruits, vegetables, and legumes.

Fiber is important in the diet because it decreases the risk for cardiovascular disease and cancer. Increased fiber intake also may lower the risk for CHD, because saturated fats often take the place of fiber in the diet, increasing the absorption and formation of cholesterol. Other health disorders that have been tied to low intake of fiber are constipation, diverticulitis, hemorrhoids, gallbladder disease, and obesity.

The recommended fiber intake for adults 50 years and younger is 25 grams per day for women and 38 grams for men. As a result of decreased food consumption in people over 50 years of age, an intake of 21 and 30 grams of fiber per day, respectively, is recommended.[1] Most people in the United States eat only 15 grams of fiber per day, putting them at increased risk for disease.

A person can increase fiber intake by eating more fruits, vegetables, legumes, whole grains, and whole-grain cereals. Research provides evidence that increasing fiber intake to 30 grams per day leads to a significant reduction in heart attacks, cancer of the colon, breast cancer, diabetes, and diverticulitis. Table 3.1 provides the fiber content of selected foods. A practical guideline to obtain your fiber intake is to eat at least five daily servings of fruits and vegetables and three servings of whole-grain foods (whole-grain bread, cereal, and rice).

Fiber is typically classified according to its solubility in water:

1. Soluble fiber dissolves in water and forms a gel-like substance that encloses food particles. This property allows soluble fiber to bind and excrete fats from the body. This type of fiber has been shown to lower blood cholesterol and blood sugar levels. Soluble fiber is found primarily in oats, fruits, barley, legumes, and psyllium (an ancient Indian grain added to some breakfast cereals).

**TABLE 3.1 Dietary Fiber Content of Selected Foods**

| Food (gm) | Serving Size | Dietary Fiber |
|---|---|---|
| Almonds, shelled | ¼ cup | 3.9 |
| Apple | 1 medium | 3.7 |
| Banana | 1 small | 1.2 |
| Beans (red kidney) | ½ cup | 8.2 |
| Blackberries | ½ cup | 4.9 |
| Beets, red, canned (cooked) | ½ cup | 1.4 |
| Brazil nuts | 1 oz | 2.5 |
| Broccoli (cooked) | ½ cup | 0.0 |
| Brown rice (cooked) | ½ cup | 1.7 |
| Carrots (cooked) | ½ cup | 3.3 |
| Cauliflower (cooked) | ½ cup | 5.0 |
| Cereal | | |
| All Bran | 1 oz | 8.5 |
| Cheerios | 1 oz | 1.1 |
| Cornflakes | 1 oz | 0.5 |
| Fruit and Fibre | 1 oz | 4.0 |
| Fruit Wheats | 1 oz | 2.0 |
| Just Right | 1 oz | 2.0 |
| Wheaties | 1 oz | 2.0 |
| Corn (cooked) | ½ cup | 2.2 |
| Eggplant (cooked) | ½ cup | 3.0 |
| Lettuce (chopped) | ½ cup | 0.5 |
| Orange | 1 medium | 4.3 |
| Parsnips (cooked) | ½ cup | 2.1 |
| Pear | 1 medium | 4.5 |
| Peas (cooked) | ½ cup | 4.4 |
| Popcorn (plain) | 1 cup | 1.2 |
| Potato (baked) | 1 medium | 4.9 |
| Strawberries | ½ cup | 1.6 |
| Summer squash (cooked) | ½ cup | 1.6 |
| Watermelon | 1 cup | 0.1 |

2. Insoluble fiber is not easily dissolved in water, and the body cannot digest it. This type of fiber is important because it binds water, causing a softer and bulkier stool that increases **peristalsis,** the involuntary muscle contractions of intestinal walls that force the stool through the intestines and enable quicker excretion of food residues. Speeding the passage of food residues through the intestines seems to lower the risk for colon cancer, mainly because it reduces the amount of time that cancer-causing agents are in contact with the intestinal wall. Insoluble fiber is also thought to bind with carcinogens (cancer-producing substances), and more water in the stool may dilute the cancer-causing agents, lessening their potency. Sources of insoluble fiber include wheat, cereals, vegetables, and skins of fruits.

The most common types of fiber are:

1. Cellulose: water-insoluble fiber found in plant cell walls
2. Hemicellulose: water-insoluble fiber found in cereal fibers
3. Pectins: water-soluble fiber found in vegetables and fruits
4. Gums and mucilages: water-soluble fiber also found in small amounts in foods of plant origin

Surprisingly, excessive fiber intake can be detrimental to health. It can produce loss of calcium, phosphorus, and iron and cause gastrointestinal discomfort. If your fiber intake is below the recommended amount, increase your intake gradually over several weeks to avoid gastrointestinal disturbances. While increasing your fiber intake, be sure to drink more water to avoid constipation and even dehydration.

**Fats (Lipids)** The human body uses **fats** as a source of energy. Also called lipids, fats are the most concentrated energy source, with each gram of fat supplying 9 calories to the body (in contrast to 4 for carbohydrates). Fats are a part of the human cell structure. Deposits of fat cells are used as stored energy and as an insulator to preserve body heat. They absorb shock, supply essential fatty acids, and carry the fat-soluble vitamins A, D, E, and K. Fats can be classified into three main groups: simple, compound, and derived (see Figure 3.3). The most familiar sources of fat are whole milk and other dairy products, meats, and meat alternatives such as eggs and nuts.

**Simple Fats** A simple fat consists of a glyceride molecule linked to one, two, or three units of fatty acids. Depending on the number of fatty acids attached, simple fats are di-

**Adipose tissue** Fat cells in the body.

**Disaccharides** Simple carbohydrates formed by two monosaccharide units linked together, one of which is glucose. The major disaccharides are sucrose, lactose, and maltose.

**Complex carbohydrates** Carbohydrates formed by three or more simple sugar molecules linked together; also referred to as polysaccharides.

**Glycogen** Form in which glucose is stored in the body.

**Dietary fiber** A complex carbohydrate in plant foods that is not digested but is essential to digestion.

**Peristalsis** Involuntary muscle contractions of intestinal walls that facilitate excretion of wastes.

**Fats** A classification of nutrients containing carbon, hydrogen, some oxygen, and sometimes other chemical elements.

## Behavior Modification Planning

### TIPS TO INCREASE FIBER IN YOUR DIET

| I PLAN TO | I DID IT | |
|---|---|---|
| ❑ | ❑ | Eat more vegetables, either raw or steamed |
| ❑ | ❑ | Eat salads daily that include a wide variety of vegetables |
| ❑ | ❑ | Eat more fruit, including the skin |
| ❑ | ❑ | Choose whole-wheat and whole-grain products |
| ❑ | ❑ | Choose breakfast cereals with more than 3 grams of fiber per serving |
| ❑ | ❑ | Sprinkle a teaspoon or two of unprocessed bran or 100 percent bran cereal on your favorite breakfast cereal |
| ❑ | ❑ | Add high-fiber cereals to casseroles and desserts |
| ❑ | ❑ | Add beans to soups, salads, and stews |
| ❑ | ❑ | Add vegetables to sandwiches: sprouts, green and red pepper strips, diced carrots, sliced cucumbers, red cabbage, onions |
| ❑ | ❑ | Add vegetables to spaghetti: broccoli, cauliflower, sliced carrots, mushrooms |
| ❑ | ❑ | Experiment with unfamiliar fruits and vegetables—collards, kale, broccoflower, asparagus, papaya, mango, kiwi, starfruit |
| ❑ | ❑ | Blend fruit juice with small pieces of fruit and crushed ice |
| ❑ | ❑ | When increasing fiber in your diet, drink plenty of fluids |

### Try It

Do you know your average daily fiber intake? If you do not know, keep a 3-day record of daily fiber intake. How do you fare against the recommended guidelines? If your intake is low, how can you change your diet to increase your daily fiber intake?

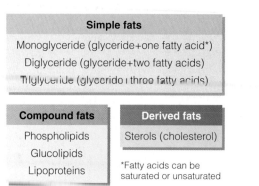

**FIGURE 3.3** Major types of fats (lipids).

vided into monoglycerides (one fatty acid), diglycerides (two fatty acids), and triglycerides (three fatty acids). More than 90 percent of the weight of fat in foods and more than 95 percent of the stored fat in the human body are in the form of triglycerides.

The length of the carbon atom chain and the amount of hydrogen saturation (i.e., the number of hydrogen molecules attached to the carbon chain) in fatty acids vary. Based on the extent of saturation, fatty acids are said to be saturated or unsaturated. Unsaturated fatty acids are classified further into monounsaturated and polyunsaturated fatty acids. Saturated fatty acids are mainly of animal origin, and unsaturated fats are found mostly in plant products.

***Saturated Fats.*** In saturated fatty acids (or "saturated fats"), the carbon atoms are fully saturated with hydrogen atoms; only single bonds link the carbon atoms on the chain (see Figure 3.4). Foods high in saturated fatty acids are meats, animal fat, lard, whole milk, cream, butter, cheese, ice cream, hydrogenated oils (hydrogenation makes oils saturated), coconut oil, and palm oils. Saturated fats typically do not melt at room temperature. Coconut and palm oils are exceptions. In general, saturated fats raise the blood cholesterol level. The data on coconut and palm oils are controversial, as some research indicates that these oils may be neutral in terms of their effects on cholesterol and actually may provide some health benefits.

***Unsaturated Fats.*** In unsaturated fatty acids (or "unsaturated fats"), double bonds form between unsaturated carbons. These healthy fatty acids (FAs) include monounsaturated and polyunsaturated fats, which are usually liquid at room temperature. Other shorter fatty acid chains also tend to be liquid at room temperature. Unsaturated fats help lower blood cholesterol. When unsaturated fats replace saturated fats in the diet, the former stimulate the liver to clear cholesterol from the blood.

In monounsaturated fatty acids (MUFAs), only one double bond is found along the chain. MUFAs are found in olive, canola, peanut, and sesame oils. They are also found in avocados, peanuts, and cashews.

FIGURE 3.4 Chemical structure of saturated and unsaturated fats.

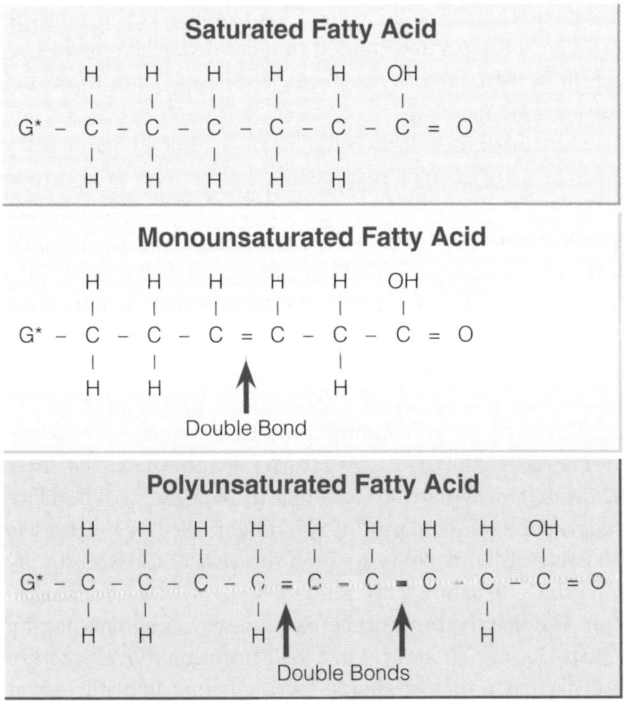

**Saturated Fatty Acid**

**Monounsaturated Fatty Acid**

Double Bond

**Polyunsaturated Fatty Acid**

Double Bonds

*Glyceride component

Polyunsaturated fatty acids (PUFAs) contain two or more double bonds between unsaturated carbon atoms along the chain. Corn, cottonseed, safflower, walnut, sunflower, and soybean oils are high in PUFAs, which are also found in fish, almonds, and pecans.

Trans Fatty Acids. Hydrogen often is added to monounsaturated and polyunsaturated fats to increase shelf life and to solidify them so they are more spreadable. During this process, called "partial hydrogenation," the position of hydrogen atoms may be changed along the carbon chain, transforming the fat into a **trans fatty acid.** Margarine and spreads, shortening, some nut butters, crackers, cookies, dairy products, meats, processed foods, and fast foods often contain trans fatty acids.

Trans fatty acids are not essential and provide no known health benefit. In truth, health-conscious people minimize their intake of these types of fats because diets high in trans fatty acids increase rigidity of the coronary arteries, elevate cholesterol, and contribute to the formation of blood clots that may lead to heart attacks and strokes.

Trans fats are found in about 40 percent of supermarket foods, including almost all cookies, 80 percent of frozen breakfast foods, 75 percent of snacks and chips, most cake mixes, and almost 50 percent of all cereals. Doughnuts, french fries, stick margarine, vegetable shortening, cookies, and crackers are all high in trans fatty acid content.[2]

Paying attention to food labels is important, because the words "partially hydrogenated" and "trans fatty acids" indicate that the product carries a health risk just as high or higher than that of saturated fat. The Food and Drug Administration now requires that food labels list trans fatty acids so consumers can make healthier choices.

Polyunsaturated Omega Fatty Acids. Omega fatty acids have gained considerable attention in recent years. These fatty acids are essential to human health and cannot be manufactured by the body (they have to be consumed in the diet). These essential fatty acids have been named based on where the first double bond appears in the carbon chain—starting from the end of the chain; hence the term "omega," from the end of the Greek alphabet. Accordingly, omega fats are classified as **omega-3 fatty acids** and **omega-6 fatty acids.**

Maintaining a balance between these fatty acids is important for good health. Excessive intake of omega-6 fatty acids tends to contribute to inflammation (a risk factor for heart disease—see Chapter 11, page 394), cancer, asthma, arthritis, and depression. A ratio of 4 to 1 omega-6 to omega-3 fatty acids is recommended to maintain and improve health.

Most critical in the diet are omega-3 fatty acids, which provide substantial health benefits. Omega-3 fatty acids tend to decrease cholesterol, triglycerides, inflammation, blood clots, abnormal heart rhythms, and high blood pressure. They also decrease the risk of heart attack, stroke, Alzheimer's disease, dementia, macular degeneration, and joint degeneration.

Unfortunately, only 25 percent of the U.S. population consumes the recommended amount (approximately 500 mg) of omega eicosapentaenoic acid (EPA) and docosahexaenoic acid (DHA) on any given day. These are two of the three major types of omega-3 fatty acids, along with alpha-linolenic acid (ALA). The evidence is strongest for EPA and DHA as being cardioprotective. Once consumed, the body converts ALA to EPA and then to DHA, but the process is not very efficient. It is best to increase consumption of EPA and DHA to obtain the greatest health benefit.

Individuals at risk for heart disease are encouraged to get an average of 500 to 1,800 grams of EPA and DHA per day.[3] These fatty acids protect against irregular heartbeats and blood clots, reduce triglycerides and blood pressure, and defend against inflammation.[4]

Fish—especially fresh or frozen salmon, mackerel, herring, tuna, and rainbow trout—are high in EPA and DHA. Table 3.2 presents a listing of total EPA plus DHA content

**Trans fatty acid** Solidified fat formed by adding hydrogen to monounsaturated and polyunsaturated fats to increase shelf life.

**Omega-3 fatty acids** Polyunsaturated fatty acids found primarily in cold-water seafood, flaxseed, and flaxseed oil; thought to lower blood cholesterol and triglycerides.

**Omega-6 fatty acids** Polyunsaturated fatty acids found primarily in corn and sunflower oils and most oils in processed foods.

**TABLE 3.2** Omega-3 Fatty Acid Content (EPA + DHA) per 100 Grams (3.5 oz) of Fish

| Type of Fish | Total EPA + DHA |
| --- | --- |
| Anchovy | 1.4 gr |
| Bluefish | 1.2 gr |
| Halibut | 0.4 gr |
| Herring | 1.7 gr |
| Mackerel | 2.4 gr |
| Sardine | 1.4 gr |
| Salmon, Atlantic | 1.0 gr |
| Salmon, Chinook | 1.9 gr |
| Salmon, Coho | 1.2 gr |
| Salmon, pink | 1.0 gr |
| Salmon, Sockeye | 1.3 gr |
| Shrimp | 0.3 gr |
| Trout, rainbow | 0.6 gr |
| Trout, lake | 1.6 gr |
| Tuna, white (Albacore) | 0.8 gr |

of selected species of fish. Canned fish is not recommended, because the canning process destroys most of the omega-3 fatty acids. Good sources of omega-3 ALA include flaxseeds, canola oil, walnuts, wheat germ, and green leafy vegetables.

The oil in flaxseeds is high in ALA and has been shown to reduce abnormal heart rhythms and prevent blood clots.[5] Flaxseeds are also high in fiber and plant chemicals known as lignans. Studies are being conducted to investigate the potential cancer-fighting ability of lignans. In one report, the addition of a daily ounce (3 to 4 tablespoons) of ground flaxseeds to the diet seemed to lead to a decrease in the onset of tumors, preventing their formation and even leading to their shrinkage.[6] Excessive flaxseed in the diet is not recommended. High doses actually may be detrimental to health. Pregnant and lactating women, especially, should not consume large amounts of flaxseed.

Because flaxseeds have a hard outer shell, they should be ground to obtain the nutrients; whole seeds will pass through the body undigested. Flavor and nutrients are best preserved by grinding the seeds just before use. Preground seeds should be kept sealed and refrigerated. Ground flaxseeds can be mixed with salad dressings, salads, wheat flour, pancakes, muffins, cereals, rice, cottage cheese, and yogurt. Flaxseed oil also may be used, but the oil has little or no fiber and lignans and must be kept refrigerated because it spoils quickly. The oil cannot be used for cooking either, because it scorches easily.

Most of the polyunsaturated fatty acid consumption in the United States comes from omega-6. Once viewed as healthy fats, we now know that excessive intake is detri-

mental to health. Omega-6 fatty acids include linoleic acid (LA), gamma linolenic acid (GLA), and arachidonic acid (AA). The typical American diet contains 10 to 20 times more omega-6 than omega-3 fatty acids. Most omega-6 fatty acids come in the form of LA from vegetable oils, the primary oil ingredient added to most processed foods. LA-rich oils include corn, soybean, sunflower, safflower, and cottonseed oils.

The imbalance between omega-3 and omega-6 fatty acids is thought to be responsible for the increased rate of inflammatory conditions seen in the United States today. Furthermore, in terms of heart health, while omega-6 fatty acids lower the "bad" low-density lipoprotein (LDL) cholesterol, they also lower the "good" high-density lipoprotein (HDL) cholesterol; thus its overall effect on cardiac health is neutral. To decrease your intake of LA, watch for corn, soybean, sunflower, and cottonseed oils in salad dressings, mayonnaise, and margarine.

The best source of omega-3 APA and DHA, the fatty acids that provide the most health benefits, is fish. Data suggest that the amount of fish oil obtained by eating two servings of fish weekly lessens the risk of CHD and may contribute to brain, joint, and vision health. A word of caution: People who have diabetes, a history of hemorrhaging or strokes, are on aspirin or blood-thinning therapy, or are presurgical patients should not consume fish oil except under a physician's instruction.

**Compound Fats** Compound fats are a combination of simple fats and other chemicals. Examples are:

1. Phospholipids: similar to triglycerides, except that choline (or another compound) and phosphoric acid take the place of one of the fatty acid units
2. Glucolipids: a combination of carbohydrates, fatty acids, and nitrogen
3. Lipoproteins: water-soluble aggregates of protein and triglycerides, phospholipids, or cholesterol

**Lipoproteins** (a combination of lipids and proteins) are especially important because they transport fats in the blood. The major forms are HDL, LDL, and very-low-density lipoprotein (VLDL). Lipoproteins play a large role in developing or in preventing heart disease. High levels of HDL ("good" cholesterol) have been associated with lower risk for CHD, whereas high levels of LDL ("bad" cholesterol) have been linked to increased risk for this disease. HDL is more than 50 percent protein and contains little cholesterol. LDL is approximately 25 percent protein and nearly 50 percent cholesterol. VLDL contains about 50 percent triglycerides, only about 10 percent protein, and 20 percent cholesterol.

**Derived Fats** Derived fats combine simple and compound fats. **Sterols** are an example. Although sterols contain no fatty acids, they are considered lipids because they do not dissolve in water. The sterol mentioned most often is cholesterol, which is found in many foods or can be manufactured in the body—primarily from saturated fats and trans fats.

**Proteins** **Proteins** are the main substances the body uses to build and repair tissues such as muscles, blood, internal organs, skin, hair, nails, and bones. They form a part of hormone, antibody, and enzyme molecules. **Enzymes** play a key role in all of the body's processes. Because all enzymes are formed by proteins, this nutrient is necessary for normal functioning. Proteins also help maintain the normal balance of body fluids.

Proteins can be used as a source of energy, too, but only if sufficient carbohydrates are not available. Each gram of protein yields 4 calories of energy (the same as carbohydrates). The main sources of protein are meats and alternatives, milk, and other dairy products. Excess proteins may be converted to glucose or fat, or even excreted in the urine.

The human body uses 20 **amino acids** to form different types of protein. Amino acids contain nitrogen, carbon, hydrogen, and oxygen. Of the 20 amino acids, 9 are called essential amino acids because the body cannot produce them. The other 11, termed "nonessential amino acids," can be manufactured in the body if food proteins in the diet provide enough nitrogen (see Table 3.3). For the body to function normally, all amino acids shown in Table 3.3 must be present in the diet.

Proteins that contain all the essential amino acids, known as "complete" or "higher-quality" protein, are usually of animal origin. If one or more of the essential amino acids are missing, the proteins are termed "incomplete" or "lower-quality" protein. Individuals have to take in enough protein to ensure nitrogen for adequate production of amino acids and also to get enough high-quality protein to obtain the essential amino acids.

Protein deficiency is not a problem in the typical U.S. diet. Two glasses of skim milk combined with about 4 ounces of poultry or fish meet the daily protein requirement. But too much animal protein can cause health problems. Some people eat twice as much protein as they need. Protein foods from animal sources are often high in fat, saturated fat, and cholesterol, which can lead to cardiovascular disease and cancer. Too much animal protein also decreases the blood enzymes that prevent precancerous cells from developing into tumors.

As mentioned earlier, a well-balanced diet contains a variety of foods from all five basic food groups, including a wise selection of foods from animal sources (see also "Balancing the Diet" on page 80). Based on current nutrition data, meat (poultry and fish included) should be replaced by grains, legumes, vegetables, and fruits as main courses. Meats should be used more for flavoring than for volume. Daily consumption of beef, poultry, or fish should be limited to 3 ounces (about the size of a deck of cards) to 6 ounces.

**Vitamins** **Vitamins** are necessary for normal bodily metabolism, growth, and development. Vitamins are classified into two types based on their solubility:

1. Fat soluble (A, D, E, and K)
2. Water soluble (B complex and C)

The body does not manufacture most vitamins, so they can be obtained only through a well-balanced diet. To decrease loss of vitamins during cooking, natural foods should be microwaved or steamed rather than boiled in water that is thrown out later.

A few exceptions, such as vitamins A, D, and K, are formed in the body. Vitamin A is produced from beta-carotene, found mainly in yellow foods such as carrots, pumpkin, and sweet potatoes. Vitamin D is created when ultraviolet light from the sun transforms 7-dehydrocholesterol, a compound in human skin. Vitamin K is created in the body by intestinal bacteria. The major functions of vitamins are outlined in Table 3.4.

Vitamins C, E, and beta-carotene also function as antioxidants, which are thought to play a key role in preventing chronic diseases. (The specific functions of these antioxidant nutrients and of the mineral selenium, also an antioxidant, are discussed under "Antioxidants," page 95.)

**TABLE 3.3** Amino Acids

| Essential Amino Acids* | Nonessential Amino Acids |
| --- | --- |
| Histidine | Alanine |
| Isoleucine | Arginine |
| Leucine | Asparagine |
| Lysine | Aspartic acid |
| Methionine | Cysteine |
| Phenylalanine | Glutamic acid |
| Threonine | Glutamine |
| Tryptophan | Glycine |
| Valine | Proline |
| | Serine |
| | Tyrosine |

*Must be provided in the diet because the body cannot manufacture them.

**Lipoproteins** Lipids covered by proteins, these transport fats in the blood. Types are LDL, HDL, and VLDL.

**Sterols** Derived fats, of which cholesterol is the best-known example.

**Proteins** A classification of nutrients consisting of complex organic compounds containing nitrogen and formed by combinations of amino acids; the main substances used in the body to build and repair tissues.

**Enzymes** Catalysts that facilitate chemical reactions in the body.

**Amino acids** Chemical compounds that contain nitrogen, carbon, hydrogen, and oxygen; the basic building blocks the body uses to build different types of protein.

**Vitamins** Organic nutrients essential for normal metabolism, growth, and development of the body.

**TABLE 3.4** Major Functions of Vitamins

| Nutrient | Good Sources | Major Functions | Deficiency Symptoms |
|---|---|---|---|
| **VITAMIN A** | Milk, cheese, eggs, liver, yellow and dark-green fruits and vegetables | Required for healthy bones, teeth, skin, gums, and hair; maintenance of inner mucous membranes, thus increasing resistance to infection, adequate vision in dim light. | Night blindness; decreased growth; decreased resistance to infection; rough, dry skin |
| **VITAMIN D** | Fortified milk, cod liver oil, salmon, tuna, egg yolk | Necessary for bones and teeth; needed for calcium and phosphorus absorption. | Rickets (bone softening), fractures, muscle spasms |
| **VITAMIN E** | Vegetable oils, yellow and green leafy vegetables, margarine, wheat germ, whole-grain breads and cereals | Related to oxidation and normal muscle and red blood cell chemistry. | Leg cramps, red blood cell breakdown |
| **VITAMIN K** | Green leafy vegetables, cauliflower, cabbage, eggs, peas, potatoes | Essential for normal blood clotting. | Hemorrhaging |
| **VITAMIN B$_1$ (THIAMIN)** | Whole-grain or enriched bread, lean meats and poultry, fish, liver, pork, poultry, organ meats, legumes, nuts, dried yeast | Assists in proper use of carbohydrates, normal functioning of nervous system, maintenance of good appetite. | Loss of appetite, nausea, confusion, cardiac abnormalities, muscle spasms |
| **VITAMIN B$_2$ (RIBOFLAVIN)** | Eggs, milk, leafy green vegetables, whole grains, lean meats, dried beans and peas | Contributes to energy release from carbohydrates, fats, and proteins; needed for normal growth and development, good vision, and healthy skin. | Cracking of the corners of the mouth, inflammation of the skin, impaired vision |
| **VITAMIN B$_6$ (PYRIDOXINE)** | Vegetables, meats, whole-grain cereals, soybeans, peanuts, potatoes | Necessary for protein and fatty acids metabolism and for normal red blood cell formation. | Depression, irritability, muscle spasms, nausea |
| **VITAMIN B$_{12}$** | Meat, poultry, fish, liver, organ meats, eggs, shellfish, milk, cheese | Required for normal growth, red blood cell formation, nervous system and digestive tract functioning. | Impaired balance, weakness, drop in red blood cell count |
| **NIACIN** | Liver and organ meats, meat, fish, poultry, whole grains, enriched breads, nuts, green leafy vegetables, and dried beans and peas | Contributes to energy release from carbohydrates, fats, and proteins; normal growth and development; and formation of hormones and nerve-regulating substances. | Confusion, depression, weakness, weight loss |
| **BIOTIN** | Liver, kidney, eggs, yeast, legumes, milk, nuts, dark-green vegetables | Essential for carbohydrate metabolism and fatty acid synthesis. | Inflamed skin, muscle pain, depression, weight loss |
| **FOLIC ACID** | Leafy green vegetables, organ meats, whole grains and cereals, dried beans | Needed for cell growth and reproduction and for red blood cell formation. | Decreased resistance to infection |
| **PANTOTHENIC ACID** | All natural foods, especially liver, kidney, eggs, nuts, yeast, milk, dried peas and beans, green leafy vegetables | Related to carbohydrate and fat metabolism. | Depression, low blood sugar, leg cramps, nausea, headaches |
| **VITAMIN C (ASCORBIC ACID)** | Fruits, vegetables | Helps protect against infection; required for formation of collagenous tissue, normal blood vessels, teeth, and bones. | Slow-healing wounds, loose teeth, hemorrhaging, rough scaly skin, irritability |

**TABLE 3.5** Major Functions of Minerals

| Nutrient | Good Sources | Major Functions | Deficiency Symptoms |
| --- | --- | --- | --- |
| **CALCIUM** | Milk, yogurt, cheese, green leafy vegetables, dried beans, sardines, salmon | Required for strong teeth and bone formation; maintenance of good muscle tone, heartbeat, and nerve function. | Bone pain and fractures, periodontal disease, muscle cramps |
| **COPPER** | Seafood, meats, beans, nuts, whole grains | Helps with iron absorption and hemoglobin formation; required to synthesize the enzyme cytochrome oxidase. | Anemia (although deficiency is rare in humans) |
| **IRON** | Organ meats, lean meats, seafood, eggs, dried peas and beans, nuts, whole and enriched grains, green leafy vegetables | Major component of hemoglobin; aids in energy utilization. | Nutritional anemia, overall weakness |
| **PHOSPHORUS** | Meats, fish, milk, eggs, dried beans and peas, whole grains, processed foods | Required for bone and teeth formation and for energy release regulation. | Bone pain and fracture, weight loss, weakness |
| **ZINC** | Milk, meat, seafood, whole grains, nuts, eggs, dried beans | Essential component of hormones, insulin and enzymes; used in normal growth and development. | Loss of appetite, slow-healing wounds, skin problems |
| **MAGNESIUM** | Green leafy vegetables, whole grains, nuts, soybeans, seafood, legumes | Needed for bone growth and maintenance, carbohydrate and protein utilization, nerve function, temperature regulation. | Irregular heartbeat, weakness, muscle spasms, sleeplessness |
| **SODIUM** | Table salt, processed foods, meat | Needed for body fluid regulation, transmission of nerve impulses, heart action. | Rarely seen |
| **POTASSIUM** | Legumes, whole grains, bananas, orange juice, dried fruits, potatoes | Required for heart action, bone formation and maintenance, regulation of energy release, acid-base regulation. | Irregular heartbeat, nausea, weakness |
| **SELENIUM** | Seafood, meat, whole grains | Component of enzymes; functions in close association with vitamin E. | Muscle pain, possible heart muscle deterioration, possible hair loss and nail loss |

**Minerals** Approximately 25 minerals have important roles in body functioning. **Minerals** are inorganic substances contained in all cells, especially those in hard parts of the body (bones, nails, teeth). Minerals are crucial to maintaining water balance and the acid–base balance. They are essential components of respiratory pigments, enzymes, and enzyme systems, and they regulate muscular and nervous tissue impulses, blood clotting, and normal heart rhythm. The four minerals mentioned most often are calcium, iron, sodium, and selenium. Calcium deficiency may result in osteoporosis, and low iron intake can induce iron-deficiency anemia (see page 107). High sodium intake may contribute to high blood pressure. Selenium seems to be important in preventing certain types of cancer. Specific functions of some of the most important minerals are given in Table 3.5.

**Water** The most important nutrient is **water**, as it is involved in almost every vital body process: in digesting and absorbing food, in producing energy, in the circulatory process, in regulating body heat, in removing waste products, in building and rebuilding cells, and in transporting other nutrients. In men, about 61 percent of total body weight is water. The proportion of body weight in women is 56 percent (see Figure 3.5). The difference is due primarily to the higher amount of muscle mass in men.

Almost all foods contain water, but it is found primarily in liquid foods, fruits, and vegetables. Although for decades the recommendation was to consume at least 8 cups of water per day, a panel of scientists of the Institute of Medicine of the National Academy of Sciences (NAS) indi-

**Minerals** Inorganic nutrients essential for normal body functions; found in the body and in food.

**Water** The most important classification of essential body nutrients, involved in almost every vital body process.

**FIGURE 3.5** Approximate proportions of nutrients in the human body.

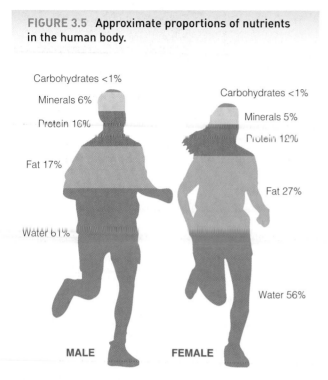

Carbohydrates <1%

Minerals 6%

Protein 16%

Fat 17%

Water 61%

**MALE**

Carbohydrates <1%

Minerals 5%

Protein 12%

Fat 27%

Water 56%

**FEMALE**

**TABLE 3.6** The American Diet: Current and Recommended Carbohydrate, Fat, and Protein Intake Expressed as a Percentage of Total Calories

|  | Current Percentage | Recommended Percentage* |
|---|---|---|
| Carbohydrates: | 50% | 45–65% |
| Simple | 26% | Less than **25%** |
| Complex | 24% | 20–40% |
| Fat: | 34% | 20–30%** |
| Monounsaturated: | 11% | Up to 20% |
| Polyunsaturated: | 10% | Up to 10% |
| Saturated: | 13% | Less than 7% |
| Protein: | 16% | 10–35% |

*Adapted from the 2002 recommended guidelines by the National Academy of Sciences.
**Up to 35% is allowed for individuals with metabolic syndrome who may need additional fat in the diet.

cated that people are getting enough water from the liquids (milk, juices, sodas, coffee) and the moisture content of solid foods. Most Americans and Canadians remain well hydrated simply by using thirst as their guide. Caffeine-containing drinks also are acceptable as a water source because data indicate that people who regularly consume such beverages do not have more 24-hour urine output than those who don't.

An exception of not waiting for the thirst signal to replenish water loss is when an individual exercises in the heat, especially for an extended time (see Chapter 9, page 334). Water lost under these conditions must be replenished regularly. If you wait for the thirst signal, you may have lost too much water already. At 2 percent of body weight lost, a person is dehydrated. At 5 percent, one may become dizzy and disoriented, have trouble with cognitive skills and heart function, and even lose consciousness.

## Balancing the Diet

One of the fundamental ways to enjoy good health and live life to its fullest is through a well-balanced diet. Several guidelines have been published to help you accomplish this. As illustrated in Table 3.6, the most recent recommended guidelines by the NAS state that daily calorie intake should be distributed so that 45 to 65 percent of the total calories come from carbohydrates (mostly complex carbohydrates and less than 25 percent from sugars), 20 to 35 percent from fat, and 10 to 35 percent from protein.[7] The recommended ranges allow for flexibility in planning diets according to individual health and physical activity needs.

In addition to the macronutrients, the diet must include all of the essential vitamins, minerals, and water. The source of fat calories is also critical. The National Cholesterol Education Program recommends that, of total calories, saturated fat should constitute less than 7 percent, polyunsaturated fat up to 10 percent, and monounsaturated fat up to 20 percent. Rating a particular diet accurately is difficult without a complete nutrient analysis. You have an opportunity to perform this analysis in Lab 3A.

The NAS guidelines vary slightly from those previously issued by major national health organizations, which recommend 50 to 60 percent of total calories from carbohydrates, less than 30 percent from fat, and about 15 percent from protein. These percentages are within the ranges recommended by NAS. The most drastic difference appears in the NAS-allowed range of fat intake, up to 35 percent of total calories. This higher percentage, however, was included to accommodate individuals with metabolic syndrome (see Chapter 11, page 409), who have an abnormal insulin response to carbohydrates and may need additional fat in the diet. For all other individuals, daily fat intake should not exceed 30 percent of total caloric intake.

The NAS recommendations will be effective only if people consistently replace saturated and trans fatty acids with unsaturated fatty acids. The latter will require changes in the typical "unhealthy" American diet, which is generally high in red meats, whole dairy products, fast foods, and processed foods—all of which are high in saturated and/or trans fatty acids.

Diets in most developed countries changed significantly after the turn of the 20th century. Today, people eat more calories and fat, fewer complex carbohydrates, and about the same amount of protein. People also weigh more than they did in 1900, an indication that we are eating more calories and are not as physically active as our forebears.

# Nutrition Standards

Nutritionists use a variety of nutrient standards, the most widely known of which is the Recommended Dietary Allowance (RDA). This, however, is not the only standard. Among others are the Dietary Reference Intakes and the Daily Values on food labels. Each standard has a different purpose and utilization in dietary planning and assessment.

Dietary Reference Intake To help people meet dietary guidelines, the NAS developed a set of **Dietary Reference Intakes (DRIs)** for healthy people in the United States and Canada. The DRIs are based on a review of the most current research on nutrient needs of healthy people. The DRI reports are written by the Food and Nutrition Board of the Institute of Medicine in cooperation with scientists from Canada.

The DRIs encompass four types of reference values for planning and assessing diets and for establishing adequate amounts and maximum safe nutrient intakes in the diet: the **Estimated Average Requirement (EAR)**, the **Recommended Dietary Allowances (RDA)**, **Adequate Intake (AI)**, and **Tolerable Upper Intake Level (UL)**. The type of reference value used for a given nutrient and a specific age/gender group is determined according to available scientific information and the intended use of the dietary standard.

*Estimated Average Requirement.* The EAR is the amount of a nutrient that is estimated to meet the nutrient requirement of half the healthy people in specific age and gender groups. At this nutrient intake level, the nutritional requirements of 50 percent of the people are not met. For example, looking at 300 healthy women at age 26, the EAR would meet the nutritional requirement for only half of these women.

*Recommended Dietary Allowance.* The RDA is the daily amount of a nutrient that is considered adequate to meet the known nutrient needs of nearly all healthy people in the United States. Because the committee must decide what level of intake to recommend for everybody, the RDA is set well above the EAR and covers about 98 percent of the population. Stated another way, the RDA recommendation for any nutrient is well above almost everyone's actual requirement. The RDA could be considered a goal for adequate intake. The process for determining the RDA depends on being able to set an EAR, because RDAs are determined statistically from the EAR values. If an EAR cannot be set, no RDA can be established.

*Adequate Intake.* When data are insufficient or inadequate to set an EAR, an AI value is determined instead of the RDA. The AI value is derived from approximations of observed nutrient intakes by a group or groups of healthy people. The AI value for children and adults is expected to meet or exceed the nutritional requirements of a corresponding healthy population.

Nutrients for which daily DRIs have been set are given in Table 3.7.

*Upper Intake Level.* The UL establishes the highest level of nutrient intake that seems to be safe for most healthy people, beyond which exists an increased risk for adverse effects. As intakes increase above the UL, so does the risk for adverse effects. In general terms, the optimum nutrient range for healthy eating is between the RDA and the UL. The established ULs are presented in Table 3.8.

Daily Values The **Daily Values (DVs)** are reference values for nutrients and food components for use on food labels. The DVs include fat, saturated fat, and carbohydrates (as a percent of total calories); cholesterol, sodium, and potassium (in milligrams); and fiber and protein (in grams). The DVs for total fat, saturated fat, and carbohydrate are expressed as percentages for a 2,000-calorie diet and therefore may require adjustments depending on an individual's daily **estimated energy requirement (EER)** in calories. For example, on a 2,000-calorie diet (the EER), the recommended carbohydrate intake is about 300 grams (about 60 percent of the EER), and the recommendation for fat is 65 grams (about 30 percent of EER). The vitamin, mineral, and protein DVs were adapted from the RDAs. The DVs also are not as specific for age and gender groups as are the DRIs. Both the DRIs and the DVs apply only to healthy adults. They are not intended for people who are ill and may require additional nutrients. Figure 3.6 shows a food label with U.S. Recommended Daily Values.

---

**Dietary Reference Intakes (DRI)** A general term that describes four types of nutrient standards that establish adequate amounts and maximum safe nutrient intakes in the diet: Estimated Average Requirements (EARs), Recommended Dietary Allowances (RDAs), Adequate Intakes (AIs), and Tolerable Upper Intake Levels (ULs).

**Estimated Average Requirement (EAR)** The amount of a nutrient that meets the dietary needs of half the people.

**Recommended Dietary Allowance (RDA)** The daily amount of a nutrient (statistically determined from the EARs) that is considered adequate to meet the known nutrient needs of almost 98 percent of all healthy people in the United States.

**Adequate Intake (AI)** The recommended amount of a nutrient intake when sufficient evidence is not available to calculate the EAR and subsequent RDA.

**Upper Intake Level (UL)** The highest level of nutrient intake that seems safe for most healthy people, beyond which exists an increased risk of adverse effects.

**Daily Values (DVs)** Reference values for nutrients and food components used in food labels.

**Estimated Energy Requirement (EER)** The average dietary energy (caloric) intake that is predicted to maintain energy balance in a healthy adult of defined age, gender, weight, height, and level of physical activity, consistent with good health.

**TABLE 3.7**  Dietary Reference Intakes (DRIs): Recommended Daily Dietary Allowances (RDA) and Adequate Intakes (AI) for Selected Nutrients

| | Recommended Dietary Allowances (RDA) | | | | | | | | | | | | | Adequate Intakes (AI) | | | | | |
|---|---|---|---|---|---|---|---|---|---|---|---|---|---|---|---|---|---|---|---|
| | Thiamin (mg) | Riboflavin (mg) | Niacin (mg NE) | Vitamin B$_6$ (mg) | Folate (mcg DFE) | Vitamin B$_{12}$ (mcg) | Phosphorus (m g) | Magnesium (mg) | Vitamin A (mcg) | Vitamin C (mg) | Vitamin E (mg) | Selenium (mcg) | Iron (mg) | Calcium (mg) | Vitamin D (mcg) | Fluoride (mg) | Pantothenic ac d (mg) | Biotin (mg) | Choline (mg) |
| **Males** | | | | | | | | | | | | | | | | | | | |
| 14–18 | 1.2 | 1.3 | 16 | 1.3 | 400 | 2.4 | 1,250 | 410 | 900 | 75 | 15 | 55 | 11 | 1,300 | 5 | 3 | 5.0 | 25 | 550 |
| 19–30 | 1.2 | 1.3 | 16 | 1.3 | 400 | 2.4 | 700 | 400 | 900 | 90 | 15 | 55 | 8 | 1,000 | 5 | 4 | 5.0 | 30 | 550 |
| 31–50 | 1.2 | 1.3 | 16 | 1.3 | 400 | 2.4 | 700 | 420 | 900 | 90 | 15 | 55 | 8 | 1,000 | 5 | 4 | 5.0 | 30 | 550 |
| 51–70 | 1.2 | 1.3 | 16 | 1.7 | 400 | 2.4 | 700 | 420 | 900 | 90 | 15 | 55 | 8 | 1,200 | 10 | 4 | 5.0 | 30 | 550 |
| >70 | 1.2 | 1.3 | 16 | 1.7 | 400 | 2.4 | 700 | 420 | 900 | 90 | 15 | 55 | 8 | 1,200 | 15 | 4 | 5.0 | 30 | 550 |
| **Females** | | | | | | | | | | | | | | | | | | | |
| 14–18 | 1.0 | 1.0 | 14 | 1.2 | 400 | 2.4 | 1,250 | 360 | 700 | 65 | 15 | 55 | 15 | 1,300 | 5 | 3 | 5.0 | 25 | 400 |
| 19–30 | 1.1 | 1.1 | 14 | 1.3 | 400 | 2.4 | 700 | 310 | 700 | 75 | 15 | 55 | 18 | 1,000 | 5 | 3 | 5.0 | 30 | 425 |
| 31–50 | 1.1 | 1.1 | 14 | 1.3 | 400 | 2.4 | 700 | 320 | 700 | 75 | 15 | 55 | 18 | 1,000 | 5 | 3 | 5.0 | 30 | 425 |
| 51–70 | 1.1 | 1.1 | 14 | 1.5 | 400 | 2.4 | 700 | 320 | 700 | 75 | 15 | 55 | 8 | 1,200 | 10 | 3 | 5.0 | 30 | 425 |
| >70 | 1.1 | 1.1 | 14 | 1.5 | 400 | 2.4 | 700 | 320 | 700 | 75 | 15 | 55 | 8 | 1,200 | 15 | 3 | 5.0 | 30 | 425 |
| Pregnant | 1.4 | 1.4 | 18 | 1.9 | 600 | 2.6 | * | +40 | 750 | 85 | 15 | 60 | 27 | * | * | 3 | 6.0 | 30 | 450 |
| Lactating | 1.5 | 1.6 | 17 | 2.0 | 500 | 2.8 | * | * | 1,300 | 120 | 19 | 70 | 10 | * | * | 3 | 7.0 | 35 | 550 |

*Values for these nutrients do not change with pregnancy or lactation. Use the value listed for women of comparable age.
**Source:** Adapted with permission from *Recommended Dietary Allowances,* 10th Edition, and the *Dietary Reference Intakes* series. Copyright © 1989 and 2002, respectively, by the National Academy of Sciences. Courtesy of the National Academies Press, Washington, DC.

**TABLE 3.8**  Tolerable Upper Intake Levels (ULs) of Selected Nutrients for Adults (19–70 years)

| Nutrient | UL per Day | Nutrient | UL per Day |
|---|---|---|---|
| Calcium | 2.5 gr | Vitamin B$_6$ | 100 mg |
| Phosphorus | 4.0 gr* | Folate | 1,000 mcg |
| Magnesium | 350 mg | Choline | 3.5 gr |
| Vitamin D | 50 mcg | Vitamin A | 3,000 mcg |
| Fluoride | 10 mg | Vitamin C | 2,000 mg |
| Niacin | 35 mg | Vitamin E | 1,000 mg |
| Iron | 45 mg | Selenium | 400 mcg |

*3.5 gr per day for pregnant women.

**FIGURE 3.6  Food label with U.S. Recommended Daily Values.**

**1** **Better by Design**
*to recognize the new food labels*
The new food labels feature a revamped nutrition panel titled "Nutrition Facts," with nutrient listings that reflect current health concerns. Now you'll be able to find information on fat, fiber, and other food components fundamental to lowering your risk of cancer and other chronic diseases. Listings for nutrients like thiamin and riboflavin will no longer be required, because Americans generally eat enough of them these days.

**2** **Size Up the Situation**
*All serving sizes are created equal*
Now you can compare similar products and know that their serving sizes are basically identical. So when you realize how much fat is packed into that carton of double-dutch chocolate caramel chunk ice cream you're eyeing, you might opt for low-fat frozen yogurt instead. Serving sizes will also be standardized, so manufacturers can't make nutrition claims for unrealistically small portions. That means a chocolate cake, for example, must be divided into 8 servings sized to satisfy the average person—not 16 servings sized to satisfy the average munchkin.

**3** **Look Before You Leap**
*Use the Daily Values*
You will find the Daily Values on the bottom half of the "Nutrition Facts" panel. Some represent maximum levels of nutrients that should be consumed each day for a healthful diet (as with fat) while others refer to minimum levels that can be exceeded (as with carbohydrates). They are based on both a 2,000 and 2,500 calorie diet. Your own needs may be more or less, but these figures give you a point from which to compare. For example, the sample label indicates that someone with a 2,000 calorie diet should eat no more than 65 grams of fat per day. This is based on a diet getting 30 percent of calories as fat. If you normally eat less calories, or want to eat less than 30 percent of calories as fat, your daily fat consumption will be lower.

**4** **Rate It Right**
*Scan the % Daily Values*
The % Daily Values make judging the nutritional quality of a food a snap. For instance, you can look at the % Daily Value column and find that a food has 25 percent of the Daily Value for fiber. This means the product will give you a substantial portion of the recommended amount of fiber for the day. You can also use this column to compare nutrients in similar products. The % Daily Values are based on a 2,000 calorie diet.

**5** **Trust Adjectives**
*Descriptors have legal definitions*
Terms like "low," "high," and "free" have long been used on food labels. What these words actually mean, however, could vary. Thanks to the new labeling laws, such descriptions must now meet legal definitions. For example, you may be shopping for foods high in vitamin A, which has been linked to lower risk of certain cancers. Under the new label laws, a food described as "high" in a particular nutrient must contain 20 percent or more of the Daily Value for that nutrient. So if the bottle of juice you're thinking of buying says "high in vitamin A," you can now feel confident that it really is a good source of the vitamin.

**6** **Read Health Claims with Confidence**
*The nutrient link to disease prevention*
You can also expect to see food packages with health claims linking certain nutrients to reduced risk of cancer and other diseases. The federal government has approved three health claims dealing with cancer prevention: a low-fat diet may reduce your risk for cancer; high fiber foods may reduce your risk for cancer; and fruits and vegetables may reduce your risk for cancer. A food may not make such a health claim for one nutrient if it contains other nutrients that undermine its health benefits. A high fiber, but high fat, jelly doughnut cannot carry a health claim!

**Nutrition Facts**
Serving Size ½ cup (91g)
Servings Per Container 5

**Amount Per Serving**
**Calories** 58          Calories from Fat 0

**% Daily Value***

| | |
|---|---|
| **Total Fat** 0g | **0%** |
| Saturated Fat 0g | **0%** |
| Trans Fat 0g | **0%** |
| **Cholesterol** 0mg | **0%** |
| **Sodium** 45mg | **2%** |
| **Total Carbohydrate** 12g | **4%** |
| Dietary Fiber 3g | **12%** |
| Sugars 3g | |
| **Protein** 3g | |

| | | | |
|---|---|---|---|
| Vitamin A | 92% | Vitamin C | 16% |
| Calcium | 2% | Iron | 5% |

* Percent Daily Values are based on a 2,000 calorie diet. Your daily values may be higher or lower depending on your calorie needs:

| | Calories | 2,000 | 2,500 |
|---|---|---|---|
| Total Fat | Less than | 65g | 80g |
| Sat Fat | Less than | 20g | 25g |
| Cholesterol | Less than | 300mg | 300mg |
| Sodium | Less than | 2,400mg | 2,400mg |
| Total Carbohydrate | | 300g | 375g |
| Fiber | | 25g | 30g |

Calories per gram:
Fat 9  •  Carbohydrates 4  •  Protein 4

Many factors affect cancer risk. Eating a diet low in fat and high in fiber may lower risk of this disease.

• GOOD SOURCE OF FIBER
• LOWFAT

Reprinted with permission from the American Institute for Cancer Research

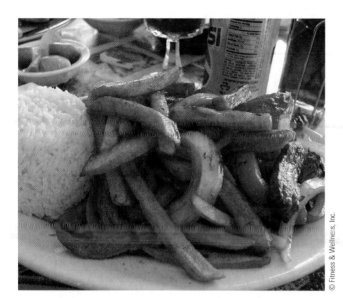

The typical American diet is too high in calories and saturated fat.

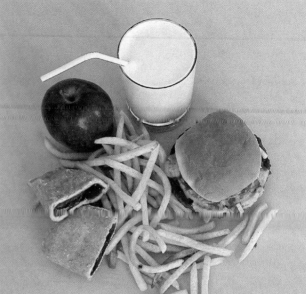

An apple a day will not keep the doctor away if most meals are high in fat content.

## Critical Thinking

What do the nutrition standards mean to you? How much of a challenge would it be to apply those standards in your daily life?

# Nutrient Analysis

The first step in evaluating your diet is to conduct a nutrient analysis. This can be quite educational, because most people do not realize how harmful and nonnutritious many common foods are. The top sources of calories in the American diet are soft drinks, sweet rolls, pastries, doughnuts, cakes, hamburgers, cheeseburgers, meatloaf, pizza, potato and corn chips, and buttered popcorn, all of which are low in essential nutrients and high in fat and/or sugar and calories.

Most nutrient analyses cover calories, carbohydrates, fats, cholesterol, and sodium, as well as eight essential nutrients: protein, calcium, iron, vitamin A, thiamin, riboflavin, niacin, and vitamin C. If the diet has enough of these eight nutrients, the foods consumed in natural form to provide these nutrients typically contain all the other nutrients the human body needs.

To do your own nutrient analysis, keep a three-day record of everything you eat using Lab 3A, Figure 3A.1 (make additional copies of this form as needed). At the end of each day, look up the nutrient content for those foods in the list of Nutritive Values of Selected Foods (in Appendix B). Record this information on the form in Lab 3A. If you do not find a food in Appendix A, the information may be on the food container itself.

When you have recorded the nutritive values for each day, add up each column and write the totals at the bottom of the chart. After the third day, fill in your totals in Lab 3A, Figure 3A.2, and compute an average for the three days. To rate your diet, compare your figures with those in the RDA (see Table 3.7). The results will give a good indication of areas of strength and deficiency in your current diet.

Some of the most revealing information learned in a nutrient analysis is the source of fat intake in the diet. The average daily fat consumption in the U.S. diet is about 34 percent of the total caloric intake, much of it from saturated and trans fatty acids, which increases the risk for inflammation and chronic diseases such as cardiovascular disease, cancer, diabetes, and obesity. Although fat provides a smaller percentage of our total daily caloric intake compared with two decades ago (37 percent), the decrease in percentage is simply because Americans now eat more calories than 20 years ago (335 additional daily calories for women and 170 for men).

As illustrated in Figure 3.7, 1 gram of carbohydrates or protein supplies the body with 4 calories, and fat provides 9 calories per gram consumed (alcohol yields 7 calories per gram). Therefore, looking at only the total grams consumed for each type of food can be misleading.

For example, a person who eats 160 grams of carbohydrates, 100 grams of fat, and 70 grams of protein has a total intake of 330 grams of food. This indicates that 30 percent of the total grams of food is in the form of fat (100 grams of fat ÷ 330 grams of total food = .30; .30 × 100 = 30 percent)—and, in reality, almost half of that diet is in the form of fat calories.

In the sample diet, 640 calories are derived from carbohydrates (160 grams × 4 calories per gram), 280 calories from protein (70 grams × 4 calories per gram), and

## Behavior Modification Planning

### CALORIC AND FAT CONTENT OF SELECTED FAST FOODS

| | Calories | Total Fat (grams) | Saturated Fat (grams) | Percent Fat Calories |
|---|---|---|---|---|
| **Burgers** | | | | |
| McDonald's Big Mac | 590 | 34 | 11 | 52 |
| McDonald's Big N' Tasty with Cheese | 590 | 37 | 12 | 56 |
| McDonald's Quarter Pounder with Cheese | 590 | 30 | 13 | 41 |
| Burger King Whopper | 760 | 46 | 15 | 54 |
| Burger King Bacon Double Cheeseburger | 580 | 34 | 18 | 53 |
| Burger King BK Smokehouse Cheddar Griller | 720 | 48 | 19 | 60 |
| Burger King Whopper with Cheese | 850 | 53 | 22 | 56 |
| Burger King Double Whopper | 1,060 | 69 | 27 | 59 |
| Burger King Double Whopper with Cheese | 1,150 | 76 | 33 | 59 |
| Wendy's Baconator | 830 | 51 | 22 | 55 |
| **Sandwiches** | | | | |
| Arby's Regular Roast Beef | 350 | 16 | 6 | 41 |
| Arby's Super Roast Beef | 470 | 23 | 7 | 44 |
| Arby's Roast Chicken Club | 520 | 28 | 7 | 48 |
| Arby's Market Fresh Roast Beef & Swiss | 810 | 42 | 13 | 47 |
| McDonald's Crispy Chicken | 430 | 21 | 8 | 43 |
| McDonald's Filet-O-Fish | 470 | 26 | 5 | 50 |
| McDonald's Chicken McGrill | 400 | 17 | 3 | 38 |
| Wendy's Chicken Club | 470 | 19 | 4 | 36 |
| Wendy's Breast Fillet | 430 | 16 | 3 | 34 |
| Wendy's Grilled Chicken | 300 | 7 | 2 | 21 |
| Burger King Specialty Chicken | 560 | 28 | 6 | 45 |
| Subway Veggie Delight* | 226 | 3 | 1 | 12 |
| Subway Turkey Breast | 281 | 5 | 2 | 16 |
| Subway Sweet Onion Chicken Teriyaki | 374 | 5 | 2 | 12 |
| Subway Steak & Cheese | 390 | 14 | 5 | 32 |
| Subway Cold Cut Trio | 440 | 21 | 7 | 43 |
| Subway Tuna | 450 | 22 | 6 | 44 |
| **Mexican** | | | | |
| Taco Bell Crunchy Taco | 170 | 10 | 4 | 53 |
| Taco Bell Taco Supreme | 220 | 14 | 6 | 57 |
| Taco Bell Soft Chicken Taco | 190 | 7 | 3 | 33 |
| Taco Bell Bean Burrito | 370 | 12 | 4 | 30 |
| Taco Bell Fiesta Steak Burrito | 370 | 12 | 4 | 29 |
| Taco Bell Grilled Steak Soft Taco | 290 | 17 | 4 | 53 |
| Taco Bell Double Decker Taco | 340 | 14 | 5 | 37 |
| **French Fries** | | | | |
| Wendy's, biggie (5½ oz) | 440 | 19 | 7 | 39 |
| McDonald's, large (6 oz) | 540 | 26 | 9 | 43 |
| Burger King, large (5½ oz) | 500 | 25 | 13 | 45 |
| **Shakes** | | | | |
| Wendy's Frosty, medium (16 oz) | 440 | 11 | 7 | 23 |
| McDonald's McFlurry, small (12 oz) | 610 | 22 | 14 | 32 |
| Burger King, Old Fashioned Ice Cream Shake, medium (22 oz) | 760 | 41 | 29 | 49 |
| **Hash Browns** | | | | |
| McDonald's Hash Browns (2 oz) | 130 | 8 | 4 | 55 |
| Burger King, Hash Browns, small (2½ oz) | 230 | 15 | 9 | 59 |

## Try It

Using the above information, record in your Online Journal or class notebook ways you can restructure fast-food consumption to decrease caloric value and fat and saturated fat content in your diet.

*6-inch sandwich with no mayo
**Source:** Adapted from *Restaurant Confidential* by Michael F. Jacobson and Jayne Hurley (Workman, 2002), by permission of Center for Science in the Public Interest.

**FIGURE 3.7** Caloric value of food (fuel nutrients).

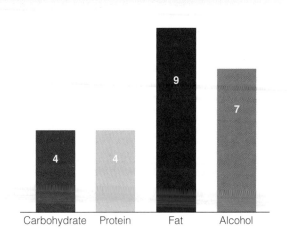

Carbohydrate 4 | Protein 4 | Fat 9 | Alcohol 7

**FIGURE 3.8** Computation for fat content in food.

## Nutrition Facts

Serving Size 1 cup (240 ml)
Servings Per Container 4

**Amount Per Serving**

**Calories** 120                    Calories from Fat 45

| | % **Daily Value*** |
|---|---|
| **Total Fat** 5g | 8% |
| Saturated Fat 3g | 15% |
| **Cholesterol** 20mg | 7% |
| **Sodium** 120mg | 5% |
| **Total Carbohydrate** 12g | 4% |
| Dietary Fiber 0g | 0% |
| Sugars 12g | |
| **Protein** 8g | |

| Vitamin A | 10% | • | Vitamin C | 4% |
|---|---|---|---|---|
| Calcium | 30% | • | Iron | 0% |

\* Percent Daily Values are based on a 2,000 calorie diet. Your daily values may be higher or lower depending on your calorie needs:

| | | Calories | 2,000 | 2,500 |
|---|---|---|---|---|
| Total Fat | Less than | 65g | 80g |
| Sat Fat | Less than | 20g | 25g |
| Cholesterol | Less than | 300mg | 300mg |
| Sodium | Less than | 2,400mg | 2,400mg |
| Total Carbohydrate | | 300g | 375g |
| Fiber | | 25g | 30g |

Calories per gram:

Fat 9   •   Carbohydrate 4   •   Protein 4

Percent fat calories = (grams of fat × 9) ÷ calories per serving × 100

5 grams of fat × 9 calories per grams of fat = 45 calories from fat

45 calories from fat ÷ 120 calories per serving × 100 = 38% fat

900 calories from fat (100 grams × 9 calories per gram), for a total of 1,820 calories. If 900 calories are derived from fat, almost half of the total caloric intake is in the form of fat (900 ÷ 1,820 × 100 = 49.5 percent).

Each gram of fat provides 9 calories—more than twice the calories of a gram of carbohydrates or protein. When figuring out the percentage of fat calories of individual foods, you may find Figure 3.8 a useful guideline. Multiply the total fat grams by 9 and divide by the total calories in that particular food (per serving). Then multiply that number by 100 to get the percentage. For example, the food label in Figure 3.8 lists a total of 120 calories and 5 grams of fat, and the equation below it shows the fat content to be 38 percent of total calories. This simple guideline can help you decrease the fat in your diet.

The fat content of selected foods, given in grams and as a percent of total calories, is presented in Figure 3.9. The percentage of fat is further subdivided into saturated, monounsaturated, polyunsaturated, and other fatty acids.

## Achieving a Balanced Diet

Anyone who has completed a nutrient analysis and has given careful attention to Tables 3.3 (vitamins) and 3.4 (minerals) probably will realize that a well-balanced diet entails eating a variety of nutrient-dense foods and monitoring total daily caloric intake. The MyPyramid healthy eating guide in Figure 3.1 contains five major food groups and oils. The food groups are grains, vegetables, fruits, milk, and meats/beans.

Whole grains, vegetables, fruits, and milk provide the nutritional base for a healthy diet. When increasing the intake of these food groups, it is important to decrease the intake of low-nutrient foods to effectively balance caloric intake with energy needs. Whole grains are a major source of fiber as well as of other nutrients. Whole grains contain the entire grain kernel (the bran, germ, and endo-

sperm). Examples include whole-wheat flour, whole cornmeal, oatmeal, cracked wheat (bulgur), and brown rice. Refined grains have been milled—a process that removes the bran and germ, along with fiber, iron, and many B vitamins. Refined grains include white flour, white bread, white rice, and degermed cornmeal. Refined grains are often enriched to add back B vitamins and iron. Fiber, however, is not added back.

In addition to providing nutrients crucial to health, fruits and vegetables are the sole source of **phytonutrients** ("phyto" comes from the Greek word for plant). These compounds show promising results in the fight against cancer

**Phytonutrients** Compounds thought to prevent and fight cancer; found in large quantities in fruits and vegetables.

**FIGURE 3.9  Fat content of selected foods.**

Fat Content of Selected Foods

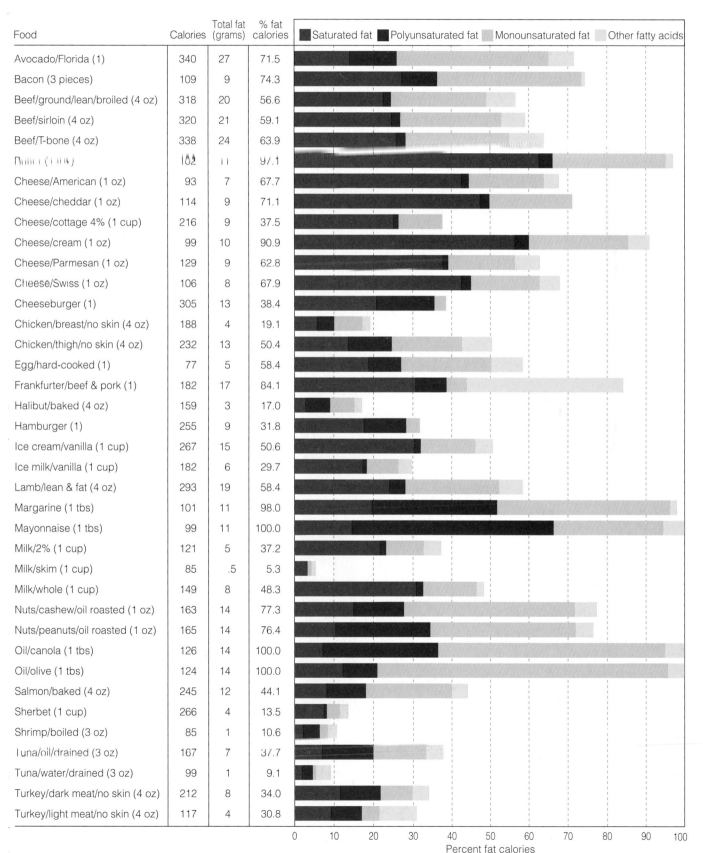

| Food | Calories | Total fat (grams) | % fat calories |
|------|----------|-------------------|----------------|
| Avocado/Florida (1) | 340 | 27 | 71.5 |
| Bacon (3 pieces) | 109 | 9 | 74.3 |
| Beef/ground/lean/broiled (4 oz) | 318 | 20 | 56.6 |
| Beef/sirloin (4 oz) | 320 | 21 | 59.1 |
| Beef/T-bone (4 oz) | 338 | 24 | 63.9 |
| Butter (1 tbs) | 102 | 11 | 97.1 |
| Cheese/American (1 oz) | 93 | 7 | 67.7 |
| Cheese/cheddar (1 oz) | 114 | 9 | 71.1 |
| Cheese/cottage 4% (1 cup) | 216 | 9 | 37.5 |
| Cheese/cream (1 oz) | 99 | 10 | 90.9 |
| Cheese/Parmesan (1 oz) | 129 | 9 | 62.8 |
| Cheese/Swiss (1 oz) | 106 | 8 | 67.9 |
| Cheeseburger (1) | 305 | 13 | 38.4 |
| Chicken/breast/no skin (4 oz) | 188 | 4 | 19.1 |
| Chicken/thigh/no skin (4 oz) | 232 | 13 | 50.4 |
| Egg/hard-cooked (1) | 77 | 5 | 58.4 |
| Frankfurter/beef & pork (1) | 182 | 17 | 84.1 |
| Halibut/baked (4 oz) | 159 | 3 | 17.0 |
| Hamburger (1) | 255 | 9 | 31.8 |
| Ice cream/vanilla (1 cup) | 267 | 15 | 50.6 |
| Ice milk/vanilla (1 cup) | 182 | 6 | 29.7 |
| Lamb/lean & fat (4 oz) | 293 | 19 | 58.4 |
| Margarine (1 tbs) | 101 | 11 | 98.0 |
| Mayonnaise (1 tbs) | 99 | 11 | 100.0 |
| Milk/2% (1 cup) | 121 | 5 | 37.2 |
| Milk/skim (1 cup) | 85 | .5 | 5.3 |
| Milk/whole (1 cup) | 149 | 8 | 48.3 |
| Nuts/cashew/oil roasted (1 oz) | 163 | 14 | 77.3 |
| Nuts/peanuts/oil roasted (1 oz) | 165 | 14 | 76.4 |
| Oil/canola (1 tbs) | 126 | 14 | 100.0 |
| Oil/olive (1 tbs) | 124 | 14 | 100.0 |
| Salmon/baked (4 oz) | 245 | 12 | 44.1 |
| Sherbet (1 cup) | 266 | 4 | 13.5 |
| Shrimp/boiled (3 oz) | 85 | 1 | 10.6 |
| Tuna/oil/drained (3 oz) | 167 | 7 | 37.7 |
| Tuna/water/drained (3 oz) | 99 | 1 | 9.1 |
| Turkey/dark meat/no skin (4 oz) | 212 | 8 | 34.0 |
| Turkey/light meat/no skin (4 oz) | 117 | 4 | 30.8 |

Legend: ■ Saturated fat  ■ Polyunsaturated fat  ▨ Monounsaturated fat  ▢ Other fatty acids

Percent fat calories

and heart disease. More than 4,000 phytonutrients have been identified. The main function of phytonutrients in plants is to protect them from sunlight. In humans, phytonutrients seem to have a powerful ability to block the formation of cancerous tumors. Their actions are so diverse

## Behavior Modification Planning

### "SUPER" FOODS

The following "super" foods that fight disease and promote health should be included often in the diet. Are you eating these foods regularly?

| I PLAN TO | I DID IT | |
|---|---|---|
| ❑ | ❑ | Avocados |
| ❑ | ❑ | Bananas |
| ❑ | ❑ | Beans |
| ❑ | ❑ | Beets |
| ❑ | ❑ | Blueberries |
| ❑ | ❑ | Broccoli |
| ❑ | ❑ | Butternut squash |
| ❑ | ❑ | Carrots |
| ❑ | ❑ | Grapes |
| ❑ | ❑ | Kale |
| ❑ | ❑ | Kiwifruit |
| ❑ | ❑ | Flaxseeds |
| ❑ | ❑ | Nuts (Brazil, walnuts) |
| ❑ | ❑ | Salmon (wild) |
| ❑ | ❑ | Soy |
| ❑ | ❑ | Oats and oatmeal |
| ❑ | ❑ | Olives and olive oil |
| ❑ | ❑ | Onions |
| ❑ | ❑ | Oranges |
| ❑ | ❑ | Peppers |
| ❑ | ❑ | Strawberries |
| ❑ | ❑ | Spinach |
| ❑ | ❑ | Tea (green, black, red) |
| ❑ | ❑ | Tomatoes |
| ❑ | ❑ | Yogurt |

### Try It

Using the above list, make a list of which super foods you can add to your diet and when you can eat them (snacks/meals). List meals that you can add these foods to.

that at almost every stage of cancer, phytonutrients have the ability to block, disrupt, slow, or even reverse the process. In terms of heart disease, they may reduce inflammation, inhibit blood clots, or prevent the oxidation of LDL cholesterol.

The consistent message is to eat a diet with ample fruits and vegetables. The daily recommended amount of fruits and vegetables has absolutely no substitute. Science has not yet found a way to allow people to eat a poor diet, pop a few pills, and derive the same benefits.

Milk and milk products (select low-fat or non-fat) can decrease the risk of low bone mass (osteoporosis) throughout life. Milk is a good source not only of calcium, but of potassium, vitamin D, and protein and may aid in managing body weight.

Foods in the meats and beans group consist of poultry, fish, eggs, nuts, legumes, and seeds. Nutrients in this group include protein, B vitamins, vitamin E, iron, zinc, and magnesium. Choose low-fat or lean meats and poultry and bake them, grill them, or broil them. Most Americans eat sufficient food in this group but need to choose leaner foods and a greater variety of fish, dry beans, nuts, and seeds. In terms of meat, poultry, and fish, the recommendation is to consume about 3 ounces but not more than 6 ounces daily. All visible fat and skin should be trimmed off meats and poultry before cooking.

Oils are fats that come from different plants and fish and are liquid at room temperature. Choose carefully and avoid oils that have trans fats (check the food label) or saturated fats. Solid fats at room temperature come from animal sources or can be made from vegetable oils through the process of hydrogenation.

As an aid to balancing your diet, the form in Lab 3B, Figure 3B.1, enables you to record your daily food intake. This record is much easier to keep than the complete di-

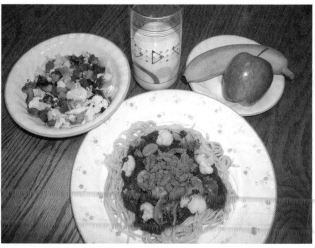

You can restructure your meals so that rice, pasta, beans, breads, and vegetables are in the center of the plate; meats are on the side and added primarily for flavoring; fruits are used for desserts; and low- or non-fat milk products are used.

etary analyses in Lab 3A. Make one copy for each day you wish to record.

To start the activity, go to http://mypyramid.gov and establish your personal MyPyramid Plan based on your age, sex, and activity level. Record this information on the form provided in Lab 3B. Next, whenever you have something to eat, record the food and the amount eaten according to the MyPyramid standard amounts (ounce, cup, or teaspoon—see Figure 3.1). Do this immediately after each meal so you will be able to keep track of your actual food intake more easily. At the end of the day, evaluate your diet by checking whether you ate the minimum required amounts for each food group. If you meet the minimum required servings at the end of each day and your caloric intake is in balance with the recommended amount, you are taking good "Steps to a Healthier You."

## Choosing Healthy Foods

Once you have completed the nutrient analysis and the healthy diet plan (Labs 3A and 3B), you may conduct a self-evaluation of your current nutritional habits. In Lab 3B, you can also assess your current stage of change regarding healthy nutrition and list strategies to help you improve your diet.

Initially, developing healthy eating habits requires a conscious effort to select nutritious foods (see box on the next page). You must learn the nutritive value of typical foods you eat. You can do so by reading food labels and looking up the nutritive values using listings such as that provided in Appendix B or by using computer software available for such purposes.

Although not a major concern, be aware that in a few cases there is label misinformation. Whether it is a simple mistake or outright deception is difficult to determine because there is little testing of food products and limited risks (penalties) if label misrepresentation occurs. The U.S. Food and Drug Administration (FDA) simply does not have the manpower to regularly check food labels.

A limited number of organizations are trying to help. For example, the Florida Department of Agriculture and Consumer Services has found a 10 percent violation rate in food products tested. As a consumer, you may never know which products are mislabeled, although in a few cases you may be able to discern the truth by yourself. If a product claims to be low in calories and fat but tastes "too good to be true," that may indeed be the case. For example, a recent independent analysis of Rising Dough Bakery cookies found that the oatmeal cranberry cookie (the size of a compact disc) had more than twice as many calories as listed on the label.

In most cases, when monitoring caloric intake, doing your own food preparation using healthy cooking methods is a better option than eating out or purchasing processed foods. Healthy eating requires proper meal planning and adequate coping strategies when one is confronted with situations that encourage unhealthy eating and overindulgence. Additional information on these topics is provided in Chapter 5, on weight management.

## Vegetarianism

More than 12 million people in the United States follow vegetarian diets. **Vegetarians** rely primarily on foods from the bread, cereal, rice, pasta, and fruit and vegetable groups and avoid most foods from animal sources in the dairy and protein groups. The five basic types of vegetarians are as follows:

1. **Vegans** eat no animal products at all.
2. **Ovovegetarians** allow eggs in the diet.
3. **Lactovegetarians** allow foods from the milk group.
4. **Ovolactovegetarians** include egg and milk products in the diet.
5. **Semivegetarians** do not eat red meat, but do include fish and poultry in addition to milk products and eggs in their diet.

Vegetarian diets can be healthful and consistent with the Dietary Guidelines for Americans and can meet the DRIs for nutrients. Vegetarians who do not select their food combinations properly, however, can develop nutritional deficiencies of protein, vitamins, minerals, and even calories. Even greater attention should be paid when planning vegetarian diets for infants and children. Unless carefully planned, a strict plant-based diet will prevent proper growth and development.

**Nutrient Concerns** In some vegetarian diets, protein deficiency can be a concern. Vegans in particular must be careful to eat foods that provide a balanced distribution of essential amino acids, such as grain products and legumes. Strict vegans also need a supplement of vitamin $B_{12}$. This vitamin is not found in plant foods; its only source is animal foods. Deficiency of this vitamin can lead to anemia and nerve damage.

The key to a healthful vegetarian diet is to eat foods that possess complementary proteins, because most plant-based products lack one or more essential amino acids in adequate amounts. For example, both grains and legumes are good protein sources, but neither provides all the essential amino acids. Grains and cereals are low in the amino acid lysine, and legumes lack methionine. Foods from these two groups—such as combinations of tortillas and beans, rice and beans, rice and soybeans, or wheat bread and peanuts—complement each other and provide all required protein nutrients. These complementary proteins may be consumed over the course of one day, but it is best if they are consumed during the same meal.

---

**Vegetarians** Individuals whose diet is of vegetable or plant origin.

**Vegans** Vegetarians who eat no animal products at all.

**Ovovegetarians** Vegetarians who allow eggs in their diet.

**Lactovegetarians** Vegetarians who eat foods from the milk group.

**Ovolactovegetarians** Vegetarians who include eggs and milk products in their diet.

**Semivegetarians** Vegetarians who include milk products, eggs, and fish and poultry in the diet.

## Behavior Modification Planning

### SELECTING NUTRITIOUS FOODS

Do you regularly follow the habits below?

**To select nutritious foods:**

PLAN TO
DID IT

☐ ☐ 1. Given the choice between whole foods and refined, processed foods, choose the former (apples rather than apple pie, potatoes rather than potato chips). No nutrients have been refined out of the whole foods, and they contain less fat, salt, and sugar.

☐ ☐ 2. Choose the leaner cuts of meat. Select fish or poultry often, beef seldom. Ask for broiled, not fried, to control your fat intake.

☐ ☐ 3. Use both raw and cooked vegetables and fruits. Raw foods offer more fiber and vitamins, such as folate and thiamin, that are destroyed by cooking. Cooking foods frees other vitamins and minerals for absorption.

☐ ☐ 4. Include milk, milk products, or other calcium sources for the calcium you need. Use low-fat or non-fat items to reduce fat and calories.

☐ ☐ 5. Learn to use margarine, butter, and oils sparingly. A little gives flavor, a lot overloads you with fat, calories, and increases disease risk.

☐ ☐ 6. Vary your choices. Eat broccoli today, carrots tomorrow, and corn the next day. Eat Chinese today, Italian tomorrow, and broiled fish with brown rice and steamed vegetables the third day.

☐ ☐ 7. Load your plate with vegetables and unrefined starchy foods. A small portion of meat or cheese is all you need for protein.

☐ ☐ 8. When choosing breads and cereals, choose the whole-grain varieties.

**To select nutritious fast foods:**

☐ ☐ 9. Choose the broiled sandwich with lettuce, tomatoes, and other goodies— and hold the mayo—rather than the fish or chicken patties coated with breadcrumbs and cooked in fat.

☐ ☐ 10. Select a salad—and use more plain vegetables than those mixed with oily or mayonnaise-based dressings.

☐ ☐ 11. Order chili with more beans than meat. Choose a soft bean burrito over tacos with fried shells.

☐ ☐ 12. Drink low-fat milk rather than a cola beverage.

**When choosing from a vending machine:**

☐ ☐ 13. Choose cracker sandwiches over chips and pork rinds (virtually pure fat). Choose peanuts, pretzels, and popcorn over cookies and candy.

☐ ☐ 14. Choose milk and juices over cola beverages.

## Try It

Based on what you have learned, list strategies you can use to increase food variety, enhance the nutritive value of your diet, and decrease fat and caloric content in your meals.

Adapted from W. W. K. Hoeger, L. W. Turner, & B. Q. Hafen. Wellness: Guidelines for a Healthy Lifestyle (Wadsworth Thomson Learning, 2007).

---

Other nutrients likely to be deficient in vegetarian diets—and ways to compensate—are as follows:

• Vitamin D can be obtained from moderate exposure to the sun or by taking a supplement.

• Riboflavin can be found in green leafy vegetables, whole grains, and legumes.

• Calcium can be obtained from fortified soybean milk or fortified orange juice, calcium-rich tofu, and selected cereals. A calcium supplement is also an option.

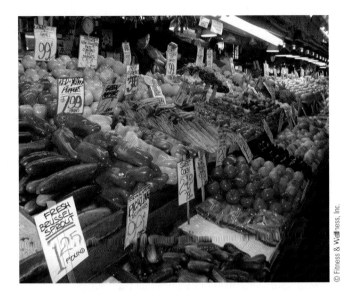

Most fruits and vegetables contain large amounts of cancer-preventing phytochemicals.

- Iron can be found in whole grains, dried fruits and nuts, and legumes. To enhance iron absorption, a good source of vitamin C should be consumed with these foods (calcium and iron are the most difficult nutrients to consume in sufficient amounts in a strict vegan diet).
- Zinc can be obtained from whole grains, wheat germ, beans, nuts, and seeds.

MyPyramid also can be used as a guide for vegetarians. The key is food variety. Most vegetarians today eat dairy products and eggs. They can replace meat with legumes, nuts, seeds, eggs, and meat substitutes (tofu, tempeh, soy milk, and commercial meat replacers such as veggie burgers and soy hot dogs). For additional MyPyramid healthy eating tips for vegetarians and how to get enough of the previously mentioned nutrients, go to http://mypyramid.gov. Those who are interested in vegetarian diets are encouraged to consult additional resources, because special vegetarian diet planning cannot be covered adequately in a few paragraphs.

**Nuts** Consumption of nuts, commonly used in vegetarian diets, has received considerable attention in recent years. A few years ago, most people regarded nuts as especially high in fat and calories. Although they are 70 to 90 percent fat, most of this is unsaturated fat. And research indicates that people who eat nuts several times a week have a lower incidence of heart disease. Eating 2 to 3 ounces (about one-half cup) of almonds, walnuts, or macadamia nuts a day may decrease high blood cholesterol by about 10 percent. Nuts can even enhance the cholesterol-lowering effects of the Mediterranean diet.

Heart-health benefits are attributed not only to the unsaturated fats but also to other nutrients found in nuts, including vitamin E and folic acid. And nuts are also packed with additional B vitamins, calcium, copper, potassium, magnesium, fiber, and phytonutrients. Many of these nutrients are cancer- and cardioprotective, help lower homocysteine levels, and act as antioxidants (discussed in "Antioxidants" [page 95] and "Folate" [page 97]).

Nuts do have a drawback: They are high in calories. A handful of nuts provides as many calories as a piece of cake, so nuts should be avoided as a snack. Excessive weight gain is a risk factor for cardiovascular disease. Nuts are recommended for use in place of high-protein foods such as meats, bacon, and eggs or as part of a meal in fruit or vegetable salads, homemade bread, pancakes, casseroles, yogurt, and oatmeal. Peanut butter is also healthier than cheese or some cold cuts in sandwiches.

**Soy Products** The popularity of soy foods, including use in vegetarian diets, is attributed primarily to Asian research that points to less heart disease and fewer hormone-related cancers in people who regularly consume soy foods. A benefit of eating soy is that it replaces unhealthy animal products high in saturated fat. Soy is rich in plant protein, unsaturated fat, and fiber, and some soy is high in calcium.

The benefits of soy lie in its high protein content and plant chemicals, known as isoflavones, that act as antioxidants and are thought to protect against estrogen-related cancers (breast, ovarian, and endometrial). The compound genistein, one of many phytonutrients in soy, may reduce the risk for breast cancer, and soy consumption also may lower the risk for prostate cancer. Limited animal studies have suggested an actual increase in breast cancer risk. Human studies are still inconclusive but tend to favor a slight protective effect in premenopausal women.

Until more data become available, the University of California Wellness Letter has issued the following recommendations:[8]

1. Do not exceed three servings of soy per day (a serving constitutes a half cup of tofu, edamame, or tempeh; one-fourth cup of roasted soy nuts; or one cup of soy yogurt or soy milk).

2. Limit soy intake to just a few servings per week if you now have or have had breast cancer.

3. Avoid soy supplements, as they may contain higher levels of isoflavones than those found in soy foods. Individuals with a history of breast cancer and pregnant and lactating women should avoid them altogether.

**Probiotics** Yogurt is rated in the "super foods" category because, in addition to being a good source of calcium, riboflavin, and protein, it contains **probiotics.** These health-promoting microorganisms live in the intestines and help break down foods and prevent disease-causing organisms from settling in. Probiotics have been found to offer protec-

---

**Probiotics** Healthy bacteria (abundant in yogurt) that help break down foods and prevent disease-causing organisms from settling in the intestines.

tion against gastrointestinal infections, boost immune activity, and even help fight certain types of cancer.

When selecting yogurt, look for products with L-acidophilus, Bifidus, and the prebiotic (substances on which probiotics feed) inulin. The latter, a soluble fiber, appears to enhance calcium absorption. Avoid yogurt with added fruit jam, sugar, and candy.

### Diets from Other Cultures

Increasingly, Americans are eating foods reflecting the ethnic composition of people from other countries. Learning how to wisely select from the wide range of options is the task of those who seek a healthy diet.

**Mediterranean Diet**  The **Mediterranean diet** has received much attention because people in that region have notably lower rates of diet-linked diseases and a longer life expectancy. The diet features olive oil, grains (whole, not refined), legumes, vegetables, fruits, and, in moderation, fish, red wine, nuts, and dairy products. Although it is a semivegetarian diet, up to 40 percent of the total daily caloric intake may come from fat—mostly monounsaturated fat from olive oil. Moderate intake of red wine is included with meals. The dietary plan also encourages regular physical activity (see Figure 3.10).

**FIGURE 3.10**  **The traditional healthy Mediterranean diet pyramid.**

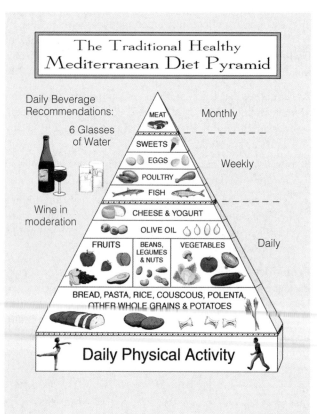

More than a "diet," the Mediterranean diet is a dietary pattern that has existed for centuries. According to the largest and most comprehensive research on this dietary pattern, the health benefits and decreased mortality are not linked to any specific component of the diet (such as olive oil or red wine) but are achieved through the interaction of all the components of the pattern.[9] Those who adhered most closely to the dietary pattern had a lower incidence of heart disease (33 percent) and deaths from cancer (24 percent). Although most people in the United States focus on the olive oil component of the diet, olive oil is used mainly as a means to increase consumption of vegetables because vegetables sautéed in oil taste better than steamed vegetables.

**Ethnic Diets**  As people migrate, they take their dietary practices with them. Many ethnic diets are healthier than the typical American diet because they emphasize consumption of complex carbohydrates and limit fat intake. The predominant minority ethnic groups in the United States are African American, Hispanic American, and Asian American. Unfortunately, the generally healthier ethnic diets quickly become Americanized when these groups adapt to the United States. Often, they cut back on vegetables and add meats and salt to the diet in conformity with the American consumer.

Ethnic dishes can be prepared at home. They are easy to make and much healthier when one uses the typical (original) variety of vegetables, corn, rice, spices, and condiments. Ethnic health recommendations also encourage daily physical activity and suggest no more than two alcoholic drinks per day. Three typical ethnic diets are as follows:

- The African American diet ("soul food") is based on the regional cuisine of the American South. Soul food includes yams, black-eyed peas, okra, and peanuts. The latter have been combined with American foods such as corn products and pork. Today, most people think of soul food as meat, fried chicken, sweet potatoes, and chitterlings.

- Hispanic foods in the United States arrived with the conquistadores and evolved through combinations with other ethnic diets and local foods available in Latin America. For example, the Cuban cuisine combined Spanish, Chinese, and native foods; Puerto Rican cuisine developed from Spanish, African, and native products; Mexican diets evolved from Spanish and native foods. Prominent in all of these diets were corn, beans, squash, chili peppers, avocados, papayas, and fish. The colonists later added rice and citrus foods. Today, the Hispanic diet incorporates a wide variety of foods, including red meat, but the staple still consists of rice, corn, and beans.

- Asian American diets are characteristically rich in vegetables and use minimal meat and fat. The Okinawan diet in Japan, where some of the healthiest and oldest people in the world live, is high in fresh (versus pickled) vegetables, high in fiber, and low in fat and salt. The Chinese cuisine includes more than 200 vegeta-

## Behavior Modification Planning

### STRATEGIES FOR HEALTHIER RESTAURANT EATING

On average, Americans eat out six times per week. Research indicates that when dining out, most people consume too many calories and too much fat. Such practice is contributing to the growing obesity epidemic and chronic conditions afflicting most Americans in the 21st century. Below are strategies that you can implement to eat healthier when dining out.

I PLAN TO

I DID IT

❑ ❑ Plan ahead. Decide before you get to the restaurant that you will select a healthy meal. Then stick to your decision. If you are unfamiliar with the menu, you may be able to access the menu at the restaurant's Internet Web site beforehand or you can obtain valuable nutrition information at HealthyDiningFinder.com. This Web site is maintained by registered dietitians and provides information on many restaurant chains located in your area.

❑ ❑ Be aware of calories in drinks. You can gulp down several hundred extra calories through drinks alone. Restaurants and beverage industries are eager to get your money, and servers wouldn't mind a larger tip by having you consume additional items on the menu. Water, sparkling soda water, or unsweetened teas are good choices.

❑ ❑ Avoid or limit appetizers, regardless of how tempting they might be. Ask your server not to bring to the table high-fat pre-meal free foods such as tortilla chips, bread and butter, or vegetables to be dipped in high-fat salad dressings. If you do munch on food freebies or appetizers (or make a meal out of them), have your server box up half or the entire meal for you to take home. If you box up an entire meal, you now have two additional meals that you can consume at home; that is because most restaurant meals can be split into two meals.

❑ ❑ Request a half-size or a child's portion If you are unable to do so, split the meal with your dining partner or box up half the meal before you start to eat.

❑ ❑ Inquire about ingredients and cooking methods. Don't be afraid to ask for healthy substitutes. For example, you may request that meat be sautéed instead of deep fried or that canola or olive oil be used instead of other oil choices. You can also request a baked potato or brown rice instead of french fries or white rice. Ask for dressing, butter, or sour cream on the side. Request whole-wheat bread for sandwiches. Furthermore, avoid high-fat foods or ingredients such as creamy or cheese sauces, butter, oils, and fatty/fried/crispy meats. When in doubt, ask the server for additional information. If the server can't answer your questions, select a different meal.

### Try It

Implement as many of the above strategies every time you dine out. Take pride in your healthy choices. Your long-term health and well-being are at stake. You will feel much better about yourself following a healthy meal than you would otherwise.

bles, and fat-free sauces and seasoning are used to enhance flavor. The Chinese diet varies somewhat within regions of China. The lowest in fat is that of southern China, with most meals containing fish, seafood, and stir-fried vegetables. Chinese food in American restaurants contains a much higher percentage of fat and protein than the traditional Chinese cuisine.

**Mediterranean diet** Typical diet of people around the Mediterranean region, focusing on olive oil, red wine, grains, legumes, vegetables, and fruits, with limited amounts of meat, fish, milk, and cheese.

**TABLE 3.9** Ethnic Eating Guide

| | Choose Often | Choose Less Often |
|---|---|---|
| **CHINESE** | Beef with broccoli<br>Chinese greens<br>Steamed rice, brown or white<br>Steamed beef with pea pods<br>Stir-fry dishes<br>Teriyaki beef or chicken<br>Wonton soup | Crispy duck<br>Egg rolls<br>Fried rice<br>Kung pao chicken (fried)<br>Peking duck<br>Pork spareribs |
| **JAPANESE** | Chiri nabe (fish stew)<br>Grilled scallops<br>Sushi, sashimi (raw fish)<br>Teriyaki<br>Yakitori (grilled chicken) | Tempura (fried chicken, shrimp, or vegetables)<br>Tonkatsu (fried pork) |
| **ITALIAN** | Cioppino (seafood stew)<br>Minestrone (vegetarian soup)<br>Pasta with marinara sauce<br>Pasta primavera (pasta with vegetables)<br>Steamed clams | Antipasto<br>Cannelloni, ravioli<br>Fettuccini alfredo<br>Garlic bread<br>White clam sauce |
| **MEXICAN** | Beans and rice<br>Black bean/vegetable soup<br>Burritos, bean<br>Chili<br>Enchiladas, bean<br>Fajitas<br>Gazpacho<br>Taco salad<br>Tamales<br>Tortillas, steamed | Chili relleno<br>Chimichangas<br>Enchiladas, beef or cheese<br>Flautas<br>Guacamole<br>Nachos<br>Quesadillas<br>Tostadas<br>Sour cream (as topping) |
| **MIDDLE EASTERN** | Tandoori chicken<br>Curry (yogurt-based)<br>Rice pilaf<br>Lentil soup<br>Shish kebab | Falafel |
| **FRENCH** | Poached salmon<br>Spinach salad<br>Consommé<br>Salad niçoise | Beef Wellington<br>Escargot<br>French onion soup<br>Sauces in general |
| **SOUL FOOD** | Baked chicken<br>Baked fish<br>Roasted pork (not smothered or "etouffe")<br>Sauteed okra<br>Baked sweet potato | Fried chicken<br>Fried fish<br>Smothered pork tenderloin<br>Okra in gumbo<br>Sweet potato casserole or pie |
| **GREEK** | Gyros<br>Pita<br>Lentil soup | Baklava<br>Moussaka |

*Source:* Adapted from P. A. Floyd, S. E. Mimms, and C. Yelding-Howard. Personal Health: Perspectives & Lifestyles (Belmont, CA: Wadsworth/Thomson Learning, 1998)

Table 3.9 provides a list of healthier foods to choose from when dining at selected ethnic restaurants. Additionally, you can consult the box on the previous page for strategies you can use to dine out healthfully.

All healthy diets have similar characteristics: They are high in fruits, vegetables, and grains and low in fat and saturated fat. Healthy diets also use low-fat or fat-free dairy products, and they emphasize portion control—essential in a healthy diet plan.

Many people now think that if a food item is labeled "low fat" or "fat free," they can consume it in large quantities. "Low fat" or "fat free" does not imply "calorie free."

Many people who consume low-fat diets eat more (and thus increase their caloric intake), which in the long term leads to obesity and its associated health problems.

# Nutrient Supplementation

Approximately half of all adults in the United States take daily nutrient **supplements.** Nutrient requirements for the body normally can be met by consuming as few as 1,200 calories per day, as long as the diet contains the recommended amounts of food from the different food groups. Still, many people consider it necessary to take vitamin supplements.

It is true that our bodies cannot retain water-soluble vitamins as long as fat-soluble vitamins. The body excretes excessive intakes readily, although it can retain small amounts for weeks or months in various organs and tissues. Fat-soluble vitamins, by contrast, are stored in fatty tissue. Therefore, daily intake of these vitamins is not as crucial.

People should not take **megadoses** of vitamins and minerals. For some nutrients, a dose of five times the RDA taken over several months may create problems. For other nutrients, it may not pose a threat to human health. Vitamin and mineral doses should not exceed the ULs. For nutrients that do not have an established UL, one day's dose should be no more than three times the RDA.

Iron deficiency (determined through blood testing) is more common in women than men. Iron supplementation is frequently recommended for women who have a heavy menstrual flow. Some pregnant and lactating women also may require supplements. The average pregnant woman who eats an adequate amount of a variety of foods should take a low dose of iron supplement daily. Women who are pregnant with more than one baby may need additional supplements. Folate supplements also are encouraged prior to and during pregnancy to prevent certain birth defects (see the following discussions of antioxidants and folate). In the above instances, individuals should take supplements under a physician's supervision.

Adults over the age of 60 are encouraged to take a daily multivitamin. Aging may decrease the body's ability to absorb and utilize certain nutrients. Nutrient deficiencies in older adults include vitamins C, D, $B_6$, $B_{12}$, folate, and the minerals calcium, zinc, and magnesium.

Other people who may benefit from supplementation are those with nutrient deficiencies, alcoholics and street-drug users who do not have a balanced diet, smokers, vegans (strict vegetarians), individuals on low-calorie diets (fewer than 1,200 calories per day), and people with disease-related disorders or who are taking medications that interfere with proper nutrient absorption.

Although supplements may help a small group of individuals, most supplements do not provide benefits to healthy people who eat a balanced diet. Supplements do not seem to prevent chronic diseases or help people run faster, jump higher, relieve stress, improve sexual prowess, cure a common cold, or boost energy levels.

**Antioxidants** Much research and discussion are taking place regarding the effectiveness of **antioxidants** in thwarting several chronic diseases. Although foods probably contain more than 4,000 antioxidants, the four most studied antioxidants are vitamins E, C, and beta-carotene (a precursor to vitamin A) and the mineral selenium (technically not an antioxidant but a component of antioxidant enzymes).

Oxygen is used during metabolism to change carbohydrates and fats into energy. During this process, oxygen is transformed into stable forms of water and carbon dioxide. A small amount of oxygen, however, ends up in an unstable form, referred to as **oxygen free radicals.** A free radical molecule has a normal proton nucleus with a single unpaired electron. Having only one electron makes the free radical extremely reactive, and it looks constantly to pair its electron with one from another molecule. When a free radical steals a second electron from another molecule, that other molecule in turn becomes a free radical. This chain reaction goes on until two free radicals meet to form a stable molecule.

Free radicals attack and damage proteins and lipids—in particular, cell membranes and DNA. This damage is thought to contribute to the development of conditions such as cardiovascular disease, cancer, emphysema, cataracts, Parkinson's disease, and premature aging. Solar radiation, cigarette smoke, air pollution, radiation, some drugs, injury, infection, chemicals (such as pesticides), and other environmental factors also seem to encourage the formation of free radicals. Antioxidants are thought to offer protection by absorbing free radicals before they can cause damage and also by interrupting the sequence of reactions once damage has begun, thwarting certain chronic diseases (see Figure 3.11).

The body's own defense systems typically neutralize free radicals so they don't cause any damage. When free radicals are produced faster than the body can neutralize them, they can damage the cells. Research, however, indicates that the body's antioxidant defense system improves as fitness improves.[10] That is, physically fit people have greater protection against free radicals.

---

**Supplements** Tablets, pills, capsules, liquids, or powders that contain vitamins, minerals, antioxidants, amino acids, herbs, or fiber that individuals take to increase their intake of these nutrients.

**Megadoses** For most vitamins, 10 times the RDA or more; for vitamins A and D, 5 and 2 times the RDA, respectively.

**Antioxidants** Compounds such as vitamins C and E, beta-carotene, and selenium that prevent oxygen from combining with other substances in the body to form harmful compounds.

**Oxygen free radicals** Substances formed during metabolism that attack and damage proteins and lipids, in particular the cell membrane and DNA, leading to diseases such as heart disease, cancer, and emphysema.

**FIGURE 3.11** Antioxidant protection: blocking and absorbing oxygen free radicals to prevent chronic disease.

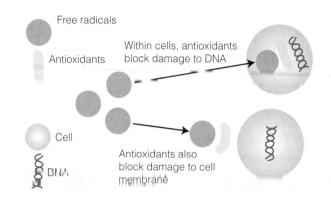

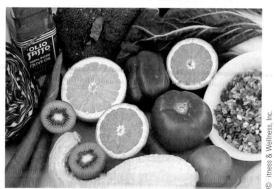

Antioxidants are found abundantly in food, especially in fruits and vegetables. Unfortunately, most Americans do not eat the minimum recommended amounts of fruits and vegetables.

Antioxidants work best in the prevention and progression of disease, but they cannot repair damage that has already occurred or cure people with disease. The benefits are obtained primarily from food sources themselves, and controversy surrounds the benefits of antioxidants taken in supplement form.

For years people believed that taking antioxidant supplements could further prevent free radical damage, but adding to the controversy, a report published in 2007 in the *Journal of the American Medical Association* indicated that antioxidant supplements actually increase the risk of death.[11] Vitamin E, beta-carotene, and vitamin A increased the risk of mortality by 4 percent, 7 percent, and 16 percent, respectively. Vitamin C had no effect on mortality, while selenium decreased risk by 9 percent. Some researchers, however, have questioned the design and conclusions of this report. More research is definitely required to settle the controversy.

**Vitamin E** Vitamin E belongs to a group of eight compounds (four tocopherols and four tocotrienols) of which alpha-tocopherol is the most active form. The RDA for vitamin E is 15 mg or 22 **international units (IU).** Vitamin E is found primarily in oil-rich seeds and vegetable oils.

Vitamin E supplements from natural sources contain d-alpha tocopherol, which is better absorbed by the body than dl-alpha tocopherol, a synthetic form composed of a variety of E compounds. Vitamin E is fat soluble, thus a supplement should be taken with a meal that has some fat in it.

Although no evidence indicates that vitamin E supplementation below the upper limit of 1,000 mg per day is harmful, little or no clinical research supports any health benefits. Foods high in vitamin E include almonds, hazelnuts, peanuts, canola oil, safflower oil, cottonseed oil, kale, sunflower seeds, shrimp, wheat germ, sweet potato, avocado, and tomato sauce. You should incorporate some of these foods regularly in the diet to obtain the RDA.

**Vitamin C** Studies have shown that vitamin C may offer benefits against heart disease, cancer, and cataracts. However, people who consume the recommended amounts of daily fruits and vegetables need no supplementation because they obtain their daily vitamin C requirements through their diet alone.

Vitamin C is water soluble, and the body eliminates it in about 12 hours. For best results, consume foods rich in vitamin C twice a day. High intake of a vitamin C supplement, above 500 mg per day, is not recommended. The body absorbs very little vitamin C beyond the first 200 mg per serving or dose. Foods high in vitamin C include oranges and other citrus fruit, kiwi fruit, cantaloupe, guava, bell peppers, strawberries, broccoli, kale, cauliflower, and tomatoes.

**Beta-Carotene** Beta-carotene supplementation was encouraged in the early 1990s, but obtaining the daily recommended dose of beta-carotene (20,000 IU) from food sources rather than supplements is preferable. Clinical trials have found that beta-carotene supplements do not offer protection against heart disease or cancer and do not provide any other health benefits. Therefore, the recommendation is to "skip the pill and eat the carrot." One medium raw carrot contains about 20,000 IU of beta-carotene. Other foods high in beta-carotene include sweet potatoes, pumpkin, cantaloupe, squash, kale, broccoli, tomatoes, peaches, apricots, mangoes, papaya, turnip greens, and spinach.

**Selenium** Adequate intake of the mineral selenium is encouraged. Data indicate that individuals who take 200 micrograms (mcg) of selenium daily decrease their risk for prostate cancer by 63 percent, for colorectal cancer by 58 percent, and for lung cancer by 46 percent.[12] Selenium also may decrease the risk of cancers of the breast, liver, and digestive tract. According to Dr. Edward Giovannucci of the Harvard Medical School, the evidence for benefits of selenium in reducing the risk for prostate cancer is so strong that public health officials should recommend that people increase their selenium intake.

One Brazil nut (unshelled) that you crack yourself provides about 100 mcg of selenium. Shelled nuts found in supermarkets average only about 20 mcg each. Other foods high in selenium include red snapper, salmon, cod, tuna, noodles, whole grains, and meats.

Based on the current body of research, 100 to 200 mcg of selenium per day seems to provide the necessary amount of antioxidant for this nutrient. A person has no reason to take more than 200 mcg daily. In fact, the UL for selenium has been set at 400 mcg. Too much selenium can damage cells rather than protect them. If you choose to take supplements, take an organic form of selenium from yeast and not selenium selenite.

Selenium may interfere with the body's absorption of vitamin C. If taken in supplemental form, the two nutrients should be taken separately. Wait about an hour following vitamin C intake before taking selenium.

## Multivitamins

Although much interest has been generated in the previously mentioned individual supplements, the American people still prefer multivitamins as supplements. A multivitamin complex that provides 100 percent of the DV for most nutrients can help fill in certain dietary deficiencies.[13] Some evidence suggests that regular intake decreases the risk for cardiovascular disease and colon cancer and improves immune function.

Multivitamins, however, are not magic pills. They may help, but they are not a license to eat carelessly. Multivitamins do not provide energy, fiber, or phytonutrients.

## Vitamin D

Vitamin D is attracting a lot of attention because current research suggests that the vitamin possesses anticancer properties (especially against breast, colon, and prostate cancers and possibly lung and digestive cancers), decreases inflammation (fighting cardiovascular disease, periodontal disease, and arthritis), strengthens the immune system, controls blood pressure, helps maintain muscle strength, and may help deter diabetes and fight depression. Vitamin D is also necessary for absorption of calcium, a nutrient critical for building and maintaining bones and teeth.

The theory that vitamin D protects against cancer is based on studies showing that people who live farther north (who have less sun exposure during the winter months) have a higher incidence of cancer. Furthermore, people diagnosed with breast, colon, or prostate cancer during the summer months, when vitamin D production by the body is at its highest, are 30 percent less likely to die from cancer, even 10 years following the initial diagnosis. Researchers believe that vitamin D level at the time of cancer onset affects survival rates.

Evidence suggests that we should get between 1,000 and 2,000 IU (25 to 50 mcg) per day.[14] Good sources of vitamin D in the diet include salmon, mackerel, tuna, and sardines. Fortified milk, yogurt, orange juice, margarines, and cereals are also good sources (see Table 3.10).

To obtain 1,000 to 2,000 IU per day from food sources alone, however, is difficult. The best source of vitamin D is sunshine. Ultraviolet rays lead to the production in the skin of an inactive form, vitamin $D_3$. The inactive form is then transformed by the liver, and subsequently the kidneys, into the active form of vitamin D. Sun-generated vitamin D is also better than that obtained from foods or supplements.

Although excessive sun exposure can lead to skin damage, you should strive for daily "safe sun" exposure, that is, up to 15 minutes of unprotected sun exposure of the face, arms, and hands during peak daylight hours a few times a week (10:00 a.m. and 4:00 p.m.). Such exposure will generate between 1,000 and 2,000 IU of vitamin D. And even though the UL has been set at 2,000 IU, experts believe that this figure needs revision because there are no data implicating toxic effects up to 10,000 IU a day.[15]

Generating too much vitamin D from the sun is impossible because the body generates only what it needs. Most people are not getting enough vitamin D. The current recommended daily intake ranges between 200 and 600 IU (5 and 15 mcg) based on your age. People at the highest risk for low vitamin D levels are older adults, those with dark skin (they make less vitamin D), and individuals who spend most of their time indoors and get little sun exposure. In the United States and Canada, most of the population cannot make vitamin D from the sun during the winter months. During periods of limited sun exposure, you should consider a daily vitamin $D_3$ supplement of up to 2,000 IU per day (some vitamins contain vitamin $D_2$, which is a less potent form of the vitamin).

## Folate

Although it is not an antioxidant, 400 mcg of **folate** (a B vitamin) is recommended for all premenopausal women. Folate helps prevent some birth defects and

**TABLE 3.10** Good Sources of Vitamin D

| Food | Amount | IU* |
|------|--------|-----|
| Multivitamins (most brands) | daily dose | 400 |
| Salmon | 3.5 oz | 360 |
| Mackerel | 3.5 oz | 345 |
| Sardines (oil/drained) | 3.5 oz | 250 |
| Shrimp | 3.5 oz | 200 |
| Orange juice (D-fortified) | 8 oz | 100 |
| Milk (any type/D-fortified) | 8 oz | 100 |
| Margarine (D-fortified) | 1 tbsp | 80 |
| Yogurt (D-fortified) | 6–8 oz | 60 |
| Cereal (D-fortified) | ¾–1 c | 40 |
| Egg | 1 | 20 |

*IU = international units

**International unit (IU)** Measure of nutrients in foods.

**Folate** One of the B vitamins.

seems to offer protection against colon and cervical cancers. Women who might become pregnant should plan to take a folate supplement, because studies have shown that folate intake (400 mcg per day) during early pregnancy can prevent serious birth defects.

Some evidence also indicates that taking 400 mcg of folate along with vitamins B$_6$ and B$_{12}$ prevents heart attacks by reducing homocysteine levels in the blood (see Chapter 12). High concentrations of homocysteine accelerate the process of plaque formation (atherosclerosis) in the arteries. Five servings of fruits and vegetables per day usually meet the needs for these nutrients. Almost 9 of 10 adults in the United States do not obtain the recommended 400 mcg of folate per day. Because of the vital role of folate in preventing heart disease, some experts recommend a daily supplement that includes 400 mcg of folate.

Side Effects Toxic effects from antioxidant supplements are rare when they are taken under the ULs. If any of the following side effects arise while taking supplements, stop supplementation and check with a physician:

- Vitamin E: gastrointestinal disturbances, increase in blood lipids (determined through blood tests)
- Vitamin C: nausea, diarrhea, abdominal cramps, kidney stones, liver problems
- Selenium: nausea, vomiting, diarrhea, irritability, fatigue, flu-like symptoms, lesions of the skin and nervous tissue, loss of hair and nails, respiratory failure, liver damage

Substantial supplementation of vitamin E is not recommended for individuals on **anticoagulant** therapy, as vitamin E is an anticoagulant itself. Therefore, if you are on this type of therapy, check with your physician. Vitamin E also may be unsafe if taken with alcohol or by people who drink more than 4 ounces of pure alcohol per day (the equivalent of eight beers). Pregnant women require a physician's approval prior to beta-carotene supplementation.

Benefits of Foods Even though you may consider taking some supplements, fruits and vegetables are the richest sources of antioxidants and phytonutrients. Re-

**Anticoagulant** Any substance that inhibits blood clotting.

**Synergy** A reaction in which the result is greater than the sum of its two parts.

**Registered dietitian (RD)** A person with a college degree in dietetics who meets all certification and continuing education requirements of the American Dietetic Association or Dietitians of Canada

**Functional foods** Foods or food ingredients containing physiologically active substances that provide specific health benefits beyond those supplied by basic nutrition.

**Fortified foods** Foods that have been modified by the addition or increase of nutrients that either were not present or were present in insignificant amounts with the intent of preventing nutrient deficiencies.

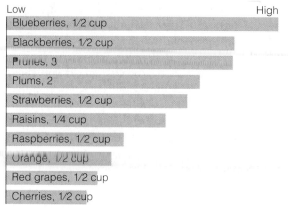

FIGURE 3.12 Top antioxidant foods.

**FRUITS**

Low — High

- Blueberries, 1/2 cup
- Blackberries, 1/2 cup
- Prunes, 3
- Plums, 2
- Strawberries, 1/2 cup
- Raisins, 1/4 cup
- Raspberries, 1/2 cup
- Orange, 1/2 cup
- Red grapes, 1/2 cup
- Cherries, 1/2 cup

**VEGETABLES**

Low — High

- Kale, 1 cup
- Beets, 1 cup
- Red bell peppers, 1/2 cup
- Brussels sprouts, 1/2 cup
- Corn, 1/2 cup
- Spinach, 1 cup
- Onions, 1/2 cup
- Broccoli, 1/2 cup
- Eggplant, 1/2 cup
- Alfalfa sprouts, 1/2 cup

*Source:* Adapted from USDA, Agricultural Research Service, *Food & Nutrition Research Briefs,* April 1999 (downloaded from www.ars.usda.gov/is/np/fnrb.)

searchers at the U.S. Department of Agriculture (USDA) compared the antioxidant effects of vitamins C and E with those of various common fruits and vegetables. The results indicated that three-fourths of a cup of cooked kale (which contains only 11 IU of vitamin E and 76 mg of vitamin C) neutralized as many free radicals as did approximately 800 IU of vitamin E or 600 mg of vitamin C. Other excellent sources of antioxidants that these researchers found are blueberries, strawberries, spinach, Brussels sprouts, plums, broccoli, beets, oranges, and grapes. A list of top antioxidant foods is presented in Figure 3.12.

Many people who eat unhealthily think that they need supplementation to balance their diets. This is a fallacy about nutrition. The problem here is not necessarily a lack of vitamins and minerals but, rather, a diet too high in calories, saturated fat, trans fatty acids, and sodium. Vitamin, mineral, and fiber supplements do not supply all of the nutrients and other beneficial substances present in food and needed for good health.

Wholesome foods contain vitamins, minerals, carbohydrates, fiber, proteins, fats, and phytonutrients, along with other substances not yet discovered. Researchers do not know whether the protective effects are caused by the antioxidants alone, in combination with other nutrients (such as phytonutrients), or by some other nutrients in food that have not been investigated yet. Many nutrients work in **synergy,** enhancing chemical processes in the body.

Supplementation will not offset poor eating habits. Pills are no substitute for common sense. If you think your diet is not balanced, you first need to conduct a nutrient analysis (see Labs 3A and 3B, pages 115–120) to determine which nutrients you lack in sufficient amounts. Eat more of them, as well as foods that are high in antioxidants and phytonutrients. Following a nutrient assessment, a **registered dietitian** can help you decide what supplement(s), if any, might be necessary.

The American Heart Association does not recommend antioxidant supplements until more definite research is available. If you take supplements in pill form, look for products that meet the disintegration standards of the U.S. Pharmacopoeia (USP) on the bottle. The USP standard suggests that the supplement should completely dissolve in 45 minutes or less. Supplements that do not dissolve, of course, cannot get into the bloodstream.

## Critical Thinking

Do you take supplements? If so, for what purposes are you taking them—and do you think you could restructure your diet so you could do without them?

## Functional Foods

**Functional foods** are foods or food ingredients that offer specific health benefits beyond those supplied by the traditional nutrients they contain. Many functional foods come in their natural forms. A tomato, for example, is a functional food because it contains the phytonutrient lycopene, thought to reduce the risk for prostate cancer. Other examples of functional foods are kale, broccoli, blueberries, red grapes, and green tea.

The term "functional food," however, has been used primarily as a marketing tool by the food industry to attract consumers. Unlike **fortified foods**, which have been modified to help prevent nutrient deficiencies, functional foods are created by the food industry by the addition of ingredients aimed at treating or preventing symptoms or disease. In functional foods, the added ingredient(s) is typically not found in the food item in its natural form but is added to allow manufacturers to make appealing health claims.

In most cases, only one extra ingredient is added (a vitamin, mineral, phytonutrient, or herb). An example is

## Behavior Modification Planning
### GUIDELINES FOR A HEALTHY DIET

| I PLAN TO | I DID IT | |
|---|---|---|
| ☐ | ☐ | Base your diet on a large variety of foods. |
| ☐ | ☐ | Consume ample amounts of green, yellow, and orange fruits and vegetables. |
| ☐ | ☐ | Eat foods high in complex carbohydrates, including at least three 1-ounce servings of whole-grain foods per day. |
| ☐ | ☐ | Obtain most of your vitamins and minerals from food sources. |
| ☐ | ☐ | Eat foods rich in vitamin D. |
| ☐ | ☐ | Maintain adequate daily calcium intake and consider a bone supplement with vitamin $D_3$. |
| ☐ | ☐ | Consume protein in moderation. |
| ☐ | ☐ | Limit daily fat, trans fat, and saturated fat intake. |
| ☐ | ☐ | Limit cholesterol consumption to less than 300 mg per day. |
| ☐ | ☐ | Limit sodium intake to 2,400 mg per day. |
| ☐ | ☐ | Limit sugar intake. |
| ☐ | ☐ | If you drink alcohol, do so in moderation (one daily drink for women and two for men). |
| ☐ | ☐ | Consider taking a daily multivitamin (preferably one that includes vitamin $D_3$). |

## Try It
Carefully analyze the above guidelines and note the areas where you can improve your diet. Work on one guideline each week until you are able to adhere to all of the above guidelines.

calcium added to orange juice to make the claim that this brand offers protection against osteoporosis. Food manufacturers now offer cholesterol-lowering margarines (enhanced with plant stanol), cancer-protective ketchup (fortified with lycopene), memory-boosting candy (with ginkgo added), calcium-fortified chips, and corn chips containing kava kava (to enhance relaxation).

The use of some functional foods, however, may undermine good nutrition. Margarines still may contain satu-

## Behavior Modification Planning

### MINIMIZING THE RISK OF FOOD CONTAMINATION AND PESTICIDE RESIDUES

Most food is safe to eat, but there is no 100 percent guarantee that all produce is free of contamination. Follow the tips below to minimize risk.

I PLAN TO

I DID IT

☐ ☐ Wash your hands thoroughly before and after touching raw produce.

☐ ☐ Do not place raw fruits and vegetables next to uncooked meat, poultry, or fish.

☐ ☐ Trim all visible fat from meat, remove the skin from poultry and fish prior to cooking (pesticides concentrate in animal fat).

☐ ☐ Use a scrub brush to wash fresh produce under running water. Pay particular attention to crevices in the produce. Washing fresh produce reduces pesticide levels but does not completely eliminate them. Eat a variety of foods to decrease exposure to any given pesticide.

☐ ☐ Select produce that is free of dirt and does not have holes or cuts or other signs of spoilage.

☐ ☐ Discard the outermost leaves of leafy vegetables such as lettuce and cabbage.

☐ ☐ Cut your own fruits and vegetables instead of getting them precut. Wash all produce thoroughly before cutting, even melons and avocados. Cutting into potentially contaminated (unwashed) inedible rinds of fruit can contaminate the inside of the fruit. Always use a knife to remove orange peels instead of biting into them. Peel waxed fruits and vegetables, and other produce as necessary (cucumbers, carrots, peaches, apples).

☐ ☐ Store produce in the refrigerator in clean containers or clean plastic bags (previously used bags that are not kept cold can grow harmful bacteria).

☐ ☐ For some produce, consider buying certified organic foods. Look for the "USDA Organic seal. According to data from the Environmental Working Group, a nonprofit consumer activist organization, conventional produce with the most pesticide residue include peaches, apples, sweet bell peppers, celery, nectarines, strawberries, cherries, grapes, lettuce, imported grapes, pears, spinach, and potatoes. Among the least contaminated are onions, avocados, sweet corn, pineapples, mangoes, sweet peas, asparagus, kiwifruit, bananas, cabbage, broccoli, and eggplant (list of foods downloaded from www.foodnews.org).

### Try It

Lifestyle behavior patterns are difficult to change. The above recommendations can minimize your risk of food contamination and ingestion of pesticide residues. Make a copy of the above recommendations and determine how many of these suggestions you are able to include in daily life over the course of the next seven days.

rated fats or partially hydrogenated oils. Regularly consuming ketchup on top of large orders of fries adds many calories and fat to the diet. Sweets are also high in calories and sugar. Chips are high in calories, salt, and fat. In all of these cases, the consumer would be better off taking the specific ingredient in a supplement form rather than consuming the functional food with its extra calories, sugar, salt, and/or fat.

Functional foods can provide added benefits if used in conjunction with a healthful diet. You may use nutrient-dense functional foods in your overall wellness plan as an adjunct to health-promoting strategies and treatments.

## Genetically Modified Crops

A genetically modified organism (GMO) has had its DNA (or basic genetic material) manipulated to obtain certain results. This is done by inserting genes with desirable traits from one plant, animal, or microorganism into another one to either introduce new traits or enhance existing traits.

Crops are genetically modified to make them better resist disease and extreme environmental conditions (such as heat and frost), require fewer fertilizers and pesticides, last longer, and improve their nutrient content and taste. GMOs could help save billions of dollars by producing more crops and helping to feed the hungry in developing countries around the world.

Concern over the safety of **genetically modified (GM) foods** has led to heated public debates in Europe and, to a lesser extent, in the United States. The concern is that genetic modifications create "transgenic" organisms that have not previously existed and that have potentially unpredictable effects on the environment and on humans. Also, there is some concern that GM foods may cause illness or allergies in humans and that cross-pollination may destroy other plants or create "super-weeds" with herbicide-resistant genes.

GM crops were first introduced into the United States in 1996. This technology is moving forward so rapidly that the USDA already has approved more than 50 GM crops. In 2003, about 40 percent of the U.S. cropland produced GM foods. Now, more than 80 percent of our soybeans, 73 percent of cotton, 50 percent of canola, and 40 percent of corn come from GM crops.

Totally avoiding GM foods is difficult because more than 60 percent of processed foods on the market today contain GM organisms. If people do not wish to consume GM foods, organic foods are an option because organic trade organizations do not certify foods with genetic modifications. Produce bought at the local farmers' market also may be an option, because small farmers are less likely to use this technology.

At this point, no evidence indicates that GM foods are harmful—but no compelling evidence guarantees that they are safe, either. Many questions remain, and much research is required in this field. As a consumer, you will have to continue educating yourself as more evidence becomes available in the next few years.

# Energy Substrates for Physical Activity

The two main fuels that supply energy for physical activity are glucose (sugar) and fat (fatty acids). The body uses amino acids, derived from proteins, as an energy substrate when glucose is low, such as during fasting, prolonged aerobic exercise, or a low-carbohydrate diet.

Glucose is derived from foods that are high in carbohydrates, such as breads, cereals, grains, pasta, beans, fruits, vegetables, and sweets in general. Glucose is stored as glycogen in muscles and the liver. Fatty acids (discussed on pages 73–76) are the product of the breakdown of fats. Unlike glucose, an almost unlimited supply of fatty acids, stored as fat in the body, can be used during exercise.

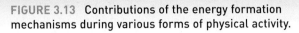

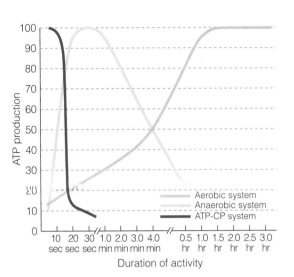

**FIGURE 3.13 Contributions of the energy formation mechanisms during various forms of physical activity.**

**Energy (ATP) Production** The energy derived from food is not used directly by the cells. It is first transformed into **adenosine triphosphate (ATP).** The subsequent breakdown of this compound provides the energy used by all energy-requiring processes of the body (see Figure 3.13).

ATP must be recycled continually to sustain life and work. ATP can be resynthesized in three ways:

1. *ATP-CP system.* The body stores small amounts of ATP and **creatine phosphate (CP).** These stores are used during all-out activities such as sprinting, long jumping, and weight lifting. The amount of stored ATP provides energy for just 1 or 2 seconds. During brief all-out efforts, ATP is resynthesized from CP, another high-energy phosphate compound. This is the ATP-CP, or phosphagen, system. Depending on the amount of physical training, the concentration of CP stored in cells is sufficient to allow maximum exertion for up to 10 seconds. Once the CP stores are depleted, the person is forced to slow down or rest to allow ATP to form through anaerobic and aerobic pathways.

2. *Anaerobic or lactic acid system.* During maximal-intensity exercise that is sustained for 10 to 180 sec-

---

**Genetically modified foods (GM foods)** Foods whose basic genetic material (DNA) is manipulated by inserting genes with desirable traits from one plant, animal, or microorganism into another one either to introduce new traits or to enhance existing ones.

**Adenosine triphosphate (ATP)** A high-energy chemical compound that the body uses for immediate energy.

**Creatine phosphate (CP)** A high-energy compound that the cells use to resynthesize ATP during all-out activities of very short duration.

onds, ATP is replenished from the breakdown of glucose through a series of chemical reactions that do not require oxygen (hence "anaerobic"). In the process, though, **lactic acid** is produced. As lactic acid accumulates, it leads to muscular fatigue. Because of the accumulation of lactic acid with high-intensity exercise, the formation of ATP during anaerobic activities is limited to about 3 minutes. A recovery period then is necessary to allow for the removal of lactic acid. Formation of ATP through the anaerobic system requires glucose (carbohydrates).

3. *Aerobic system.* The production of energy during slow-sustained exercise is derived primarily through aerobic metabolism. Glucose (carbohydrates), fatty acids (fat), and oxygen (hence "aerobic") are required to form ATP using this process; and under steady-state exercise conditions, lactic acid accumulation is minimal. Because oxygen is required, a person's capacity to utilize oxygen is crucial for successful athletic performance in aerobic events. The higher one's maximal oxygen uptake ($VO_{2max}$—see pages 201–209), the greater is one's capacity to generate ATP through the aerobic system—and the better the athletic performance in long-distance events. From the previous discussion, it becomes evident that for optimal performance, both recreational and highly competitive athletes make the required nutrients a part of their diet.

# Nutrition for Athletes

During resting conditions, fat supplies about two-thirds of the energy to sustain the body's vital processes. During exercise, the body uses both glucose (glycogen) and fat in combination to supply the energy demands. The proportion of fat to glucose changes with the intensity of exercise. When a person is exercising below 60 percent of his or her maximal work capacity ($VO_{2max}$), fat is used as the primary energy substrate. As the intensity of exercise increases, so does the percentage of glucose utilization—up to 100 percent during maximal work that can be sustained for only 2 to 3 minutes.

In general, athletes do not require special supplementation or any other special type of diet. Unless the diet is deficient in basic nutrients, no special secret or magic diet will help people perform better or develop faster as a result of what they eat. As long as they eat a balanced diet—that is, based on a large variety of nutrients from all basic food groups—athletes do not require additional supplements. Even in strength training and body building, protein in excess of 20 percent of total daily caloric intake is not necessary. The recommended daily protein intake ranges from 0.8 gram per kilogram of body weight for sedentary people to 1.5 grams per kilogram for extremely active individuals (Table 3.11).

The main difference between a sensible diet for a sedentary person and a sensible diet for a highly active individual is the total number of calories required daily and

**TABLE 3.11** Recommended Daily Protein Intake

| Activity Level | Intake in Grams per kg (2.2 lb) of Body Weight |
| --- | --- |
| Sedentary | 0.8 |
| Lightly active | 0.9 |
| Moderately active | 1.1 |
| Very active | 1.3 |
| Extremely active | 1.5 |

the amount of carbohydrate intake needed during prolonged physical activity. People in training consume more calories because of their greater energy expenditure—which is required as a result of intense physical training.

**Carbohydrate Loading** On a regular diet, the body is able to store between 1,500 and 2,000 calories in the form of glycogen. About 75 percent of this glycogen is stored in muscle tissue. This amount, however, can be increased greatly through **carbohydrate loading.**

A regular diet should be altered during several days of heavy aerobic training or when a person is going to participate in a long-distance event of more than 90 minutes (for example, marathon, triathlon, road cycling). For events shorter than 90 minutes, carbohydrate loading does not seem to enhance performance.

During prolonged exercise, glycogen is broken down into glucose, which then is readily available to the muscles for energy production. In comparison with fat, glucose frequently is referred to as the "high-octane fuel," because it provides about 6 percent more energy per unit of oxygen consumed.

Heavy training over several consecutive days leads to depletion of glycogen faster than it can be replaced through the diet. Glycogen depletion with heavy training is common in athletes. Signs of depletion include chronic fatigue, difficulty in maintaining accustomed exercise intensity, and lower performance.

On consecutive days of exhaustive physical training (this means several hours daily), a carbohydrate-rich diet—70 percent of total daily caloric intake or 8 grams of carbohydrate per kilogram (2.2 pounds) of body weight—is recommended. This diet often restores glycogen levels in 24 hours. Along with the high-carbohydrate diet, a day of rest often is needed to allow the muscles to recover from glycogen depletion following days of intense training. For people who exercise less than an hour a day, a 60 percent carbohydrate diet, or 6 grams of carbohydrate per kilogram of body weight, is enough to replenish glycogen stores.

Following an exhaustive workout, eating a combination of carbohydrates and protein (such as a tuna sandwich) within 30 minutes of exercise seems to speed up glycogen storage even more. Protein intake increases insulin activity, thereby enhancing glycogen replenishment. A 70 percent carbohydrate intake then should be maintained throughout the rest of the day.

By following a special diet and exercise regimen five days before a long-distance event, highly (aerobically) trained individuals are capable of storing two to three times the amount of glycogen found in the average person. Athletic performance may be enhanced for long-distance events of more than 90 minutes by eating a regular balanced diet (50 to 60 percent carbohydrates), along with vigorous physical training the fifth and fourth days before the event, followed by a diet high in carbohydrates (about 70 percent) and a gradual decrease in training intensity over the last three days before the event.

The amount of glycogen stored as a result of a carbohydrate-rich diet does not seem to be affected by the proportion of complex and simple carbohydrates. The intake of simple carbohydrates (sugars) can be raised while on a 70 percent carbohydrate diet, as long as it doesn't exceed 25 percent of the total calories. Complex carbohydrates provide more nutrients and fiber, making them a better choice for a healthier diet.

On the day of the long-distance event, carbohydrates are still the recommended choice of substrate. As a general rule, athletes should consume 1 gram of carbohydrate for each kilogram (2.2 pounds) of body weight 1 hour prior to exercise (that is, if you weigh 160 pounds, you should consume 160 ÷ 2.2 = 72 grams). If the pre-event meal is eaten earlier, the amount of carbohydrate can be increased to 2, 3, or 4 grams per kilogram of weight two, three, or four hours, respectively, before exercise.

During the long-distance event, researchers recommend that the athlete consume 30 to 60 grams of carbohydrates (120 to 240 calories) every hour. This is best accomplished by drinking 8 ounces of a 6 to 8 percent carbohydrate sports drink every 15 minutes (check labels to ensure proper carbohydrate concentration). This also lessens the chance of dehydration during exercise, which hinders performance and endangers health. The percentage of the carbohydrate drink is determined by dividing the amount of carbohydrate (in grams) by the amount of fluid (in milliliters) and then multiplying by 100. For example, 18 grams of carbohydrate in 240 milliliters (8 ounces) of fluid yields a drink that is 7.5 percent (18 ÷ 240 × 100) carbohydrate.

**Hyponatremia** In some cases, athletes participating in long- or ultra-long-distance races may suffer from **hyponatremia,** or low sodium concentration in the blood. The longer the race, the greater the risk for hyponatremia. This condition occurs as lost sweat, which contains salt and water, and is replaced only by water (no salt) during a very long distance race. Although the athlete is overhydrated, blood sodium is diluted and hyponatremia occurs. Typical symptoms are similar to those of heat illness and include fatigue, weakness, disorientation, muscle cramps, bloating, nausea, dizziness, confusion, slurred speech, fainting, and even seizures and coma in severe cases.

Based on estimates, about 30 percent of the participants in the Hawaii Ironman Triathlon suffer from hyponatremia. The condition, however, is rare in the everyday exerciser. To help prevent hyponatremia, athletes should ingest extra sodium prior to the event and then adequately monitor fluid intake during the race to prevent overhydration. Sports drinks that contain sodium (ingest about 1 gram of sodium per hour) should be used during the race to replace **electrolytes** lost in sweat and to prevent blood sodium dilution.

## Creatine Supplementation
**Creatine** is an organic compound obtained in the diet primarily from meat and fish. In the human body, creatine combines with inorganic phosphate to form the high-energy compound CP, which is then used to resynthesize ATP during short bursts of all-out physical activity. Individuals on a normal mixed diet consume an average of 1 gram of creatine per day. Each day, 1 additional gram is synthesized from various amino acids. One pound of meat or fish provides approximately 2 grams of creatine.

Creatine supplementation is popular among individuals who want to increase muscle mass and improve athletic performance. Creatine monohydrate—a white, tasteless powder that is mixed with fluids prior to ingestion—is

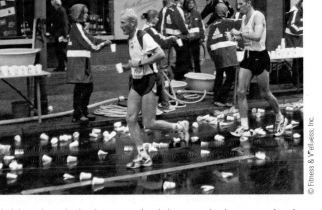

Fluid and carbohydrate replenishment during exercise is essential when participating in long-distance aerobic endurance events, such as a marathon or a triathlon.

© Fitness & Wellness, Inc.

**Lactic acid** End product of anaerobic glycolysis (metabolism).

**Carbohydrate loading** Increasing intake of carbohydrates during heavy aerobic training or prior to aerobic endurance events that last longer than 90 minutes.

**Hyponatremia** A low sodium concentration in the blood caused by overhydration with water.

**Electrolytes** Substances that become ions in solution and are critical for proper muscle and neuron activation (include sodium, potassium, chloride, calcium, magnesium, phosphate, and bicarbonate among others).

**Creatine** An organic compound derived from meat, fish, and amino acids that combines with inorganic phosphate to form creatine phosphate.

the form most popular among people who use the supplement. Supplementation can result in an approximate 20 percent increase in the amount of creatine that is stored in muscles. Most of this creatine binds to phosphate to form CP, and 30 to 40 percent remains as free creatine in the muscle. Increased creatine storage is believed to enable individuals to train more intensely—thereby building more muscle mass and enhancing performance in all-out activities of very short duration (less than 30 seconds).

Creatine supplementation has two phases: the loading phase and the maintenance phase. During the loading phase, the person consumes between 20 and 25 grams (1 teaspoonful is about 5 grams) of creatine per day for 5 to 6 days, divided into four or five dosages of 5 grams each throughout the day (this amount represents the equivalent of consuming 10 or more pounds of meat per day). Research also suggests that the amount of creatine stored in muscle is enhanced by taking creatine in combination with a high-carbohydrate food. Once the loading phase is complete, taking 2 grams per day seems to be sufficient to maintain the increased muscle stores.

To date, no serious side effects have been documented in people who take up to 25 grams of creatine per day for five days. Stomach distress and cramping have been reported only in rare instances. The 2 grams taken per day during the maintenance phase is just slightly above the average intake in our daily diet. Long-term effects of creatine supplementation on health, however, have not been established.

A frequently documented result following five to six days of creatine loading is an increase of 2 to 3 pounds in body weight. This increase appears to be related to the increased water retention necessary to maintain the additional creatine stored in muscles. Some data, however, suggest that the increase in stored water and CP stimulates protein synthesis, leading to an increase in lean body mass.

The benefits of elevated creatine stores may be limited to high-intensity/short-duration activities such as sprinting, strength training (weight lifting), and sprint cycling. Supplementation is most beneficial during exercise training itself, rather than as an aid to enhance athletic performance a few days before competition.

Enhanced creatine stores do not benefit athletes competing in aerobic endurance events, because CP is not used in energy production for long-distance events. Actually, the additional weight can be detrimental in long-distance running and swimming events, because the athlete must expend more energy to carry the extra weight during competition.

**Amino Acid Supplements** A myth regarding athletic performance is that protein (amino acid) supplements will increase muscle mass. The RDA for protein is 0.8 gram per kilogram of body weight per day. That is, if you weigh 154 pounds (70 kilograms, 154 ÷ 2.2), you should consume 56 grams (70 × 0.8) of protein.

Most athletes, including weight lifters and body builders, increase their caloric intake automatically during intense training. As caloric intake increases, so does the intake of protein, often approaching 2 or more grams per kilogram of body weight. This amount is more than enough to build and repair muscle tissue. Typically, athletes in strength training consume between 3 and 4 grams per kilogram of body weight. In response, manufacturers of supplements have created expensive "free amino acid supplements."

People who buy costly free amino acid supplements are led to believe that these contribute to the development of muscle mass. The human body, however, cannot distinguish between amino acids obtained from food and those obtained through supplements. Excess protein either is used for energy or is turned into fat. With amino acid supplements, each capsule provides about 500 mg of amino acids and no additional nutrients. In contrast, 3 ounces of meat or fish provide more than 20,000 mg of amino acids, along with other essential nutrients such as iron, niacin, and thiamin. The benefits of natural foods to health and budget are clear.

Proponents of free amino acid supplements further claim that only a small amount of amino acids in food is absorbed and that free amino acids are absorbed more readily than protein foods. Neither claim is correct. The human body absorbs and utilizes between 85 and 99 percent of all protein from food intake. The body handles whole, natural proteins better than single amino acids that have been predigested in the laboratory setting.

Amino acid supplementation can even be dangerous: An excess of a single amino acid or a group of chemically similar amino acids often prevents the absorption of other amino acids. Needed amino acids then pass through the body unabsorbed, potentially causing critical imbalances and toxicities.

The advertised rate of absorption provides no additional benefit, because building muscle takes hours, not minutes. Muscle overload through heavy training, not supplementation, builds muscle.

# Bone Health and Osteoporosis

**Osteoporosis,** literally meaning "porous bones," is a condition in which bones lack the minerals required to keep them strong. In osteoporosis, bones—primarily of the hip, wrist, and spine—become so weak and brittle that they fracture readily. The process begins slowly in the third and fourth decades of life. Women are especially susceptible after menopause because of the accompanying loss of estrogen, which increases the rate at which bone mass is broken down.

Approximately 22 million U.S. women have osteoporosis, and 16 million don't know they have this disease. About 30 percent of postmenopausal women have osteoporosis, but only about 2 percent are actually diagnosed and treated for this condition.[16]

Osteoporosis is the leading cause of serious morbidity and functional loss in the elderly population. One of every

FIGURE 3.14 Threats to bone health (osteoporosis).

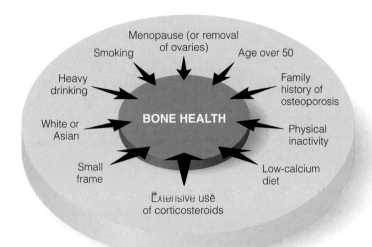

two women and one in eight men over age 50 will have an osteoporotic-related fracture at some point in their lives. The chances of a postmenopausal woman developing osteoporosis are much greater than her chances of developing breast cancer or incurring a heart attack or stroke.

According to the National Osteoporosis Foundation, an estimated 10 million Americans (8 million women and 2 million men) had osteoporosis in 2006. Up to 20 percent of people who have a hip fracture die within a year because of complications related to the fracture. As alarming as these figures are, they do not convey the pain and loss of quality of life in people who suffer the crippling effects of osteoporotic fractures.

Although osteoporosis is viewed primarily as a woman's disease, more than 30 percent of all men will be affected by age 75. About 100,000 of the yearly 300,000 hip fractures in the United States occur in men.

Despite the strong genetic component, osteoporosis is preventable. Maximizing bone density at a young age and subsequently decreasing the rate of bone loss later in life are critical factors in preventing osteoporosis.

Normal hormone levels prior to menopause and adequate calcium intake and physical activity throughout life cannot be overemphasized. These factors are all crucial in preventing osteoporosis. The absence of any one of these three factors leads to bone loss for which the other two factors never completely compensate. Smoking and excessive use of alcohol and corticosteroid drugs also accelerate the rate of bone loss in women and men alike. And osteoporosis is more common in whites, Asians, and people with small frames. Figure 3.14 depicts these variables.

Bone health begins at a young age. Some experts have called osteoporosis a "pediatric disease." Bone density can be promoted early in life by making sure the diet has sufficient calcium and participating in weight-bearing activities. Adequate calcium intake in women and men alike is also associated with a reduced risk for colon cancer.[17] The RDA for calcium is between 1,000 and 1,300 mg per day, but leading researchers in this area recommend higher

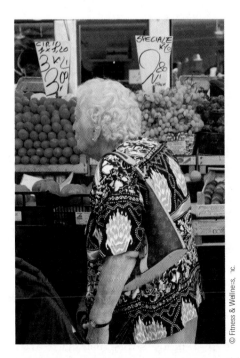

Osteoporosis is the leading cause of serious morbidity and functional loss in the elderly.

**Osteoporosis** A condition of softening, deterioration, or loss of bone mineral density that leads to disability, bone fractures, and even death from medical complications.

**Estrogen** Female sex hormone essential for bone formation and conservation of bone density.

**TABLE 3.12  Recommended Daily Calcium Intake**

| Age | Amount (mg) |
| --- | --- |
| 1–8 | 800 |
| 9–24 | 1,300 |
| 25–50 | 1,000 |
| Women over 50 | 1,500 |
| Men 51–65 | 1,200 |
| Men over 65 | 1,500 |

**TABLE 3.13  Low-Fat Calcium-Rich Foods**

| Food | Amount | Calcium (mg) | Calories |
| --- | --- | --- | --- |
| Beans, red kidney, cooked | 1 cup | 70 | 218 |
| Beet, greens, cooked | ½ cup | 82 | 19 |
| Bok choy (Chinese cabbage) | 1 cup | 158 | 20 |
| Broccoli, cooked, drained | 1 cup | 72 | 44 |
| Burrito, bean (no cheese) | 1 | 57 | 225 |
| Cottage cheese, 2% low-fat | ½ cup | 78 | 103 |
| Ice milk (vanilla) | ½ cup | 102 | 100 |
| Instant Breakfast, non-fat milk | 1 cup | 407 | 216 |
| Kale, cooked, drained | 1 cup | 94 | 36 |
| Milk, non-fat, powdered | 1 tbs | 52 | 15 |
| Milk, skim | 1 cup | 296 | 88 |
| Oatmeal, instant, fortified, plain | ½ cup | 109 | 70 |
| Okra, cooked, drained | ½ cup | 74 | 23 |
| Orange juice, fortified | 1 cup | 300 | 110 |
| Soy milk, fortified, fat-free | 1 cup | 400 | 110 |
| Spinach, raw | 1 cup | 56 | 12 |
| Turnip greens, cooked | 1 cup | 197 | 29 |
| Tofu (some types) | ½ cup | 138 | 76 |
| Yogurt, fruit | 1 cup | 372 | 250 |
| Yogurt, low-fat, plain | 1 cup | 448 | 155 |

intakes (see Table 3.12). Although the recommended daily intakes can be met easily through diet alone, some experts recommend calcium supplements even for children before puberty.

To obtain your daily calcium requirement, get as much calcium as possible from calcium-rich foods, including calcium-fortified foods. If you don't get enough (most people don't), take calcium supplements.

Supplemental calcium can be obtained in the form of calcium citrate and calcium carbonate. Calcium citrate seems to be equally well absorbed with or without food, whereas calcium carbonate is not well absorbed without food. Thus, if your supplement contains calcium carbonate, always take the supplement with meals. Do not take more than 500 mg at a time, because larger amounts are not well absorbed. And don't forget vitamin D, which is vital for calcium absorption.

Avoid taking calcium supplements with an iron-rich meal or in conjunction with an iron-containing multivitamin. Because calcium interferes with iron absorption, the intake of these two minerals should be separated. The benefit of taking a calcium supplement without food (calcium citrate) is that, in a young menstruating woman who needs iron, calcium won't interfere with the absorption of iron.

Table 3.13 provides a list of selected foods and their calcium contents. Along with having an adequate calcium intake, taking 400 to 800 IU of vitamin D daily is recommended for optimal calcium absorption. People over age 50 may require 800 to 1,000 IU of calcium. About 40 percent of these adults are deficient in vitamin D.[18]

Vitamin $B_{12}$ may also be a key nutrient in the prevention of osteoporosis. Several reports have shown an association between low vitamin $B_{12}$ and lower bone mineral density in both men and women. Vitamin $B_{12}$ is found primarily in dairy products, meats, poultry, fish, and some fortified cereals.

Excessive protein intake also may affect the body's absorption of calcium. The more protein we eat, the higher the calcium content in the urine (that is, the more calcium excreted). This might be the reason that countries with a high protein intake, including the United States, also have the highest rates of osteoporosis. Individuals should aim to

achieve the RDA for protein nonetheless, because people who consume too little protein (less than 35 grams per day) lose more bone mass than those who eat too much (more than 100 grams per day). The RDA for protein is about 50 grams per day for women and 63 grams for men.

Soft drinks, coffee, and alcoholic beverages also can contribute to a loss in bone density if consumed in large quantities. Although they may not cause the damage directly, they often take the place of dairy products in the diet.

Exercise plays a key role in preventing osteoporosis by decreasing the rate of bone loss following the onset of menopause. Active people are able to maintain bone density much more effectively than their inactive counterparts. A combination of weight-bearing exercises, such as walking or jogging and weight training, is especially helpful.

The benefits of exercise go beyond maintaining bone density. Exercise strengthens muscles, ligaments, and tendons—all of which provide support to the bones (skeleton). Exercise also improves balance and coordination, which can help prevent falls and injuries.

People who are active have higher bone mineral density than inactive people. Similar to other benefits of participating in exercise, there is no such thing as "bone in the bank." To have good bone health, people need to participate in a regular lifetime exercise program.

Prevailing research also tells us that estrogen is the most important factor in preventing bone loss. Lumbar bone density in women who have always had regular menstrual cycles exceeds that of women with a history of **oligomenorrhea** and **amenorrhea** interspersed with regular cycles. Furthermore, the lumbar density of these two groups of women is higher than that of women who have never had regular menstrual cycles.

For instance, athletes with amenorrhea (who have lower estrogen levels) have lower bone mineral density than even nonathletes with normal estrogen levels. Studies have shown that amenorrheic athletes at age 25 have the bones of women older than 50. It has become clear that sedentary women with normal estrogen levels have better bone mineral density than active amenorrheic athletes. Many experts believe the best predictor of bone mineral content is the history of menstrual regularity.

As a baseline, women age 65 and older should have a bone density test to establish the risk for osteoporosis. Younger women who are at risk for osteoporosis should discuss a bone density test with their physician at menopause. The test also can be used to monitor changes in bone mass over time and to predict the risk of future fractures. The bone density test is a painless scan requiring only a small amount of radiation to determine bone mass of the spine, hip, wrist, heel, or fingers. The amount of radiation is so low that technicians administering the test can sit next to the person receiving it. The procedure often takes less than 10 minutes.

Following menopause, every woman should consider some type of therapy to prevent bone loss. The various therapy modalities available should be discussed with a physician.

## Hormone-Replacement Therapy

For decades, hormone-replacement therapy (HRT) was the most common treatment modality to prevent bone loss following menopause. A large study (16,000 healthy women, ages 50 to 79) was terminated three years early because the results showed that taking estrogen and progestin, a common form of HRT, actually increased the risk for disease.[19] The study was the first major long-term (eight years) clinical trial investigating the association between HRT and age-related diseases, including cardiovascular disease, cancer, and osteoporosis. Although the risk for hip fractures and colorectal cancer decreased, the risk for developing breast cancer, blood clots, strokes, and heart attacks increased.

HRT may still be the most effective treatment to relieve acute (short-term) symptoms of menopause, such as hot flashes, mood swings, sleep difficulties, and vaginal dryness. Researchers and physicians, however, now must determine how long women can remain on HRT, how to best taper off treatment to provide maximal physical and emotional relief, and how to protect women from osteoporosis and other age-related diseases. Women who believed that HRT would help their bones become stronger and would ward off age-related diseases now must seek other treatments.

Alternative treatments to prevent bone loss are being developed. Miacalcin, a synthetic form of the hormone calcitonin, is FDA-approved for women who have osteoporosis and are at least five years postmenopausal. Calcitonin is a thyroid hormone that helps maintain the body's delicate balance of calcium by taking calcium from the blood and depositing it in the bones. Though it is effective in preventing bone loss, it does not help much in rebuilding bone. The drug seems to have no side effects and is available in injectable and nasal spray forms.

Two promising nonhormonal drugs, alendronate (Fosamax) and risedronate (Actonel), prevent bone loss and, furthermore, actually help increase bone mass. Alendronate (recommended for women who already have osteoporosis) is used primarily for bone health and does not provide benefits to the cardiovascular system. Although the research is limited, this drug seems to be safe and effective.

Selective estrogen receptor modulators (SERMs) also are used to prevent bone loss. These compounds have a positive effect on blood lipids and pose no risk to breast and uterine tissue. Data indicate that SERMs contribute a 1 to 2 percent increase in bone density over a period of four years but that they are less effective against osteoporosis than alendronate and risedronate. One SERM used currently to prevent osteoporosis is raloxifene (Evista).

## Iron Deficiency

Iron is a key element of **hemoglobin** in blood. The RDA for iron for adult women is between 15 and 18 mg per day (8 to 11 mg for men). Inadequate iron intake is often seen in children, teenagers, women of childbearing age, and endurance athletes. If iron absorption does not compensate for losses or if dietary intake is low, iron deficiency develops. As many as half of American women have an iron deficiency. Over time, excessive depletion of iron stores in the body leads to iron-deficiency anemia, a condition in which the concentration of hemoglobin in the red blood cells is lower than it should be.

Physically active individuals, in particular women, have a greater than average need for iron. Heavy training

---

**Oligomenorrhea** Irregular menstrual cycles.

**Amenorrhea** Cessation of regular menstrual flow.

**Hemoglobin** Protein–iron compound in red blood cells that transports oxygen in the blood.

creates a demand for iron that is higher than the recommended intake because small amounts of iron are lost through sweat, urine, and stools. Mechanical trauma, caused by the pounding of the feet on the pavement during extensive jogging, may also lead to destruction of iron-containing red blood cells.

A large percentage of female endurance athletes are reported to have iron deficiency. The blood **ferritin** levels of women who participate in intense physical training should be checked frequently.

The rates of iron absorption and iron loss vary from person to person. In most cases, though, people can get enough iron by eating more iron-rich foods such as beans, peas, green leafy vegetables, enriched grain products, egg yolk, fish, and lean meats. Although organ meats, such as liver, are especially good sources, they also are high in cholesterol. A list of foods high in iron is given in Table 3.14.

**TABLE 3.14  Iron-Rich Foods**

| Food | Amount | Iron (mg) | Calories | % Calories From Fat |
|---|---|---|---|---|
| Beans, red kidney, cooked | 1 cup | 3.2 | 218 | 4 |
| Beef, ground lean (21% fat) | 3 oz | 2.1 | 237 | 57 |
| Beef, sirloin, lean only | 3 oz | 2.9 | 171 | 36 |
| Beef, liver, fried | 3 oz | 5.3 | 184 | 33 |
| Beet, greens, cooked | ½ cup | 1.4 | 19 | — |
| Broccoli, cooked, drained | 1 cup | 1.3 | 44 | — |
| Burrito, bean (no cheese) | 1 | 2.3 | 225 | 28 |
| Egg, hard-cooked | 1 | .7 | 77 | 58 |
| Farina (Cream of Wheat), cooked | ½ cup | 5.2 | 65 | — |
| Instant Breakfast, nonfat milk | 1 cup | 4.8 | 216 | 4 |
| Peas, frozen, cooked, drained | ½ cup | 1.3 | 62 | — |
| Shrimp, boiled | 3 oz | 2.7 | 87 | 10 |
| Spinach, raw | 1 cup | 1.5 | 12 | — |
| Vegetables, mixed, cooked | 1 cup | 1.5 | 108 | — |

# 2005 Dietary Guidelines for Americans

The *Dietary Guidelines for Americans, 2005* (6th edition) provides science-based advice to promote health and to reduce risk for major chronic diseases through diet and physical activity. The secretaries of the Department of Health and Human Services (DHHS) and the USDA appoint an expert Dietary Guidelines advisory committee at least every five years to issue a report and make recommendations concerning Dietary Guidelines for Americans.

The topics that the committee addressed in depth included meeting recommended nutrient intakes; physical activity; energy balance; relationships of fats, carbohydrates, selected food groups, and alcohol with health; and consumer aspects of food safety. The committee was especially interested in finding strong scientific support for dietary and physical activity measures that could reduce the nation's major diet-related health problems: overweight and obesity, hypertension, abnormal blood lipids, diabetes, CHD, certain types of cancer, and osteoporosis.

The recommendations are designated for the general public age 2 years and older and are based on the preponderance of scientific and medical knowledge that is current at the time the committee's report is published. The Dietary Guidelines describe a healthy diet as one that:

- Emphasizes fruits, vegetables, whole grains, and fat-free or low-fat milk products
- Includes lean meats, poultry, fish, beans, eggs, and nuts
- Is low in saturated fats, trans fatty acids, cholesterol, salt (sodium), and added sugars

The committee's extensive review of the evidence led to the development of the following set of nine key messages[20] (see Figure 3.15):

1. *Consume a variety of foods within and among the basic food groups while staying within energy needs.* The recommendations for nutrient intakes consider the prevention of chronic disease as well as basic nutrient needs. Meeting those recommendations provides a firm foundation for health and for reducing chronic disease risk. For most nutrients, intakes by Americans appear adequate. Still, efforts are warranted to promote increased dietary intakes of vitamin E, calcium, magnesium, potassium, and fiber by children and adults and to promote increased dietary intakes of vitamins A and C by adults. A basic premise of dietary guidance is to meet the recommended nutrient intakes while staying within energy needs.

2. *Control calorie intake to manage body weight.* Calorie intake and physical activity go hand in hand in controlling a person's weight. To stem the obesity epidemic, most Americans need to consume fewer calories. In weight control, calories do count. Limiting portion sizes

**FIGURE 3.15** 2005 Dietary Guidelines for Americans.

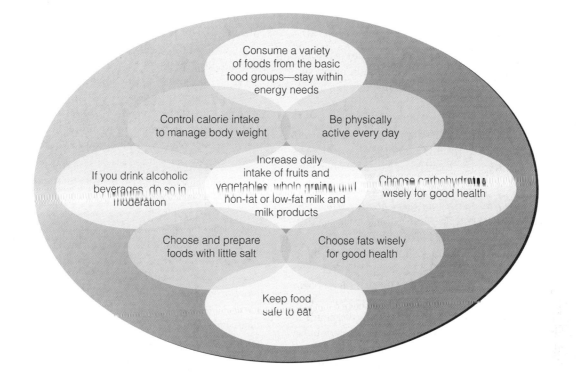

and monitoring weight regularly to adjust food intake as necessary are recommended.

3. *Be physically active every day.* Making moderate physical activity a part of an adult's daily routine for at least 30 minutes per day promotes fitness and reduces the risk of acquiring chronic health conditions. Moderate physical activity for an hour each day can increase energy expenditure by about 150 to 200 calories, depending on body size. According to the committee, many adults need to participate in up to 60 minutes of moderate to vigorous physical activity on most days to prevent unhealthy weight gain; adults who previously have lost weight may need 60 and up to 90 minutes of moderate physical activity daily to avoid regaining weight. Compared with moderate physical activity, vigorous physical activity provides greater benefits for physical fitness and burns more calories per unit of time.

4. *Increase daily intake of fruits and vegetables, whole grains, and non-fat or low-fat milk and milk products.* Fruits contain glucose, fructose, sucrose, and fiber, and most fruits are relatively low in calories. Also, fruits are important sources of at least eight additional nutrients, including vitamin C, folate, and potassium. Many vegetables provide only small amounts of sugars and/or starch, some are high in starch, and all provide fiber. Vegetables are important sources of 19 or more nutrients, including potassium, folate, and vitamins A and E.

Moreover, increased consumption of fruits and vegetables may be a useful component of programs designed to achieve and sustain weight loss. Consuming a variety of fruits and vegetables daily is recommended (choose among citrus fruits, melons, and berries; other fruits; dark-green leafy vegetables; bright-orange vegetables; legumes; starchy vegetables; and other vegetables). Whole grains are high in starch, and they are important sources of 14 nutrients, including fiber. Important sources of whole grains include whole wheat, oatmeal, popcorn, bulgur, and brown rice. The goal is to eat at least three 1 ounce equivalents per day of whole-grain foods, preferably in place of refined grains.

Milk and milk products are important sources of at least 12 nutrients, including calcium, magnesium, potassium, and vitamin D. Diets that provide three cups (or the equivalent) of non-fat or low-fat milk and/or milk products per day can improve bone mass and are not associated with weight gain.

5. *Choose fats wisely for good health.* Keeping a low intake of saturated fat, trans fat, and cholesterol can reduce the risk for CHD. The lower the combined intake of saturated and trans fat and the lower the dietary cholesterol intake, the greater the cardiovascular benefit will be. The main way to keep saturated fat low is to limit one's intake of animal fats (such as those in cheese, milk, butter, ice cream, and other full-fat dairy products; fatty meat; bacon and sausage; and poultry skin and fat). The major way to limit trans fat intake is

**Ferritin** Iron stored in the body.

to limit the intake of foods made with partially hydrogenated vegetable oils. To limit dietary intake of cholesterol, a person has to limit the intake of eggs and organ meats especially, as well as limit the intake of meat, shellfish, poultry, and dairy products that contain fat.

A total fat intake of 20 to 35 percent of calories is recommended for all Americans age 18 years and older. Intakes of fat outside of this range are not recommended for most Americans because of the potential adverse effects on achieving recommended nutrient intakes and on risk factors for chronic diseases. The lower limit of fat intake is higher for children: 30 percent of calories from fat for children age 2 and 3 years, and 25 percent of calories from fat for those age 4 to 10 years.

6. *Choose carbohydrates wisely for good health.* When selecting foods from the fruit, vegetable, and grains groups, frequent fiber-rich choices are beneficial. This means, for example, choosing whole fruits rather than juices, and whole grains rather than refined grains. Following the guidelines to increase the intake of fruits, vegetables, whole grains, and non-fat or low-fat milk and milk products is a healthful way to obtain the recommended amounts of carbohydrates. Compared with individuals who consume small amounts of foods and beverages that are high in added sugars, those who consume large amounts tend to consume more calories but smaller amounts of vitamins and minerals. A reduced intake of added sugars (especially sugar-sweetened beverages) may be helpful in achieving the recommended intakes of nutrients and in controlling weight.

7. *Choose and prepare foods with little salt.* Reducing salt (sodium chloride) intake is one of several ways by which people can lower their blood pressure. Reducing blood pressure, ideally to the normal range, decreases the chance of developing a stroke, heart disease, heart failure, and kidney disease. The relationship between salt intake and blood pressure is direct and progressive without an apparent threshold. The goal is to consume less than 2,300 mg of sodium per day. On average, the higher a person's salt intake, the higher the blood pressure. Thus, reducing salt intake as much as possible is one way to lower blood pressure.

8. *If you drink alcoholic beverages, do so in moderation.* Among middle-aged and older adults, the lowest all-cause mortality occurs at the level of one or two drinks per day. The mortality reduction likely stems from the protective effects of moderate alcohol consumption on CHD, primarily among males older than 45 years of age and women older than 55 years. Among younger people, alcohol consumption seems to provide little, if any, health benefit. Alcohol use among young adults is associated with increased risk for traumatic injury and death. Heavy drinking is hazardous, contributing to automobile injuries and deaths, assault, liver disease, and other health problems. Abstention is an important option.

The goal for adults who choose to drink is to do so in moderation, defined as consuming up to one drink per day for women and two drinks per day for men. One drink is defined as 12 ounces of regular beer, 5 ounces of wine (12 percent alcohol), or 1.5 ounces of 80-proof distilled spirits. Among those who should not consume alcoholic beverages are individuals who cannot restrict their drinking to moderate levels, children and adolescents, and individuals taking medications that can interact with alcohol or who have specific medical conditions. Alcoholic beverages should be avoided by women who may become pregnant or who are pregnant, by breastfeeding women, and by individuals who plan to drive or take part in other activities that require attention, skill, or coordination.

9. *Keep food safe to eat.* According to the 2005 Dietary Guidelines report, foodborne diseases cause approximately 76 million illnesses, 325,000 hospitalizations, and 5,000 deaths in the United States each year. Three pathogens (salmonella, listeria, and toxoplasma) are responsible for more than 75 percent of these deaths. Actions by consumers can reduce the occurrence of foodborne illness substantially. The behaviors in the home that are most likely to prevent a problem with foodborne illnesses are:

(a) Cleaning hands, contact surfaces, and fruits and vegetables (This does not apply to meat and poultry, which should not be washed.)
(b) Separating raw, cooked, and ready-to-eat foods while shopping, preparing, or storing
(c) Cooking foods to a safe temperature
(d) Chilling (refrigerating) perishable foods promptly
(e) Avoiding higher-risk foods (e.g., deli meats and frankfurters that have not been reheated to a safe temperature and thus may contain listeria). This is especially important for high-risk groups (the very young, pregnant women, the elderly, and those who are immunocompromised).

Additional information on these guidelines is posted at www.health.gov/dietaryguidelines.

# Proper Nutrition: A Lifetime Prescription for Healthy Living

The three factors that do the most for health, longevity, and quality of life are proper nutrition, a sound exercise program, and quitting (or never starting) smoking. Achieving and maintaining a balanced diet is not as difficult as most people think. If everyone were more educated about their own nutrition habits and the nutrition habits of their children, the current magnitude of nutrition-related health problems would be much smaller. Although treatment of obesity is important, we should place far greater emphasis on preventing obesity in youth and adults in the first place.

Children tend to eat the way their parents do. If parents adopt a healthy diet, children most likely will follow.

The difficult part for most people is to retrain themselves—to closely examine the eating habits they learned from their parents—to follow a lifetime healthy nutrition plan that includes lots of grains, legumes, fruits, vegetables, and low-fat dairy products, with moderate use of animal protein, junk food, sodium, and alcohol.

### Critical Thinking

What factors in your life and the environment have contributed to your current dietary habits? Do you need to make changes? What may prevent you from doing so?

In spite of the ample scientific evidence linking poor dietary habits to early disease and mortality rates, many people remain precontemplators: They are not willing to change their eating patterns. Even when faced with obesity, elevated blood lipids, hypertension, and other nutrition-related conditions, people do not change. The motivating factor to change one's eating habits seems to be a major health breakdown, such as a heart attack, a stroke, or cancer—by which time the damage has been done already. In many cases it is irreversible and, for some, fatal.

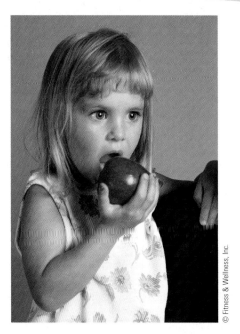

© Fitness & Wellness, Inc.

Positive nutrition habits should be taught and reinforced in early youth.

An ounce of prevention is worth a pound of cure. The sooner you implement the dietary guidelines presented in this chapter, the better your chances of preventing chronic diseases and reaching a higher state of wellness.

## ASSESS YOUR BEHAVIOR

Log on to http://www.cengage.com/sso/ to assess your eating habits and create a plan for healthier eating.

1. Are whole grains, fruits, and vegetables the staple of your diet?

2. Are you meeting your personal MyPyramid recommendations for daily fruits, vegetables, grains, meat (or substitutes) and legumes, and milk?

3. Will the information presented in this chapter change in any manner the way you eat?

4. Are there dietary changes that you need to implement to meet energy, nutrition, and disease risk-reduction guidelines and improve health and wellness? If so, list these changes and indicate what you will do to make it happen.

## ASSESS YOUR KNOWLEDGE

Log on to http://www.cengage.com/sso/ to assess your understanding of this chapter's topics by taking the Student Practice Test and exploring the modules recommended in your Personalized Study Plan.

1. The science of nutrition studies the relationship of
   a. vitamins and minerals to health.
   b. foods to optimal health and performance.
   c. carbohydrates, fats, and proteins to the development and maintenance of good health.
   d. the macronutrients and micronutrients to physical performance.
   e. kilocalories to calories in food items.

2. Faulty nutrition often plays a crucial role in the development and progression of which disease?
   a. Cardiovascular disease
   b. Cancer
   c. Osteoporosis
   d. Diabetes
   e. All are correct choices.

3. According to MyPyramid, daily vegetable consumption is measured in
   a. servings.
   b. ounces.
   c. cups.
   d. calories.
   e. all of the above.

4. The recommended amount of fiber intake for adults 50 years and younger is
   a. 10 grams per day for women and 12 grams for men.
   b. 21 grams per day for women and 30 grams for men.
   c. 20 grams per day for women and 35 grams for men.
   d. 25 grams per day for women and 38 grams for men.
   e. 45 grams per day for women and 50 grams for men.

5. Unhealthy fats include
   a. unsaturated fatty acids.
   b. monounsaturated fats.
   c. polyunsaturated fatty acids.
   d. saturated fats.
   e. all of the above.

6. The daily recommended carbohydrate intake is
   a. 45 to 65 percent of the total calories.
   b. 10 to 35 percent of the total calories.
   c. 20 to 35 percent of the total calories.
   d. 60 to 75 percent of the total calories.
   e. 35 to 50 percent of the total calories.

7. The amount of a nutrient that is estimated to meet the nutrient requirement of half the healthy people in specific age and gender groups is known as the
   a. Estimated Average Requirement.
   b. Recommended Dietary Allowance.
   c. Daily Values.
   d. Adequate Intake.
   e. Dietary Reference Intake.

8. The percent fat intake for an individual who on a given day consumes 2,385 calories with 106 grams of fat is
   a. 44 percent of total calories.
   b. 17.7 percent of total calories.
   c. 40 percent of total calories.
   d. 31 percent of total calories.
   e. 22.5 percent of total calories.

9. Carbohydrate loading is beneficial for
   a. endurance athletes.
   b. people with diabetes.
   c. strength athletes.
   d. sprinters.
   e. All of the above are correct.

10. Osteoporosis is
   a. a crippling disease.
   b. more prevalent in women.
   c. more prevalent in people who were calcium deficient at a young age.
   d. linked to heavy drinking and smoking.
   e. All are correct choices.

Correct answers can be found at the back of the book.

# MEDIA MENU

You can find the links below at the book companion site: www.cengage.com/health/hoeger/plfw10e

- Analyze your eating habits.
- Check how well you understand the chapter's concepts.

### Internet Connections

- American Dietetic Association. This comprehensive site features daily food tips, frequently asked questions, nutrition resources, and links to other reliable Web sites on nutrition. *http://www.eatright.org*

- U.S. Department of Agriculture Center for Nutrition Policy and Promotion. The Center for Nutrition Policy and Promotion is the national organization that links scientific research to the nutritional needs of the American public. This site includes "The Interactive Healthy Eating Index," an online dietary assessment tool that includes nutrition messages. After providing a day's worth of dietary information, you will receive a score on the overall quality of your diet, based on the types and amounts of food compared with those recommended by the Food Guide Pyramid. *http://www.cnpp.usda.gov*

- Dietary Guidelines for Americans 2005—A Brochure for Consumers. Dietary Guidelines for Americans, published jointly by the Department of Health and Human Services (DHHS) and the U.S. Department of Agriculture (USDA), provides advice about how good dietary habits for people aged 2 years and older can promote health and reduce risk for major chronic diseases. *http://www.health.gov/dietaryguidelines/dga2005/document/default.htm*

- Cyber Kitchen. This interactive site helps you discover how much you are really eating through an activity that compares standard serving sizes with real serving sizes. If you provide information regarding your age, gender, height, weight, and activity level, the Cyber Kitchen will provide you with a healthy diet plan to meet your weight management goals. It's fun and educational. *http://www.nhlbisupport.com/chd1/Tipsheets/cyberkit.htm*

## NOTES

1. National Academy of Sciences, Institute of Medicine, *Dietary Reference Intakes for Energy, Carbohydrates, Fiber, Fat, Protein and Amino Acids (Macronutrients)* (Washington, DC: National Academy Press, 2002).

2. M. Enig, "The Deadliest Fats," *Bottom Line/Health*, Sept. 2005.

3. Editors of *Environmental Nutrition,* "Healthy Eating: Essential Information for Living Longer and Living Better." Norwalk, CT: Belvoir Media Group LLC, 2008.

4. J. L. Breslow, "n-3 Fatty Acids and Cardiovascular Disease," *American Journal of Clinical Nutrition* 83 (2006): 1477S–1482S.

5. "Is There Flaxseed in Your Fridge Yet?" *Tufts University Health & Nutrition Letter* (September 2002).

6. P. E. Bowen, "Evaluating the Health Claim of Flaxseed and Cancer Prevention," *Nutrition Today* 36 (2001): 144–158; "Flax Facts," *University of California at Berkeley Wellness Letter* (May 2002).

7. See note 1.

8. "Soy and Breast Cancer," *University of California at Berkeley Wellness Letter* (June 2007).

9. A. Trichopoulou, et al., "Adherence to a Mediterranean Diet and Survival in a Greek Population," *New England Journal of Medicine* 348 (2000). 2599–2608.

10. G. Kojda and R. Hambrecht, "Molecular Mechanism of Vascular Adaptations to Exercise: Physical Activity as an Effective Antioxidant Therapy?" *Cardiovascular Research* 67 (2005): 187–197.

11. G. Bjelakovic, et al., "Mortality in Randomized Trials of Antioxidant Supplements for Primary and Secondary Prevention," *Journal of the American Medical Association* 297 (2007): 842–857.

12. L. C. Clark, et al., "Effects of Selenium Supplementation for Cancer Prevention in Patients with Carcinoma of the Skin: A Randomized Controlled Trial," *Journal of the American Medical Association* 276 (1996): 1957–1963.

13. "The Merits of Multivitamins: EN's Guide to Choosing a Supplement," *Environmental Nutrition* 24, no. 6 (2001): 1.

14. "Vitamin D May Help You Dodge Cancer: How to Be Sure You Get Enough," *Environmental Nutrition* 30, no. 6 (2007): 1, 4.

15. "Ride the D Train: Research Finds Even More Reasons to Get Vitamin D," *Environmental Nutrition* 28, no. 9 (2005): 1, 4.

16. "New Advice About Bone Density Tests," *University of California at Berkeley Wellness Letter* 18, no. 10 (2002): 1–2.

17. M. T. Goodman, et al., "Association of Dairy Products, Lactose, and Calcium with the Risk of Ovarian Cancer," *American Journal of Epidemiology* 156 (2002): 148–157.

18. "How to Build Better Bones: Overview of All the New Osteoporosis Options," *Environmental Nutrition* 24, no. 9 (2001): 1, 4–5.

19. Writing Group for the Women's Health Initiative, "Risks and Benefits of Combined Estrogen and Progestin in Healthy Postmenopausal Women: Principal Results from the Women's Health Initiative Randomized Controlled Trial," *Journal of the American Medical Association* 288 (2002): 321–333.

20. U.S. Department of Health and Human Services and U.S. Department of Agriculture, *Dietary Guidelines for Americans 2005* (Washington, DC: U.S. Government Printing Office, 2005).

## SUGGESTED READINGS

Coleman, E. *Eating for Endurance.* Palo Alto, CA: Bull Publishing, 2003.

Clark, N. *Nancy Clark's Sports Nutrition Guidebook.* Champaign, IL: Human Kinetics, 2008.

Editors of *Environmental Nutrition.* "Healthy Eating: Essential Information for Living Longer and Living Better." Norwalk, CT: Belvoir Media Group LLC, 2008.

McArdle, W. D., F. I. Katch, and V. L. Katch. *Sports & Exercise Nutrition.* Baltimore: Lippincott Williams & Wilkins, 2005.

National Academy of Sciences, Institute of Medicine. *Dietary Reference Intakes for Energy, Carbohydrates, Fiber, Fat, Protein and Amino Acids (Macronutrients).* Washington, DC: National Academy Press, 2002.

S. R. Rolfes, K. Pinna, and E. N. Whitney. *Understanding Normal and Clinical Nutrition.* Belmont, CA: Wadsworth/Cengage Learning, 2009.

Sizer, F. S., and E. N. Whitney. *Nutrition: Concepts and Controversies.* Belmont, CA: Wadsworth/Cengage Learning, 2008.

Whitney, E. N., and S. R. Rolfes. *Understanding Nutrition.* Belmont, CA: Wadsworth/Cengage Learning, 2008.

# LAB 3A: Nutrient Analysis

Name _____ Date _____ Grade _____

Instructor _____ Course _____ Section _____

### Necessary Lab Equipment
Appendix A (Nutritive Value of Selected Foods) and a small calculator.

### Objective
To evaluate your present diet using the Recommended Dietary Allowances (RDA).

### Instructions
To conduct the nutrient analysis, record all the foods eaten during a 3-day period using the list of Nutritive Value of Selected Foods provided in Appendix A. Record this information prior to this lab session in the form provided in Figure 3A.1 (make additional copies for a 3-day record). After recording the nutritive values for each day, add up the values in each column and record the totals at the bottom of the form. During your lab, proceed to compute an average for the 3 days. The percentages of carbohydrates, fat, saturated fat, and the protein requirements can be computed by using the instructions at the bottom of Figure 3A.2. The results can then be compared against the Recommended Dietary Allowances.

FIGURE 3A.1 Daily nutrient intake

| Foods | Amount | Calories | Protein (g) | Fat (total g) | Sat. Fat (g) | Cho- lesterol (mg) | Carbo- hydrates (g) | Dietary Fiber (g) | Calcium (mg) | Iron (mg) | Sodium (mg) | Vit. E (mg) | Folate (mcg) | Vit. C (mg) | Selenium (mcg) |
|-------|--------|----------|-------------|---------------|--------------|---------------------|----------------------|--------------------|---------------|------------|--------------|--------------|---------------|--------------|------------------|
| | | | | | | | | | | | | | | | |
| | | | | | | | | | | | | | | | |
| | | | | | | | | | | | | | | | |
| | | | | | | | | | | | | | | | |
| | | | | | | | | | | | | | | | |
| | | | | | | | | | | | | | | | |
| | | | | | | | | | | | | | | | |
| | | | | | | | | | | | | | | | |
| | | | | | | | | | | | | | | | |
| | | | | | | | | | | | | | | | |
| | | | | | | | | | | | | | | | |
| | | | | | | | | | | | | | | | |
| | | | | | | | | | | | | | | | |
| | | | | | | | | | | | | | | | |
| | | | | | | | | | | | | | | | |
| | | | | | | | | | | | | | | | |
| | | | | | | | | | | | | | | | |
| | | | | | | | | | | | | | | | |
| | | | | | | | | | | | | | | | |
| | | | | | | | | | | | | | | | |
| | | | | | | | | | | | | | | | |
| Totals | | | | | | | | | | | | | | | |

FIGURE 3A.2 Daily nutrient intake

| Day | Calories | Protein (g) | Fat (g) | Sat. Fat (g) | Cho-lesterol (mg) | Carbo-hydrates (g) | Dietary Fiber (g) | Calcium (mg) | Iron (mg) | Sodium (mg) | Vit. E (mg) | Folate (mcg) | Vit. C (mg) | Selenium (mcg) |
|---|---|---|---|---|---|---|---|---|---|---|---|---|---|---|
| One | | | | | | | | | | | | | | |
| Two | | | | | | | | | | | | | | |
| Three | | | | | | | | | | | | | | |
| Totals | | | | | | | | | | | | | | |
| Average[a] | | | | | | | | | | | | | | |
| Percentages[b] | | | | | | | | | | | | | | |
| **Recommended Dietary Allowances*** | | | | | | | | | | | | | | |
| **Men** | See below[c] | See below[d] | | | | | | | | | | | | |
| 14–18 yrs. | | | 20–30%[e] | 7% | <300 | 45–65% | 38 | 1,300 | 12 | 2,400 | 15 | 400 | 75 | 55 |
| 19–30 yrs. | | | 20–30%[e] | 7% | <300 | 45–65% | 38 | 1,000 | 10 | 2,400 | 15 | 400 | 90 | 55 |
| 31–50 yrs. | | | 20–30%[e] | 7% | <300 | 45–65% | 38 | 1,000 | 10 | 2,400 | 15 | 400 | 90 | 55 |
| 51+ yrs. | | | 20–30%[e] | 7% | <300 | 45–65% | 30 | 1,200 | 10 | 2,400 | 15 | 400 | 90 | 55 |
| **Women** | | | | | | | | | | | | | | |
| 14–18 yrs. | | | 20–30%[e] | 7% | <300 | 45–65% | 25 | 1,300 | 15 | 2,400 | 15 | 400 | 65 | 55 |
| 19–30 yrs. | | | 20–30%[e] | 7% | <300 | 45–65% | 25 | 1,000 | 15 | 2,400 | 15 | 400 | 75 | 55 |
| 31–50 yrs. | | | 20–30%[e] | 7% | <300 | 45–65% | 25 | 1,000 | 15 | 2,400 | 15 | 400 | 75 | 55 |
| 51+ yrs. | | | 20–30%[e] | 7% | <300 | 45–65% | 21 | 1,200 | 10 | 2,400 | 15 | 400 | 75 | 55 |
| Pregnant | | | 20–30%[e] | 7% | <300 | 45–65% | 25 | 1,200 | 30 | 2,400 | 15 | 600 | 85 | 60 |
| Lactating | | | 20–30%[e] | 7% | <300 | 45–65% | 25 | 1,200 | 15 | 2,400 | 19 | 500 | 120 | 70 |

[a] Divide totals by 3 or number of days assessed.

[b] Percentages: Protein and carbohydrates = multiply average by 4, divide by average calories, and multiply by 100.
Fat and saturated fat = multiply average by 9, divide by average calories, and multiply by 100.

[c] Use Table 5.3 (page 172) for all categories.

[d] Protein intake should be .8 grams per kilogram of body weight. Pregnant women should consume an additional 15 grams of daily protein, and lactating women should have an extra 20 grams.

[e] Based on recommendations by nutrition experts. Up to 35% is allowed for individuals who suffer from metabolic syndrome.

*Adapted from *Recommended Dietary Allowances,* 10th Edition, and the Dietary Reference Intakes series, National Academy Press, © National Academy of Sciences 1989, 1997, 1998, 2000, 2001. Washington, DC.

# LAB 3B: MyPyramid Record Form

## Homework Assignment

Name _____  Date _____  Grade _____

Instructor _____  Course _____  Section _____

### Assignment

This laboratory experience should be carried out as a homework assignment to be completed over the next 7 days.

### Lab Resources    "MyPyramid" at http://mypyramid.gov

### Instructions

Keep a 7-day record of your food consumption using the MyPyramid guidelines in Figure 3.1. Whenever you have something to eat, record the food item, the number of calories, the grams of fat (use the Nutritive Value of Selected Foods list given in Appendix A), and the amounts eaten based on the MyPyramid guidelines. If a particular food item is not listed in the Nutritive Value of Selected Foods list, the information can be obtained from the food container itself.

Record all information immediately after each meal, because it will be easier to keep track of foods and amounts eaten. If twice the amount of a particular serving is eaten, the calories, grams of fat, and amounts must be doubled as well.

### Objective

To meet the minimum daily required amounts of the basic food groups and monitor total daily fat intake.

At the end of the day, evaluate the diet by checking whether the minimum required amounts for each food group were met, and by total amount of calories and fat consumed. If you meet the required food group amounts and your daily caloric intake recommendation, you are well on your way to achieving a well-balanced diet. In addition, fat intake should not exceed 30 percent of the daily caloric consumption (may be up to 35 percent for individuals who suffer from metabolic syndrome—see Table 3.5, page 79). If you are on a diet, you may want to reduce fat intake to less than 20 percent of total daily calories (see Table 5.5, page 173).

### II. Nutrition Stage of Change

Using Figure 2.5 (page 57) and Table 2.3 (page 57) identify your current stage of change for nutrition (healthy diet):

[                                    ]

### III. What I Learned and What I Can Do to Improve My Nutrition:

Based on the nutrient analysis conducted in Lab 3A and your daily diet analysis conducted in this lab, explain what these experiences have taught you and list specific changes and strategies that you can use to improve your present nutrition habits. Use an extra blank sheet of paper as needed.

I have learned the following about myself/my current diet: _____

_____

_____

Specific changes I plan to make: _____

_____

_____

Strategies I will use: _____    _____    _____

_____

_____

IV. Current number of daily steps: [          ]    Category (Use Table 1.2, page 10): _____

FIGURE 3B.1 MyPyramid Record Form

Name _____ Section _____ Date _____

Course _____ Gender _____ Age _____

| No. | Food* | Calories | Fat (gm)** | Food Groups Number of Recommended Daily Amounts (see Figure 3.1) | | | | | |
| --- | --- | --- | --- | --- | --- | --- | --- | --- | --- |
| | | | | Grains | Vegetables | Fruits | Oils | Milk | Meats and Beans |
| 1 | | | | | | | | | |
| 2 | | | | | | | | | |
| 3 | | | | | | | | | |
| 4 | | | | | | | | | |
| 5 | | | | | | | | | |
| 6 | | | | | | | | | |
| 7 | | | | | | | | | |
| 8 | | | | | | | | | |
| 9 | | | | | | | | | |
| 10 | | | | | | | | | |
| 11 | | | | | | | | | |
| 12 | | | | | | | | | |
| 13 | | | | | | | | | |
| 14 | | | | | | | | | |
| 15 | | | | | | | | | |
| 16 | | | | | | | | | |
| 17 | | | | | | | | | |
| 18 | | | | | | | | | |
| 19 | | | | | | | | | |
| 20 | | | | | | | | | |
| 21 | | | | | | | | | |
| 22 | | | | | | | | | |
| 23 | | | | | | | | | |
| 24 | | | | | | | | | |
| 25 | | | | | | | | | |
| 26 | | | | | | | | | |
| 27 | | | | | | | | | |
| 28 | | | | | | | | | |
| 29 | | | | | | | | | |
| 30 | | | | | | | | | |
| Totals | | | | | | | | | |
| Recommended Amount: Obtain online at http://mypyramid.gov based on age, sex, and activity level | | | | | | | | | |
| Deficiencies/Excesses | | | | | | | | | |

*See "List of Nutritive Value of Selected Foods" in Appendix A.
**Multiply the recommended amount of calories by .30 (30%) and divide by 9 to obtain the recommended amount of grams of fat (if on a diet, multiply by .20 or .10—see Table 5.5, page 173)

# Body Composition

© Fitness & Wellness, Inc.

## Objectives

- Define body composition and understand its relationship to assessment of recommended body weight
- Explain the difference between essential fat and storage fat
- Describe various techniques used to assess body composition
- Be able to assess body composition using hydrostatic weighing, girth measurements, and skinfold thickness
- Understand the importance of body mass index (BMI) and waist circumference in the assessment of risk for disease
- Be able to determine recommended weight according to recommended percent body fat values and BMI

**CENGAGENOW™**

Learn how to measure body composition.
Assess your risks for potential disease.
Check your understanding of the chapter contents by logging on to CengageNOW and accessing the pre-test, personalized learning plan, and post-test for this chapter.

# FAQ

### What constitutes ideal body weight?

There is no such thing as "ideal" body weight. Health/fitness professionals prefer to use the terms "recommended" or "healthy" body weight. Let's examine the question in more detail. For instance, 25 percent body fat is the recommended health fitness standard for a 40-year-old man. For the average "apparently healthy" individual, this body fat percentage does not constitute a threat to good health. Due to genetic and lifestyle conditions, however, if a person this same age at 25 percent body fat is prediabetic and prehypertensive, with abnormal blood lipids (cholesterol and triglycerides—see Chapter 11), weight (fat) loss and a lower percent body fat may be recommended. Thus, what will work as recommended weight for most individuals may not be the best standard for individuals with disease risk factors. The current recommended or healthy weight standards (based on percent body fat or BMI) are established at the point where there appears to be a lower incidence for overweight-related conditions for most people. Individual differences have to be taken into consideration when making a final recommendation, especially in people with risk factors or a personal and family history of chronic conditions.

### How accurate are body composition assessments?

Most of the techniques to determine body composition require proper training on the part of the technician administering the test (skinfolds, hydrostatic weighing, DXA) and, in the case of hydrostatic weighing, proper performance on the part of the person being tested. As detailed in this chapter, body composition assessment is not a precise science. Some of the procedures are more accurate than others. Before undergoing body composition testing, make sure that you understand the accuracy of the technique (see SFEs included under the description of each technique); and even more important, inquire about the training and experience of the person administering the test. We often encounter individuals who have been tested elsewhere by any number of assessments, particularly skinfolds, who come to our laboratory in disbelief (and rightfully so) because of the results that were given to them. To obtain the best possible results, look for trained and experienced technicians.

### Is there a future trend in body composition assessment?

Results of research data indicate that the area of the body where people store fat is more critical than how much is stored. Individuals with a higher amount of intra-abdominal or abdominal visceral fat (located around internal organs), as opposed to primarily abdominal fat stored beneath the skin (subcutaneous fat), are at greater risk for disease. Thus, to increase disease risk evaluation, future body composition tests will be designed to get a clearer view of where the abdominal fat lies.

Additionally, although not a body composition assessment, BMI guidelines to detect thinness and excessive fatness (see BMI section on page 130) will most likely change based on age, gender, and physical activity patterns. BMIs of 25 or greater are not accurate predictors of excessive fatness in younger people and in athletic populations. Furthermore, because of differences in essential fat between men and women, the same standard may not apply for men and women alike.

**Body composition** is used in reference to the fat and nonfat components of the human body. The fat component is called fat mass or **percent body fat.** The non-fat component is termed **lean body mass.**

To determine **recommended body weight,** we need to find out what percent of total body weight is fat and what amount is lean tissue—in other words, assess body composition. Body composition should be assessed by a well-trained technician who understands the procedure being used.

Once the fat percentage is known, recommended body weight can be calculated from recommended body fat. Recommended body weight, also called "healthy weight," implies the absence of any medical condition that would improve with weight loss and a fat distribution pattern that is not associated with higher risk for illness.

Formerly, people relied on simple height/weight charts to determine their recommended body weight, but these tables can be highly inaccurate and fail to identify critical fat values associated with higher risk for disease.

Standard height/weight tables, first published in 1912, were based on average weights (including shoes and clothing) for men and women who obtained life insurance policies between 1888 and 1905—a notably unrepresentative population. The recommended body weight on these tables was obtained according to sex, height, and frame size. Currently, because no scientific guidelines are given to determine frame size, most people choose their frame size based on the column in which the weight comes closest to their own!

The best way to determine whether people are truly **overweight** or falsely at recommended body weight is through assessment of body composition. **Obesity** is an excess of body fat. If body weight is the only criterion, an individual might easily appear to be overweight according to height/weight charts, yet not have too much body fat. Typical examples are football players, body builders, weight lifters, and other athletes with large muscle size. Some athletes who appear to be 20 or 30 pounds overweight really have little body fat.

The inaccuracy of height/weight charts was illustrated clearly when a young man who weighed about 225 pounds applied to join a city police force but was turned down without having been granted an interview. The reason? He was "too fat," according to the height/weight charts. When this young man's body composition was assessed at a preventive medicine clinic, it was determined that only 5 percent of his total body weight was in the form of fat—considerably less than the recommended standard. In the words of the director of the clinic, "The only way this fellow could come down to the chart's target weight would have been through surgical removal of a large amount of his muscle tissue."

At the other end of the spectrum, some people who weigh very little (and may be viewed as skinny or underweight) actually can be classified as overweight because of their high body fat content. People who weigh as little as 120 pounds but are more than 30 percent fat (about one-third of their total body weight) are not rare. These cases are found more readily in the sedentary population and among people who are always dieting. Physical inactivity and a constant negative caloric balance both lead to a loss in lean body mass (see Chapter 5). These examples illustrate that body weight alone clearly does not tell the whole story.

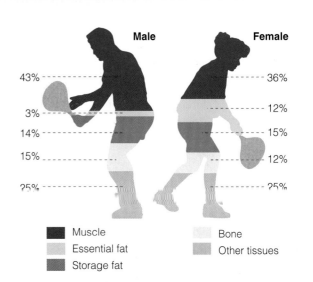

**FIGURE 4.1 Typical body composition of an adult man and woman.**

Male — 43%, 3%, 14%, 15%, 25%
Female — 36%, 12%, 15%, 12%, 25%

- Muscle
- Essential fat
- Storage fat
- Bone
- Other tissues

# Essential and Storage Fat

Total fat in the human body is classified into two types: **essential fat** and **storage fat.** Essential fat is needed for normal physiological function. Without it, human health and physical performance deteriorate. This type of fat is found within tissues such as muscles, nerve cells, bone marrow, intestines, heart, liver, and lungs. Essential fat constitutes about 3 percent of the total weight in men and 12 percent in women (Figure 4.1). The percentage is higher in women because it includes sex-specific fat, such as that found in the breast tissue, the uterus, and other sex-related fat deposits.

**Body composition** The fat and non-fat components of the human body; important in assessing recommended body weight.

**Percent body fat** Proportional amount of fat in the body based on the person's total weight; includes both essential fat and storage fat; also termed "fat mass."

**Lean body mass** Body weight without body fat.

**Recommended body weight** Body weight at which there seems to be no harm to human health; healthy weight.

**Overweight** An excess amount of weight against a given standard, such as height or recommended percent body fat.

**Obesity** An excessive accumulation of body fat, usually at least 30 percent above recommended body weight.

**Essential fat** Minimal amount of body fat needed for normal physiological functions; constitutes about 3 percent of total weight in men and 12 percent in women.

**Storage fat** Body fat in excess of essential fat; stored in adipose tissue.

Storage fat is the fat stored in adipose tissue, mostly just beneath the skin (subcutaneous fat) and around major organs in the body. This fat serves three basic functions:

1. as an insulator to retain body heat,
2. as energy substrate for metabolism, and
3. as padding against physical trauma to the body.

The amount of storage fat does not differ between men and women, except that men tend to store fat around the waist and women around the hips and thighs.

## Critical Thinking

Mary is a cross-country runner whose coach has asked her to decrease her total body fat to 7 percent. Will Mary's performance increase at this lower percent body fat? How would you respond to this coach?

# Techniques to Assess Body Composition

Body composition can be estimated through the several procedures described in the following pages. Each procedure includes a *standard error of estimate* (SEE), a measure of the accuracy of the prediction made through the regression equation for that specific technique. For example, if the SEE for a given technique is ±3.0 and the individual is given a fat percentage of 18.0, this indicates that the actual fat percentage may range from 15 to 21 percent.

### Dual Energy X-Ray Absorptiometry **Dual energy X-ray absorptiometry (DXA)** is a method to assess body composition that is used most frequently in research and by medical facilities. A radiographic technique, DXA uses very low-dose beams of X-ray energy (hundreds of times lower than a typical body X-ray) to measure total body fat mass, fat distribution pattern (see waist circumference on page 135), and bone density. Bone density is measured to assess the risk for osteoporosis. The procedure itself is simple and takes less than 15 minutes to administer. Many exercise scientists consider DXA to be the standard technique to assess body composition. The SEE for this technique is ±1.8 percent.

Because DXA is not readily available to most fitness participants, other methods to estimate body composition are used. The most common of these are:

1. Hydrostatic, or underwater, weighing
2. Air displacement

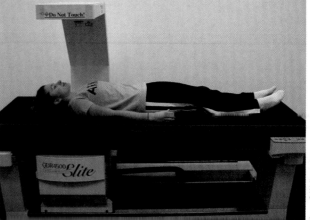

Dual energy X-ray absorptiometry (DXA) technique to assess body composition and bone density.

3. Skinfold thickness
4. Girth measurements
5. Bioelectrical impedance

Because these procedures yield estimates of body fat, each technique may yield slightly different values. Therefore, when assessing changes in body composition, be sure to use the same technique for pre- and post-test comparisons.

The most accurate technique presently available in fitness laboratories is still hydrostatic weighing. Other techniques to assess body composition are available, but the equipment is costly and not easily accessible to the general population. In addition to percentages of lean tissue and body fat, some of these methods also provide information on total body water and bone mass. These techniques include air displacement, magnetic resonance imaging (MRI), computed tomography (CT), and total body electrical conductivity (TOBEC). In terms of predicting percent body fat, these techniques are not more accurate than hydrostatic weighing.

### Hydrostatic Weighing For decades, **hydrostatic weighing** has been the most common technique used in determining body composition in exercise physiology laboratories. In essence, a person's "regular" weight is compared with a weight taken underwater. Because fat is more buoyant than lean tissue, comparing the two weights can determine a person's percent of fat. Almost all other indirect techniques to assess body composition have been validated against hydrostatic weighing. The procedure requires a considerable amount of time, skill, space, and equipment and must be administered by a well-trained technician. The SEE for hydrostatic weighing is 2.5 percent.

This technique has several drawbacks. First, because each individual assessment can take as long as 30 minutes, hydrostatic weighing is not feasible when testing a lot of

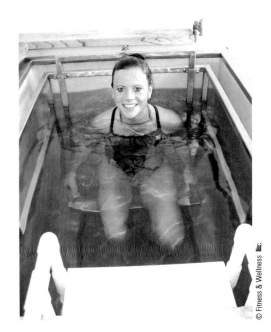

Hydrostatic, or underwater, weighing technique.

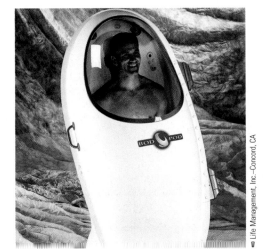

The BOD POD, used for assessment of body composition.

people. Furthermore, the person's residual lung volume (amount of air left in the lungs following complete forceful exhalation) should be measured before testing. If residual volume cannot be measured, as is the case in some laboratories and health/fitness centers, it is estimated using the predicting equations—which may decrease the accuracy of hydrostatic weighing. Also, the requirement of being completely under water makes hydrostatic weighing difficult to administer to **aquaphobic** people. For accurate results, the individual must be able to perform the test properly.

As described in Figure 4.2 and in Lab 4A, for each underwater weighing trial, the person has to (a) force out all of the air in the lungs, (b) lean forward and completely submerge underwater for about 5 to 10 seconds (long enough to get the underwater weight), and (c) remain as calm as possible (chair movement makes reading the scale difficult). This procedure is repeated 8 to 10 times.

Forcing all of the air out of the lungs is not easy for everyone but is important to obtain an accurate reading. Leaving additional air (beyond residual volume) in the lungs makes a person more buoyant. Because fat is less dense than water, overweight individuals weigh less in water. Additional air in the lungs makes a person lighter in water, yielding a false, higher body fat percentage.

## Air Displacement

**Air displacement** (also known as air displacement plethysmography) is a newer technique that holds considerable promise. With this method, an individual sits inside a small chamber, commercially known as the **Bod Pod**. Computerized pressure sensors determine the amount of air displaced by the person inside the chamber. Body volume is calculated by subtracting the air volume with the person inside the chamber from the volume of the empty chamber. The amount of air in the person's lungs also is taken into consideration when

determining the actual body volume. Body density and percent body fat then are calculated from the obtained body volume.

Initial research has shown that this technique compares favorably with hydrostatic weighing and is less cumbersome to administer. The procedure takes only about 5 minutes. Additional research is needed, however, to determine its accuracy among different age groups, ethnic backgrounds, and athletic populations. The published SEE for air displacement as compared with hydrostatic weighing is approximately ±2.2 percent; however, the SEE may actually be higher. Administering this assessment is relatively simple, but because of the high cost, the Bod Pod is not readily available in fitness centers and exercise laboratories.

## Skinfold Thickness

Because of the cost, time, and complexity of hydrostatic weighing and the expense of Bod Pod equipment, most health and fitness programs use **anthropometric measurement** techniques. These techniques, primarily skinfold thickness and girth measure-

**Dual energy X-ray absorptiometry (DXA)** Method to assess body composition that uses very low-dose beams of X-ray energy to measure total body fat mass, fat distribution pattern, and bone density.

**Hydrostatic weighing** Underwater technique to assess body composition; considered the most accurate of the body composition assessment techniques.

**Aquaphobic** Having a fear of water.

**Air displacement** Technique to assess body composition by calculating the body volume from the air replaced by an individual sitting inside a small chamber.

**Bod Pod** Commercial name of the equipment used to assess body composition through the air displacement technique.

**Anthropometric measurement** Techniques to measure body girths at different sites.

**FIGURE 4.2** Hydrostatic weighing procedure.

A small tank or pool, an autopsy scale, and a submersible chair are needed. The scale should measure up to about 10 kilograms (kg) and should be readable to the nearest .01 kilogram. The chair is suspended from the scale and submerged in a tank of water or pool measuring at least 5 × 5 × 5 feet. A swimming pool can be used in place of the tank.

The procedure for the technician is

1. Ask the person to be weighed to fast for approximately 6 to 8 hours and to have a bladder and bowel movement prior to underwater weighing.

2. Measure the individual's residual lung volume (RV, or amount of air left in the lungs following complete exhalation). If no equipment (spirometer) is available to measure the residual volume, estimate it using the following predicting equations* (to convert inches to centimeters, multiply inches by 2.54):

Men: $RV = [(0.027 \times \text{height in centimeters}) + (0.017 \times \text{age})] - 3.447$

Women: $RV = [(0.032 \times \text{height in centimeters}) + (0.009 \times \text{age})] - 3.9$

3. Have the person remove all jewelry prior to weighing. Weigh the person on land in a swimsuit and subtract the weight of the suit. Convert the weight from pounds to kilograms (divide pounds by 2.2046).

4. Record the water temperature in the tank in degrees Centigrade. Use that temperature to obtain the water density factor provided below, which is required in the formula to compute body density.

| Temp (°C) | Water Density (gr/ml) | Temp (°C) | Water Density (gr/ml) |
|---|---|---|---|
| 28 | 0.99626 | 35 | 0.99406 |
| 29 | 0.99595 | 36 | 0.99371 |
| 30 | 0.99567 | 37 | 0.99336 |
| 31 | 0.99537 | 38 | 0.99299 |
| 32 | 0.99505 | 39 | 0.99262 |
| 33 | 0.99473 | 40 | 0.99224 |
| 34 | 0.99440 | | |

5. After the person is dressed in the swimsuit, have him or her enter the tank and completely wipe off all air clinging to the skin. Have the person sit in the chair with the water at about chin level (raise or lower the chair as needed). If you do not have a system that uses computerized electronic sensors, make sure the water and scale remain as still as possible during the entire procedure, because this allows for a more accurate reading. (During underwater weighing, you can decrease scale movement by holding and slowly releasing the neck of the scale until the subject is floating freely in the water.)

ments, allow quick, simple, and inexpensive estimates of body composition.

Assessing body composition using **skinfold thickness** is based on the principle that the amount of **subcutaneous fat** is proportional to total body fat. Valid and reliable measurements of this tissue give a good indication of percent body fat. The SEE for skinfold analysis is ±3.5 percent.

The skinfold test is done with the aid of pressure calipers. Several techniques requiring measurement of three to seven sites have been developed. The following three-site procedure is the most commonly used technique. The sites measured are as follows (also see Figure 4.3):

- Women: triceps, suprailium, and thigh skinfolds
- Men: chest, abdomen, and thigh

All measurements should be taken on the right side of the body.

With the skinfold technique, training is necessary to obtain accurate measurements. In addition, different technicians may produce slightly different measurements of the same person. Therefore, the same technician should take pre- and post-test measurements.

Measurements should be done at the same time of the day—preferably in the morning—because changes in water hydration from activity and exercise can affect skinfold girth. The procedure is given in Figure 4.4. If skinfold calipers are available, you may assess your percent body

**Skinfold thickness** Technique to assess body composition by measuring a double thickness of skin at specific body sites.

**Subcutaneous fat** Deposits of fat directly under the skin.

**Girth measurements** Technique to assess body composition by measuring circumferences at specific body sites.

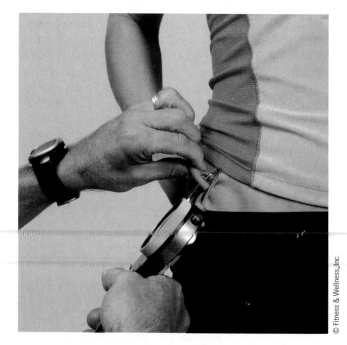

Skinfold thickness technique.

6. Now have the person forcefully exhale all of the air out of the lungs. The individual then totally submerges underwater. Make sure that all the air is exhaled from the lungs prior to submerging. Record the reading on the scale. Repeat this procedure 8 to 10 times, because practice and experience increase the accuracy of the underwater weight. Use the average of the three heaviest underwater weights as the gross underwater weight.

7. Because tare weight (the weight of the chair and chain or rope used to suspend the chair) accounts for part of the gross underwater weight, subtract this weight to obtain the person's net underwater weight. To determine tare weight, place a clothespin on the chain or rope at the water level when the ▊▊▊▊▊ ▊▊▊▊▊▊▊▊▊▊ ▊▊▊▊▊▊▊ ▊▊▊▊ ▊▊▊ ▊▊▊▊▊▊ ▊▊▊▊▊▊▊▊▊ ▊▊ the water, lower the chair into the water to the pin level. Now record tare weight. Determine the net underwater weight by subtracting the tare weight from the gross underwater weight.

8. Compute body density and percent fat using the following equations:

$$\text{Body density} = \frac{BW}{\dfrac{BW - UW}{WD} - RV - .1}$$

$$\text{Percent fat**} = \frac{495}{BD} - 450$$

**Where:**
BW = body weight in kg
UW = net underwater weight
WD = water density (determined by water temperature)
RV = residual volume
BD = body density

A sample computation for body fat assessment according to hydrostatic weighing is provided in Lab 4A.

*From H. L. Goldman and M. R. Becklake, "Respiratory function tests: normal values at medium altitudes and the prediction of normal results," in *American Review of Tuberculosis* 79 (1959): 457–467.
**From W. E. Siri, Body Composition from Fluid Spaces and Density (Berkeley: University of California, Donner Laboratory of Medical Physics, March 19, 1956.)

fat with the help of your instructor or an experienced technician (also see Lab 4B). Then locate the percent fat estimates on Table 4.1, 4.2, or 4.3, as appropriate.

## Girth Measurements
Another method that is frequently used to estimate body fat is to measure circumferences, or **girth measurements,** at various body sites. This technique requires only a standard measuring tape. The limitation is that it may not be valid for athletic individuals (men or women) who participate actively in strenuous physical activity or for people who can be classified

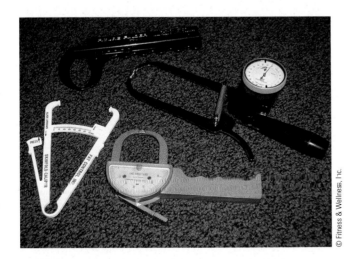

Various types of calipers used to assess skinfold thickness.

**FIGURE 4.3 Anatomical landmarks for skinfold measurements.**

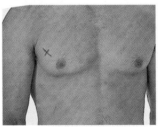
Chest (men)

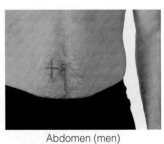
Abdomen (men)

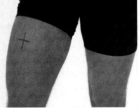
Thigh (men and women)

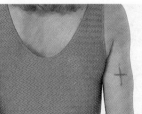
Triceps (women)

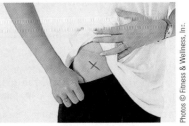
Suprailium (women)

© Fitness & Wellness, Inc.

Photos © Fitness & Wellness, Inc.

**FIGURE 4.4** Procedure for body fat assessment using skinfold thickness technique.

1. Select the proper anatomical sites. For men, use chest, abdomen, and thigh skinfolds. For women, use triceps, suprailium, and thigh skinfolds. Take all measurements on the right side of the body with the person standing. The correct anatomical landmarks for skinfolds are

Chest: a diagonal fold halfway between the shoulder crease and the nipple.

Abdomen: a vertical fold taken about one inch to the right of the umbilicus.

Triceps: a vertical fold on the back of the upper arm, halfway between the shoulder and the elbow.

Thigh: a vertical fold on the front of the thigh, midway between the knee and the hip.

Suprailium: a diagonal fold above the crest of the ilium (on the side of the hip).

2. Measure each site by grasping a double thickness of skin firmly with the thumb and forefinger, pulling the fold slightly away from the muscular tissue. Hold the calipers perpendicular to the fold and take the measurement ½ inch below the finger hold. Measure each site three times and read the values to the nearest .1 to .5 mm. Record the average of the two closest readings as the final value. Take the readings without delay to avoid excessive compression of the skinfold. Releasing and refolding the skinfold is required between readings.

3. When doing pre- and post-assessments, conduct the measurement at the same time of day. The best time is early in the morning to avoid hydration changes resulting from activity or exercise.

4. Obtain percent fat by adding the three skinfold measurements and looking up the respective values on Table 4.1 for women, Table 4.2 for men under age 40, and Table 4.3 for men over 40.

For example, if the skinfold measurements for an 18-year-old female are (a) triceps = 16, (b) suprailium = 4, and (c) thigh = 30 (total = 50), the percent body fat is 20.6%.

**TABLE 4.1** Skinfold Thickness Technique: Percent Fat Estimates for Women Calculated from Triceps, Suprailium, and Thigh

| Sum of 3 Skinfolds | Age at Last Birthday | | | | | | | | |
|---|---|---|---|---|---|---|---|---|---|
| | 22 or Under | 23 to 27 | 28 to 32 | 33 to 37 | 38 to 42 | 43 to 47 | 48 to 52 | 53 to 57 | 58 and Over |
| 23–25 | 9.7 | 9.9 | 10.2 | 10.4 | 10.7 | 10.9 | 11.2 | 11.4 | 11.7 |
| 26–28 | 11.0 | 11.2 | 11.5 | 11.7 | 12.0 | 12.3 | 12.5 | 12.7 | 13.0 |
| 29–31 | 12.3 | 12.5 | 12.8 | 13.0 | 13.3 | 13.5 | 13.8 | 14.0 | 14.3 |
| 32–34 | 13.6 | 13.8 | 14.0 | 14.3 | 14.5 | 14.8 | 15.0 | 15.3 | 15.5 |
| 35–37 | 14.8 | 15.0 | 15.3 | 15.5 | 15.8 | 16.0 | 16.3 | 16.5 | 16.8 |
| 38–40 | 16.0 | 16.3 | 16.5 | 16.7 | 17.0 | 17.2 | 17.5 | 17.7 | 18.0 |
| 41–43 | 17.2 | 17.4 | 17.7 | 17.9 | 18.2 | 18.4 | 18.7 | 18.9 | 19.2 |
| 44–46 | 18.3 | 18.6 | 18.8 | 19.1 | 19.3 | 19.6 | 19.8 | 20.1 | 20.3 |
| 47–49 | 19.5 | 19.7 | 20.0 | 20.2 | 20.5 | 20.7 | 21.0 | 21.2 | 21.5 |
| 50–52 | 20.6 | 20.8 | 21.1 | 21.3 | 21.6 | 21.8 | 22.1 | 22.3 | 22.6 |
| 53–55 | 21.7 | 21.9 | 22.1 | 22.4 | 22.6 | 22.9 | 23.1 | 23.4 | 23.6 |
| 56–58 | 22.7 | 23.0 | 23.2 | 23.4 | 23.7 | 23.9 | 24.2 | 24.4 | 24.7 |
| 59–61 | 23.7 | 24.0 | 24.2 | 24.5 | 24.7 | 25.0 | 25.2 | 25.5 | 25.7 |
| 62–64 | 24.7 | 25.0 | 25.2 | 25.5 | 25.7 | 26.0 | 26.2 | 26.4 | 26.7 |
| 65–67 | 25.7 | 25.9 | 26.2 | 26.4 | 26.7 | 26.9 | 27.2 | 27.4 | 27.7 |
| 68–70 | 26.6 | 26.9 | 27.1 | 27.4 | 27.6 | 27.9 | 28.1 | 28.4 | 28.6 |
| 71–73 | 27.5 | 27.8 | 28.0 | 28.3 | 28.5 | 28.8 | 29.0 | 29.3 | 29.5 |
| 74–76 | 28.4 | 28.7 | 28.9 | 29.2 | 29.4 | 29.7 | 29.9 | 30.2 | 30.4 |
| 77–79 | 29.3 | 29.5 | 29.8 | 30.0 | 30.3 | 30.5 | 30.8 | 31.0 | 31.3 |
| 80–82 | 30.1 | 30.4 | 30.6 | 30.9 | 31.1 | 31.4 | 31.6 | 31.9 | 32.1 |
| 83–85 | 30.9 | 31.2 | 31.4 | 31.7 | 31.9 | 32.2 | 32.4 | 32.7 | 32.9 |
| 86–88 | 31.7 | 32.0 | 32.2 | 32.5 | 32.7 | 32.9 | 33.2 | 33.4 | 33.7 |
| 89–91 | 32.5 | 32.7 | 33.0 | 33.2 | 33.5 | 33.7 | 33.9 | 34.2 | 34.4 |
| 92–94 | 33.2 | 33.4 | 33.7 | 33.9 | 34.2 | 34.4 | 34.7 | 34.9 | 35.2 |
| 95–97 | 33.9 | 34.1 | 34.4 | 34.6 | 34.9 | 35.1 | 35.4 | 35.6 | 35.9 |
| 98–100 | 34.6 | 34.8 | 35.1 | 35.3 | 35.5 | 35.8 | 36.0 | 36.3 | 36.5 |
| 101–103 | 35.2 | 35.4 | 35.7 | 35.9 | 36.2 | 36.4 | 36.7 | 36.9 | 37.2 |
| 104–106 | 35.8 | 36.1 | 36.3 | 36.6 | 36.8 | 37.1 | 37.3 | 37.5 | 37.8 |
| 107–109 | 36.4 | 36.7 | 36.9 | 37.1 | 37.4 | 37.6 | 37.9 | 38.1 | 38.4 |
| 110–112 | 37.0 | 37.2 | 37.5 | 37.7 | 38.0 | 38.2 | 38.5 | 38.7 | 38.9 |
| 113–115 | 37.5 | 37.8 | 38.0 | 38.2 | 38.5 | 38.7 | 39.0 | 39.2 | 39.5 |
| 116–118 | 38.0 | 38.3 | 38.5 | 38.8 | 39.0 | 39.3 | 39.5 | 39.7 | 40.0 |
| 119–121 | 38.5 | 38.7 | 39.0 | 39.2 | 39.5 | 39.7 | 40.0 | 40.2 | 40.5 |
| 122–124 | 39.0 | 39.2 | 39.4 | 39.7 | 39.9 | 40.2 | 40.4 | 40.7 | 40.9 |
| 125–127 | 39.4 | 39.6 | 39.9 | 40.1 | 40.4 | 40.6 | 40.9 | 41.1 | 41.4 |
| 128–130 | 39.8 | 40.0 | 40.3 | 40.5 | 40.8 | 41.0 | 41.3 | 41.5 | 41.8 |

Body density is calculated based on the generalized equation for predicting body density of women developed by A. S. Jackson, M. L. Pollock, and A. Ward and published in *Medicine and Science in Sports and Exercise* 12 (1980): 175–182. Percent body fat is determined from the calculated body density using the Siri formula.

visually as thin or obese. The SEE for girth measurements is approximately 4 percent.

The required procedure for girth measurements is given in Figure 4.5; conversion factors are in Tables 4.4 and 4.5. Measurements for women are the upper arm, hip, and wrist; for men, the waist and wrist.

# Bioelectrical Impedance The **bioelectrical impedance** technique is much simpler to administer, but its accuracy is questionable. In this technique, sensors are applied to the skin, and a weak (totally painless) electrical current is run through the body to estimate body fat, lean body mass, and body water. The technique is based on the principle that fat tissue is a less efficient conductor of electrical current than is lean tissue. The easier the conductance, the leaner the individual. Body weight scales

**Bioelectrical impedance** Technique to assess body composition by running a weak electrical current through the body.

**TABLE 4.2** Skinfold Thickness Technique: Percent Fat Estimates for Men Under 40 Calculated from Chest, Abdomen, and Thigh

| Sum of 3 Skinfolds | 19 or Under | 20 to 22 | 23 to 25 | 26 to 28 | 29 to 31 | 32 to 34 | 35 to 37 | 38 to 40 |
|---|---|---|---|---|---|---|---|---|
| | | | | Age at Last Birthday | | | | |
| 8–10 | .9 | 1.3 | 1.6 | 2.0 | 2.3 | 2.7 | 3.0 | 3.3 |
| 11–13 | 1.9 | 2.3 | 2.6 | 3.0 | 3.3 | 3.7 | 4.0 | 4.3 |
| 14–16 | 2.9 | 3.3 | 3.6 | 3.9 | 4.3 | 4.6 | 5.0 | 5.3 |
| 17–19 | 3.9 | 4.2 | 4.6 | 4.9 | 5.3 | 5.6 | 6.0 | 6.3 |
| 20–22 | 4.8 | 5.2 | 5.5 | 5.9 | 6.2 | 6.6 | 6.9 | 7.3 |
| 23–25 | 5.8 | 6.2 | 6.5 | 6.9 | 7.2 | 7.5 | 7.9 | 8.2 |
| 26–28 | 6.8 | 7.1 | 7.5 | 7.8 | 8.1 | 8.5 | 8.8 | 9.2 |
| 29–31 | 7.7 | 8.0 | 8.4 | 8.7 | 9.1 | 9.4 | 9.8 | 10.1 |
| 32–34 | 8.6 | 9.0 | 9.3 | 9.7 | 10.0 | 10.4 | 10.7 | 11.1 |
| 35–37 | 9.5 | 9.9 | 10.2 | 10.6 | 10.9 | 11.3 | 11.6 | 12.0 |
| 38–40 | 10.5 | 10.8 | 11.2 | 11.5 | 11.8 | 12.2 | 12.5 | 12.9 |
| 41–43 | 11.4 | 11.7 | 12.1 | 12.4 | 12.7 | 13.1 | 13.4 | 13.8 |
| 44–46 | 12.2 | 12.6 | 12.9 | 13.3 | 13.6 | 14.0 | 14.3 | 14.7 |
| 47–49 | 13.1 | 13.5 | 13.8 | 14.2 | 14.5 | 14.9 | 15.2 | 15.5 |
| 50–52 | 14.0 | 14.3 | 14.7 | 15.0 | 15.4 | 15.7 | 16.1 | 16.4 |
| 53–55 | 14.8 | 15.2 | 15.5 | 15.9 | 16.2 | 16.6 | 16.9 | 17.3 |
| 56–58 | 15.7 | 16.0 | 16.4 | 16.7 | 17.1 | 17.4 | 17.8 | 18.1 |
| 59–61 | 16.5 | 16.9 | 17.2 | 17.6 | 17.9 | 18.3 | 18.6 | 19.0 |
| 62–64 | 17.4 | 17.7 | 18.1 | 18.4 | 18.8 | 19.1 | 19.4 | 19.8 |
| 65–67 | 18.2 | 18.5 | 18.9 | 19.2 | 19.6 | 19.9 | 20.3 | 20.6 |
| 68–70 | 19.0 | 19.3 | 19.7 | 20.0 | 20.4 | 20.7 | 21.1 | 21.4 |
| 71–73 | 19.8 | 20.1 | 20.5 | 20.8 | 21.2 | 21.5 | 21.9 | 22.2 |
| 74–76 | 20.6 | 20.9 | 21.3 | 21.6 | 22.0 | 22.2 | 22.7 | 23.0 |
| 77–79 | 21.4 | 21.7 | 22.1 | 22.4 | 22.8 | 23.1 | 23.4 | 23.8 |
| 80–82 | 22.1 | 22.5 | 22.8 | 23.2 | 23.5 | 23.9 | 24.2 | 24.6 |
| 83–85 | 22.9 | 23.2 | 23.6 | 23.9 | 24.3 | 24.6 | 25.0 | 25.3 |
| 86–88 | 23.6 | 24.0 | 24.3 | 24.7 | 25.0 | 25.4 | 25.7 | 26.1 |
| 89–91 | 24.4 | 24.7 | 25.1 | 25.4 | 25.8 | 26.1 | 26.5 | 26.8 |
| 92–94 | 25.1 | 25.5 | 25.8 | 26.2 | 26.5 | 26.9 | 27.2 | 27.5 |
| 95–97 | 25.8 | 26.2 | 26.5 | 26.9 | 27.2 | 27.6 | 27.9 | 28.3 |
| 98–100 | 26.6 | 26.9 | 27.3 | 27.6 | 27.9 | 28.3 | 28.6 | 29.0 |
| 101–103 | 27.3 | 27.6 | 28.0 | 28.3 | 28.6 | 29.0 | 29.3 | 29.7 |
| 104–106 | 27.9 | 28.3 | 28.6 | 29.0 | 29.3 | 29.7 | 30.0 | 30.4 |
| 107–109 | 28.6 | 29.0 | 29.3 | 29.7 | 30.0 | 30.4 | 30.7 | 31.1 |
| 110–112 | 29.3 | 29.6 | 30.0 | 30.3 | 30.7 | 31.0 | 31.4 | 31.7 |
| 113–115 | 30.0 | 30.3 | 30.7 | 31.0 | 31.3 | 31.7 | 32.0 | 32.4 |
| 116–118 | 30.6 | 31.0 | 31.3 | 31.6 | 32.0 | 32.3 | 32.7 | 33.0 |
| 119–121 | 31.3 | 31.6 | 32.0 | 32.3 | 32.6 | 33.0 | 33.3 | 33.7 |
| 122–124 | 31.9 | 32.2 | 32.6 | 32.9 | 33.3 | 33.6 | 34.0 | 34.3 |
| 125–127 | 32.5 | 32.9 | 33.2 | 33.5 | 33.9 | 34.2 | 34.6 | 34.9 |
| 128–130 | 33.1 | 33.5 | 33.8 | 34.2 | 34.5 | 34.9 | 35.2 | 35.5 |

**TABLE 4.3** Skinfold Thickness Technique: Percent Fat Estimates for Men over 40 Calculated from Chest, Abdomen, and Thigh

| Sum of 3 Skinfolds | 41 to 43 | 44 to 46 | 47 to 49 | 50 to 52 | 53 to 55 | 56 to 58 | 59 to 61 | 62 and Over |
|---|---|---|---|---|---|---|---|---|
| | | | | Age at Last Birthday | | | | |
| 8–10 | 3.7 | 4.0 | 4.4 | 4.7 | 5.1 | 5.4 | 5.8 | 6.1 |
| 11–13 | 4.7 | 5.0 | 5.4 | 5.7 | 6.1 | 6.4 | 6.8 | 7.1 |
| 14–16 | 5.7 | 6.0 | 6.4 | 6.7 | 7.1 | 7.4 | 7.8 | 8.1 |
| 17–19 | 6.7 | 7.0 | 7.4 | 7.7 | 8.1 | 8.4 | 8.7 | 9.1 |
| 20–22 | 7.6 | 8.0 | 8.3 | 8.7 | 9.0 | 9.4 | 9.7 | 10.1 |
| 23–25 | 8.6 | 8.9 | 9.3 | 9.6 | 10.0 | 10.3 | 10.7 | 11.0 |
| 26–28 | 9.5 | 9.9 | 10.2 | 10.6 | 10.9 | 11.3 | 11.6 | 12.0 |
| 29–31 | 10.5 | 10.8 | 11.2 | 11.5 | 11.9 | 12.2 | 12.6 | 12.9 |
| 32–34 | 11.4 | 11.8 | 12.1 | 12.4 | 12.8 | 13.1 | 13.5 | 13.8 |
| 35–37 | 12.3 | 12.7 | 13.0 | 13.4 | 13.7 | 14.1 | 14.4 | 14.8 |
| 38–40 | 13.2 | 13.6 | 13.9 | 14.3 | 14.6 | 15.0 | 15.3 | 15.7 |
| 41–43 | 14.1 | 14.5 | 14.8 | 15.2 | 15.5 | 15.9 | 16.2 | 16.6 |
| 44–46 | 15.0 | 15.4 | 15.7 | 16.1 | 16.4 | 16.8 | 17.1 | 17.5 |
| 47–49 | 15.9 | 16.2 | 16.6 | 16.9 | 17.3 | 17.6 | 18.0 | 18.3 |
| 50–52 | 16.8 | 17.1 | 17.5 | 17.8 | 18.2 | 18.5 | 18.8 | 19.2 |
| 53–55 | 17.6 | 18.0 | 18.3 | 18.7 | 19.0 | 19.4 | 19.7 | 20.1 |
| 56–58 | 18.5 | 18.8 | 19.2 | 19.5 | 19.9 | 20.2 | 20.6 | 20.9 |
| 59–61 | 19.3 | 19.7 | 20.0 | 20.4 | 20.7 | 21.0 | 21.4 | 21.7 |
| 62–64 | 20.1 | 20.5 | 20.8 | 21.2 | 21.5 | 21.9 | 22.2 | 22.6 |
| 65–67 | 21.0 | 21.3 | 21.7 | 22.0 | 22.4 | 22.7 | 23.0 | 23.4 |
| 68–70 | 21.8 | 22.1 | 22.5 | 22.8 | 23.2 | 23.5 | 23.9 | 24.2 |
| 71–73 | 22.6 | 22.9 | 23.3 | 23.6 | 24.0 | 24.3 | 24.7 | 25.0 |
| 74–76 | 23.4 | 23.7 | 24.1 | 24.4 | 24.8 | 25.1 | 25.4 | 25.8 |
| 77–79 | 24.1 | 24.5 | 24.8 | 25.2 | 25.5 | 25.9 | 26.2 | 26.6 |
| 80–82 | 24.9 | 25.3 | 25.6 | 26.0 | 26.3 | 26.6 | 27.0 | 27.3 |
| 83–85 | 25.7 | 26.0 | 26.4 | 26.7 | 27.1 | 27.4 | 27.8 | 28.1 |
| 86–88 | 26.4 | 26.8 | 27.1 | 27.5 | 27.8 | 28.2 | 28.5 | 28.9 |
| 89–91 | 27.2 | 27.5 | 27.9 | 28.2 | 28.6 | 28.9 | 29.2 | 29.6 |
| 92–94 | 27.9 | 28.2 | 28.6 | 28.9 | 29.3 | 29.6 | 30.0 | 30.3 |
| 95–97 | 28.6 | 29.0 | 29.3 | 29.7 | 30.0 | 30.4 | 30.7 | 31.1 |
| 98–100 | 29.3 | 29.7 | 30.0 | 30.4 | 30.7 | 31.1 | 31.4 | 31.8 |
| 101–103 | 30.0 | 30.4 | 30.7 | 31.1 | 31.4 | 31.8 | 32.1 | 32.5 |
| 104–106 | 30.7 | 31.1 | 31.4 | 31.8 | 32.1 | 32.5 | 32.8 | 33.2 |
| 107–109 | 31.4 | 31.8 | 32.1 | 32.4 | 32.8 | 33.1 | 33.5 | 33.8 |
| 110–112 | 32.1 | 32.4 | 32.8 | 33.1 | 33.5 | 33.8 | 34.2 | 34.5 |
| 113–115 | 32.7 | 33.1 | 33.4 | 33.8 | 34.1 | 34.5 | 34.8 | 35.2 |
| 116–118 | 33.4 | 33.7 | 34.1 | 34.4 | 34.8 | 35.1 | 35.5 | 35.8 |
| 119–121 | 34.0 | 34.4 | 34.7 | 35.1 | 35.4 | 35.8 | 36.1 | 36.5 |
| 122–124 | 34.7 | 35.0 | 35.4 | 35.7 | 36.1 | 36.4 | 36.7 | 37.1 |
| 125–127 | 35.3 | 35.6 | 36.0 | 36.3 | 36.7 | 37.0 | 37.4 | 37.7 |
| 128–130 | 35.9 | 36.2 | 36.6 | 36.9 | 37.3 | 37.6 | 38.0 | 38.5 |

Body density is calculated based on the generalized equation for predicting body density of men developed by A. S. Jackson and M. L. Pollock and published in the *British Journal of Nutrition* 40 (1978): 497–504. Percent body fat is determined from the calculated body density using the Siri formula.

**FIGURE 4.5  Procedure for body fat assessment according to girth measurements.**

### Girth Measurements for Women*

1. Using a regular tape measure, determine the following girth measurements in centimeters (cm):

   Upper arm:  Take the measure halfway between the shoulder and the elbow.

   Hip:  Measure at the point of largest circumference.

   Wrist:  Take the girth in front of the bones where the wrist bends.

2. Obtain the person's age.

3. Using Table 4.4, find the subject's age, girth measurement for each site in the left column below, then look up the constant values for each. These values will allow you to derive body density (BD) by substituting the constants in the following formula:

   BD = A − B − C + D

4. Using the derived body density, calculate percent body fat (%F) according to the following equation:

   %F = (495 ÷ BD) − 450**

**Example:** Jane is 20 years old, and the following girth measurements were taken: biceps = 27 cm, hip = 99.5 cm, wrist = 15.4 cm

| Data | Constant |
|---|---|
| Upper arm = 27 cm | A = 1.0813 |
| Age = 20 | B = .0102 |
| Hip = 99.5 cm | C = .1206 |
| Wrist = 15.4 cm | D = .0971 |

BD = A − B − C + D
BD = 1.0813 − .0102 − .1206 + .0971 = 1.0476

%F = (495 ÷ BD) − 450
%F = (495 ÷ 1.0476) − 450 = 22.5

### Girth Measurements for Men***

1. Using a regular tape measure, determine the following girth measurements in inches (the men's measurements are taken in inches, as opposed to centimeters for women):

   Waist:  Measure at the umbilicus (belly button).

   Wrist:  Measure in front of the bones where the wrist bends.

2. Subtract the wrist from the waist measurement.

3. Obtain the weight of the subject in pounds.

4. Look up the percent body fat (%F) in Table 4.5 by using the difference obtained in number 2 above and the person's body weight.

**Example:** John weighs 160 pounds, and his waist and wrist girth measurements are 36.5 and 7.5 inches, respectively.

Waist girth = 36.5 inches
Wrist girth = 7.5 inches
Difference = 29.0 inches
Body weight = 160.0 lbs.
%F = 22

---

*From R. B. Lambson, "Generalized body density prediction equations for women using simple anthropometric measurements." Unpublished doctoral dissertation, Brigham Young University, Provo, UT, August 1987. Reproduced by permission.
**From W. E. Siri, Body Composition from Fluid Spaces and Density (Berkeley: University of California, Donner Laboratory of Medical Physics, March 19, 1956.)
***From A. G. Fisher and P. E. Allsen, Jogging, Dubuque, IA: Wm. C. Brown, 1987. This table was developed according to "Generalized body composition equation for men using simple measurement techniques," by K. W. Penrouse, A. G. Nelson, and A. G. Fisher, *Medicine and Science in Sports and Exercise* 17, no. 2 (1985): 189. © American College of Sports Medicine, 1985.

with sensors on the surface also are available to conduct this procedure.

The accuracy of equations used to estimate percent body fat with this technique is questionable. A single equation cannot be used for everyone, but rather valid and accurate equations to estimate body fat for the specific population (age, gender, and ethnicity) being tested are required. Following all manufacturers' instructions will ensure the most accurate result, but even then percent body fat may be off by as much as 10 percentage points (or even more on some scales).

---

**Body mass index (BMI)** Technique to determine thinness and excessive fatness that incorporates height and weight to estimate critical fat values at which the risk for disease increases.

## Body Mass Index

The most common technique to determine thinness and excessive fatness is the **body mass index (BMI).** BMI incorporates height and weight to estimate critical fat values at which the risk for disease increases.

BMI is calculated by either (a) dividing the weight in kilograms by the square of the height in meters or (b) multiplying body weight in pounds by 705 and dividing this figure by the square of the height in inches. For example, the BMI for an individual who weighs 172 pounds (78 kg) and is 67 inches (1.7 m) tall would be 27: $[78 ÷ (1.7)^2]$ or $[172 × 705 ÷ (67)^2]$. You also can look up your BMI in Table 4.6 according to your height and weight.

Because of its simplicity and measurement consistency across populations, BMI is the most widely used measure to determine overweight and obesity. Due to the various

**TABLE 4.5  Girth Measurement Technique: Estimated Percent Body Fat for Men**

Waist Minus Wrist Girth Measurement (inches)

| Body Weight (pounds) | Estimated Percent Body Fat |
|---|---|
| 120 | 4  8  10  14  16  18  20  21  23  25  27  29  31  33  35  37  39  41  43  45  47  49  50  52  54  56  58 |
| 125 | 4  6  7  9  13  15  17  19  20  22  24  26  28  30  32  33  35  37  39  41  43  45  46  48  50  52  54  56  58 |
| 130 | 3  5  7  9  12  14  16  18  20  21  23  25  27  28  30  32  34  36  37  39  41  43  44  46  48  50  52  53  55  57 |
| 135 | 3  5  7  8  12  13  15  17  19  20  22  24  26  27  29  31  32  34  36  38  39  41  43  44  46  48  50  51  53  55  56 |
| 140 | 3  5  6  8  11  13  15  16  18  19  21  23  24  26  28  29  31  33  34  36  38  39  41  43  44  46  48  49  51  53  54  56 |
| 145 | 3  4  6  7  11  12  14  15  17  19  20  22  23  25  27  28  30  31  33  35  36  38  39  41  43  44  46  47  49  51  52  54  55 |
| 150 | 2  4  6  7  10  12  13  15  16  18  19  21  23  24  26  27  29  30  32  33  35  36  38  40  41  43  44  46  47  49  50  52  53  55 |
| 155 | 2  4  5  7  10  11  13  14  16  17  19  20  22  23  25  26  28  29  31  32  34  35  37  38  40  41  43  44  46  47  49  50  52  53  55 |
| 160 | 2  4  5  6  10  11  12  14  15  17  18  19  21  22  24  25  27  28  30  31  33  34  36  37  39  40  41  43  44  46  47  48  50  51  53  54 |
| 165 | 2  3  5  6  9  10  12  13  15  16  17  19  20  22  23  25  26  27  29  30  32  33  34  36  37  39  40  41  43  44  45  47  48  50  51  52  54 |
| 170 | 2  3  4  6  9  10  11  13  14  15  17  18  20  21  22  24  25  26  28  29  31  32  33  35  36  37  39  40  41  43  44  45  47  48  49  51  52  54 |
| 175 | 2  3  4  6  8  10  11  12  13  15  16  17  19  20  21  23  24  25  27  28  29  31  32  33  35  36  37  39  40  41  43  44  45  47  48  49  50  52  53 |
| 180 | 3  4  5  9  10  12  13  14  16  17  18  19  21  22  23  25  26  27  28  30  31  32  34  35  36  38  39  40  41  43  44  45  47  48  49  50  52  53 |
| 185 | 3  4  5  9  10  11  13  14  15  16  18  19  20  21  23  24  25  27  28  29  30  32  33  34  36  37  38  39  41  42  43  44  46  47  48  49  50  51  53 |
| 190 | 2  4  5  8  10  11  12  13  15  16  17  18  20  21  22  24  25  26  27  29  30  31  33  34  35  37  38  39  40  41  43  44  45  46  47  49  50  51  52 |
| 195 | 2  3  5  8  9  11  12  13  14  16  17  18  19  21  22  23  24  26  27  28  29  31  32  33  34  36  37  38  39  40  42  43  44  45  46  47  49  50  51  52 |
| 200 | 2  3  4  7  8  9  11  12  13  14  16  17  18  19  20  22  23  24  25  26  28  29  30  31  32  34  35  36  37  38  40  41  42  43  44  45  46  47  49  50  51  52 |
| 205 | 2  3  4  7  8  9  10  11  12  14  15  16  17  18  20  21  22  23  24  25  26  28  29  30  31  32  33  35  36  37  38  39  40  42  43  44  45  46  47  48  49  51  52 |
| 210 | 2  3  4  7  8  9  10  11  12  13  14  16  17  18  19  20  21  22  23  25  26  27  28  29  30  31  32  33  35  36  37  38  39  40  41  42  43  44  45  46  47  48  49  50  51 |
| 215 | 2  3  4  6  8  9  9  11  12  13  14  15  16  17  18  19  20  22  23  24  25  26  27  28  29  30  31  32  33  34  35  36  37  38  39  40  42  43  44  45  46  47  48  49  50  51 |
| 220 | 2  3  6  7  8  9  10  11  12  13  14  15  16  18  19  20  21  22  23  24  25  26  27  28  29  30  31  32  33  34  35  36  37  38  39  40  41  42  43  44  45  46  47  48  49  50 |
| 225 | 2  3  6  7  8  9  10  11  12  13  14  15  16  17  18  19  20  21  22  23  24  25  26  27  28  29  30  31  32  33  34  35  36  37  38  39  40  41  42  43  44  45  46  47  48  49  50 |
| 230 | 2  3  5  6  7  8  9  10  11  12  13  14  15  16  17  18  19  20  21  22  23  24  25  26  27  28  29  30  31  32  33  34  35  36  37  38  39  40  41  42  43  44  44  45  46  47  48  49  50 |
| 235 | 2  3  5  6  7  8  9  10  11  12  13  14  15  16  17  18  19  20  21  22  23  24  24  25  26  27  28  29  30  31  32  33  34  35  36  37  38  39  40  41  42  43  44  45  46  47  48  49  50 |
| 240 | 2  3  5  6  7  8  9  10  11  12  13  14  15  16  17  18  19  20  20  21  22  23  24  25  26  27  28  29  30  31  32  33  34  35  36  37  38  39  40  41  42  43  44  44  45  46  47  48  49  50 |
| 245 | 2  3  4  6  7  8  9  9  10  11  12  13  14  15  16  17  18  19  20  21  22  23  24  24  25  26  27  28  29  30  31  32  33  34  35  36  36  37  38  39  40  41  42  43  44  44  45  46  47  48  49  50 |
| 250 | 2  3  4  5  6  7  8  9  10  11  12  13  14  15  16  17  18  19  20  21  22  23  24  25  25  26  27  28  29  30  31  32  33  34  35  36  37  38  38  39  40  41  42  43  44  44  45  46  47  48  49  50 |
| 255 | 2  3  4  5  6  7  8  9  10  11  12  13  14  15  16  17  18  18  19  20  21  22  23  24  25  26  26  27  28  29  30  31  32  33  34  35  36  36  37  38  39  40  41  42  43  43  44  45  46  47  48  49 |
| 260 | 2  3  4  5  6  7  8  9  10  11  11  12  13  14  15  16  17  18  19  20  21  22  23  23  24  25  26  27  28  29  30  31  32  33  33  34  35  36  37  38  39  40  41  42  42  43  44  45  46  47  48  49 |
| 265 | 2  3  4  5  6  7  8  9  10  11  12  13  14  15  16  16  17  18  19  20  21  22  23  23  24  25  26  27  28  29  30  31  32  32  33  34  35  36  37  38  39  40  41  41  42  43  44  45  46  47  48 |
| 270 | 2  3  4  5  6  7  8  8  9  10  11  12  13  14  15  16  17  18  19  20  20  21  22  23  24  25  26  26  27  28  29  30  31  32  33  34  34  35  36  37  38  39  40  41  41  42  43  44  45  46  47  48 |
| 275 | 2  3  4  5  6  7  8  9  10  11  12  13  14  15  16  17  18  19  19  20  21  22  23  24  25  26  26  27  28  29  30  31  32  32  33  34  35  36  37  38  39  40  41  42  43  44  45  46 |
| 280 | 2  3  4  4  5  6  7  8  9  10  11  12  13  14  15  16  16  17  18  19  20  21  22  23  24  24  25  26  27  28  29  30  31  31  32  33  34  35  36  37  38  39  40  41  42  43  44  45  46 |
| 285 | 2  3  4  5  6  7  8  8  9  10  11  12  13  14  15  16  17  18  19  19  20  21  22  23  24  24  25  26  27  28  29  30  30  31  32  33  34  35  36  37  38  39  40  41  42  43  44  45 |
| 290 | 2  3  4  5  6  6  7  8  9  10  11  12  13  14  15  15  16  17  18  19  20  21  22  23  23  24  25  26  27  28  29  30  31  31  32  33  34  35  36  37  38  39  40  41  42  43  44 |
| 295 | 2  3  4  5  6  6  7  8  9  10  11  12  13  14  14  15  16  17  18  19  20  21  22  22  23  24  25  26  27  28  29  30  31  31  32  33  34  35  36  37  38  39  40  41  42  43 |
| 300 | 2  3  4  5  5  6  7  8  9  10  11  12  13  14  15  16  17  18  19  20  21  22  23  24  25  26  27  28  29  30  31  32  33  34  35  36  37  38  39  40  41  42  43 |

PRINCIPLES AND LABS

**TABLE 4.6  Determination of Body Mass Index (BMI)**

Determine your BMI by looking up the number where your weight and height intersect on the table. According to the results, look up your disease risk in Tables 4.7 and 4.9.

| HEIGHT | 110 | 115 | 120 | 125 | 130 | 135 | 140 | 145 | 150 | 155 | 160 | 165 | 170 | 175 | 180 | 185 | 190 | 195 | 200 | 205 | 210 | 215 | 220 | 225 | 230 | 235 | 240 | 245 | 250 |
|---|---|---|---|---|---|---|---|---|---|---|---|---|---|---|---|---|---|---|---|---|---|---|---|---|---|---|---|---|---|
| 5'0" | 21 | 22 | 23 | 24 | 25 | 26 | 27 | 28 | 29 | 30 | 31 | 32 | 33 | 34 | 35 | 36 | 37 | 38 | 39 | 40 | 41 | 42 | 43 | 44 | 45 | 46 | 47 | 48 | 49 |
| 5'1" | 21 | 22 | 23 | 24 | 25 | 26 | 26 | 27 | 28 | 29 | 30 | 31 | 32 | 33 | 34 | 35 | 36 | 37 | 38 | 39 | 40 | 41 | 42 | 43 | 43 | 44 | 45 | 46 | 47 |
| 5'2" | 20 | 21 | 22 | 23 | 24 | 25 | 26 | 27 | 27 | 28 | 29 | 30 | 31 | 32 | 33 | 34 | 35 | 36 | 37 | 37 | 38 | 39 | 40 | 41 | 42 | 43 | 44 | 45 | 46 |
| 5'3" | 19 | 20 | 21 | 22 | 23 | 24 | 25 | 26 | 27 | 27 | 28 | 29 | 30 | 31 | 32 | 33 | 34 | 35 | 35 | 36 | 37 | 38 | 39 | 40 | 41 | 42 | 43 | 43 | 44 |
| 5'4" | 19 | 20 | 21 | 21 | 22 | 23 | 24 | 25 | 26 | 27 | 27 | 28 | 29 | 30 | 31 | 32 | 33 | 33 | 34 | 35 | 36 | 37 | 38 | 39 | 39 | 40 | 41 | 42 | 43 |
| 5'5" | 18 | 19 | 20 | 21 | 22 | 22 | 23 | 24 | 25 | 26 | 27 | 27 | 28 | 29 | 30 | 31 | 32 | 32 | 33 | 34 | 35 | 36 | 37 | 37 | 38 | 39 | 40 | 41 | 42 |
| 5'6" | 18 | 19 | 19 | 20 | 21 | 22 | 23 | 23 | 24 | 25 | 26 | 27 | 27 | 28 | 29 | 30 | 31 | 31 | 32 | 33 | 34 | 35 | 36 | 36 | 37 | 38 | 39 | 40 | 40 |
| 5'7" | 17 | 18 | 19 | 20 | 20 | 21 | 22 | 23 | 23 | 24 | 25 | 26 | 27 | 27 | 28 | 29 | 30 | 31 | 31 | 32 | 33 | 34 | 34 | 35 | 36 | 37 | 38 | 38 | 39 |
| 5'8" | 17 | 17 | 18 | 19 | 20 | 21 | 21 | 22 | 23 | 24 | 24 | 25 | 26 | 27 | 27 | 28 | 29 | 30 | 30 | 31 | 32 | 33 | 33 | 34 | 35 | 36 | 36 | 37 | 38 |
| 5'9" | 16 | 17 | 18 | 18 | 19 | 20 | 21 | 21 | 22 | 23 | 24 | 24 | 25 | 26 | 27 | 27 | 28 | 29 | 30 | 30 | 31 | 32 | 32 | 33 | 34 | 35 | 35 | 36 | 37 |
| 5'10" | 16 | 17 | 17 | 18 | 19 | 19 | 20 | 21 | 22 | 22 | 23 | 24 | 24 | 25 | 26 | 27 | 27 | 28 | 29 | 29 | 30 | 31 | 32 | 32 | 33 | 34 | 34 | 35 | 36 |
| 5'11" | 15 | 16 | 17 | 17 | 18 | 19 | 20 | 20 | 21 | 22 | 22 | 23 | 24 | 24 | 25 | 26 | 26 | 27 | 28 | 29 | 29 | 30 | 31 | 31 | 32 | 33 | 33 | 34 | 35 |
| 6'0" | 15 | 16 | 16 | 17 | 18 | 18 | 19 | 20 | 20 | 21 | 22 | 22 | 23 | 24 | 24 | 25 | 26 | 26 | 27 | 28 | 28 | 29 | 30 | 31 | 31 | 32 | 33 | 33 | 34 |
| 6'1" | 15 | 15 | 16 | 16 | 17 | 18 | 18 | 19 | 20 | 20 | 21 | 22 | 22 | 23 | 24 | 24 | 25 | 26 | 26 | 27 | 28 | 28 | 29 | 30 | 30 | 31 | 32 | 32 | 33 |
| 6'2" | 14 | 15 | 15 | 16 | 17 | 17 | 18 | 19 | 19 | 20 | 21 | 21 | 22 | 22 | 23 | 24 | 24 | 25 | 26 | 26 | 27 | 28 | 28 | 29 | 30 | 30 | 31 | 31 | 32 |
| 6'3" | 14 | 14 | 15 | 16 | 16 | 17 | 17 | 18 | 19 | 19 | 20 | 21 | 21 | 22 | 22 | 23 | 24 | 24 | 25 | 26 | 26 | 27 | 27 | 28 | 29 | 29 | 30 | 31 | 31 |
| 6'4" | 13 | 14 | 15 | 15 | 16 | 16 | 17 | 18 | 18 | 19 | 19 | 20 | 21 | 21 | 22 | 23 | 23 | 24 | 24 | 25 | 26 | 26 | 27 | 27 | 28 | 29 | 29 | 30 | 30 |

**FIGURE 4.6  Mortality risk versus body mass index (BMI).**

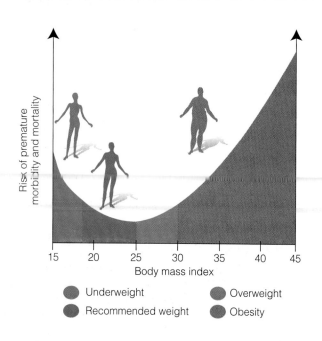

Risk of premature morbidity and mortality

Body mass index

- Underweight
- Recommended weight
- Overweight
- Obesity

limitations of previously mentioned body composition techniques—including cost, availability to the general population, lack of consistency among technicians and laboratories, inconsistent results between techniques, and standard error of measurement of the procedures—BMI is used almost exclusively to determine health risks and mortality rates associated with excessive body weight.

Scientific evidence indicates that the risk for disease starts to increase when BMI exceeds 25.[1] Although a BMI index between 18.5 and 25 is considered normal (see Tables 4.7 and 4.9), the lowest risk for chronic disease is in the 22-to-25 range.[2] Individuals are classified as overweight if their indexes lie between 25 and 30. BMIs above 30 are defined as obese, and those below 18.5 as **underweight.** Scientific evidence has shown that even though the risk for premature illness and death is greater for those who are overweight, the risk also increases for individuals who are underweight[3] (Figure 4.6).

Compared with individuals with BMIs between 22 and 25, people with BMIs between 25 and 30 (overweight) exhibit mortality rates up to 25 percent higher; rates for those with BMIs above 30 (obese) are 50 to 100 percent higher.[4] Table 4.7 provides disease risk categories when BMI is used as the sole criterion to identify people at risk. More than one-fifth of the U.S. adult population has a BMI

**FIGURE 4.7** Overweight and Obesity Trends in the United States, 1960–2000.

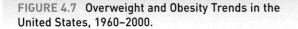
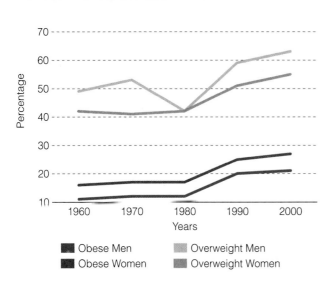

Legend: Obese Men · Overweight Men · Obese Women · Overweight Women

Adapted from the National Center for Health Statistics, Centers for Disease Control and Prevention, and the *Journal of the American Medical Association.*

**TABLE 4.7** Disease Risk According to Body Mass Index (BMI)

| BMI | Disease Risk | Classification |
| --- | --- | --- |
| <18.5 | Increased | Underweight |
| 18.5–21.99 | Low | Acceptable |
| 22.0–24.99 | Very Low | Acceptable |
| 25.0–29.99 | Increased | Overweight |
| 30.0–34.99 | High | Obesity I |
| 35.0–39.99 | Very High | Obesity II |
| ≥40.00 | Extremely High | Obesity III |

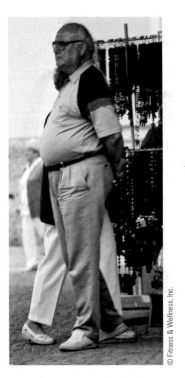

Individuals who accumulate body fat around the midsection are at greater risk for disease than those who accumulate body fat in other areas.

of 30 or more. Overweight and obesity trends starting in 1960 according to BMI are given in Figure 4.7.

BMI is a useful tool to screen the general population, but its one weakness is that it fails to differentiate fat from lean body mass or note where most of the fat is located (waist circumference—see discussion that follows). Using BMI, athletes with a large amount of muscle mass (such as body builders and football players) can easily fall in the moderate- or even high-risk categories.

**Waist Circumference** Scientific evidence suggests that the way people store fat affects their risk for disease. The total amount of body fat by itself is not the best predictor of increased risk for disease but, rather, the location of the fat. **Android obesity** is seen in individuals who tend to store fat in the trunk or abdominal area (which produces the "apple" shape). **Gynoid obesity** is seen in people who store fat primarily around the hips and thighs (which creates the "pear" shape).

Obese individuals with abdominal fat are clearly at higher risk for heart disease, hypertension, type 2 diabetes ("non-insulin-dependent" diabetes), and stroke than are obese individuals with similar amounts of body fat that is stored primarily in the hips and thighs.[5] Evidence also indicates that among individuals with a lot of abdominal fat, those whose fat deposits are located around internal organs (intra-abdominal or abdominal visceral fat) have an even greater risk for disease than those with fat mainly just beneath the skin (subcutaneous fat).[6]

Complex scanning techniques to identify individuals at risk because of high intra-abdominal fatness are costly, so a simple **waist circumference (WC)** measure, designed by the National Heart, Lung, and Blood Institute, is used to assess this risk.[7] WC seems to predict abdominal visceral fat as accurately as the DXA technique.[8] A waist circumference of more than 40 inches in men and 35 inches in women indicates a higher risk for cardiovascular disease, hypertension, and type 2 diabetes (see Table 4.8). Weight loss is encouraged when individuals exceed these measurements.

**Underweight** Extremely low body weight.

**Android obesity** Obesity pattern seen in individuals who tend to store fat in the trunk or abdominal area.

**Gynoid obesity** Obesity pattern seen in people who store fat primarily around the hips and thighs.

**Waist circumference (WC)** A waist girth measurement to assess potential risk for disease based on intra-abdominal fat content.

**TABLE 4.8** Disease Risk According to Waist Circumference (WC)

| Men | Women | Disease Risk |
|---|---|---|
| <35.5 | <32.5 | Low |
| 35.5–40.0 | 32.5–35.0 | Moderate |
| >40.0 | >35.0 | High |

**TABLE 4.9** Disease Risk According to Body Mass Index (BMI) and Waist Circumference (WC)

| | | Disease Risk Relative to Normal Weight and WC | |
|---|---|---|---|
| Classification | BMI (kg/m²) | Men ≤40″ (102 cm) Women <35″ (88 cm) | Men >40″ (102 cm) Women >35″ (88 cm) |
| Underweight | <18.5 | Increased | Low |
| Normal | 18.5–24.9 | Very low | Increased |
| Overweight | 25.0–29.9 | Increased | High |
| Obesity Class I | 30.0–34.9 | High | Very high |
| Obesity Class II | 35.0–39.9 | Very high | Very high |
| Obesity Class III | ≥40.0 | Extremely high | Extremely high |

Adapted from Expert Panel, *Executive Summary of the Clinical Guidelines on the Identification, Evaluation, and Treatment of Overweight and Obesity in Adults,* Archives of Internal Medicine 158:1855–1867, 1998.

Research indicates that WC may be a better predictor than BMI of the risk for disease.[9] Thus, BMI in conjunction with WC provides the best combination to identify individuals at higher risk resulting from excessive body fat. Table 4.9 provides guidelines to identify people at risk according to BMI and WC.

A second procedure that was used for years to identify health risk based on the pattern of fat distribution is the waist-to-hip ratio (WHR) test. In recent years, however, several studies have found that WC is a better indicator than WHR of abdominal visceral obesity.[10] Thus, a combination of BMI and WC, rather than WHR, is now recommended by health care professionals to assess potential risk for disease.

# Determining Recommended Body Weight

After finding out your percent body fat, you can determine your current body composition classification by consulting Table 4.10, which presents percentages of fat according to both the health fitness standard and the high physical fitness standard (see discussion in Chapter 1).

For example, the recommended health fitness fat percentage for a 20-year-old female is 28 percent or less. Although there are no clearly identified percent body fat levels at which the risk for disease definitely increases, the health fitness standard in Table 4.10 is currently the best estimate of the point at which there seems to be no harm to health.

According to Table 4.10, the high physical fitness range for this same 20-year-old woman would be between 18 and 23 percent. The high physical fitness standard does not mean that you cannot be somewhat below this number. Many highly trained male athletes are as low as 3 percent, and some female distance runners have been measured at 6 percent body fat (which may not be healthy).

People generally agree that the mortality rate is higher for obese people, and some evidence indicates that the same is true for underweight people. "Underweight" and "thin" do not necessarily mean the same thing. The body fat of a healthy thin person is near the high physical fitness standard, whereas an underweight person has extremely low body fat, even to the point of compromising the essential fat.

The 3 percent essential fat for men and 12 percent for women seem to be the lower limits for people to maintain good health. Below these percentages, normal physiological functions can be seriously impaired. Some experts point out that a little storage fat (in addition to the essential fat) is better than none at all. As a result, the health and high fitness standards for percent fat in Table 4.10 are set higher than the minimum essential fat requirements, at a point beneficial to optimal health and well-being. Finally, because lean tissue decreases with age, one extra percentage point is allowed for every additional decade of life.

## Critical Thinking

Do you think you have a weight problem? Do your body composition results make you think differently about the way you perceive your current body weight and image?

Your recommended body weight is computed based on the selected health or high fitness fat percentage for your age and sex. Your decision to select a "desired" fat percentage should be based on your current percent body fat and your personal health/fitness objectives. Following are steps to compute your own recommended body weight:

**TABLE 4.10** Body Composition Classification According to Percent Body Fat

| MEN | | | | | | |
|---|---|---|---|---|---|---|
| Age | Underweight | Excellent | Good | Moderate | Overweight | Significantly Overweight |
| ≤19 | <3 | 12.0 | 12.1–17.0 | 17.1–22.0 | 22.1–27.0 | ≥27.1 |
| 20–29 | <3 | 13.0 | 13.1–18.0 | 18.1–23.0 | 23.1–28.0 | ≥28.1 |
| 30–39 | <3 | 14.0 | 14.1–19.0 | 19.1–24.0 | 24.1–29.0 | ≥29.1 |
| 40–49 | <3 | 15.0 | 15.1–20.0 | 20.1–25.0 | 25.1–30.0 | ≥30.1 |
| ≥50 | <3 | 16.0 | 16.1–21.0 | 21.1–26.0 | 26.1–31.0 | ≥31.1 |
| WOMEN | | | | | | |
| Age | Underweight | Excellent | Good | Moderate | Overweight | Significantly Overweight |
| ≤19 | <12 | 17.0 | 17.1–22.0 | 22.1–27.0 | 27.1–32.0 | ≥32.1 |
| 20–29 | <12 | 18.0 | 18.1–23.0 | 23.1–28.0 | 28.1–33.0 | ≥33.1 |
| 30–39 | <12 | 19.0 | 19.1–24.0 | 24.1–29.0 | 29.1–34.0 | ≥34.1 |
| 40–49 | <12 | 20.0 | 20.1–25.0 | 25.1–30.0 | 30.1–35.0 | ≥35.1 |
| ≥50 | <12 | 21.0 | 21.1–26.0 | 26.1–31.0 | 31.1–36.0 | ≥36.1 |

☐ High physical fitness standard          ☐ Health fitness standard

1. Determine the pounds of body weight that are fat (FW) by multiplying your body weight (BW) by the current percent fat (%F) expressed in decimal form (FW = BW × %F).

2. Determine lean body mass (LBM) by subtracting the weight in fat from the total body weight (LBM = BW − FW). (Anything that is not fat must be part of the lean component.)

3. Select a desired body fat percentage (DFP) based on the health or high fitness standards given in Table 4.10.

4. Compute recommended body weight (RBW) according to the formula RBW = LBM ÷ (1.0 − DFP).

As an example of these computations, a 19-year-old female who weighs 160 pounds and is 30 percent fat would like to know what her recommended body weight would be at 22 percent:

> Sex: Female
> Age: 19
> BW: 160 lbs
> %F: 30% (.30 in decimal form)

1. FW = BW × %F
   FW = 160 × .30 = 48 lbs
2. LBM = BW − FW
   LBM = 160 − 48 = 112 lbs
3. DFP: 22% (.22 in decimal form)
4. RBW = LBM ÷ (1.0 − DFP)
   RBW = 112 ÷ (1.0 − .22)
   RBW = 112 ÷ .78 = 143.6 lbs

In Lab 4B, you will have the opportunity to determine your own body composition and recommended body weight. A second column is provided in the activity for a follow-up assessment at a future date. The disease risk according to BMI and WC and recommended body weight according to BMI also are determined in Lab 4B.

Other than hydrostatic weighing and air displacement, skinfold thickness seems to be the most practical and valid technique to estimate body fat. If skinfold calipers are available, use this technique to assess your percent body fat. If none of these techniques is available to you, estimate your percent fat according to girth measurements (or another technique available to you). You also may wish to use several techniques and compare the results.

## Critical Thinking

How do you feel about your current body weight, and what influence does society have on the way you perceive yourself in terms of your weight? Do your body composition results make you think differently about the way you see your current body weight and image?

## Behavior Modification Planning

**TIPS FOR LIFETIME WEIGHT MANAGEMENT**

Maintenance of recommended body composition is one of the most significant health issues of the 21st century. If you are committed to lifetime weight management, the following strategies will help:

**I PLAN TO**

**I DID IT**

☐ ☐ Accumulate 60 to 90 minutes of physical activity daily.

☐ ☐ Exercise at a vigorous aerobic pace for a minimum of 20 minutes three times per week.

☐ ☐ Strength train two to three times per week.

☐ ☐ Use common sense and moderation in your daily diet.

☐ ☐ Manage daily caloric intake by keeping in mind long-term benefits (recommended body weight) instead of instant gratification (overeating).

☐ ☐ "Junior-size" instead of "super-size."

☐ ☐ Regularly monitor body weight, body composition, body mass index, and waist circumference.

☐ ☐ Do not allow increases in body weight (percent fat) to accumulate; deal immediately with the problem through moderate reductions in caloric intake and maintenance of physical activity and exercise habits.

### Try It

In your Online Journal or your class notebook, note which of these tips you are already using and which ones you can incorporate into your daily habits right away.

# Importance of Regular Body Composition Assessment

Children in the United States do not start with a weight problem. Although a few struggle with weight throughout life, most are not overweight in the early years of life.

Trends indicate that starting at age 25, the average person in the United States gains 1 to 2 pounds of weight per year. Thus, by age 65, the average American will have gained 40 to 80 pounds. Because of the typical reduction in physical activity in our society, however, the average person also loses 1/2 pound of lean tissue each year. Therefore, this span of 40 years has produced an actual fat gain of 60 to 100 pounds accompanied by a 20-pound loss of lean body mass[11] (Figure 4.8). These changes cannot be detected without assessing body composition periodically.

If you are on a diet/exercise program, you should repeat your percent body fat assessment and recommended weight computations about once a month. This is important because lean body mass is affected by weight-reduction programs and amount of physical activity. As lean body mass changes, so will your recommended body weight. To make valid comparisons, use the same technique for both pre- and post-program assessments. Knowing your percent body fat also is useful to identify fad diets that promote water loss and lean body mass, especially muscle mass (also see "Diet Crazes" in Chapter 5, page 152).

Changes in body composition resulting from a weight control/exercise program were illustrated in a co-ed aerobic dance course taught during a six-week summer term.

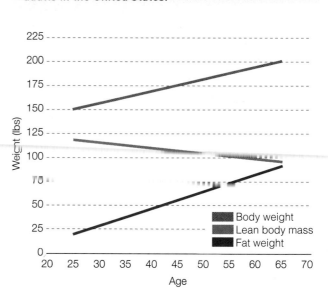

**FIGURE 4.8  Typical body composition changes for adults in the United States.**

Students participated in a 60-minute dance aerobics class four times a week. On the first and last days of class, several physiological parameters, including body composition, were assessed. Students also were given information on diet and nutrition, but they followed their own dietary program.

At the end of the six weeks, the average weight loss for the entire class was 3 pounds (Figure 4.9). But, because body composition was assessed, class members were surprised to find that the average fat loss was actually 6 pounds, accompanied by a 3-pound increase in lean body mass.

When dieting, have your body composition reassessed periodically because of the effects of negative caloric balance on lean body mass. As discussed in Chapter 5, dieting does decrease lean body mass. This loss of lean body mass can be offset or eliminated by combining a sensible diet with exercise.

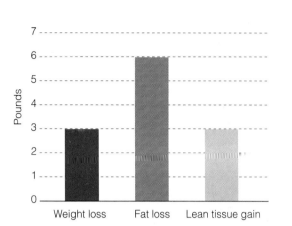

**FIGURE 4.9 Effects of a 6-week aerobics exercise program on body composition.**

*Source:* W. W. K. Hoeger, data collected at the University of Texas of the Permian Basin, 1985.

# ASSESS YOUR BEHAVIOR

 Log on to http://www.cengage.com/sso/ and take a wellness inventory to assess the behaviors that might benefit most from healthy change.

1. Do you know what your percent body fat is according to a reliable body composition assessment technique administered by a qualified technician?

2. Do you know your disease risk according to BMI and WC parameters?

3. Have you been able to maintain your body weight at a stable level during the past 12 months?

# ASSESS YOUR KNOWLEDGE

 Log on to http://www.cengage.com/sso/ to assess your understanding of this chapter's topics by taking the Student Practice Test and exploring the modules recommended in your Personalized Study Plan.

1. Body composition incorporates
   a. a fat component.
   b. a non-fat component.
   c. percent body fat.
   d. lean body mass.
   e. all of the four components above.

2. Recommended body weight can be determined through
   a. waist-to-hip ratio.
   b. body composition analysis.
   c. lean body mass assessment.
   d. waist circumference.
   e. all of the above.

3. Essential fat in women is
   a. 3 percent.
   b. 5 percent.
   c. 10 percent.
   d. 12 percent.
   e. 17 percent.

4. Which of the following is *not* a technique to assess body fat?
   a. Body mass index
   b. Skinfold thickness
   c. Hydrostatic weighing
   d. Circumference measurements
   e. Air displacement

5. Which of the following sites is used to assess percent body fat according to skinfold thickness in men?
   a. Suprailium
   b. Chest
   c. Scapular
   d. Triceps
   e. All four sites are used.

6. Which variable is *not* used to assess percent body fat in women according to girth measurements?
   a. Age
   b. Hip
   c. Wrist
   d. Upper arm
   e. Height

7. Waist circumference can be used to
   a. determine percent body fat.
   b. assess risk for disease.
   c. measure lean body mass.
   d. identify underweight people.
   e. All of the above.

8. An acceptable BMI is between
   a. 15 and 18.49.
   b. 18.5 and 24.99.
   c. 25 and 29.99.
   d. 30 and 34.99.
   e. 35 and 39.99.

9. The health fitness percent body fat for women of various ages is in the range of
   a. 3 to 7 percent.
   b. 7 to 12 percent.
   c. 12 to 20 percent.
   d. 20 to 27 percent.
   e. 27 to 31 percent

10. When a previously inactive individual starts an exercise program, the person may
   a. lose weight.
   b. gain weight.
   c. improve body composition.
   d. lose more fat pounds than total weight pounds.
   e. do all of the above.

Correct answers can be found at the back of the book.

# MEDIA MENU

You can find the links below at the book companion site: www.cengage.com/health/hoeger/plfw10e

- Learn how to measure body composition.
- Check how well you understand the chapter's concepts.

## Internet Connections

- Body Composition Laboratory. The Body Composition Laboratory at the Children's Nutrition Research Center in Houston, Texas, sponsors this informative Web site, which explains the techniques for and applications of body composition measurements in all populations, ranging from low–birth weight infants to adults. Learn how high-precision instruments are used to measure total body levels of body water, mineral, protein, and fat. *http://www.bcm.tmc.edu/bodycomplab*

- The Exercise and Physical Fitness Laboratory at Georgia State University. This site, from the GSU Department of Kinesiology and Health, describes six methods for measuring body composition and provides information regarding procedure description, accuracy, and relative cost, as well as a list of advantages and disadvantages for each. *http://www.gsu.edu/~wwwfit/bodycomp.html*

- Cornell University Research on Body Composition and Metabolic Rate. This instructional Web site describes methods used to calculate basal metabolic rate and body composition. *http://instruct1.cit.cornell.edu/Courses/ns421/BMR.html*

# NOTES

1. J. Stevens, J. Cai, E. R. Pamuk, D. F. Williamson, M. J. Thun, and J. L. Wood, "The Effect of Age on the Association Between Body Mass Index and Mortality," *New England Journal of Medicine* 338 (1998): 1–7.

2. E. E. Calle, M. J. Thun, J. M. Petrelli, C. Rodriguez, and C. W. Heath, "Body-Mass Index and Mortality in a Prospective Cohort of U.S. Adults," *New England Journal of Medicine* 341 (1999): 1097–1105.

3. American College of Sports Medicine, "Position Stand: Appropriate Intervention Strategies for Weight Loss and Prevention for Weight Regain for Adults," *Medicine and Science in Sports and Exercise* 33 (2001): 2145–2156.

4. K. M. Flegal, M. D. Carrol, R. J. Kuczmarski, and C. L. Johnson, "Overweight and Obesity in the United States: Prevalence and Trends, 1960–1994," *International Journal of Obesity and Related Metabolic Disorders* 22 (1998): 39–47.

5. "Comparing Apples and Pears," *University of California at Berkeley Wellness Letter* (Palm Coast, FL: The Editors, March 2004).

6. C. Bouchard, G. A. Bray, and V. S. Hubbard, "Basic and Clinical Aspects of Regional Fat Distribution," *American Journal of Clinical Nutrition* 52 (1990): 946–950; J. P. Després, I. Lemieux, and D. Prudhomme, "Treatment of Obesity: Need to Focus on High Risk Abdominally Obese Patients," *British Medical Journal* 322 (2001): 716–720; M. C. Pouliot et al., "Waist Circumference and Abdominal Sagittal Diameter: Best Simple An-

thropometric Indexes of Abdominal Visceral Adipose Tissue Accumulation and Related Cardiovascular Risk in Men and Women," *American Journal of Cardiology* 73 (1994): 460–468.

7. National Heart, Lung, and Blood Institute, National Institutes of Health, *The Practical Guide: Identification, Evaluation, and Treatment of Overweight and Obesity in Adults* (NIH Publication no. 00–4084) (Washington DC: Government Printing Office, 2000).

8. M. B. Snijder et al., "The Prediction of Visceral Fat by Dual-Energy X-ray Absorptiometry in the Elderly: A Comparison with Computed Tomography and Anthropometry," *International Journal of Obesity* 26 (2002): 984–993.

9. I. Janssen, P. T. Katzmarzyk, and R. Ross, "Waist Circumference and Not Body Mass Index Explains Obesity-Related Health Risk," *American Journal of Clinical Nutrition* 79 (2004): 379–384.

10. P. M. Ribisl, "Toxic 'Waist' Dump: Our Abdominal Visceral Fat," *ACSM's Health & Fitness Journal* 8, no. 4 (2004): 22–25.

11. J. H. Wilmore, "Exercise and Weight Control: Myths, Misconceptions, and Quackery," lecture given at annual meeting of American College of Sports Medicine, Indianapolis, June 1994.

## SUGGESTED READINGS

Heymsfield, S. B., T. G. Lohman, Z. Wang, and S. B. Going. *Human Body Composition*. Champaign, IL: Human Kinetics, 2005.

Heyward, V. H., and D. Wagner. *Applied Body Composition Assessment*. Champaign, IL: Human Kinetics, 2004.

# LAB 4A: Hydrostatic Weighing for Body Composition Assessment

Name _____  Date _____  Grade _____

Instructor _____  Course _____  Section _____

### Necessary Lab Equipment
Hydrostatic or underwater weighing tank and residual volume spirometer (if no spirometer is available, predicting equations can be used to determine this volume—see Figure 4.2, pages 126–127).

### Objective
To determine body density and percent body fat according to hydrostatic weighing.

### Lab Preparation
Bring a swimsuit and towel to this lab. A 6- to 8-hour fast and bladder and bowel movements are recommended prior to underwater weighing.

### Instructions
Follow the procedure outlined in Figure 4.2. If time is a factor, assess only the body composition of one or two participants in the course and compute the results using the form provided below. A sample of the computations is provided on the back of this page.

### I. Hydrostatic Weighing

Name: _____  Age: _____  Weight: _____ lbs

Height: _____ inches × 2.54 = _____ cm  Water temperature: _____ °C  Water density (WD): _____ gr/ml

Residual volume (RV): _____ lt  (See Figure 4.2)

Body weight (BW) in kg = weight in pounds ÷ 2.2046

BW in kg = _____ ÷ 2.2046 = _____ kg

Gross underwater weights:

1. _____ kg   2. _____ kg   3. _____ kg   4. _____ kg   5. _____ kg

6. _____ kg   7. _____ kg   8. _____ kg   9. _____ kg   10. _____ kg

Average of three heaviest underwater weights (AUW): _____ kg

Tare weight (TW): _____ kg

Net underwater weight (UW) = AUW − TW

Net underwater weight (UW) = _____ − _____ = _____ kg

Body density (BD):

$$BD = \dfrac{BW}{\dfrac{BW - UW}{WD} - RV - .1}$$

$$BD = \dfrac{\rule{2cm}{0.4pt}}{\dfrac{\rule{1.5cm}{0.4pt}}{\rule{1cm}{0.4pt}} - \rule{1cm}{0.4pt} - .1}$$

Percent body fat (%Fat):

$$\%Fat = \frac{495}{BD} - 450 = \frac{495}{\rule{1.5cm}{0.4pt}} - 450 = \rule{1.5cm}{0.4pt} \%$$   **Follow-up** percent body fat: _____ %

Sample computation for percent body fat according to hydrostatic weighing

Name: _____ Jane Doe _____  Age: ____20____  Weight: ___148.5___ lbs

Height: ___67___ inches × 2.54 = ___170.2___ cm  Water temperature: ___33___ °C  Water density (WD): __.99473__ gr/ml

Residual volume (RV). ___1.73___ lt  (See Figure 4.2)

Body weight (BW) in kg = weight in pounds ÷ 2.2046

BW in kg = ___148.5___ ÷ 2.2046 = ___67.36___ kg

Gross underwater weights:

1. ___6.15___ kg  2. ___6.12___ kg  3. ___6.24___ kg  4. ___6.26___ kg  5. ___6.21___ kg

6. ___6.26___ kg  7. ___6.29___ kg  8. ___6.28___ kg  9. ___6.24___ kg  10. ___6.27___ kg

Average of three heaviest underwater weights (AUW): ___6.28___ kg

Tare weight (TW): 5.154 kg

Net underwater weight (UW) = AUW − TW

Net underwater weight (UW) = 6.28 − 5.154 = 1.126 kg

Body density (BD):

$$BD = \frac{BW}{\dfrac{BW - UW}{WD} - RV - .1} \qquad BD = \frac{67.36}{\dfrac{67.36 - 1.126}{.99473} - 1.73 - .1} = 1.0402301$$

Percent body fat (%Fat):

$$\%Fat = \frac{495}{BD} - 450 = \frac{495}{1.0402301} - 450 = 25.9\%$$  **Follow-up** percent body fat: _____ %

II. What I learned from the underwater weighing procedure.

Describe the experience of being weighed underwater. Do you feel that the results of the test were accurate?

_____

_____

_____

_____

_____

_____

_____

_____

_____

_____

# LAB 4B: Body Composition, Disease Risk Assessment, and Recommended Body Weight Determination

Name _____     Date _____     Grade _____

Instructor _____     Course _____     Section _____

### Necessary Lab Equipment
Skinfold calipers and standard measuring tapes.

### Objective
To assess percent body fat according to skinfold thickness or girth measurements; disease risk according to body mass index and waist circumference; and recommended body weight.

### Instructions
If skinfold calipers are available, use this technique to assess your percent body fat (see Figure 4.4, page 128).

Otherwise, estimate the percent fat according to the girth measurements technique. You may wish to use both techniques and compare the results. Next, compute your recommended body weight according to your current percent body fat and the recommended percent body fat guidelines provided in Table 4.10, page 137. Determine also your waist circumference, body mass index, and recommended weight using the guidelines provided in this lab.

### I. Percent Body Fat According to Skinfold Thickness

| Men | Women | |
| --- | --- | --- |

**Men**

Chest (mm): _____

Abdomen (mm): _____

Thigh (mm): _____

Total (mm): _____

% Fat: _____

**Women**

Triceps (mm): _____

Suprailium (mm): _____

Thigh (mm): _____

Total (mm): _____

% Fat: _____

**Follow-up**

Date _____

% Fat _____ %

### II. Percent Fat According to Girth Measurements (Follow the instructions in Fig 4.5 on page 130 to obtain percent body fat, using Table 4.4 (women) or 4.5 (men).)

Men    Waist (in): [ ]    Wrist (in): [ ]    Body weight: [ ] lb    Percent body fat [ ] %

Women    Upper arm (cm): [ ]    Hip (cm): [ ]    Wrist (cm): [ ]    Age: [ ]

Percent body fat [ ] %

### III. Recommended Body Weight Determination

**Follow Up**

A. Body weight (BW): [ ] lb

B. Current %F*: [ ] %

C. Fat weight (FW) = BW × %F

    FW = [ ] × [ ] = [ ] lb

D. Lean body mass (LBM) = BW − FW = [ ] − [ ] = [ ] lb

E. Age: [ ]

F. Desired fat percent (DFP − see Table 4.10, page 137): [ ] %

G. Recommended body weight (RBW) = LBM ÷ (1.0 − DFP*)

    RBW = [ ] ÷ (1.0 − [ ]) = [ ] lb

Date: [ ]

A. BW: [ ] lbs

B. %F: [ ] %

C. FW: [ ]

D. LBM: [ ] lbs

E. Age: [ ]

F. DFP: [ ] %

G. RBW: [ ] lbs

*Express percentages in decimal form (for example, 25% 5 .25).

### IV. Body Mass Index

Weight: ☐ lb ☐ kg

Height: ☐ in ☐ m

BMI = Weight (lb) × 705 ÷ Height (in) ÷ Height (in)

BMI = ☐ (lb) ÷ 705 ÷ ☐ (in) ÷ ☐ (in)

BMI = ☐ Disease Risk: (use Table 4.7, page 135): ☐

**Follow-up**  Date ☐  BMI = ☐  Disease Risk (use Table 4.7, page 135): ☐

### V. Waist Circumference

Follow Up

Waist (in): ☐

Disease Risk (use Table 4.8, page 136): ☐

☐

☐

### VI. Disease Risk According to BMI and WC (use Table 4.9, page 136): ☐

### VII. Recommended Body Weight (RBW) According to BMI

RBW based on BMI = Desired BMI × height (in) × height (in) ÷ 705

RBW at BMI of 25 = 25 × ☐ × ☐ ÷ 705 = ☐ lb

RBW at BMI of 22 = 22 × ☐ × ☐ ÷ 705 = ☐ lb

### VIII. Determining Body Composition Results and Goals

Briefly state your feelings about your body composition results and your recommended body weight using both percent body fat and BMI. Do you plan to reduce your percent body fat and increase your lean body mass? Write the goal(s) you want to achieve by the end of the term and indicate how you plan to achieve them.

_____

_____

_____

_____

_____

_____

_____

_____

_____

_____

# Weight Management

5

If you are unwilling to increase daily physical activity, do not attempt to lose weight, because most likely you won't be able to keep it off.

## Objectives

- Describe the health consequences of obesity
- Expose some popular fad diets and myths and fallacies regarding weight control
- Describe eating disorders and their associated medical problems and behavior patterns, and outline the need for professional help in treating these conditions
- Explain the physiology of weight loss, including setpoint theory and the effects of diet on basal metabolic rate
- Explain the role of a lifetime exercise program as the key to a successful weight loss and weight maintenance program
- Be able to implement a physiologically sound weight reduction and weight maintenance program

- Describe behavior modification techniques that help support adherence to a lifetime weight maintenance program

CENGAGENOW™

On your exercise log, check your progress.

Check your understanding of the chapter contents by logging on to CengageNOW and accessing the pre-test, personalized learning plan, and post-test for this chapter.

# FAQ

**What is more important for weight loss: a negative caloric balance (diet) or increased physical activity?**

Most of the research shows that weight loss is more effective when cutting back on calories (dieting), as opposed to only increasing physical activity in caloric. Weight loss is accelerated, nonetheless, when physical activity is added to dieting. Body composition changes, however, are much more effective when dieting and exercise are combined while attempting to lose body weight. Most of the weight loss when dieting with exercise comes in the form of body fat and not lean body tissue, a desirable outcome. Weight loss maintenance, however, in most cases is possible only with 60 to 90 minutes of sustained daily physical activity or exercise.

**Does the time of day when calories are consumed matter in a weight loss program?**

The time of day when a person eats food appears to play a part in weight reduction. When attempting to lose weight, intake should consist of a minimum of 25 percent of the total daily calories for breakfast, 50 percent for lunch, and 25 percent or less for dinner. Also, try not to eat within 3 hours of going to bed. This is the time of day when your metabolism is slowest. Your caloric intake is less likely to be used for energy and more likely to be stored as fat.

**Are some diet plans more effective than others?**

The term "diet" implies a negative caloric balance. A negative caloric balance means that you are consuming fewer calories than those required to maintain your current weight. When energy output surpasses energy intake, weight loss will occur. Popular diets differ widely in the food choices that you are allowed to have. The more limited the choices, the lower the chances to overeat, and thus you will have a lower caloric intake. And the fewer the calories that you consume, the

greater the weight loss. For health reasons, to obtain the variety of nutrients the body needs, even during weight loss periods, women should not consume fewer than 1,200 calories per day, and men no less than 1,500 calories per day. These calories should be distributed over a wide range of foods, emphasizing grains, fruits, vegetables, and small amounts of low-fat animal products or fish.

**Why is it so difficult to change dietary habits?**

In most developed countries, there is an overabundance of food and practically an unlimited number of food choices. With unlimited supply and choices, most people do not have the willpower, stemming from their core values, to avoid overconsumption.

Our bodies were not created to go hungry or to overeat. We are uncomfortable overeating and we feel even worse when we have to go hungry. Our health values, however, are not strong enough to prevent overconsumption. The end result: weight gain. Next, we restrict calories (go on a diet), we feel hungry, and we have a difficult time adhering to the diet. Stated quite simply, going hungry is an uncomfortable and unpleasant experience.

To avoid this vicious cycle, our dietary habits (and most likely physical activity habits) must change. A question you need to ask yourself is: Do you value health and quality of life more than food overindulgence? If you do not, then the achievement and maintenance of recommended body weight and good health is a moot point. If you desire to avoid disease and increase quality of life, you have to value health more than food overconsumption. If we have spent the last 20 years tasting and "devouring" every food item in sight, it is now time to make healthy choices and consume only moderate amounts of food at a time (portion control). You do not have to taste and eat everything that is placed before your eyes. If you can make such a change in your eating habits, you may not have to worry about another diet for the rest of your life.

Obesity is a health hazard of epidemic proportions in most developed countries around the world. According to the World Health Organization, an estimated 35 percent of the adult population in industrialized nations is obese. Obesity has been defined as a body mass index (BMI) of 30 or higher. The obesity level is the point at which excess body fat can lead to serious health problems.

The number of people who are obese and overweight in the United States has increased dramatically in the past few years, a direct result of physical inactivity and poor dietary habits. The average weight of American adults between the ages of 20 and 74 has increased by 25 pounds or more since 1965 (Figure 5.1). About one-half of all adults in the United States do not achieve the minimum recommended amount of physical activity (see Chapter 1, Figure 1.7). In 2004, American women consumed 335 more calories daily than they had 20 years earlier, and men an additional 170 calories per day.[1]

More than 66 percent of U.S. adults age 20 and older are overweight (have a BMI greater than 25), and 32 percent are obese (Figure 5.2).[2] More than 120 million people are overweight and 30 million are obese. Between 1960 and 2002, the overall (men and women combined) prevalence of adult obesity increased from about 13 percent to 30 percent. Most of this increase occurred in the 1990s.

As illustrated in Figure 5.3, the obesity epidemic continues to escalate. Before 1990, not a single state reported an obesity rate above 15 percent of the state's total population (including both adults and children). By the year 2007, only one state had a prevalence of less than 20 per-

cent. Thirty states had a prevalence equal to or greater than 25 percent, and three of these states had reached a rate above 30 percent.

In the last decade alone, the average weight of American adults increased by about 15 pounds. The prevalence of obesity is even higher in ethnic groups, especially African Americans and Hispanic Americans. Further, as the nation continues to evolve into a more mechanized and automated society (relying on escalators, elevators, remote controls, computers, electronic mail, cell phones, and automatic-sensor doors), the amount of required daily physical activity continues to decrease. We are being lulled into a high-risk sedentary lifestyle.

About 44 percent of all women and 29 percent of all men are on a diet at any given moment.[3] People spend about $40 billion yearly attempting to lose weight, with more than $10 billion going to memberships in weight reduction centers and another $30 billion to diet food sales. Furthermore, the total cost attributable to treating obesity-related diseases is estimated at $100 billion per year.[4]

Excessive body weight and physical inactivity are the second leading cause of preventable death in the United States, causing more than 112,000 deaths each year.[5] Furthermore, obesity is more prevalent than smoking (19 percent), poverty (14 percent), and problem drinking (6 percent).[6] Obesity and unhealthy lifestyle habits are the most critical public health problems we face in the 21st century.

Excessive body weight and obesity are associated with poor health status and are risk factors for many physical ailments, including cardiovascular disease and cancer. Evidence indicates that health risks associated with increased body weight start at a BMI over 25 and are enhanced greatly at a BMI over 30.

The American Heart Association has identified obesity as one of the six major risk factors for coronary heart disease. Estimates also indicate that 14 percent of all cancer

---

**FIGURE 5.1** Average weight of Americans between 1963–1965 and 1999–2002.

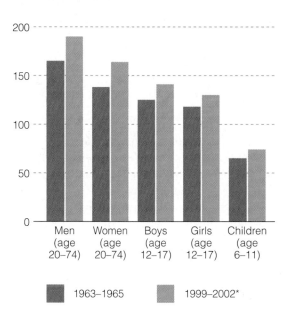

1963–1965 ■ 1999–2002*

*Adults are about an inch taller and children about half an inch taller as compared with the early 1960s. The height difference accounts for about 3 to 6 extra pounds.

*Source:* "It's gaining on us." *UC Berkeley Wellness Letter,* May 2005.

---

**FIGURE 5.2** Percentage of the adult population that is overweight (BMI ≥ 25) and obese (BMI ≥ 30) and in the United States.

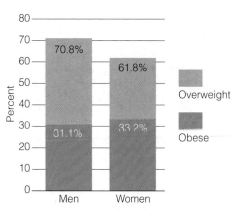

*Source:* "Prevalence of overweight and obesity in the US," by C. L. Ogden et al., *Journal of the American Medical Association* 295 (2006): 1549–1555.

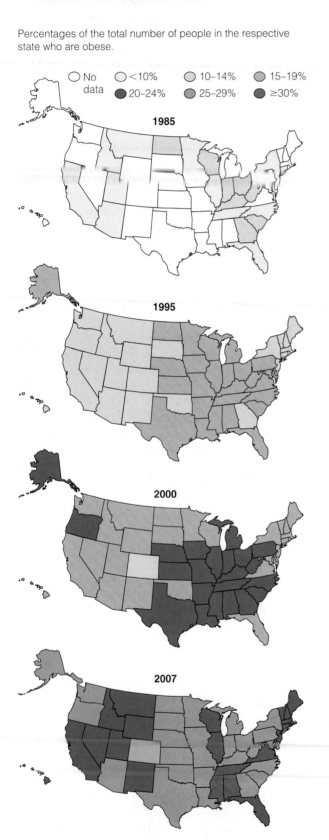

**FIGURE 5.3** Obesity trends in the United States, 1985–2007, based on BMI ≥ 30 or 30 pounds overweight.

Percentages of the total number of people in the respective state who are obese.

○ No data   ○ <10%   ○ 10–14%   ○ 15–19%
● 20–24%   ● 25–29%   ● ≥30%

1985

1995

2000

2007

***Source:*** Obesity Trends Among U.S. Adults Between 1985 and 2007. (Atlanta: Centers for Disease Control and Prevention, 2008).

## Health Consequences of Excessive Body Weight

Being overweight or obese increases the risk for

- high blood pressure
- elevated blood lipids (high blood cholesterol and triglycerides)
- type 2 (non-insulin-dependent) diabetes
- insulin resistance, glucose intolerance
- coronary heart disease
- angina pectoris
- congestive heart failure
- stroke
- gallbladder disease
- gout
- osteoarthritis
- obstructive sleep apnea and respiratory problems
- some types of cancer (endometrial, breast, prostate, and colon)
- complications of pregnancy (gestational diabetes, gestational hypertension, preeclampsia, and complications during C-sections)
- poor female reproductive health (menstrual irregularities, infertility, irregular ovulation)
- bladder control problems (stress incontinence)
- psychological disorders (depression, eating disorders, distorted body image, discrimination, and low self-esteem)
- shortened life expectancy
- decreased quality of life

***Source:*** Centers for Disease Control and Prevention, downloaded September 30, 2008.

deaths in men and 20 percent in women are related to current overweight and obesity patterns in the United States.[7] Furthermore, excessive body weight is implicated in psychological maladjustment and a higher accidental death rate. Extremely obese people have a lower mental health–related quality of life.

# Overweight Versus Obesity

Overweight and obesity are not the same thing. Many overweight people (people who weigh about 10 to 20 pounds over the recommended weight) are not obese. Although a few pounds of excess weight may not be harmful to most people,

Obesity is a health hazard of epidemic proportions in industrialized nations.

this is not always the case. People with excessive body fat who have type 2 diabetes and other cardiovascular risk factors (elevated blood lipids, high blood pressure, physical inactivity, and poor eating habits) benefit from losing weight. People who have a few extra pounds of weight but are otherwise healthy and physically active, exercise regularly, and eat a healthy diet may not be at higher risk for early death. Such is not the case, however, with obese individuals.

Research indicates that individuals who are 30 or more pounds overweight during middle age (30 to 49 years of age) lose about 7 years of life, whereas being 10 to 30 pounds overweight decreases the lifespan by about 3 years.[8] These decreases are similar to those seen with tobacco use. Severe obesity (BMI greater than 45) at a young age, nonetheless, may cut up to 20 years off one's life.[9]

Although the loss of years of life is significant, decreased life expectancy doesn't even begin to address the loss in quality of life and the increase in illness and disability throughout the years. Even a modest reduction of 5 to 10 percent can reduce the risk for chronic diseases, including heart disease, high blood pressure, high cholesterol, and diabetes.[10]

A primary objective to achieve overall physical fitness and enhanced quality of life is to attain recommended body composition. Individuals at recommended body weight are able to participate in a wide variety of moderate to vigorous activities without functional limitations. These people have the freedom to enjoy most of life's recreational activities to their fullest potential. Excessive body weight does not afford an individual the fitness level to enjoy many lifetime activities such as basketball, soccer, racquetball, surfing, mountain cycling, or mountain climbing. Maintaining high fitness and recommended body weight gives a person a degree of independence throughout life that most people in developed nations no longer enjoy.

Scientific evidence also recognizes problems with being underweight. Although the social pressure to be thin has declined slightly in recent years, the pressure to attain model-like thinness is still with us and contributes to the gradual increase in the number of people who develop eat-

ing disorders (anorexia nervosa and bulimia, discussed under "Eating Disorders" on pages 157–160).

Extreme weight loss can lead to medical conditions such as heart damage, gastrointestinal problems, shrinkage of internal organs, abnormalities of the immune system, disorders of the reproductive system, loss of muscle tissue, damage to the nervous system, and even death. About 14 percent of people in the United States are underweight.

## Critical Thinking

Do you consider yourself overweight? If so, how long have you had a weight problem, what attempts have you made to lose weight, and what has worked best for you?

**Tolerable Weight** Many people want to lose weight so they will look better. That's a noteworthy goal. The problem, however, is that they have a distorted image of what they would really look like if they were to reduce to what they think is their ideal weight. Hereditary factors play a big role, and only a small fraction of the population has the genes for a "perfect body."

The media have the greatest influence on people's perception of what constitutes "ideal" body weight. Most people consult fashion, fitness, and beauty magazines to determine what they should look like. The "ideal" body shapes, physiques, and proportions illustrated in these magazines are rare and are achieved mainly through airbrushing and medical reconstruction.[11] Many individuals, primarily young women, go to extremes in attempts to achieve these unrealistic figures. Failure to attain a "perfect body" may lead to eating disorders in some individuals.

When people set their own target weight, they should be realistic. Attaining the "Excellent" percent of body fat shown in Table 4.8 in Chapter 4 is extremely difficult for some. It is even more difficult to maintain over time, unless the person makes a commitment to a vigorous lifetime exercise program and permanent dietary changes. Few people are willing to do that. The "Moderate" percent body fat category may be more realistic for many people.

The question you should ask yourself is: Am I happy with my weight? Part of enjoying a higher quality of life is being happy with yourself. If you are not, you need to either do something about it or learn to live with it.

If your percent of body fat is higher than those in the Moderate category of Table 4.8, you should try to reduce it and stay in this category, for health reasons. This is the category that seems to pose no detriment to health.

If you are in the Moderate category but would like to reduce your percent of body fat further, you need to ask yourself a second question: How badly do I want it? Do I

FIGURE 5.4 Differences between self-reported and actual daily caloric intake and exercise in obese individuals attempting to lose weight.

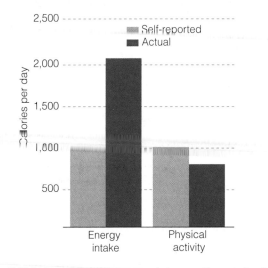

*Source:* S. W. Lichtman et al., "Discrepancy between self-reported and actual caloric intake and exercise in obese subjects," *New England Journal of Medicine* 327 (1992): 1893–1898.

want it badly enough to implement lifetime exercise and dietary changes? If you are not willing to change, you should stop worrying about your weight and deem the Moderate category "tolerable" for you.

The Weight Loss Dilemma Yo-yo dieting carries as great a health risk as being overweight and remaining overweight in the first place. Epidemiological data show that frequent fluctuations in weight (up or down) markedly increase the risk of dying from cardiovascular disease. Based on the findings that constant losses and regains can be hazardous to health, quick-fix diets should be replaced by a slow but permanent weight loss program (as described under "Losing Weight the Sound and Sensible Way," page 169). Individuals reap the benefits of recommended body weight when they get to that weight and stay there throughout life.

Unfortunately, only about 10 percent of all people who begin a traditional weight loss program without exercise are able to lose the desired weight. Worse, only 5 in 100 are able to keep the weight off. The body is highly resistant to permanent weight changes through caloric restrictions alone.

Traditional diets have failed because few of them incorporate permanent behavioral changes in food selection and an overall increase in physical activity and exercise as fundamental to successful weight loss and weight maintenance. When the diet stops, weight gain begins. The $40 billion diet industry tries to capitalize on the false idea that a person can lose weight quickly without considering the consequences of fast weight loss or the importance of lifetime behavioral changes to ensure proper weight loss and maintenance.

In addition, various studies indicate that most people, especially obese people, underestimate their energy intake. Those who try to lose weight but apparently fail to do so are often described as "diet resistant." One study found that while on a "diet," a group of obese individuals with a self-reported history of diet resistance underreported their average daily caloric intake by almost 50 percent (1,028 self-reported versus 2,081 actual calories) (Figure 5.4).[12] These individuals also overestimated their amount of daily physical activity by about 25 percent (1,022 self-reported versus 771 actual calories). These differences represent an additional 1,304 calories of energy per day unaccounted for by the subjects in the study. The findings indicate that failing to lose weight often is related to misreports of actual food intake and level of physical activity.

# Diet Crazes

Capitalizing on hopes that the latest diet to hit the market will really work this time, fad diets continue to appeal to people of all shapes and sizes. These diets may work for a while, but their success is usually short-lived. Regarding their effectiveness, Dr. Kelly Brownell, one of the foremost researchers in the field of weight management, has stated: "When I get the latest diet fad, I imagine a trick birthday cake candle that keeps lighting up and we have to keep blowing it out."

Fad diets deceive people and claim that dieters will lose weight by following all instructions. Many diets are very low in calories and deprive the body of certain nutrients, generating a metabolic imbalance. Under these conditions, a lot of the weight lost is in the form of water and protein, not fat. Most fad diets create a nutritional deficiency, which can be detrimental to health.

On average, a 150-pound person stores about 1.3 pounds of glycogen (carbohydrate or glucose storage) in the body. This amount of glycogen is higher in aerobically trained individuals, as intense training (elite athletes) can more than double the body's capacity to store glycogen. About 80 percent of the glycogen is stored in muscles and the remaining 20 percent in the liver. Water, however, is required to store glycogen. A 2.6 to 1 water to glycogen ratio is necessary to store glycogen.[13] Thus, our 150-pound person stores about 3.4 pounds of water (1.3 × 2.6), along with the 1.3 pounds of glycogen, accounting for a total of 4.7 pounds of the person's normal body weight.

When fasting or on a crash diet (defined as less than 500 calories per day), glycogen storage can be completely depleted in just a few days. This loss of weight is not in the form of body fat and is typically used to promote and guarantee rapid weight loss with many fad diets on the market today. When the person resumes a normal eating plan, the body will again store its glycogen, along with the water required to do so, and subsequent weight gain.

Furthermore, on a crash diet, close to half the weight loss is in lean (protein) tissue. When the body uses protein instead of a combination of fats and carbohydrates as a source of energy, weight is lost as much as 10 times faster. This is because a gram of protein produces half the amount of energy that fat does. In the case of muscle protein, one fifth of protein is mixed with four fifths water. Therefore, each pound of muscle yields only one tenth the amount of energy of a pound of fat. As a result, most of the weight lost is in the form of water, which on the scale, of course, looks good.

Diet books are frequently found on best-seller lists. The market is flooded with these books. Examples include the Volumetrics Eating Plan, the Ornish Diet, the Atkins Diet, the Zone Diet, the South Beach Diet, the Best Life Diet, the Abs Diet, and You on a Diet. Some of these popular diets are becoming more nutritionally balanced and encourage consumption of fruits and vegetables, whole grains, some lean meat and fish, and low-fat milk and dairy products. Such plans reduce the risk for chronic diseases, including cardiovascular diseases and cancer.

While it is clear that some types of diet are healthier than others, strictly from a weight loss point of view, it doesn't matter what diet plan you follow: If caloric intake is lower than your caloric output, weight will come off. Dropout rates for many popular diets, however, are high because of the difficulty in long-term adherence to limited dietary plans.

## Low-Carb Diets

Among the most popular diets on the market in recent years were the low-carbohydrate/high-protein (LCHP) diet plans. Although they vary slightly, low-carb diets, in general, limit the intake of carbohydrate-rich foods—bread, potatoes, rice, pasta, cereals, crackers, juices, sodas, sweets (candy, cake, cookies), and even fruits and vegetables. Dieters are allowed to eat all the protein-rich foods they desire, including steak, ham, chicken, fish,

## Popular Diets

### The Volumetrics Eating Plan

Diet plan that focuses on maximizing the volume of food and limiting calories by emphasizing high-water-content/low-fat foods (lower energy density), low-fat cooking techniques, and extensive use of vegetables. The average daily caloric intake is reduced by 500–1,000 calories, with a macronutrient composition of approximately 55% carbohydrates, less than 20–30% fat, and more than 20% protein.

### The Best Life Diet

The initial phase of the diet plan encourages exercise and a recommended eating schedule. The second phase requires a reduction in caloric intake through consumption of healthful foods to satisfy hunger. The plan deals extensively with "emotional eating." Caloric intake averages about 1,700 with maintenance of daily moderate physical activity. The diet composition is about 50% carbohydrates, 30% fat, and 20% protein.

### Ornish Diet

Very low fat, vegetarian-type diet. Dieters are not allowed to drink alcohol or eat meat, fish, oils, sugar, or white flour. Data indicate that strict adherence to the Ornish Diet can prevent and reverse heart disease. An average daily caloric intake is about 1,500, composed of approximately 75% carbohydrates, 15% protein, and less than 10% fat.

### The Zone Diet

The diet proposes that proper macronutrient (carbohydrate/fat/protein) distribution is critical to keep blood sugar and hormones in balance to prevent weight gain and disease. All meals need to provide 40% carbohydrate calories, 30% fat calories, and 30% protein calories. Daily caloric allowance is about 1,100 for women and 1,400 for men.

### Atkins Diet

A low-carbohydrate/high-protein diet. Practically all carbohydrates are eliminated the first two weeks of the diet. Thereafter, very small amounts of carbohydrates are allowed, primarily in the form of limited fruits, vegetables, and wine. No caloric guidelines are given, but a typical daily diet plan is about 1,500 calories, extremely high in fat (about 60% of calories), followed by protein (about 30% of calories), and limited carbohydrates (about 10% of calories). Dieters may not be as hungry on the Atkins Diet, but they tend to find it too restrictive for long-term adherence.

### The South Beach Diet

Also a low-carbohydrate/high-protein diet, but not as restrictive as the Atkins Diet. Emphasizes low-glycemic foods thought to decrease cravings for sugar and refined carbohydrates. Sugar, fruits, and grains are initially eliminated. In phase 2, some high-fiber grains, fruit, and dark chocolate are permitted. No caloric guidelines are given, but a typical dietary plan provides about 1,400 calories per day composed of 40% fat, 40% carbohydrate, and 20% protein.

bacon, eggs, nuts, cheese, tofu, high-fat salad dressings, butter, and small amounts of a few fruits and vegetables. Typically, these diets also are high in fat content. Examples of these diets are the Atkins Diet, the Zone, Protein Power, the Scarsdale Diet, the Carb Addict's Diet, the South Beach Diet, and Sugar Busters.

During digestion, carbohydrates are converted into glucose, a basic fuel used by every cell in the body. As blood glucose rises, the pancreas releases insulin. Insulin is a hormone that facilitates the entry of glucose into the cells, thereby lowering the glucose level in the bloodstream. A rapid rise in glucose also causes a rapid spike in insulin, which is followed by a rapid removal and drop in blood glucose that leaves you hungry again. A slower rise in blood glucose is desirable because the level is kept constant longer, delaying the onset of hunger. If the cells don't need the glucose for normal cell functions or to fuel physical activity, and if cellular glucose stores are already full, glucose is converted to, and stored as, body fat.

Not all carbohydrates cause a similar rise in blood glucose. The rise in glucose is based on the speed of digestion, which depends on a number of factors, including the size of the food particles. Small-particle carbohydrates break down rapidly and cause a quick, sharp rise in blood glucose. Thus, to gauge a food's effect on blood glucose, carbohydrates are classified by their **glycemic index.**

A high glycemic index signifies a food that causes a quick rise in blood glucose. At the top of the 100-point scale is glucose itself. This index is not directly related to simple and complex carbohydrates, and the glycemic values are not always what one might expect. Rather, the index is based on the actual laboratory-measured speed of absorption. Processed foods generally have a high glycemic index, whereas high-fiber foods tend to have a lower index (Table 5.1). Other factors that affect the index are the amount of

**TABLE 5.1  Glycemic Index of Selected Foods**

| Item | Index | Item | Index |
|---|---|---|---|
| All-Bran cereal | 46 | Honey | 58 |
| Apples | 40 | Milk, chocolate | 43 |
| Bagel, white | 72 | Milk, skim | 32 |
| Banana | 56 | Milk, whole | 30 |
| Bread, French | 95 | Jelly beans | 80 |
| Bread, wheat | 69 | Oatmeal | 54 |
| Bread, white | 69 | Oranges | 40 |
| Carrots, boiled (Australia) | 41 | Pasta, white | 50 |
| Carrots, boiled (Canada) | 92 | Pasta, wheat | 42 |
| Carrots, raw | 47 | Peanuts | 20 |
| Cherries | 20 | Peas | 50 |
| Colas | 65 | Pizza, cheese | 60 |
| Corn, sweet | 55 | Potato, baked | 56–100 |
| Corn Flakes | 83 | Potato, French fries | 75 |
| Doughnut | 76 | Potato, sweet | 51 |
| Frosted Flakes | 55 | Rice, white | 45–70 |
| Fruit cocktail | 55 | Sugar, table | 65 |
| Gatorade | 78 | Watermelon | 72 |
| Glucose | 100 | Yogurt, low-fat | 30 |

## Are Low-Carb/High-Protein Diets More Effective?

A few studies suggest that, at least over the short-term, low-carb/high-protein (LCHP) diets are more effective in producing weight loss than carbohydrate-based diets. These results are preliminary and controversial. In LCHP diets:

- A large amount of weight loss is water and muscle protein, not body fat. Some of this weight is quickly regained when regular dietary habits are resumed.
- Few people are able to stay with LCHP diets for more than a few weeks at a time. The majority stop dieting before the targeted program completion.
- LCHP dieters are rarely found in a national weight loss registry of people who have lost 30 pounds and kept them off for a minimum of 6 years.
- Food choices are severely restricted in LCHP diets. With less variety, individuals tend to eat less (800 to 1,200 calories/day) and thus lose more weight.
- LCHP diets may promote heart disease, cancer, and increase the risk for osteoporosis.
- LCHP diets are fundamentally high in fat (about 60% fat calories).
- LCHP diets are not recommended for people with diabetes, high blood pressure, heart disease, or kidney disease.
- LCHP diets do not promote long-term healthy eating patterns.

**FIGURE 5.5** Effects of high- and low-glycemic carbohydrate intake on blood glucose levels.

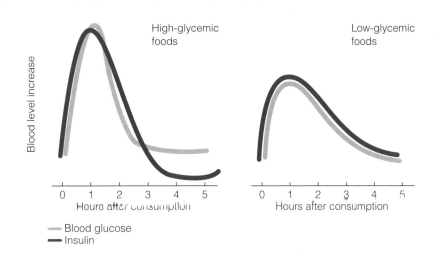

High-glycemic foods

Low-glycemic foods

Blood level increase

Hours after consumption

Hours after consumption

— Blood glucose
— Insulin

carbohydrate, fat, and protein in the food; how refined the ingredients are; and whether the food was cooked.

The body functions best when blood sugar remains at a constant level. Although this is best accomplished by consuming foods with a low glycemic index (nuts, apples, oranges, low-fat yogurt), a person does not have to eliminate all high-glycemic-index foods (sugar, potatoes, bread, white rice, soda drinks) from the diet. Foods with a high glycemic index along with some protein are useful to replenish depleted glycogen stores following prolonged or exhaustive aerobic exercise. Combining high- with low-glycemic-index items or with some fat and protein brings down the average index.

Regular consumption of high-glycemic foods by themselves may increase the risk of cardiovascular disease, especially in people at risk for diabetes. A person does not need to plan the diet around the index itself, as many popular diet programs indicate. The glycemic index deals with single foods eaten alone. Most people eat high-glycemic-index foods in combination with other foods as part of a meal. In combination, these foods have a lower effect on blood sugar. Even people at risk for diabetes or who have the disease can use high-glycemic foods in moderation.

Low-glycemic foods may also aid in weight loss and weight maintenance. As blood sugar levels drop between snacks and meals, hunger increases. Keeping blood sugar levels constant by including low-glycemic foods in the diet helps stave off hunger, appetite, and overeating (Figure 5.5).

Proponents of LCHP diets claim that if a person eats fewer carbohydrates and more protein, the pancreas will produce less insulin, and as insulin drops, the body will turn to its own fat deposits for energy. There is no scientific proof, however, that high levels of insulin lead to weight gain. None of the authors of these diets have published any studies validating their claims. Yet, these authors base their diets on the faulty premise that high insulin leads to obesity. We know the opposite to be true:

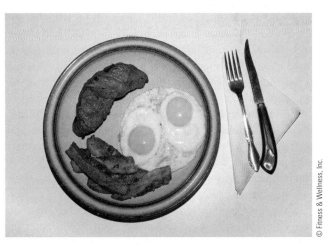

Low-carbohydrate/high-protein diets create nutritional deficiencies and may contribute to the development of cardiovascular disease, cancer, and osteoporosis.

Excessive body fat causes insulin levels to rise, thereby increasing the risk for developing diabetes.

The reason for rapid weight loss in LCHP dieting is that a low carbohydrate intake causes glycogen depletion and forces the liver to produce glucose. The source for most of this glucose is body proteins—your lean body mass, including muscle. As indicated earlier, protein is mostly water; thus, weight is lost rapidly. When a person terminates the diet, the body restores glycogen stores and rebuilds some of the protein tissue and quickly regains some weight.

**Glycemic index** A measure that is used to rate the plasma glucose response of carbohydrate-containing foods with the response produced by the same amount of carbohydrate from a standard source, usually glucose or white bread.

Research studies have indicated that individuals on an LCHP (Atkins) diet lose slightly more weight in the first few months than those on a low-fat diet.[14] The effectiveness of the diet, however, seemed to dwindle over time. In one of the studies, at 12 months into the diet, participants in the LCHP diet had regained more weight than those on the low-fat diet plan.

Years of research will be required to determine the extent to which adhering over the long term to LCHP diets will have an effect on heart disease, cancer, kidney, or bone damage. Low-carb diets are contrary to the nutrition advice of most national leading health organizations (which recommend a diet lower in saturated fat and trans fats and high in complex carbohydrates). Without fruits, vegetables, and whole grains, high-protein diets lack many vitamins, minerals, antioxidants, phytonutrients, and fiber—all dietary factors that protect against an array of ailments and diseases.

The major increased risk associated with long-term adherence to LCHP diets could be for heart disease, because high-protein foods are also high in fat content (see Chapter 11). Research shows that up to two years' adherence to LCHP diets does not appear to increase heart disease risk.[15] The long-term (many years) effects of these types of diet, nonetheless, have not been evaluated by scientific research. A possible long-term adverse effect of adherence to an LCHP diet is a potential increase in cancer risk. Phytonutrients found in fruits, vegetables, and whole grains protect against certain types of cancer. A low carbohydrate intake also produces a loss of vitamin B, calcium, and potassium. Potential bone loss can accentuate the risk for osteoporosis.

Side effects commonly associated with LCHP diets include weakness, nausea, bad breath, constipation, irritability, lightheadedness, and fatigue. If you choose to go on an LCHP diet for longer than a few weeks, let your physician know so he or she may monitor your blood lipids, bone density, and kidney function.

The benefit of adding extra protein to a weight loss program may be related to the hunger-suppressing effect of protein. Data suggest that protein curbs hunger more effectively than do carbohydrates or fat. Dieters feel less hungry when caloric intake from protein is increased to about 30 percent of total calories and fat intake is cut to about 20 percent (while carbohydrate intake is kept constant at 50 percent of total calories). Thus, if you struggle with frequent hunger pangs, try to include 10 to 15 grams of lean protein with each meal. This amount of protein is the equivalent of one and a half ounces of lean meat (beef, fowl, or fish), two tablespoons of natural peanut butter, or eight ounces of plain low-fat yogurt.

The reason why many of these diets succeed is because they restrict a large number of foods. Thus, people tend to eat less food overall. With the extraordinary variety of foods available to us, it is unrealistic to think that people will adhere to these diets for very long. People eventually get tired of eating the same thing day in and day out and start eating less, leading to weight loss. If they happen to

## How to Recognize Fad Diets

Fad diets have characteristics in common. These diets typically

- are nutritionally unbalanced.
- rely primarily on a single food (for example, grapefruit).
- are based on testimonials.
- were developed according to "confidential research."
- are based on a "scientific breakthrough."
- promote rapid and "painless" weight loss.
- promise miraculous results.
- restrict food selection.
- are based on pseudo claims that excessive weight is related to a specific condition such as insulin resistance, combinations or timing of nutrient intake, food allergies, hormone imbalances, certain foods (fruits, for example).
- require the use of selected products.
- use liquid formulas instead of foods.
- misrepresent salespeople as individuals qualified to provide nutrition counseling.
- fail to provide information on risks associated with weight loss and of the diet use.
- do not involve physical activity.
- do not encourage healthy behavioral changes.
- are not supported by the scientific community or national health organizations.
- fail to provide information for weight maintenance upon completion of diet phase.

achieve the lower weight but do not make permanent dietary changes, they regain the weight quickly once they go back to their previous eating habits.

A few diets recommend exercise along with caloric restrictions—the best method for weight reduction, of course. People who adhere to these programs will succeed, so the diet has achieved its purpose. Unfortunately, if the people do not change their food selection and activity level permanently, they gain back the weight once they discontinue dieting and exercise.

If people only accepted that no magic foods will provide all of the necessary nutrients, that a person has to eat a variety of foods to be well nourished, dieters would be more successful and the diet industry would go broke. Also, let's not forget that we eat for pleasure and for health. Two of the most essential components of a well-

## Behavior Modification Planning

### CALCIUM AND WEIGHT MAINTENANCE

Initial research stated that eating calcium-rich foods—especially from dairy products—may help control or reduce body weight. Women with a high calcium intake were found to gain less weight and body fat than those with a lower intake. Furthermore, women on low-calcium diets more than double the risk of becoming overweight. The data also indicate that even in the absence of caloric restriction, obese women with high dietary calcium intake (the equivalent of 3 to 4 cups of milk per day) lose body fat and weight. And dieters who consume calcium-rich dairy foods lose more fat and less lean body mass than those who consume less dairy products. Researchers believe that

- calcium regulates fat storage inside the cell.
- calcium helps the body break down fat or cause fat cells to produce less fat.
- high calcium intake converts more calories into heat rather than fat.
- adequate calcium intake contributes to a decrease in intra-abdominal (visceral) fat.

The data in women also seem to indicate that calcium from dairy sources is more effective in attenuating weight and fat gain and accelerating fat loss than calcium obtained from other sources. Most likely other nutrients found in dairy products may enhance the weight-regulating action of calcium.

More recent data in a 12-year weight change study in men, however, do not support the theory that an increase in calcium intake or dairy foods leads to lower long-term weight gain in men.

Although additional research is needed, the best recommendation at this point is that if you are attempting to lose or maintain weight loss, do not eliminate dairy foods from your diet. Substitute non fat (skim milk) or low-fat dairy products for other drinks and foods in your diet to enhance nutrition, and possibly, to help you manage weight.

***Sources:*** M. B. Zemel, "Role of Dietary Calcium and Dairy Products in Modulating Adiposity" *Lipids* 38, no. 2 (2003): 139–146; "A Nice Surprise from Calcium," *University of California Berkeley Wellness Letter,* 19, no. 11 (August 2003). 1, 3. N. Rajpathak et al., "Calcium and Dairy Intakes in Relation to Long-term Weight Gain in US Men," *The American Journal of Clinical Nutrition* 83, no. 3 (2006): 559–566.

## Try It

If you limit dairy products in your regular diet or while on a negative caloric balance, record in your Online Journal or class notebook what effects such a practice might have on your weight management and overall health. What is one thing you could change in your diet to increase your intake of dairy products?

---

ness lifestyle are healthy eating and regular physical activity, and they provide the best weight management program available today.

# Eating Disorders

Eating disorders are medical illnesses that involve critical disturbances in eating behaviors thought to stem from some combination of environmental pressures. These disorders are characterized by an intense fear of becoming fat, which does not disappear even when the person is losing weight in extreme amounts. The three most common types of eating disorders are **anorexia nervosa, bulimia nervosa,** and **binge-eating disorder.** Another eating behavior, **emotional eating,** can also be listed as an eating disorder.

Most people who have eating disorders are afflicted by significant family and social problems. They may lack fulfillment in many areas of their lives. The eating disorder then becomes the coping mechanism to avoid dealing with these problems. Taking control of their body weight helps them believe that they are restoring some sense of control over their lives.

---

**Anorexia nervosa** An eating disorder characterized by self-imposed starvation to lose and maintain very low body weight.

**Bulimia nervosa** An eating disorder characterized by a pattern of binge eating and purging in an attempt to lose weight and maintain low body weight.

**Binge-eating disorder** An eating disorder characterized by uncontrollable episodes of eating excessive amounts of food within a relatively short time.

**Emotional eating** The consumption of large quantities of food to suppress negative emotions.

Anorexia nervosa and bulimia nervosa are common in industrialized nations where society encourages low-calorie diets and thinness. The female role in society has changed rapidly, which makes women more susceptible to eating disorders. Although frequently seen in young women, the disorder is most prevalent among individuals between the ages of 25 and 50. Surveys, nonetheless, indicate that as many as 40 percent of college-age women are struggling with an eating disorder.

Eating disorders are not limited to women. Every 1 in 10 cases occurs in men. But because men's role and body image are viewed differently in our society, these cases often go unreported.

Although genetics may play a role in the development of eating disorders, most cases are environmentally related. Individuals who have clinical depression and obsessive-compulsive behavior are more susceptible. About half of all people with eating disorders have some sort of chemical dependency (alcohol and drugs), and most of them come from families with alcohol- and drug-related problems. Of reported cases of eating disorders, a large number come from individuals who are, or have been, victims of sexual molestation.

Eating disorders develop in stages. Typically, individuals who are already dealing with significant issues in life start a diet. At first they feel in control and are happy about the weight loss, even if they are not overweight. Encouraged by the prospect of weight loss and the control they can exert over their own weight, the dieting becomes extreme and often is combined with exhaustive exercise and the overuse of laxatives and diuretics.

The syndrome typically emerges following emotional issues or a stressful life event and the uncertainty about one's ability to cope efficiently. Life experiences that can trigger the syndrome might be: gaining weight, starting the menstrual period, beginning college, losing a boyfriend, having poor self-esteem, being socially rejected, starting a professional career, or becoming a wife or a mother. The eating disorder then takes on a life of its own and becomes the primary focus of attention for the individual afflicted with it. Self worth revolves around what the scale reads every day, one's relationship with food, and one's perception of how one looks each day.

**Anorexia Nervosa** An estimated 1 percent of the population in the United States has the eating disorder anorexia nervosa. Anorexic individuals seem to fear weight gain more than death from starvation. Furthermore, they have a distorted image of their bodies and think of themselves as being fat even when they are emaciated.

Anorexic patients commonly develop obsessive and compulsive behaviors and emphatically deny their condition. They are preoccupied with food, meal planning, and grocery shopping, and they have unusual eating habits. As they lose weight and their health begins to deteriorate, they feel weak and tired. They might realize they have a problem, but they will not stop the starvation, and they refuse to consider the behavior abnormal.

Once they have lost a lot of weight and malnutrition sets in, the physical changes become more visible. Typical changes are amenorrhea (absence of menstruation); digestive problems; extreme sensitivity to cold; fluid and electrolyte abnormalities (which may lead to an irregular heartbeat and sudden stopping of the heart); injuries to nerves and tendons; abnormalities of immune function; anemia; growth of fine body hair, dry skin, lowered skin/body temperature, and other hair and skin problems; mental confusion; inability to concentrate; lethargy and depression; and osteoporosis.

Diagnostic criteria for anorexia nervosa are:[16]

- Refusal to maintain body weight over a minimal normal weight for age and height (weight loss leading to maintenance of body weight less than 85 percent of that expected, or failure to make expected weight gain during periods of growth, leading to body weight less than 85 percent of that expected)
- Intense fear of gaining weight or becoming fat, even though one is underweight
- Disturbance in the way in which one's body weight, size, or shape is perceived, undue influences of body weight or shape on self-evaluation, or denial of the seriousness of the current low body weight
- In postmenarchal females, amenorrhea (absence of at least three consecutive menstrual cycles) (A woman is

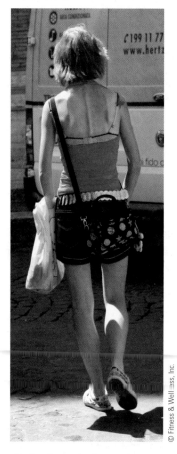

Society's unrealistic view of what constitutes recommended weight and "ideal" body image contributes to the development of eating disorders.

considered to have amenorrhea if her periods occur only following estrogen therapy.)

Many of the changes induced by anorexia nervosa can be reversed. Individuals with this condition can get better with professional therapy. Unfortunately, sometimes they turn to bulimia nervosa or they die from the disorder. Anorexia nervosa has the highest mortality rate of all psychosomatic illnesses today—20 percent of anorexic individuals die as a result of their condition. The disorder is 100 percent curable, but treatment almost always requires professional help. The sooner it is obtained, the better are the chances for reversibility and cure. Therapy consists of a combination of medical and psychological techniques to restore proper nutrition, prevent medical complications, and modify the environment or events that triggered the syndrome.

Seldom can anorexia sufferers overcome the problem by themselves. They strongly deny their condition. They are able to hide it and deceive friends and relatives. Based on their behavior, many of them meet all of the characteristics of anorexia nervosa, but it goes undetected because both thinness and dieting are socially acceptable. Only a well-trained clinician is able to diagnose anorexia nervosa.

### Bulimia Nervosa
Bulimia nervosa is more prevalent than anorexia nervosa. As many as 1 in every 5 women on college campuses may be bulimic, according to some estimates. Bulimia nervosa also is more prevalent than anorexia nervosa in males, although bulimia is still much more prevalent in females.

People with bulimia usually are healthy looking, well educated, and near recommended body weight. They seem to enjoy food and often socialize around it. In actuality, they are emotionally insecure, rely on others, and lack self-confidence and self-esteem. Recommended weight and food are important to them.

The binge–purge cycle usually occurs in stages. As a result of stressful life events or the simple compulsion to eat, bulimic individuals engage periodically in binge eating that may last an hour or longer. With some apprehension, bulimics anticipate and plan the cycle. Next they feel an urgency to binge, followed by large and uncontrollable food consumption, during which time they may eat several thousand calories (up to 10,000 calories in extreme cases). After a short period of relief and satisfaction, feelings of deep guilt, shame, and intense fear of gaining weight emerge. Purging seems to be an easy answer, as the bingeing cycle can continue without fear of gaining weight.

The diagnostic criteria for bulimia nervosa are:[17]

- Recurrent episodes of binge eating. An episode of binge eating is characterized by both of the following:
    - (a) Eating in a discrete period of time (for example, within any 2-hour period) an amount of food that is definitely more than most people would eat during a similar period and under similar circumstances

    - (b) A sense of lack of control over eating during the episode (a feeling that one cannot stop eating or control what or how much one is eating)
- Recurring inappropriate compensatory behaviors to prevent weight gain, such as self-induced vomiting; misuse of laxatives, diuretics, other medications, or enemas; fasting; or excessive exercise
- Binge eating and inappropriate compensatory behaviors that both occur, on average, at least twice a week for 3 months
- Self-evaluation unduly influenced by body shape and weight

The most typical form of purging is self-induced vomiting. Bulimics, too, frequently ingest strong laxatives and emetics. Near-fasting diets and strenuous bouts of exercise are common. Medical problems associated with bulimia nervosa include cardiac arrhythmias, amenorrhea, kidney and bladder damage, ulcers, colitis, tearing of the esophagus or stomach, tooth erosion, gum damage, and general muscular weakness.

Unlike anorexics, bulimia sufferers realize that their behavior is abnormal and feel shame about it. Fearing social rejection, they pursue the binge–purge cycle in secrecy and at unusual hours of the day. Bulimia nervosa can be treated successfully when the person realizes that this destructive behavior is not the solution to life's problems. A change in attitude can prevent permanent damage or death.

### Binge-Eating Disorder
Binge-eating disorder is probably the most common of the three main eating disorders. About 2 percent of American adults are afflicted with binge-eating disorder in any 6-month period. Although most people think they overeat from time to time, eating more than one should now and then does not mean that the individual has a binge-eating disorder. The disorder is slightly more common in women than in men; three women for every two men have it.

Binge-eating disorder is characterized by uncontrollable episodes of eating excessive amounts of food within a relatively short time. The causes of binge-eating disorder are unknown, although depression, anger, sadness, boredom, and worry can trigger an episode. Unlike bulimic sufferers, binge eaters do not purge; thus, most people with this disorder are either overweight or obese.

Typical symptoms of binge-eating disorder include:

- Eating what most people think is an unusually large amount of food
- Eating until uncomfortably full
- Eating out of control
- Eating much faster than usual during binge episodes
- Eating alone because of embarrassment of how much food one is consuming
- Feeling disgusted, depressed, or guilty after overeating

### Emotional Eating
In addition to physiological purposes, eating also fulfills psychological, social, and cultural purposes. We eat to sustain our daily energy

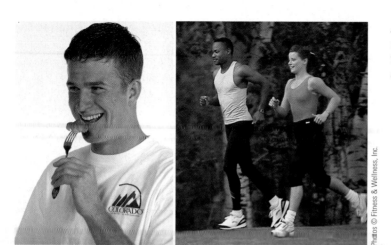

Achieving and maintaining a high physical fitness percent body fat standard requires a lifetime commitment to regular physical activity and proper nutrition.

requirements, but we also eat at family celebrations, national holidays, social gatherings, sporting events (as spectators), and even when we become very emotional (some people stop eating when emotional). Emotional eating involves the consumption of large quantities of food, mostly "comfort" and junk food, to suppress negative emotions. Such emotions include stress, anxiety, uncertainty, guilt, anger, pain, depression, loneliness, sadness, or boredom. In such circumstances, people eat for comfort when they are at their weakest point emotionally. Comfort foods often include calorie-dense, sweet, salty, and fatty foods. Excessive emotional eating hinders proper weight management.

Some palatable foods, such as chocolate, cause the body to release small amounts of mood-elevating opiates, helping to offset negative emotions. A preference for certain foods is also present when one experiences specific feelings (loneliness, anxiety, fear). Eating helps to divert the stressor away for a while, but the distraction is only temporary. The emotions return and may be compounded by feelings of guilt from overeating.

If you are an emotional overeater, you can always seek help from a therapist at your school's counseling center. The following list of suggestions may also help:

1. Learn to differentiate between emotional and physical hunger.
2. Avoid storing and snacking on unhealthy foods.
3. Keep healthy snacks handy.
4. Use countering techniques (go for a walk instead of reaching for the ice cream, listen to music instead of eating the candy bar).
5. Keep a "trigger log" and get to know what triggers your emotional food consumption.
6. Work it out with exercise instead of food.

## Treatment

Treatment for eating disorders is available on most school campuses through the school's counseling center or health center. Local hospitals also offer treatment for these conditions. Many communities have support groups, frequently led by professional personnel and often free of charge. All information and the individual's identity are kept confidential, so the person need not fear embarrassment or repercussions when seeking professional help.

# The Physiology of Weight Loss

Traditional concepts related to weight control have centered on three assumptions:

1. Balancing food intake against output allows a person to achieve recommended weight.
2. All fat people simply eat too much.
3. The human body doesn't care how much (or little) fat it stores.

Although these statements contain some truth, they are open to much debate and research. We now know that the causes of obesity are complex, involving a combination of genetics, behavior, and lifestyle factors.

## Energy-Balancing Equation

The principle embodied in the **energy-balancing equation** is simple: As long as caloric input equals caloric output, the person will not gain or lose weight. If caloric intake exceeds output, the person gains weight; when output exceeds input, the person loses weight. If daily energy requirements could be determined accurately, caloric intake could be balanced against output. This is not always the case, though, because genetic and lifestyle-related individual differences determine the number of calories required to maintain or lose body weight.

Table 5.3 (page 171) offers general guidelines to determine the **estimated energy requirement (EER)** in calories per day. This is an estimated figure and (as discussed under "Losing Weight the Sound and Sensible

Way," page 169) serves only as a starting point from which individual adjustments have to be made.

The total daily energy requirement has three basic components (Figure 5.6):

1. Resting metabolic rate
2. Thermic effect of food
3. Physical activity

The **resting metabolic rate (RMR)**—the energy requirement to maintain the body's vital processes in the resting state—accounts for approximately 60 to 70 percent of the total daily energy requirement. The thermic effect of food—the energy required to digest, absorb, and store food—accounts for about 5 to 10 percent of the total daily requirement. Physical activity accounts for 15 to 30 percent of the total daily requirement.

One pound of fat is the equivalent of 3,500 calories. If a person's EER is 2,500 calories and that person were to decrease intake by 500 calories per day, it should result in a loss of 1 pound of fat in 7 days (500 × 7 = 3,500). But research has shown—and many people have experienced that even when dieters carefully balance caloric input against caloric output, weight loss does not always result as predicted. Furthermore, two people with similar measured caloric intakes and outputs seldom lose weight at the same rate.

The most common explanation for individual differences in weight loss and weight gain has been variation in human metabolism from one person to another. We are all familiar with people who can eat "all day long" and not gain an ounce of weight, while others cannot even "dream about food" without gaining weight. Because experts did not believe that human metabolism alone could account for such extreme differences, they developed other theories that might better explain these individual variations.

**Setpoint Theory** Results of several research studies point toward a **weight-regulating mechanism (WRM)** that has a **setpoint** for controlling both appetite and the amount of fat stored. Setpoint is hypothesized to work like a thermostat for body fat, maintaining fairly constant body weight, because it "knows" at all times the exact amount of adipose tissue stored in the fat cells. Some people have high settings; others have low settings.

If body weight decreases (as in dieting), the setpoint senses this change and triggers the WRM to increase the person's appetite or make the body conserve energy to maintain the "set" weight. The opposite also may be true. Some people have a hard time gaining weight. In this case, the WRM decreases appetite or causes the body to waste energy to maintain the lower weight.

Every person has his or her own certain body fat percentage (as established by the setpoint) that the body attempts to maintain. The genetic instinct to survive tells the body that fat storage is vital, and therefore it sets an acceptable fat level. This level may remain somewhat constant or may climb gradually because of poor lifestyle habits.

For instance, under strict calorie reduction, the body may make extreme metabolic adjustments in an effort to maintain its setpoint for fat. The **basal metabolic rate (BMR),** the lowest level of caloric intake necessary to sustain life, may drop dramatically when operating under a consistent negative caloric balance, and that person's weight loss may plateau for days or even weeks. A low metabolic rate compounds a person's problems in maintaining recommended body weight.

These findings were substantiated by research conducted at Rockefeller University in New York.[18] The authors showed that the body resists maintaining altered weight. Obese and lifetime nonobese individuals were used in the investigation. Following a 10 percent weight loss, the body, in an attempt to regain the lost weight, compensated by burning up to 15 percent fewer calories than expected for the new re-

---

**FIGURE 5.6  Components of Total Daily Energy Requirement.**

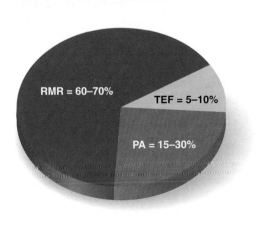

RMR = resting metabolic rate
TEF = thermic effect of food
PA = physical activity

---

**Energy-balancing equation**  A principle holding that as long as caloric input equals caloric output, the person will not gain or lose weight. If caloric intake exceeds output, the person gains weight; when output exceeds input, the person loses weight.

**Estimated energy requirement (EER)**  The average dietary energy (caloric) intake that is predicted to maintain energy balance in a healthy adult of defined age, gender, weight, height, and level of physical activity, consistent with good health.

**Resting metabolic rate (RMR)**  The energy requirement to maintain the body's vital processes in the resting state

**Weight-regulating mechanism (WRM)**  A feature of the hypothalamus of the brain that controls how much the body should weigh.

**Setpoint**  Weight control theory that the body has an established weight and strongly attempts to maintain that weight.

**Basal metabolic rate (BMR)**  The lowest level of oxygen consumption necessary to sustain life.

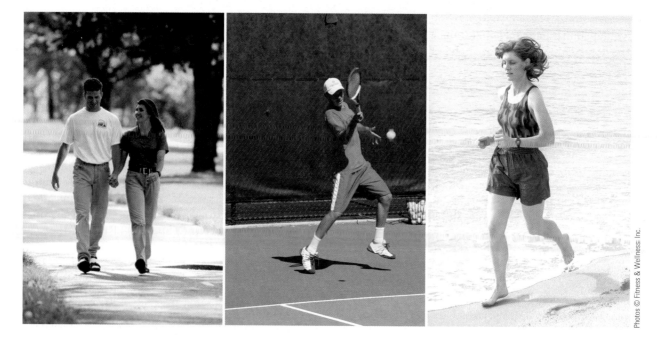

Exercising with other people and in different places helps people maintain exercise regularity.

Photos © Fitness & Wellness, Inc.

duced weight (after accounting for the 10 percent loss). The effects were similar in the obese and nonobese participants. These results imply that after a 10 percent weight loss, a person would have to eat even less or exercise even more to compensate for the estimated 15 percent slowdown (a difference of about 200 to 300 calories).

In this same study, when the participants were allowed to increase their weight to 10 percent above their "normal" body (pre–weight loss) weight, the body burned 10 to 15 percent more calories than expected—attempting to waste energy and maintain the preset weight. This is another indication that the body is highly resistant to weight changes unless additional lifestyle changes are incorporated to ensure successful weight management. (These methods are discussed under "Losing Weight the Sound and Sensible Way," page 169.)

## Critical Thinking

Do you see a difference in the amount of food that you are now able to eat compared with the amount that you ate in your mid- to late-teen years? If so, to what do you attribute these differences? What actions are you taking to account for the difference?

**Very low calorie diet** A diet that allows an energy intake (consumption) of only 800 calories or less per day.

Dietary restriction alone will not lower the setpoint, even though the person may lose weight and fat. When the dieter goes back to the normal or even below-normal caloric intake (at which the weight may have been stable for a long time), he or she quickly regains the lost fat as the body strives to regain a comfortable fat store.

**An Example** Let's use a practical illustration. A person would like to lose some body fat and assumes that his or her current stable body weight has been reached at an average daily caloric intake of 1,800 calories (no weight gain or loss occurs at this daily intake). In an attempt to lose weight rapidly, this person now goes on a **very low calorie diet** (defined as 800 calories per day or less), or, even worse, a near-fasting diet. This immediately activates the body's survival mechanism and readjusts the metabolism to a lower caloric balance. After a few weeks of dieting at the 800-calories-per-day level, the body now can maintain its normal functions at 1,300 calories per day. This new figure (1,300) represents a drop of 500 calories per day in the metabolic rate.

Having lost the desired weight, the person terminates the diet but realizes that the original intake of 1,800 calories per day will have to be lower to maintain the new lower weight. To adjust to the new lower body weight, the person restricts intake to about 1,600 calories per day. The individual is surprised to find that even at this lower daily intake (200 fewer calories), the weight comes back at a rate of 1 pound every one to two weeks. After the diet is over, this new lowered metabolic rate may take several months to kick back up to its normal level.

Based on this explanation, individuals clearly should not go on very low calorie diets. This will slow the resting metabolic rate and also will deprive the body of basic daily nutrients required for normal function. Very low calorie diets should be used only in conjunction with dietary supplements and under proper medical supervision.[19] Furthermore, people who use very low calorie diets are not as effective in keeping the weight off once the diet is terminated.

**Recommendation** Daily caloric intakes of 1,200 to 1,500 calories provide the necessary nutrients if they are distributed properly over the basic food groups (meeting the daily recommended amounts from each group). Of course, the individual will have to learn which foods meet the requirements and yet are low in fat and sugar.

Under no circumstances should a person go on a diet that calls for a level of 1,200 calories or less for women or 1,500 calories or less for men. Weight (fat) is gained over months and years, not overnight. Likewise, weight loss should be gradual, not abrupt.

A second way in which the setpoint may work is by keeping track of the nutrients and calories consumed daily. It is thought that the body, like a cash register, records the daily food intake and that the brain will not feel satisfied until the calories and nutrients have been "registered."

This setpoint for calories and nutrients seems to operate even when people participate in moderately intense exercise. Some evidence suggests that people do not become hungrier with moderate physical activity. Therefore, people can choose to lose weight either by going hungry or by combining a sensible calorie-restricted diet with an increase in daily physical activity. Burning more calories through physical activity helps to lower body fat.

**Lowering the Setpoint** The most common question regarding the setpoint is how to lower it so the body will feel comfortable at a reduced fat percentage. The factors that seem to affect the setpoint directly by lowering the fat thermostat are:

- Exercise
- A diet high in complex carbohydrates
- Nicotine
- Amphetamines

The last two are more destructive than the extra fat weight, so they are not reasonable alternatives (as far as the extra strain on the heart is concerned, smoking one pack of cigarettes per day is said to be the equivalent of carrying 50 to 75 pounds of excess body fat). A diet high in fats and refined carbohydrates, near-fasting diets, and perhaps even use of artificial sweeteners seem to raise the setpoint. Therefore, the only practical and sensible way to lower the setpoint and lose fat weight is a combination of exercise and a diet high in complex carbohydrates and only moderate amounts of fat.

Because of the effects of proper food management on the body's setpoint, most of the successful dieter's effort should be spent in re-forming eating habits, increasing the intake of complex carbohydrates and high-fiber foods, and decreasing the consumption of processed foods that are high in

## Behavior Modification Planning

### EATING RIGHT WHEN ON THE RUN

Current lifestyles often require people to be on the run. We don't seem to have time to eat right, but fortunately it doesn't have to be that way. If you are on the run, it is even more critical to make healthy choices to keep up with a challenging schedule. Do you regularly consume the following foods when you are eating on the run?

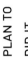

| I PLAN TO | I DID IT | |
|:---:|:---:|:---|
| ❏ | ❏ | Water |
| ❏ | ❏ | Whole-grain cereal and skim milk |
| ❏ | ❏ | Whole-grain bread and bagels |
| ❏ | ❏ | Whole-grain bread with peanut butter |
| ❏ | ❏ | Non-fat or low-fat yogurt |
| ❏ | ❏ | Fresh fruits |
| ❏ | ❏ | Frozen fresh fruit (grapes, cherries, banana slices) |
| ❏ | ❏ | Dried fruits |
| ❏ | ❏ | Raw vegetables (carrots, red peppers, cucumbers, radishes, cauliflower, asparagus) |
| ❏ | ❏ | Crackers |
| ❏ | ❏ | Pretzels |
| ❏ | ❏ | Bread sticks |
| ❏ | ❏ | Low-fat cheese sticks |
| ❏ | ❏ | Granola bars |
| ❏ | ❏ | Snack-size cereal boxes |
| ❏ | ❏ | Nuts |
| ❏ | ❏ | Trail mix |
| ❏ | ❏ | Plain popcorn |
| ❏ | ❏ | Vegetable soups |

### Try It

In your Online Journal or class notebook, plan your fast-meal menus for the upcoming week. It may require extra shopping and some food preparation (for instance, cutting vegetables to place in snack plastic bags). At the end of the week, evaluate how many days you had a "healthy eating on the run day." What did you learn from the experience?

refined carbohydrates (sugars) and fats. This change in eating habits will bring about a decrease in total daily caloric intake. Because 1 gram of carbohydrates provides only 4 calories, as opposed to 9 calories per gram of fat, you could eat twice the volume of food (by weight) when substituting carbohydrates for fat. Some fat, however, is recommended in the diet—preferably polyunsaturated and monounsaturated fats. These so-called good fats do more than help protect the heart, they help delay hunger pangs.

A "diet" should not be viewed as a temporary tool to aid in weight loss but, instead, as a permanent change in eating behaviors to ensure weight management and better health. The role of increased physical activity also must be considered, because successful weight loss, maintenance, and recommended body composition are seldom attained without a moderate reduction in caloric intake combined with a regular exercise program.

# Diet and Metabolism

Fat can be lost by selecting the proper foods, exercising, or restricting calories. However, when dieters try to lose weight by dietary restrictions alone, they also lose lean body mass (muscle protein, along with vital organ protein). The amount of lean body mass lost depends entirely on caloric limitation. When people go on a near-fasting diet, up to half of the weight loss is lean body mass and the other half is actual fat loss (Figure 5.7).[20] When diet is combined with exercise, close to 100 percent of the weight loss is in the form of fat, and lean tissue actually may increase. Loss of lean body mass is never good, because it weakens the organs and muscles and slows metabolism. Large losses in lean tissue can cause disturbances in heart function and damage to other organs. Equally important is not to overindulge (binge) following a very low calorie diet, as this may cause changes in metabolic rate and electrolyte balance, which could trigger fatal cardiac arrhythmias.

Contrary to some beliefs, aging is not the main reason for the lower metabolic rate. It is not so much that metabolism slows down as that people slow down. As people age, they tend to rely more on the amenities of life (remote controls, cell phones, intercoms, single-level homes, riding lawnmowers) that lull a person into sedentary living.

Basal metabolism also is related to lean body weight. More lean tissue yields a higher metabolic rate. As a consequence of sedentary living and less physical activity, the lean component decreases and fat tissue increases. The human body requires a certain amount of oxygen per pound of lean body mass. Given that fat is considered metabolically inert from the point of view of caloric use, the lean tissue uses most of the oxygen, even at rest. As muscle and organ mass (lean body mass) decrease, so do the energy requirements at rest.

Diets with intakes below 1,200 to 1,500 calories cannot guarantee the retention of lean body mass. Even at this intake level, some loss is inevitable unless the diet is combined with exercise. Despite the claims of many diets that they do not alter the lean component, the simple truth is that regardless of what nutrients may be added to the diet, severe caloric restrictions always prompt the loss of

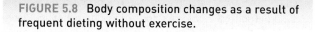

**FIGURE 5.8** Body composition changes as a result of frequent dieting without exercise.

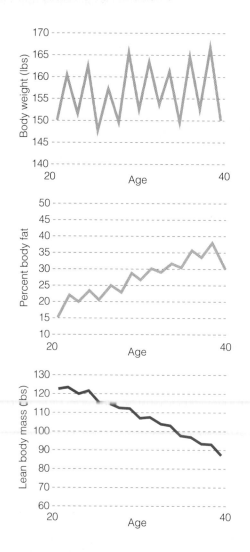

**FIGURE 5.7** Outcome of three forms of diet on fat loss.

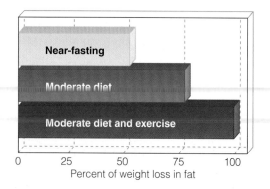

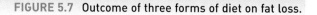

***Source:*** Adapted from R. J. Shephard, *Alive Man: The Physiology of Physical Activity* (Springfield, IL: Charles C. Thomas, 1975): 484–488.

lean tissue. Sadly, many people go on very low calorie diets constantly. Every time they do, their metabolic rate slows as more lean tissue is lost.

People in their 40s and older who weigh the same as they did when they were 20 tend to think they are at recommended body weight. During this span of 20 years or more, though, they may have dieted many times without participating in an exercise program. After they terminate each diet, they regain the weight, and much of that gain is additional body fat. Maybe at age 20 they weighed 150 pounds, of which only 15 percent was fat. Now at age 40, even though they still weigh 150 pounds, they might be 30 percent fat (Figure 5.8). At recommended body weight, they wonder why they are eating very little and still having trouble staying at that weight.

# Exercise: The Key to Weight Management

A more effective way to tilt the energy-balancing equation in your favor is by burning calories through physical activity. Research shows that the combination of diet and exercise leads to greater weight loss. Further, exercise seems to be the best predictor of long-term maintenance of weight loss.[21]

Exercise seems to exert control over how much a person weighs. On the average, starting at age 25, the typical American gains 1 to 2 pounds of weight per year. A 1-pound weight gain represents a simple energy surplus of under 10 calories per day. The additional weight accumulated in middle age comes from people becoming less physically active and increasing caloric intake. Dr. Jack

Wilmore, a leading exercise physiologist and expert weight management researcher, stated:

> Physical inactivity is certainly a major, if not the primary, cause of obesity in the United States today. A certain minimal level of activity might be necessary for us to accurately balance our caloric intake to our caloric expenditure. With too little activity, we appear to lose the fine control we normally have to maintain this incredible balance. This fine balance amounts to less than 10 calories per day, or the equivalent of one potato chip.[22]

Exercise enhances the rate of weight loss and is vital in maintaining the lost weight. Not only will exercise maintain lean tissue, but advocates of the setpoint theory say that exercise resets the fat thermostat to a new, lower level. This change may be rapid, or it may take time.

Although a few individuals lose weight by participating in 30 minutes of exercise per day, many overweight people need 60 to 90 minutes of daily physical activity to effectively manage body weight (the 30 minutes of exercise are included as part of the 60 to 90 minutes of physical activity).

Accumulating 30 minutes of moderate-intensity activity per day provides substantial health benefits. From a weight management point of view, however, the Institute of Medicine of the National Academy of Sciences recommends that people accumulate 60 minutes of moderate-intensity physical activity most days of the week.[23] The evidence shows that people who maintain recommended weight typically accumulate an hour or more of daily physical activity.

As illustrated in Figure 5.9, greater weight loss is achieved by combining a diet with an exercise program. Of even greater significance, however, only individuals who remain physically active for 60 or more minutes per day are able to keep the weight off (Figure 5.10).

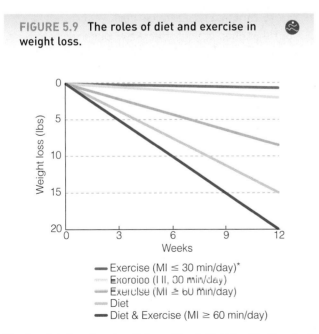

FIGURE 5.9 The roles of diet and exercise in weight loss.

- Exercise (MI ≤ 30 min/day)*
- Exercise (MI 30 min/day)
- Exercise (MI ≥ 60 min/day)
- Diet
- Diet & Exercise (MI ≥ 60 min/day)

Based on data from American College of Sports Medicine, "Position stand: appropriate intervention strategies for weight loss and prevention for weight regain for adults," *Medicine and Science in Sports and Exercise* 33 (2001): 2145–2156.

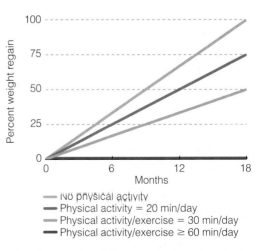

FIGURE 5.10 Effects of different amounts of daily energy expenditure on weight maintenance following a weight reduction program.

- No physical activity
- Physical activity = 20 min/day
- Physical activity/exercise = 30 min/day
- Physical activity/exercise ≥ 60 min/day

Based on data from American College of Sports Medicine, "Position stand: appropriate intervention strategies for weight loss and prevention for weight regain for adults," *Medicine and Science in Sports and Exercise* 33 (2001): 2145–2156.

Further, data from the National Weight Control Registry (http://www.nwcr.ws) indicate that individuals who have lost at least 30 pounds and kept them off for a minimum of 6 years typically accumulate 90 minutes of daily activity. Those who are less active gradually regain the lost weight. Individuals who completely stop physical activity regain almost 100 percent of the weight within 18 months of discontinuing the weight loss program (see Figure 5.10). Thus, if weight management is not a consideration, 30 minutes of daily activity five days per week provides health benefits. To prevent weight gain, 60 minutes of daily activity is recommended; to maintain substantial weight loss, 90 minutes may be required.

If a person is trying to lose weight, a combination of aerobic and strength-training exercises works best. Aerobic exercise is the best to offset the setpoint, and the continuity and duration of these types of activities cause many calories to be burned in the process. The role of aerobic exercise in successful lifetime weight management cannot be overestimated. Strength training is critical in helping maintain lean body mass. Unfortunately, of those individuals who are attempting to lose weight, only 19 percent of women and 22 percent of men decrease their caloric intake and exercise above an average of 25 or more minutes per day.[24]

The number of calories burned during a typical hour-long strength-training session is much less than during an hour of aerobic exercise. Because of the high intensity of strength training, the person needs frequent rest intervals to recover from each set of exercises. The average person actually lifts weights only 10 to 12 minutes during each hour of exercise. In the long run, however, the person enjoys the benefits of gains in lean tissue. Guidelines for developing aerobic and strength-training programs are given in Chapters 6 and 7.

Weight loss might be more rapid if aerobic exercise is combined with a strength-training program. Although the increase in BMR through increased muscle mass is being debated in the literature and merits further research, data indicate that each additional pound of muscle tissue raises the BMR in the range of 6 to 35 calories per day.[25]

The latter figure is based on calculations that an increase of 3 to 3.5 pounds of lean tissue through strength training increases BMR by about 105 to 120 calories per day.[26] Most likely, the benefit of strength training goes beyond the new muscle tissue itself. Maybe a pound of muscle tissue requires only 6 calories per day to sustain itself, but as all muscles undergo strength training, they also undergo increased protein synthesis to build and repair themselves, resulting in increased energy expenditure of 1 to 1.5 calories per pound in all trained muscle tissue. Such an increase would explain the BMR increase of 105 to 120 calories per day in some research studies.

To examine the effects of a small increase in BMR on long-term body weight, let's use a very conservative estimate of an additional 50 calories per day as a result of a regular strength-training program. An increase of 50 calories represents an additional 18,250 calories per year (50 ×

## Behavior Modification Planning

### PHYSICAL ACTIVITY GUIDELINES FOR WEIGHT MANAGEMENT

The following physical activity guidelines are recommended to effectively manage body weight:

☐ I PLAN TO  ☐ I DID IT

☐ ☐ 30 minutes of physical activity on most days of the week if you do not have difficulty maintaining body weight (more minutes and/or higher intensity if you choose to reach a high level of physical fitness).

☐ ☐ 60 minutes of daily activity if you want to prevent weight gain.

☐ ☐ Between 60 and 90 minutes each day if you are trying to lose weight or attempting to keep weight off following extensive weight loss (30 pounds of weight loss or more). Be sure to include some high-intensity/low-impact activities at least twice a week in your program.

### Try It

In your Behavior Change Planner Progress Tracker, Online Journal, or class notebook, record how many minutes of daily physical activity you accumulate on a regular basis and record your thoughts on how effectively your activity has helped you manage your body weight. Is there one thing you could do today to increase your physical activity?

365), or the equivalent of 5.2 pounds of fat (18,250 ÷ 3,500). This increase in BMR would more than offset the typical adult weight gain of 1 to 2 pounds per year.

This figure of 18,250 calories per year does not include the actual energy cost of the strength-training workout. If we use an energy expenditure of only 150 calories per strength-training session, done twice per week, over a year's time it would represent 15,600 calories (150 × 2 × 52), or the equivalent of another 4.5 pounds of fat (15,600 ÷ 3,500).

In addition, although the amounts seem small, the previous calculations do not account for the increase in metabolic rate following the strength-training workout

## Behavior Modification Planning

### WEIGHT-MAINTENANCE BENEFITS OF LIFETIME AEROBIC EXERCISE

The authors of this book have been jogging together a minimum of 15 miles per week (3 miles/5 times per week) for the past 32 years. Without considering the additional energy expenditure from their regular strength-training program and 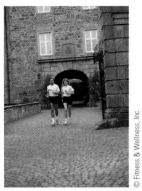 their many other sport and recreational activities, the energy cost of this regular jogging program over 32 years has been approximately 2,496,000 calories (15 miles × 100 calories/mile × 52 weeks × 32 years), or the equivalent of 713 pounds of fat (2,496,000 ÷ 3,500). In essence, without this 30-minute workout 5 times per week, the authors would weigh 855 and 829 pounds respectively!

### Try It

Ask yourself whether a regular aerobic exercise program is part of your long-term gratification and health enhancement program. If the answer is no, are you ready to change your behavior? Use the Behavior Change Planner to help you answer the question.

(the time it takes the body to return to its preworkout resting rate—about 2 hours). Depending on the training volume (see Chapter 7), this recovery energy expenditure ranges from 20 to 100 calories following each strength-training workout.[27] All these "apparently small" changes make a big difference in the long run.

Although size (inches) and percent body fat both decrease when sedentary individuals begin an exercise program, body weight often remains the same or may even increase during the first couple of weeks of the program. Exercise helps to increase muscle tissue, connective tissue, blood volume (as much as 500 mL, or the equivalent of 1 pound, following the first week of aerobic exercise), enzymes and other structures within the cell, and glycogen (which binds water). All of these changes lead to a higher functional capacity of the human body. With exercise, most of the weight loss becomes apparent after a few weeks of training, when the lean component has stabilized.

We know that a negative caloric balance of 3,500 calories does not always result in a loss of exactly 1 pound of fat, but the role of exercise in achieving a negative balance by burning additional calories is significant in weight reduction and maintenance programs. Sadly, some individuals claim that the number of calories burned during exercise is hardly worth the effort. They think that cutting their daily intake by 300 calories is easier than participating in some sort of exercise that would burn the same amount of calories. The problem is that the willpower to cut those 300 calories lasts only a few weeks, and then the person goes back to the old eating patterns.

If a person gets into the habit of exercising regularly, say three times a week, jogging 3 miles per exercise session (about 300 calories burned), this represents 900 calories in one week, about 3,600 calories in one month, or 46,800 calories per year. This minimal amount of exercise represents as many as 13.5 extra pounds of fat in one year, 27 in two, and so on.

We tend to forget that our weight creeps up gradually over the years, not just overnight. Hardly worth the effort? And we have not even taken into consideration the increase in lean tissue, possible resetting of the setpoint, benefits to the cardiovascular system, and, most important, the improved quality of life. Fundamental reasons for overfatness and obesity, few could argue, are sedentary living and lack of a regular exercise program.

In terms of preventing disease, many of the health benefits that people seek by losing weight are reaped through exercise alone, even without weight loss. Exercise offers protection against premature morbidity and mortality for everyone, including people who already have risk factors for disease.

### Low-Intensity Versus Vigorous-Intensity Exercise for Weight Loss

Some individuals promote low-intensity over vigorous-intensity exercise for weight loss purposes. Compared with vigorous intensity, a greater proportion of calories burned during low-intensity exercise are derived from fat. The lower the intensity of exercise, the higher the percentage of fat used as an energy source. In theory, if you are trying to lose fat, this principle makes sense, but in reality it is misleading. The bottom line when you are trying to lose weight is to burn more calories. When your daily caloric expenditure exceeds your intake, you lose weight. The more calories you burn, the more fat you lose.

During low-intensity exercise, up to 50 percent of the calories burned may be derived from fat (the other 50 percent from glucose [carbohydrates]). With intense exercise, only 30 to 40 percent of the caloric expenditure comes from fat. Overall, however, you can burn twice as many calories during vigorous-intensity exercise and, subsequently, more fat as well.

## "Alli" Weight Loss Drug

"Alli" is an over-the-counter weight loss drug that promises 50 percent greater weight loss than achieved through diet and exercise alone. Alli is not a miracle weight loss pill but may enhance the rate of weight loss.

Alli contains orlistat, the same active ingredient found in the prescription weight loss drug Xenical, but only at half the dose of Xenical. Alli is recommended for overweight people who are not obese and who are willing to commit to a rigorous online diet and exercise program. Orlistat works by preventing the absorption of about 25 percent of all fat in the diet. Along with unhealthy fat, the drug also blocks essential fatty acids (omega-3) and fat-soluble nutrients (such as vitamins A, E, and D) needed for good health. A daily multivitamin is encouraged to offset the loss of fat-soluble nutrients. Alli is not recommended for people with an organ transplant (it interferes with antirejection drugs) or those with health problems that prevent nutrient absorption.

Unpleasant and uncomfortable side effects include gas with oily spotting, loose stools, more frequent stools, and urgent, uncontrollable bowel movements. The magnitude of the side effects increases with increased fat intake. To reduce side effects, the manufacturer recommends consumption of less than 15 grams of fat per meal. At 15 grams of fat per meal, one consumes 45 grams of fat per day, for a total of 405 fat calories, or 20 percent fat calories based on a 2,000-calorie daily diet (405 ÷ 2000). Such a low-fat diet, in and of itself (without the drug), combined with exercise, leads to healthy weight loss in most individuals.

Alli is marketed under the slogan "If you have the will, we have the power." Alli costs about $2 per day. If you have the will to commit to a "rigorous diet and exercise program," lifetime weight management will be accomplished without the need of expensive drugs with undesirable and potentially embarrassing side effects.

Let's look at a practical illustration (also see Table 5.2). If you exercised for 30 to 40 minutes at moderate intensity and burned 200 calories, about 100 of those calories (50 percent) would come from fat. If you exercised at a vigorous intensity during those same 30 to 40 minutes, you could burn 400 calories, with 120 to 160 of the calories (30 to 40 percent) coming from fat. Thus, even though it is true that the percentage of fat used is greater during low intensity exercise, the overall amount of fat used is still less during low-intensity exercise. Plus, if you were to exercise at a low intensity, you would have to do so twice as long to burn the same amount of calories. Another benefit is that the metabolic rate remains at a slightly higher level longer after vigorous-intensity exercise, so you continue to burn a few extra calories following exercise.

Moreover, vigorous-intensity exercise by itself seems to trigger more fat loss than low-intensity exercise. Research conducted at Laval University in Quebec, Canada, showed that subjects who performed a vigorous-intensity intermittent-training program lost more body fat than participants in a low- to moderate-intensity continuous aerobic endurance group.[28] Even more surprisingly, this finding occurred despite the fact that the vigorous-intensity group burned fewer total calories per exercise session. The results support the notion that vigorous exercise is more conducive to weight loss than low- to moderate-intensity exercise.

Before you start vigorous-intensity exercise sessions, a word of caution is in order: Be sure that it is medically safe for you to participate in such activities and that you build up gradually to that level. If you are cleared to participate in vigorous-intensity exercise, do not attempt to do too much too quickly, because you may incur injuries and become discouraged. You must allow your body a proper conditioning period of 8 to 12 weeks, or even longer for people with a moderate-to-serious weight problem. Vigorous intensity also does not mean high impact. High-impact activities are the most common cause of exercise-related injuries. Additional information on these topics is presented in Chapter 6.

The previous discussion on vigorous- versus low-intensity exercise does not mean that low intensity is ineffective. Low-intensity exercise provides substantial health benefits, and people who initiate exercise programs are more willing to participate and stay with low-intensity programs. Low-intensity exercise does promote weight loss, but it is not as effective. You will have to exercise longer to obtain the same results.

### Healthy Weight Gain

"Skinny" people, too, should realize that the only healthy way to gain weight is through exercise (mainly strength-training exercises) and a slight increase in caloric intake. Attempting to gain weight by overeating alone will raise the fat component and not the lean component—which is not the path to better health. Exercise is the best solution to weight (fat) reduction and weight (lean) gain alike.

A strength-training program such as the one outlined in Chapter 7 is the best approach to add body weight. The

**TABLE 5.2** Comparison of Energy Expenditure Between 30 and 40 Minutes of Low-Intensity vs. Vigorous-Intensity Exercise

| Exercise Intensity | Total Energy Expenditure (Calories) | Percent Calories From Fat | Total Fat Calories | Percent Calories From CHO* | Total CHO Calories | Calories Burned Per Minute | Calories Per Pound Per Minute |
| --- | --- | --- | --- | --- | --- | --- | --- |
| Low Intensity | 200 | 50% | 100 | 50% | 100 | 6.67 | 0.045 |
| Vigorous Intensity | 400 | 30% | 120 | 70% | 280 | 13.5 | 0.090 |

*CHO = Carbohydrates

training program should include at least two exercises of one to three sets for each major body part. Each set should consist of about 8 to 12 repetitions maximum.

Even though the metabolic cost of synthesizing a pound of muscle tissue is still unclear, consuming an estimated 500 additional calories per day is recommended to gain an average of 1 pound of muscle tissue per week. Your diet should include a daily total intake of about 1.5 grams of protein per kilogram of body weight. If your daily protein intake already exceeds 1.5 grams per day, the extra 500 calories should be primarily in the form of complex carbohydrates. The higher caloric intake must be accompanied by a strength-training program, otherwise the increase in body weight will be in the form of fat, not muscle tissue (Lab 5D can be used to monitor your caloric intake for healthy weight gain). Additional information on nutrition to optimize muscle growth and strength development is provided in Chapter 7 in the section "Dietary Guidelines for Strength Development," page 252.

**Weight Loss Myths** Cellulite and **spot reducing** are mythical concepts. **Cellulite** is nothing but enlarged fat cells that bulge out from accumulated body fat.

Doing several sets of daily sit-ups will not get rid of fat in the midsection of the body. When fat comes off, it does so throughout the entire body, not just the exercised area. The greatest proportion of fat may come off the biggest fat deposits, but the caloric output of a few sets of sit-ups has practically no effect on reducing total body fat. A person has to exercise much longer to see results.

Other touted means toward quick weight loss, such as rubberized sweat suits, steam baths, and mechanical vibrators, are misleading. When a person wears a sweat suit or steps into a sauna, the weight lost is not fat but merely a significant amount of water. Sure, it looks nice when you step on the scale immediately afterward, but this represents a false loss of weight. As soon as you replace body fluids, you gain back the weight quickly.

Wearing rubberized sweat suits hastens the rate of body fluid that is lost—fluid that is vital during prolonged exercise—and raises core temperature at the same time. This combination puts a person in danger of dehydration, which impairs cellular function and, in extreme cases, can even cause death.

Similarly, mechanical vibrators are worthless in a weight-control program. Vibrating belts and turning roll-

ers may feel good, but they require no effort whatsoever. Fat cannot be shaken off. It is lost primarily by burning it in muscle tissue.

# Losing Weight the Sound and Sensible Way

Dieting never has been fun and never will be. People who are overweight and are serious about losing weight, however, have to include regular exercise in their lives, along with proper food management and a sensible reduction in caloric intake.

Because excessive body fat is a risk factor for cardiovascular disease, some precautions are in order. Depending on the extent of the weight problem, getting a medical examination and possibly a stress ECG (see "Abnormal Electrocardiograms" in Chapter 11, pages 397–398) may be a good idea before undertaking the exercise program. Consult a physician in this regard. Significantly overweight individuals may have to choose activities in which they will not have to support their own body weight but that will still be effective in burning calories. Injuries to joints and muscles are common in excessively overweight individuals who participate in weight-bearing exercises such as walking, jogging, and aerobics.

Swimming may not be a good weight loss exercise either. More body fat makes a person more buoyant, and many people are not at the skill level required to swim fast enough to get the best training effect, thus limiting the number of calories burned as well as the benefits to the cardiorespiratory system.

During the initial stages of exercise, better alternatives include riding a bicycle (either road or stationary), walking in a shallow pool, doing water aerobics, or running in place in deep water (treading water). The latter forms of

---

**Spot reducing** Fallacious theory proposing that exercising a specific body part will result in significant fat reduction in that area.

**Cellulite** Term frequently used in reference to fat deposits that "bulge out"; these deposits are nothing but enlarged fat cells from excessive accumulation of body fat.

water exercise are gaining popularity and have proven to be effective in reducing weight without fear of injuries.

How long should each exercise session last? The amount of exercise needed to lose weight and maintain the weight loss is different from the amount of exercise needed to improve fitness. For health fitness, accumulating 30 minutes of physical activity a minimum of five days per week is recommended. To develop and maintain cardiorespiratory fitness, 20 to 60 minutes of exercise at the recommended target rate, three to five times per week, is suggested (see Chapter 6). For successful weight loss, however, 60 to 90 minutes of physical activity on most days of the week is recommended.

A person should not try to do too much too fast. Unconditioned beginners should start with about 15 minutes of aerobic activity three times a week, and during the next 3 to 4 weeks gradually increase the duration by approximately 5 minutes per week and the frequency by one day per week.

One final benefit of long-duration exercise for weight control is that fat-burning enzymes increase with aerobic training. Fat is lost primarily by burning it in muscle. Therefore, as the concentration of the enzymes increases, so does the ability to burn fat.

In addition to exercise and food management, a sensible reduction in caloric intake and careful monitoring of this intake are recommended. Most research finds that a negative caloric balance is required to lose weight because:

1. Most people underestimate their caloric intake and are eating more than they should.

2. Developing new behaviors takes time, and most people have trouble changing and adjusting to new eating habits.

3. Many individuals are in such poor physical condition that they take a long time to increase their activity

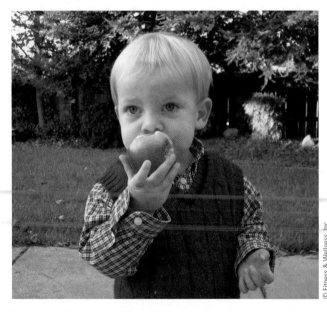

The establishment of healthy eating patterns starts at a young age.

level enough to offset the setpoint and burn enough calories to aid in losing body fat.

4. Most successful dieters carefully monitor their daily caloric intake.

5. A few people simply will not alter their food selection. For those who will not (which will increase their risk for chronic diseases), the only solution to lose weight successfully is a large increase in physical activity, a negative caloric balance, or a combination of the two.

Perhaps the only exception to a decrease in caloric intake for weight loss purposes is in people who already are eating too few calories. A nutrient analysis (see Chapter 3) often reveals that long-term dieters are not consuming enough calories. These people actually need to increase their daily caloric intake and combine it with an exercise program to get their metabolism to kick back up to a normal level.

You also must learn to make wise food choices. Think in terms of long-term benefits (weight management) instead of instant gratification (unhealthy eating and subsequent weight gain). Making healthful choices allows you to eat more food, eat more nutritious food, and ingest fewer calories. For example, instead of eating a high-fat, 700-calorie scone, you could eat as much as 1 orange, 1 cup of grapes, a hard-boiled egg, 2 slices of whole-wheat toast, 2 teaspoons of jam, ½ cup of honey-sweetened oatmeal, and 1 glass of skim milk (Figure 5.11).

You can estimate your daily energy (caloric) requirement by consulting Tables 5.3 and 5.4 and completing Lab 5A. Given that this is only an estimated value, individual adjustments related to many of the factors discussed in this chapter may be necessary to establish a more precise value. Nevertheless, the estimated value does offer beginning guidelines for weight control or reduction.

The EER without additional planned activity and exercise is based on age, total body weight, and gender. Individuals who hold jobs that require a lot of walking or heavy manual labor burn more calories during the day than those who have sedentary jobs (such as working behind a desk). To estimate your EER, refer to Table 5.3. For example, the EER computation for a 20-year-old man, 71 inches tall, who weighs 160 pounds, would be as follows:

1. Body weight in kilograms = 72.6 kg (160 lbs ÷ 2.2046)

   Height in meters = 1.8 m (71 × 0.0254)

2. EER = 662 − (9.53 × age) + (15.91 × body weight) + (539 × height)

   EER = 662 − (9.53 × 20) = (15.91 × 72.6) + (539 × 1.8)

   EER = 662 − 190.6 + 1155 + 970

   EER = 2,596 calories/day

Thus, the EER to maintain body weight for this individual would be 2,596 calories per day.

To determine the average number of calories you burn daily as a result of exercise, figure out the total number of

**FIGURE 5.11  Making wise food choices.**

These illustrations provide a comparison of how much more food you can eat when you make healthy choices. You also get more vitamins, minerals, phytochemicals, antioxidants, and fiber by making healthy choices.

| **Breakfast** | **Lunch** | **Dinner** |
|---|---|---|

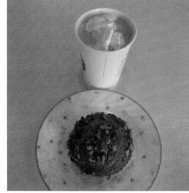

1 banana nut muffin, 1 cafe mocha
Calories: 940
Percent fat calories: 48%

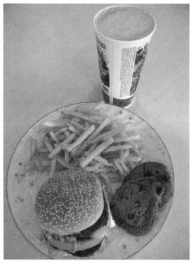

1 double-decker cheeseburger, 1 serving medium French fries, 2 chocolate chip cookies, 1 medium strawberry milkshake
Calories: 1790
Percent fat calories: 37%

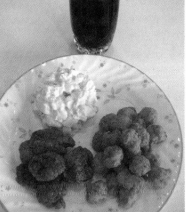

6 oz. popcorn chicken, 3 oz. barbecue chicken wings, 1 cup potato salad, 1 12-oz. cola drink
Calories: 1250
Percent fat calories: 42%

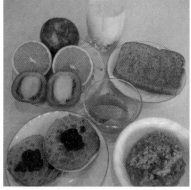

1 cup oatmeal, 1 English muffin with jelly, 1 slice whole wheat bread with honey, ½ cup peaches, 1 kiwi fruit, 1 orange, 1 apple, 1 cup skim milk
Calories: 900
Percent fat calories: 5%

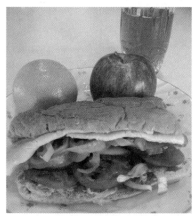

6-inch turkey breast/vegetable sandwich, 1 apple, 1 orange, 1 cup sweetened green tea
Calories: 500
Percent fat calories: 10%

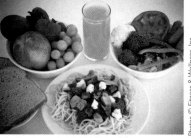

2 cups spaghetti with tomato sauce and vegetables, a 2-cup salad bowl with two tablespoons Italian dressing, 2 slices whole wheat bread, 1 cup grapes, 3 large strawberries, 1 kiwi fruit, 1 peach, 1 12-oz. fruit juice drink
Calories: 1240
Percent fat calories: 14%

Photos © Fitness & Wellness, Inc.

**TABLE 5.3  Estimated Energy Requirement (EER) Based on Age, Body Weight, and Height**

| | |
|---|---|
| **MEN** | $\text{EER} = 662 - (9.53 \times \text{Age}) + (15.91 \times \text{BW}) + (539 \times \text{HT})$ |
| **WOMEN** | $\text{EER} = 354 - (6.91 \times \text{Age}) + (9.36 \times \text{BW}) + (726 \times \text{HT})$ |

Note: Includes activities of independent living only and no moderate physical activity or exercise.
BW = body weight in kilograms (divide BW in pounds by 2.2046),
HT = height in meters (multiply HT in inches by .0254).

**TABLE 5.4  Caloric Expenditure of Selected Physical Activities**

| Activity* | Cal/lb/min | Activity* | Cal/lb/min |
|---|---|---|---|
| Aerobics | | 8.5 min/mile | 0.090 |
|   Moderate | 0.065 | 7.0 min/mile | 0.102 |
|   Vigorous | 0.095 | 6.0 min/mile | 0.114 |
|   Step aerobics | 0.070 | Deep water** | 0.100 |
| Archery | 0.030 | Skating (moderate) | 0.038 |
| Badminton | | Skiing | |
|   Recreation | 0.038 |   Downhill | 0.060 |
|   Competition | 0.065 |   Level (5 mph) | 0.078 |
| Baseball | 0.031 | Soccer | 0.059 |
| Basketball | | Stairmaster | |
|   Moderate | 0.046 |   Moderate | 0.070 |
|   Competition | 0.063 |   Vigorous | 0.090 |
| Bowling | 0.030 | Stationary Cycling | |
| Calisthenics | 0.033 |   Moderate | 0.055 |
| Cycling (on a level surface) | |   Vigorous | 0.070 |
|   5.5 mph | 0.033 | Strength Training | 0.050 |
|   10.0 mph | 0.050 | Swimming (crawl) | |
|   13.0 mph | 0.071 |   20 yds/min | 0.031 |
| Dance | |   25 yds/min | 0.040 |
|   Moderate | 0.030 |   45 yds/min | 0.057 |
|   Vigorous | 0.055 |   50 yds/min | 0.070 |
| Golf | 0.030 | Table Tennis | 0.030 |
| Gymnastics | | Tennis | |
|   Light | 0.030 |   Moderate | 0.045 |
|   Heavy | 0.056 |   Competition | 0.064 |
| Handball | 0.064 | Volleyball | 0.030 |
| Hiking | 0.040 | Walking | |
| Judo/Karate | 0.086 |   4.5 mph | 0.045 |
| Racquetball | 0.065 |   Shallow pool | 0.090 |
| Rope Jumping | 0.060 | Water Aerobics | |
| Rowing (vigorous) | 0.090 |   Moderate | 0.050 |
| Running (on a level surface) | |   Vigorous | 0.070 |
|   11.0 min/mile | 0.070 | Wrestling | 0.085 |

*Values are for actual time engaged in the activity.
**Treading water

Adapted from:
P. E. Allsen, J. M. Harrison, and B. Vance, *Fitness for Life: An Individualized Approach* (Dubuque, IA: Wm. C. Brown, 1989).
C. A. Bucher and W. E. Prentice, *Fitness for College and Life* (St. Louis: Times Mirror/Mosby College Publishing, 1989).
C. F. Consolazio, R. E. Johnson, and L. J. Pecora, *Physiological Measurements of Metabolic Functions in Man* (New York: McGraw-Hill, 1963).
R. V. Hockey, *Physical Fitness: The Pathway to Healthful Living* (St. Louis: Times Mirror/Mosby College Publishing, 1989).
W. W. K. Hoeger et al., Research conducted at Boise State University, 1986–1993.

minutes you exercise weekly, then figure the daily average exercise time. For instance, a person cycling at 10 miles per hour five times a week, 60 minutes each time, exercises 300 minutes per week (5 × 60). The average daily exercise time, therefore, is 42 minutes (300 ÷ 7, rounded off to the lowest unit).

Next, from Table 5.4, find the energy expenditure for the activity (or activities) chosen for the exercise program. In the case of cycling (10 miles per hour), the expenditure is .05 calorie per pound of body weight per minute of activity (cal/lb/min). With a body weight of 160 pounds, this man would burn 8 calories each minute (body weight × .05, or 160 × .05). In 42 minutes he would burn approximately 336 calories (42 × 8).

Now you can obtain the daily energy requirement, with exercise, needed to maintain body weight. To do this, add the EER obtained from Table 5.3 and the average calories burned through exercise. In our example, it is 2,932 calories (2,596 + 336).

If a negative caloric balance is recommended to lose weight, this person has to consume fewer than 2,932 calories daily to achieve the objective. Because of the many factors that play a role in weight control, this 2,932-calorie value is only an estimated daily requirement. Furthermore, we cannot predict that you will lose exactly 1 pound of fat in 1 week if you cut your daily intake by 500 calories (500 × 7 = 3,500 calories, or the equivalent of 1 pound of fat).

The daily energy requirement figure is only a target guideline for weight control. Periodic readjustments are necessary because individuals differ, and the daily requirement changes as you lose weight and modify your exercise habits.

To determine the target caloric intake to lose weight, multiply your current weight by 5 and subtract this amount from the total daily energy requirement (2,932 in our example) with exercise. For our example, this would mean 2,132 calories per day to lose weight (160 × 5 = 800 and 2,932 − 800 = 2,132 calories).

This final caloric intake to lose weight should never be below 1,200 calories for women and 1,500 for men. If distributed properly over the various food groups, these figures are the lowest caloric intakes that provide the necessary nutrients the body needs. In terms of percentages of total calories, the daily distribution should be approximately 60 percent carbohydrates (mostly complex carbohydrates), less than 30 percent fat, and about 12 percent protein.

Many experts believe that a person can take off weight more efficiently by reducing the amount of daily fat intake to about 20 percent of the total daily caloric intake. Because 1 gram of fat supplies more than twice the amount of calories that carbohydrates and protein do, the tendency when someone eats less fat is to consume fewer calories. With fat intake at 20 percent of total calories, the individual will have sufficient fat in the diet to feel satisfied and avoid frequent hunger pangs.

Further, it takes only 3 to 5 percent of ingested calories to store fat as fat, whereas it takes approximately 25 percent of ingested calories to convert carbohydrates to fat. Some evidence indicates that if people eat the same number of calories as carbohydrate or as fat, those on the fat diet will store more fat. Long-term successful weight loss and weight management programs are low in fat content.

Many people have trouble adhering to a low-fat-calorie diet. During times of weight loss, however, you are strongly encouraged to do so. Refer to Table 5.5 to aid you in determining the grams of fat at 20 percent of the total calories for selected energy intakes. Also, use the form provided in Lab 3A in Chapter 3 to monitor your daily fat intake. For weight maintenance, individuals who have been successful in maintaining an average weight loss of 30 pounds for more than 6 years are consuming about 24 percent of calories from fat, 56 percent from carbohydrates, and 20 percent from protein.[29]

Breakfast is a critical meal while you are on a weight loss program. Many people skip breakfast because it's the easiest meal to skip. Evidence indicates that people who skip breakfast are hungrier later in the day and end up consuming more total daily calories than those who eat breakfast. Furthermore, regular breakfast eaters have less of a weight problem, lose weight more effectively, and have less difficulty maintaining the weight loss.

**TABLE 5.5** Grams of Fat at 10%, 20%, and 30% of Total Calories for Selected Energy Intakes

| Caloric Intake | Grams of Fat | | |
| | 10% | 20% | 30% |
| --- | --- | --- | --- |
| 1,200 | 13 | 27 | 40 |
| 1,300 | 14 | 29 | 43 |
| 1,400 | 16 | 31 | 47 |
| 1,500 | 17 | 33 | 50 |
| 1,600 | 18 | 36 | 53 |
| 1,700 | 19 | 38 | 57 |
| 1,800 | 20 | 40 | 60 |
| 1,900 | 21 | 42 | 63 |
| 2,000 | 22 | 44 | 67 |
| 2,100 | 23 | 47 | 70 |
| 2,200 | 24 | 49 | 73 |
| 2,300 | 26 | 51 | 77 |
| 2,400 | 27 | 53 | 80 |
| 2,500 | 28 | 56 | 83 |
| 2,600 | 29 | 58 | 87 |
| 2,700 | 30 | 60 | 90 |
| 2,800 | 31 | 62 | 93 |
| 2,900 | 32 | 64 | 97 |
| 3,000 | 33 | 67 | 100 |

## Behavior Modification Planning

### HEALTHY BREAKFAST CHOICES

Breakfast is the most important meal of the day. Skipping breakfast makes you hungrier later in the day and leads to overconsumption and greater caloric intake throughout the rest of the day. Regular breakfast eaters have less of a weight problem, lose weight more effectively, have less difficulty maintaining lost weight, and live longer. Skipping breakfast also temporarily raises LDL (bad) cholesterol and lowers insulin sensitivity, changes that may increase the risk for heart disease and diabetes. Below are some healthy breakfast food choices. Have you tried these options for breakfast?

| I PLAN TO | I DID IT | |
| --- | --- | --- |
| ❑ | ❑ | Fresh fruit |
| ❑ | ❑ | Low-fat or skim milk |
| ❑ | ❑ | Low-fat yogurt |
| ❑ | ❑ | Whole-grain cereal |
| ❑ | ❑ | Whole-grain bread or bagel with fat-free cream cheese and slices of red or green pepper |
| ❑ | ❑ | Hummus over a whole-grain bagel |
| ❑ | ❑ | Peanut butter with whole-grain bread or bagel |
| ❑ | ❑ | Low-fat cottage cheese with fruit |
| ❑ | ❑ | Oatmeal |
| ❑ | ❑ | Reduced-fat cheese |
| ❑ | ❑ | Egg Beaters with salsa |
| ❑ | ❑ | An occasional egg |

### Try It

Select a healthy breakfast choice each day for the next 7 days. Evaluate how you feel the rest of the morning. What effect did eating breakfast have on your activities of daily living and daily caloric intake? Be sure to record your food choices, how you felt, and what activities you engaged in.

If most of the daily calories are consumed during one meal (as in the typical evening meal), the body may perceive that something is wrong and will slow the metabolism so it can store more calories in the form of fat. Also, eating most of the calories during one meal causes a person to go hungry the rest of the day, making it more difficult to adhere to the diet.

Consuming most of the calories earlier in the day seems helpful in losing weight and also in managing atherosclerosis. The time of day when most of the fats and cholesterol are consumed can influence blood lipids and coronary heart disease. Peak digestion time following a heavy meal is about seven hours after that meal. If most lipids are consumed during the evening meal, digestion peaks while the person is sound asleep, when the metabolism is at its lowest rate. Consequently, the body may not metabolize fats and cholesterol as well, leading to a higher blood lipid count and increasing the risk for atherosclerosis and coronary heart disease.

Before you proceed to develop a thorough weight loss program, take a moment to identify, in Lab 5B, your current stage of change as it pertains to your recommended body weight. If applicable—that is, if you are not at recommended weight—list also the processes and techniques for change that you will use to accomplish your goal. In Lab 5B, you also outline your exercise program for weight management.

## Monitoring Your Diet with Daily Food Logs

To help you monitor and adhere to a weight loss program, use the daily food logs provided in Lab 5C. If the goal is to maintain or increase body weight, use Lab 5D.

Evidence indicates that people who monitor daily caloric intake are more successful at weight loss than those who don't self-monitor. Before using the forms in Lab 5C, make a master copy for your files so you can make future copies as needed. Guidelines are provided for 1,200-, 1,500-, 1,800-, and 2,000-calorie diet plans. These plans have been developed based on MyPyramid and the Dietary Guidelines for Americans to meet the Recommended Dietary Allowances.[30] The objective is to meet (not exceed) the number of servings allowed for each diet plan. Each time you eat a serving of a certain food, record it in the appropriate box.

To lose weight, you should use the diet plan that most closely approximates your target caloric intake. The plan is based on the following caloric allowances for these food groups:

- Grains: 80 calories per serving
- Fruits: 60 calories per serving
- Vegetables: 25 calories per serving
- Milk (use low-fat products): 120 calories per serving
- Meat and beans: 300 calories per serving (use low-fat frozen entrees or an equivalent amount if you prepare your own main dish; see the following discussion)

As you start your diet plan, pay particular attention to food serving sizes. Take care with cup and glass sizes. A standard cup is 8 ounces, but most glasses nowadays contain between 12 and 16 ounces. If you drink 12 ounces of fruit juice, in essence you are getting two servings of fruit because a standard serving is ¾ cup of juice.

Read food labels carefully to compare the caloric value of the serving listed on the label with the caloric guidelines provided on the previous page. Here are some examples:

- One slice of standard white bread has about 80 calories. A plain bagel may have 200 to 350 calories. Although it is low in fat, a 350-calorie bagel is equivalent to almost 4 servings in the grains group.
- The standard serving size listed on the food label for most cereals is 1 cup. As you read the nutrition information, however, you will find that for the same cup of cereal, one type of cereal has 120 calories and another cereal has 200 calories. Because a standard serving in the grains group is 80 calories, the first cereal would be 1½ servings and the second one 2½ servings.
- A medium-size fruit is usually considered to be 1 serving. A large fruit could provide as many as 2 or more servings.
- In the milk group, 1 serving represents 120 calories. A cup of whole milk has about 160 calories, compared with a cup of skim milk, which contains 88 calories. A cup of whole milk, therefore, would provide 1⅓ servings in this food group.

**Using Low-Fat Entrees** To be more accurate with caloric intake and to simplify meal preparation, use commercially prepared low-fat frozen entrees as the main dish for lunch and dinner meals (only one entree per meal for the 1,200-calorie diet plan; see Lab 5C). Look for entrees that provide about 300 calories and no more than 6 grams of fat per entree. These two entrees can be used as selections for the meat and beans group and will provide most of your daily protein requirement. Supplement the entree with some of your servings from the other food groups. This diet plan has been used successfully in weight loss research programs.[31] If you choose not to use these low-fat entrees, prepare a similar meal using 3 ounces (cooked) of lean meat, poultry, or fish with additional vegetables, rice, or pasta that will provide 300 calories with fewer than 6 grams of fat per dish.

In your daily logs, be sure to record the precise amount in each serving. You also can run a computerized nutrient analysis to verify your caloric intake and food distribution pattern (percent of total calories from carbohydrate, fat, and protein).

# Behavior Modification and Adherence to a Weight Management Program

Achieving and maintaining recommended body composition is certainly possible, but it does require desire and commitment. If weight management is to become a prior-

ity, people must realize that they have to transform their behavior to some extent.

Modifying old habits and developing new, positive behaviors take time. Individuals who apply the management techniques provided in the Behavior Modification Planning box (pages 176–177) are more successful at changing detrimental behavior and adhering to a positive lifetime weight control program. In developing a retraining program, you are not expected to incorporate all of the strategies given but should note the ones that apply to you. The form provided in Lab 5E will allow you to evaluate and monitor your own weight management behaviors.

During the weight loss process, surround yourself with people who have the same weight loss goals as you do. Data released in 2007 showed that obesity can spread through "social networks."[32] That is, if your friends, siblings, or spouse gains weight, you are more likely to gain weight as well. People tend to accept a higher weight standard if someone they are close to or care about gains weight.

In the study, the social ties of more than 12,000 people were examined over 32 years. The findings revealed that if a close friend becomes obese, your risk of becoming obese during the next 2 to 4 years increases 171 percent. The risk also increases 57 percent for casual friends, 40 percent for siblings, and 37 percent for the person's spouse. The reverse was also found to be true. When a person loses weight, the likelihood of friends, siblings, or spouse to lose weight is also enhanced.

Furthermore, the research found that gender plays a role in social networks. A male's weight has a greater effect on the weight of male friends and brothers than on female friends or sisters. Similarly, a woman's weight has a far greater influence on sisters and girlfriends than on brothers or male friends. Thus, if you are trying to lose weight, choose your friendships carefully: Do not surround yourself with people who either have a weight problem or are still gaining weight.

## Critical Thinking

What behavioral strategies have you used to properly manage your body weight? How do you think those strategies would work for others?

# The Simple Truth

There is no quick and easy way to take off excess body fat and keep it off for good. Weight management is accomplished by making a lifetime commitment to physical ac-

# Behavior Modification Planning

## WEIGHT LOSS STRATEGIES

☐ I PLAN TO  ☐ I DID IT

☐ ☐ 1. Make a commitment to change. The first necessary ingredient is the desire to modify your behavior. You have to stop precontemplating or contemplating change and get going! You must accept that you have a problem and decide by yourself whether you really want to change. Sincere commitment increases your chances for success.

☐ ☐ 2. Set realistic goals. The weight problem developed over several years. Similarly, new lifetime eating and exercise habits take time to develop. A realistic long-term goal also will include short-term objectives that allow for regular evaluation and help maintain motivation and renewed commitment to attain the long-term goal.

☐ ☐ 3. Incorporate exercise into the program. Choosing enjoyable activities, places, times, equipment, and people to work out with will help you adhere to an exercise program. (See Chapters 6, 7, 8, and 9.)

☐ ☐ 4. Differentiate hunger and appetite. Hunger is the actual physical need for food. Appetite is a desire for food, usually triggered by factors such as stress, habit, boredom, depression, availability of food, or just the thought of food itself. Developing and sticking to a regular meal pattern will help control hunger.

☐ ☐ 5. Eat less fat. Each gram of fat provides 9 calories, and protein and carbohydrates provide only 4. In essence, you can eat more food on a low-fat diet because you consume fewer calories with each meal. Most of your fat intake should come from unsaturated sources.

☐ ☐ 6. Pay attention to calories. Just because food is labeled "low-fat" does not mean you can eat as much as you want. When reading food labels—and when eating—don't just look at the fat content. Pay attention to calories as well. Many low-fat foods are high in calories.

☐ ☐ 7. Cut unnecessary items from your diet. Substituting water for a daily can of soda would cut 51,100 (140 × 365) calories yearly from the diet—the equivalent of 14.6 (51,000 ÷ 3,500) pounds of fat.

☐ ☐ 8. Maintain a daily intake of calcium-rich foods, especially low-fat or non-fat dairy products.

☐ ☐ 9. Add foods to your diet that reduce cravings, such as eggs; small amounts of red meat, fish, poultry, tofu, oils, fats; and nonstarchy vegetables such as lettuce, green beans, peppers, asparagus, broccoli, mushrooms, and Brussels sprouts. Also increasing the intake of low-glycemic carbohydrates with your meals helps you go longer before you feel hungry again.

☐ ☐ 10. Avoid automatic eating. Many people associate certain daily activities with eating, for example, cooking, watching television, or reading. Most foods consumed in these situations lack nutritional value or are high in sugar and fat.

☐ ☐ 11. Stay busy. People tend to eat more when they sit around and do nothing. Occupying the mind and body with activities not associated with eating helps take away the desire to eat. Some options are walking; cycling; playing sports; gardening; sewing; or visiting a library, a museum, or a park. You also might develop other skills and interests not associated with food.

☐ ☐ 12. Plan meals and shop sensibly. Always shop on a full stomach, because hungry shoppers tend to buy unhealthy foods impulsively—and then snack on the way home. Always use a shopping list, which should include whole-grain breads and cereals, fruits and vegetables, low-fat milk and dairy products, lean meats, fish, and poultry.

☐ ☐ 13. Cook wisely:
- ☐ Use less fat and fewer refined foods in food preparation.
- ☐ Trim all visible fat from meats and remove skin from poultry before cooking.
- ☐ Skim the fat off gravies and soups.
- ☐ Bake, broil, boil, or steam instead of frying.
- ☐ Sparingly use butter, cream, mayonnaise, and salad dressings.
- ☐ Avoid coconut oil, palm oil, and cocoa butter.
- ☐ Prepare plenty of foods that contain fiber.
- ☐ Include whole-grain breads and cereals, vegetables, and legumes in most meals.
- ☐ Eat fruits for dessert.

❑ Stay away from soda pop, fruit juices, and fruit-flavored drinks.

❑ Use less sugar, and cut down on other refined carbohydrates, such as corn syrup, malt sugar, dextrose, and fructose.

❑ Drink plenty of water—at least six glasses a day.

❑ ❑ 14. Do not serve more food than you should eat. Measure the food in portions and keep serving dishes away from the table. Do not force yourself or anyone else to "clean the plate" after they are satisfied (including children after they already have had a healthy, nutritious serving).

❑ ❑ 15. Try "junior size" instead of "super size." People who are served larger portions eat more, whether they are hungry or not. Use smaller plates, bowls, cups, and glasses. Try eating half as much food as you commonly eat. Watch for portion sizes at restaurants as well: Supersized foods create supersized people.

❑ ❑ 16. Eat out infrequently. The more often people eat out, the more body fat they have. People who eat out six or more times per week consume an average of about 300 extra calories per day and 30 percent more fat than those who eat out less often.

❑ ❑ 17. Eat slowly and at the table only. Eating on the run promotes overeating because the body doesn't have enough time to "register" consumption and people overeat before the body perceives the fullness signal. Eating at the table encourages people to take time out to eat and deters snacking between meals. After eating, do not sit around the table but, rather, clean up and put away the food to avoid snacking.

❑ ❑ 18. Avoid social binges. Social gatherings tend to entice self-defeating behavior. Use visual imagery to plan ahead. Do not feel pressured to eat or drink and don't rationalize in these situations. Choose low-calorie foods and entertain yourself with other activities, such as dancing and talking.

❑ ❑ 19. Do not place unhealthy foods within easy reach. Ideally, avoid bringing high-calorie, high-sugar, or high-fat foods into the house. If they are there already, store them where they are hard to get to or see—perhaps the garage or basement.

❑ ❑ 20. Avoid evening food raids. Most people do really well during the day but then "lose it" at night. Take control. Stop and think. To avoid excessive nighttime snacking, stay busy after your evening meal. Go for a short walk; floss and brush your teeth, and get to bed earlier. Even better, close the kitchen after dinner and try not to eat anything 3 hours prior to going to sleep.

❑ ❑ 21. Practice stress management techniques (discussed in Chapter 10). Many people snack and increase their food consumption in stressful situations.

❑ ❑ 22. Get support. People who receive support from friends, relatives, and formal support groups are much more likely to lose and maintain weight loss than those without such support. The more support you receive, the better off you will be.

❑ ❑ 23. Monitor changes and reward accomplishments. Being able to exercise without interruption for 15, 20, 30, or 60 minutes; swimming a certain distance; running a mile—all these accomplishments deserve recognition. Create rewards that are not related to eating: new clothing, a tennis racquet, a bicycle, exercise shoes, or something else that is special and you would not have acquired otherwise.

❑ ❑ 24. Prepare for slip-ups. Most people will slip and occasionally splurge. Do not despair and give up. Reevaluate and continue with your efforts. An occasional slip won't make much difference in the long run.

❑ ❑ 25. Think positive. Avoid negative thoughts about how difficult changing past behaviors might be. Instead, think of the benefits you will reap, such as feeling, looking, and functioning better, plus enjoying better health and improving the quality of life. Avoid negative environments and unsupportive people.

## Try It

In your Online Journal or class notebook, answer the following questions: How many of the above strategies do you use to help you maintain recommended body weight? Do you feel that any of these strategies specifically help you manage body weight more effectively? If so, explain why.

PRINCIPLES AND LABS

tivity and proper food selection. When taking part in a weight (fat) reduction program, people also have to decrease their caloric intake moderately, be physically active, and implement strategies to modify unhealthy eating behaviors.

During the process, relapses into past negative behaviors are almost inevitable. The three most common reasons for relapse are:

1. Stress-related factors (such as major personal-life changes, depression, job changes, illness)

2. Social reasons (entertaining, eating out, business travel)

3. Self-enticing behaviors (placing yourself in a situation to see how much you can get away with: "One small taste won't hurt" leads to "I'll eat just one slice" and finally to "I haven't done well, so I might as well eat some more")

Making mistakes is human and does not necessarily mean failure. Failure comes to those who give up and do not build upon previous experiences to develop skills that will prevent self-defeating behaviors. Where there's a will, there's a way, and those who persist will reap the rewards.

## ASSESS YOUR BEHAVIOR

Log on to http://www.cengage.com/sso/ to update your pedometer log if you are tracking your steps.

1. Are you satisfied with your current body composition (including body weight) and quality of life? If not, are you willing to do something about it to properly resolve the problem?

2. Are physical activity, aerobic exercise, and strength training a regular part of your lifetime weight management program?

3. Do you weigh yourself regularly and make adjustments in energy intake and physical activity habits if your weight starts to slip upward?

4. Do you exercise portion control, watch your overall fat intake, and plan ahead before you eat out or attend social functions that entice overeating?

## ASSESS YOUR KNOWLEDGE

Log on to http://www.cengage.com/sso/ to assess your understanding of this chapter's topics by taking the Student Practice Test and exploring the modules recommended in your Personalized Study Plan.

1. During the last decade, the rate of obesity in the United States has
   a. been on the decline.
   b. increased at an alarming rate.
   c. increased slightly.
   d. remained steady.
   e. increased in men and decreased in women.

2. Obesity is defined as a body mass index (BMI) equal to or above
   a. 10.
   b. 25.
   c. 30.
   d. 45.
   e. 50.

3. Obesity increases the risk for
   a. hypertension.
   b. congestive heart failure.
   c. atherosclerosis.
   d. type 2 diabetes.
   e. All of the above

4. Tolerable weight is a body weight
   a. that is not ideal but one that you can live with.
   b. that will tolerate the increased risk for chronic diseases.

   c. with a BMI range between 25 and 30.
   d. that meets both ideal values for percent body weight and BMI.
   e. All are correct choices.

5. When the body uses protein instead of a combination of fats and carbohydrates as a source of energy,
   a. weight loss is very slow.
   b. a large amount of weight loss is in the form of water.
   c. muscle turns into fat.
   d. fat is lost very rapidly.
   e. fat cannot be lost.

6. Eating disorders
   a. are characterized by an intense fear of becoming fat.
   b. are physical and emotional conditions.
   c. almost always require professional help for successful treatment of the disease.
   d. are common in societies that encourage thinness.
   e. All are correct choices.

7. The mechanism that seems to regulate how much a person weighs is known as
   a. setpoint.
   b. weight factor.

c. basal metabolic rate.

d. metabolism.

e. energy-balancing equation.

8. The key to maintaining weight loss successfully is
   a. frequent dieting.
   b. very low calorie diets when "normal" dieting doesn't work.
   c. a lifetime physical activity program.
   d. regular high-protein/low-carbohydrate meals.
   e. All are correct choices.

9. The daily amount of physical activity recommended for weight loss purposes is
   a. 15 to 20 minutes.
   b. 20 to 30 minutes.

c. 30 to 60 minutes.

d. 60 to 90 minutes.

e. Any amount is sufficient as long as it is done daily.

10. A daily energy expenditure of 300 calories through physical activity is the equivalent of approximately _____ pounds of fat per year.
    a. 12
    b. 15
    c. 22
    d. 27
    e. 31

Correct answers can be found at the back of the book.

# MEDIA MENU

You can find the links below at the book companion site: www.cengage.com/health/hoeger/plfw10e

- Check your progress in your exercise log.
- Check how well you understand the chapter's concepts.

## Internet Connections

- Shape Up America! This excellent fitness and weight management site is endorsed by former U.S. Surgeon General C. Everett Koop, M.D. *http://www.shapeup.org*

- Eating Disorders. This award-winning site, by MentalHelp Net, features links describing symptoms, possible causes, consequences, treatment, online resources, organizations, online support, and research. *http://eatingdisorder.mentalhelp.net*

- Mayo Clinic Food and Nutrition Center. This site features a wealth of reliable nutrition information, including different food pyramids and the benefits and dangers of herbs, vitamins, and mineral supplements. *http://www.mayoclini.com/health/food-and-nutrition/NU99999*

- USDA Center for Nutrition Policy and Promotion My-Pyramid Tracker. MyPyramid Tracker is an online dietary and physical activity assessment tool that provides information on your diet quality, physical activity status, related nutrition messages, and links to nutrient and physical activity information. *http://www.mypyramidtracker.gov*

- HealthyDiningFinder.com. An exceptional website run by registered dietitians that lists healthful menu choices and nutrient information for many restaurants. You can personalize it by typing in your own zip code and price range for restaurants in your area.

# NOTES

1. "Wellness Facts," *University of California at Berkeley Wellness Letter* (Palm Coast, FL: The Editors, May 2004).

2. Centers for Disease Control and Prevention, *Fast Stats A to Z: Overweight,* http://www.cdc.gov/nchs/faststats/overwt.htm; downloaded July 5, 2007.

3. M. K. Serdula, et al., "Prevalence of Attempting Weight Loss and Strategies for Controlling Weight," *Journal of the American Medical Association* 282 (1999): 1353–1358.

4. A. M. Wolf and G. A. Colditz, "Current Estimates of the Economic Cost of Obesity in the United States," *Obesity Research* 6 (1998): 97–106.

5. A. H. Mokdad, J. S. Marks, D. F. Stroup, and J. L. Gerberding, "Actual Causes of Death in the United States, 2000," *Journal of the American Medical Association* 291 (2004): 1238–1241.

6. R. Sturm and K. B. Wells, "Does Obesity Contribute as Much to Morbidity as Poverty or Smoking?" *Public Health* 115 (2001): 229–235.

7. E. E. Calle, et al., "Overweight, Obesity, and Mortality from Cancer in a Prospectively Studied Cohort of U.S. Adults," *New England Journal of Medicine* 348 (2003): 1625–1638.

8. A. Peeters, et al., "Obesity in Adulthood and Its Consequences for Life Expectancy: A Life-Table Analysis," *Annals of Internal Medicine* 138 (2003): 2432.

9. K. R. Fontaine, et al., "Years of Life Lost Due to Obesity," *Journal of the American Medical Association* 289 (2003): 187–193.

10. R. R. Wing, E. Venditti, J. M. Jakicic, B. A. Polley, and W. Lang, "Lifestyle Intervention in Overweight Individuals with a Family History of Diabetes," *Diabetes Care* 21 (1998): 350–359.

11. S. Thomsen, "A Steady Diet of Images," *BYU Magazine* 57, no. 3 (2003): 20–21.

12. S. Lichtman, et al., "Discrepancy Between Self-Reported and Actual Caloric Intake and Exercise in Obese Subjects," *New England Journal of Medicine* 327 (1992): 1893–1898.

13. J. H. Wilmore, D. L. Costill, and W. L. Kenney, *Physiology of Sport and Exercise* (Champaign, IL: Human Kinetics, 2008).

14. C. D. Gardner, et al., "Comparison of the Atkins, Zone, Ornish, and LEARN Diets for Change in Weight and Related Risk Factors Among Overweight Premenopausal Women," *Journal of the American Medical Association* 297 (2007): 969-977; G. D. Foster et al., "A Randomized Trial of a Low-Carbohydrate Diet for Obesity," *New England Journal of Medicine* 348 (2003): 2082–2090.

15. I. Shai, et al., "Weight Loss with a Low-Carbohydrate, Mediterranean, or Low-Fat Diet," *New England Journal of Medicine* 359 (2008): 229–241.

16. American Psychiatric Association, *Diagnostic and Statistical Manual of Mental Disorders* (Washington, DC: APA, 1994).

17. See note 16.

18. R. L. Leibel, M. Rosenbaum, and J. Hirsh, "Changes in Energy Expenditure Resulting from Altered Body Weight," *New England Journal of Medicine* 332 (1995): 621–628.

19. American College of Sports Medicine, "Position Stand: Appropriate Intervention Strategies for Weight Loss and Prevention for Weight Regain for Adults," *Medicine and Science in Sports and Exercise* 33 (2001): 2145–2156.

20. R. J. Shepard, *Alive Man: The Physiology of Physical Activity* (Springfield, IL: Charles C. Thomas, 1975): 484–488.

21. W. C. Miller, D. M. Koceja, and E. J. Hamilton, "A Meta-Analysis of the Past 25 Years of Weight Loss Research Using Diet, Exercise, or Diet Plus Exercise Intervention," *International Journal of Obesity* 21 (1997): 941–947.

22. J. H. Wilmore, "Exercise, Obesity, and Weight Control," *Physical Activity and Fitness Research Digest* (Washington, DC: President's Council on Physical Fitness & Sports, 1994).

23. National Academy of Sciences, Institute of Medicine, *Dietary Reference Intakes for Energy, Carbohydrates, Fiber, Fat, Protein and Amino Acids (Macronutrients)* (Washington, DC: National Academy Press, 2002).

24. See note 3.

25. E. T. Poehlman, et al., "Effects of Endurance and Resistance Training on Total Daily Energy Expenditure in Young Women: A Controlled Randomized Trial," *Journal of Clinical Endocrinology and Metabolism* 87 (2002): 1004–1009; L. M. Van Etten, et al., "Effect of an 18-wk Weight-training Program on Energy Expenditure and Physical Activity," *Journal of Applied Physiology* 82 (1997): 298–304; W. W. Campbell, M. C. Crim, V. R. Young, and W. J. Evans, "Increased Energy Requirements and Changes in Body Composition with Resistance Training in Older Adults," *American Journal of Clinical Nutrition* 60 (1994): 167–175; Z. Wang, et al., "Resting Energy Expenditure: Systematic Organization and Critique of Prediction Methods," *Obesity Research* 9 (2001): 331–336.

26. J. R. Karp and W. L. Wescott, "The Resting Metabolic Rate Debate," *Fitness Management* 23, no. 1 (2007): 44–47.

27. American College of Sports Medicine, *ACSM's Guidelines for Exercise Testing and Prescription* (Baltimore: Williams & Wilkins, 2006).

28. A. Tremblay, J. A. Simoneau, and C. Bouchard, "Impact of Exercise Intensity on Body Fatness and Skeletal Muscle Metabolism," *Metabolism* 43 (1994): 814 818.

29. M. L. Klem, R. R. Wing, M. T. McGuire, H. M. Seagle, and J. O. Hill, "A Descriptive Study of Individuals Successful at Long-Term Maintenance of Substantial Weight Loss," *American Journal of Clinical Nutrition* 66 (1997): 239–246.

30. See note 22; U.S. Department of Health and Human Services, Department of Agriculture, *Dietary Guidelines for Americans* 2005 (Washington, DC: DHHS, 2005).

31. W. W. K. Hoeger, C. Harris, E. M. Long, and D. R. Hopkins, "Four-Week Supplementation with a Natural Dietary Compound Produces Favorable Changes in Body Composition," *Advances in Therapy* 15, no. 5 (1998): 305–313; W. W. K. Hoeger, C. Harris, E. M. Long, R. L. Kjorstad, M. Welch, T. L. Hafner, and D. R. Hopkins, "Dietary Supplementation with Chromium Picolinate/L-Carnitine Complex in Combination with Diet and Exercise Enhances Body Composition," *Journal of the American Nutraceutical Association* 2, no. 2 (1999): 40–45.

32. N. A. Christakis and J. H. Fowler, "The Spread of Obesity in a Large Social Network over 32 Years," *New England Journal of Medicine* 357 (2007): 370–379.

# SUGGESTED READINGS

*ACSM's Health and Fitness Journal*, Vol. 9, issue 1, January/February 2005.

American College of Sports Medicine. "Effective Weight Management." *ACSM Fit Society Page* (http://acsm.org/health1fitness/fit_society.htm), Summer 2004.

American College of Sports Medicine. "Position Stand: Appropriate Intervention Strategies for Weight Loss and Prevention for Weight Regain for Adults." *Medicine and Science in Sports and Exercise* 33 (2001): 2145–2156.

American Diabetes Association and American Dietetic Association. *Exchange Lists for Meal Planning*. Chicago: American Dietetic Association and American Diabetes Association, 2008.

Mokdad, A. H., et al. "The Spread of the Obesity Epidemic in the United States, 1991–1998." *Journal of the American Medical Association* 282 (1999): 1519–1522.

National Academy of Sciences, Institute of Medicine. *Dietary Reference Intakes for Energy Carbohydrates, Fiber, Fat, Protein and Amino Acids (Macronutrients)*. Washington, DC: National Academy Press, 2002.

National Institutes of Health. *Clinical Guidelines on the Identification, Evaluation, and Treatment of Overweight and Obesity in Adults* (NIH Publication No. 98-4083). Washington, DC: NIH, 1998.

# LAB 5A: Computing Your Daily Caloric Requirement

Name _____  Date _____  Grade _____

Instructor _____  Course _____  Section _____

### Necessary Lab Equipment
Tables 5.3 (page 171) and 5.4 (page 172).

### Objective
To estimate your daily caloric requirement for weight maintenance or reduction and to select fitness activities for your exercise program.

### Instructions
Complete all of the sections provided in this lab.

A. Current body weight (BW) in kilograms (body weight in pounds ÷ 2.2046) ............................. ☐

B. Current height (HT) in meters (HT in inches × .0254) ......................................................... ☐

C. Estimated energy requirement (EER) (Table 5.3, page 171)

  Men:    $EER = 663 - (9.53 \times Age) + (15.91 \times BW) + (539.6 \times HT)$

  Women:  $EER = 354 - (6.91 \times Age) + (9.36 \times BW) + (726 \times HT)$

  EER = ☐ − ( ☐ × ☐ ) + ( ☐ × ☐ ) + ( ☐ × ☐ )

  EER = ☐ − ☐ + ☐ + ☐ = ☐ calories

D. Selected physical activity (e.g., jogging)[a] .......................................... ☐

E. Number of exercise sessions per week .................................................. ☐

F. Duration of exercise session (in minutes) ............................................. ☐

G. Total weekly exercise time in minutes (E × F) ...................................... ☐

H. Average daily exercise time in minutes (G ÷ 7) ..................................... ☐

I. Caloric expenditure per pound per minute (cal/lb/min) of physical activity (use Table 5.4, page 172) ........ ☐

J. Total calories burned per minute of physical activity (A × I) ................... ☐

K. Average daily calories burned as a result of the exercise program (H × J) ... ☐

L. Total daily energy requirement with exercise to maintain body weight (C + K) ... ☐

**Stop here if no weight loss is required, otherwise proceed to items M and N.**

M. Number of calories to subtract from daily requirement to achieve a negative caloric balance
   (multiply current body weight by 5) .................................................... ☐

N. Target caloric intake to lose weight (L − M)[b] ...................................... ☐

---

[a]If more than one physical activity is selected, you will need to estimate the average daily calories burned as a result of each additional activity (steps D through K) and add all of these figures to L above.
[b]This figure should never be below 1,200 calories for women or 1,500 calories for men. See Activity 5.3 for the 1,200-, 1,500-, 1,800-, and 2,000-calorie diet plans.

# LAB 5B: Weight-Loss Behavior Modification Plan

Name _____ Date _____ Grade _____

Instructor _____ Course _____ Section _____

### Necessary Lab Equipment
Tables 5.3 (page 171) and 5.4 (page 172).

### Instructions
Complete all of the sections provided in this lab.

### Objective
To estimate your daily caloric requirement for weight management and to select fitness activities for your exercise program.

1. Using Figure 2.5 (page 57) and Table 2.3 (page 57), identify your current stage of change regarding **recommended body weight:** [                    ]

2. How much weight do you want to lose? [                    ] Is it a realistic goal? [                    ]

3. Target caloric intake to lose weight (diet plan—see Lab 5A, item N) [                    ].

4. Based on the processes and techniques of change discussed in Chapter 2, indicate what you can do to help yourself implement a weight management program.

   _____

   _____

5. How much effort are you willing to put into reaching your weight loss goal? _____

   Indicate your feelings about participating in an exercise program.

   _____

6. Will you commit to participate in a combined aerobic and strength-training program?* Yes [    ] No [    ]

   If your answer is "Yes," proceed to the next question; if you answered "No," please read Chapters 3–9.

7. Select one or two aerobic activities in which you will participate regularly: [                    ]

   List facilities available to you where you can carry out the aerobic and strength-training programs.

   _____

8. Indicate days and times you will set aside for your aerobic and strength-training program (5 or 6 days per week should be devoted to aerobic exercise and 1 to 3 nonconsecutive days per week to strength training).

   | | |
   |---|---|
   | Monday: | |
   | Tuesday: | |
   | Wednesday: | |
   | Thursday: | |
   | Friday: | |
   | Saturday: | |

   Sunday:  A complete day of rest once a week is recommended to allow your body to fully recover from exercise.

### Behavior Modification

Briefly describe whether you think you can meet the goals of your aerobic and strength-training program. What obstacles will you have to overcome, and how will you overcome them?

   _____

   _____

---

*Flexibility programs are necessary for adequate fitness, possible injury prevention, and good health but do not help with weight loss. Stretching exercises can be conducted regularly during the cool-down phase of your aerobic and strength-training programs (see Chapter 8).

# LAB 5C: Calorie-Restricted Diet Plans

Name _____  Date _____  Grade _____

Instructor _____  Course _____  Section _____

**Necessary Lab Equipment**
None required.

**Objective**
To help you implement a calorie-restricted diet plan according to your target caloric intake obtained in Lab 5A.

**Lab Preparation**
Read Chapter 5 prior to this lab and make additional copies (as needed) of your selected diet plan.

**1,200 Calorie Diet Plan**

The objective of the diet plan is to meet (not exceed) the number of servings allowed for the food groups listed. Each time that you eat a particular food, record it in the space provided for each group along with the amount you ate. Refer to the Food Guide Pyramid (Figure 3.1, page 70) to find out what counts as one serving for each group listed. Instead of the meat, poultry, fish, dry beans, eggs, and nuts group, you are allowed to have a commercially available low-fat frozen entree for your main meal (this entree should provide no more than 300 calories and less than 6 grams of fat). You can make additional copies of this form as needed.

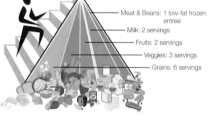

Meat & Beans: 1 low-fat frozen entree
Milk: 2 servings
Fruits: 2 servings
Veggies: 3 servings
Grains: 6 servings

**Bread, Cereal, Rice, Pasta Group** (80 calories/serving): 6 servings

| 1 | |
|---|---|
| 2 | |
| 3 | |
| 4 | |
| 5 | |
| 6 | |

**Vegetable Group** (25 calories/serving): 3 servings

| 1 | |
|---|---|
| 2 | |
| 3 | |

**Fruit Group** (60 calories/serving): 2 servings

| 1 | |
|---|---|
| 2 | |

**Milk Group** (120 calories/serving, use low-fat milk and milk products): 2 servings

| 1 | |
|---|---|
| 2 | |

**Low-fat Frozen Entree** (300 calories and less than 6 grams of fat): 1 serving

| 1 | |
|---|---|

Today's physical activity: [     ]   Intensity: [  ]   Duration: [  ] min   Number of steps: [        ]

## 1,500 Calorie Diet Plan

**Instructions:**

The objective of the diet plan is to meet (not exceed) the number of servings allowed for the food groups listed. Each time that you eat a particular food, record it in the space provided for each group along with the amount you ate. Refer to the Food Guide Pyramid (Figure 3.1, page 70) to find out what counts as one serving for each group listed. Instead of the meat, poultry, fish, dry beans, eggs, and nuts group, you are allowed to have two commercially available low-fat frozen entrees for your main meal (these entrees should provide no more than 300 calories and less than 6 grams of fat). You can make additional copies of this form as needed.

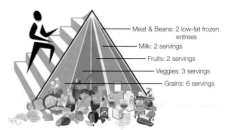

Meat & Beans: 2 low-fat frozen entrees
Milk: 2 servings
Fruits: 2 servings
Veggies: 3 servings
Grains: 6 servings

**Bread, Cereal, Rice, Pasta Group** (80 calories/serving): 6 servings

| 1 | |
|---|---|
| 2 | |
| 3 | |
| 4 | |
| 5 | |
| 6 | |

**Vegetable Group** (25 calories/serving): 3 servings

| 1 | |
|---|---|
| 2 | |
| 3 | |

**Fruit Group** (60 calories/serving): 2 servings

| 1 | |
|---|---|
| 2 | |

**Milk Group** (120 calories/serving, use low-fat milk and milk products): 2 servings

| 1 | |
|---|---|
| 2 | |

**Two Low-fat Frozen Entree** (300 calories and less than 6 grams of fat): 2 servings

| 1 | |
|---|---|
| 2 | |

Today's physical activity: _____ Intensity: _____ Duration: _____ min Number of steps: _____

1,800 Calorie Diet Plan

**Instructions:**
The objective of the diet plan is to meet (not exceed) the number of servings allowed for the food groups listed. Each time that you eat a particular food, record it in the space provided for each group along with the amount you ate. Refer to the Food Guide Pyramid (Figure 3.1, page 70) to find out what counts as one serving for each group listed. Instead of the meat, poultry, fish, dry beans, eggs, and nuts group, you are allowed to have two commercially available low-fat frozen entrees for your main meal (these entrees should provide no more than 300 calories and less than 6 grams of fat). You can make additional copies of this form as needed.

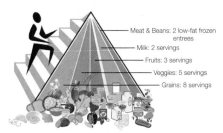

Meat & Beans: 2 low-fat frozen entrees
Milk: 2 servings
Fruits: 3 servings
Veggies: 5 servings
Grains: 8 servings

**Bread, Cereal, Rice, Pasta Group** (80 calories/serving): 8 servings

| 1 | |
|---|---|
| 2 | |
| 3 | |
| 4 | |
| 5 | |
| 6 | |
| 7 | |
| 8 | |

**Vegetable Group** (25 calories/serving): 5 servings

| 1 | |
|---|---|
| 2 | |
| 3 | |
| 4 | |
| 5 | |

**Fruit Group** (60 calories/serving): 3 servings

| 1 | |
|---|---|
| 2 | |
| 3 | |

**Milk Group** (120 calories/serving, use low-fat milk and milk products): 2 servings

| 1 | |
|---|---|
| 2 | |

**Two Low-fat Frozen Entree** (300 calories and less than 6 grams of fat): 2 servings

| 1 | |
|---|---|
| 2 | |

Today's physical activity: [        ]   Intensity: [    ]   Duration: [    ] min   Number of steps: [        ]

2.000 Calorie Diet Plan

**Instructions:**
The objective of the diet plan is to meet (not exceed) the number of servings allowed for the food groups listed. Each time that you eat a particular food, record it in the space provided for each group along with the amount you ate. Refer to the Food Guide Pyramid (Figure 3.1, page 70) to find out what counts as one serving for each group listed. Instead of the meat, poultry, fish, dry beans, eggs, and nuts group, you are allowed to have two commercially available low-fat frozen entrees for your main meal (these entrees should provide no more than 300 calories and less than 6 grams of fat). You can make additional copies of this form as needed.

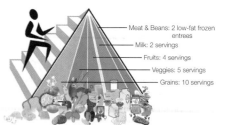

Meat & Beans: 2 low-fat frozen entrees
Milk: 2 servings
Fruits: 4 servings
Veggies: 5 servings
Grains: 10 servings

**Bread, Cereal, Rice, Pasta Group** (80 calories/serving): 10 servings

| 1 | |
|----|----|
| 2 | |
| 3 | |
| 4 | |
| 5 | |
| 6 | |
| 7 | |
| 8 | |
| 9 | |
| 10 | |

**Vegetable Group** (25 calories/serving): 5 servings

| 1 | |
|----|----|
| 2 | |
| 3 | |
| 4 | |
| 5 | |

**Fruit Group** (60 calories/serving): 4 servings

| 1 | |
|----|----|
| 2 | |
| 3 | |
| 4 | |

**Milk Group** (120 calories/serving, use low-fat milk and milk products): 2 servings

| 1 | |
|----|----|
| 2 | |

**Two Low-fat Frozen Entree** (300 calories and less than 6 grams of fat): 2 servings

| 1 | |
|----|----|
| 2 | |

Today's physical activity: ☐   Intensity: ☐   Duration: ☐ min   Number of steps: ☐

# LAB 5D: Healthy Plan for Weight Maintenance or Gain

Name _____     Date _____     Grade _____

Instructor _____     Course _____     Section _____

**Necessary Lab Equipment**
None.

**Lab Preparation**
Read Chapters 3, 4, and 5 prior to this lab.

**Objective**
To design a sample daily healthy diet plan to maintain current body weight or increase body weight.

## I. Daily Caloric Requirement

A. Current body weight in pounds ................................................................. ☐

B. Current percent body fat ....................................................................... ☐

C. Current body composition classification (Table 4.10, page 137) ................. ☐

D. Total daily energy requirement with exercise to maintain body weight (use item L from Activity 5.1). Use this figure and stop further computations if the goal is to maintain body weight ................. ☐

E. Target body weight to increase body weight ............................................ ☐

F. Number of additional daily calories to increase body weight (500 calories are recommended—combine this increased caloric intake with a strength-training program, see Chapter 7) ........................................... ☐

G. Total daily energy (caloric) requirement with exercise to increase body weight (D + F) ........................... ☐

## II. Strength-Training Program

For weight gain purposes, indicate three days during the week and the time when you will engage in a strength-training program.

_____

_____

## III. Healthy Diet Plan

Design a sample healthy daily diet plan according to the total daily energy requirement computed in D (maintenance) or G (weight gain) above. Using Appendix A, list all individual food items that you can consume on that day, along with their caloric, carbohydrate, fat, protein content. Be sure that the diet meets the recommended number of servings from the five food groups.

**Breakfast**

| | Food item | Serving Size | Calories | Carbohydrates (gr) | Fat (gr) | Protein (gr) |
|---|---|---|---|---|---|---|
| 1. | | | | | | |
| 2. | | | | | | |
| 3. | | | | | | |
| 4. | | | | | | |
| 5. | | | | | | |

**Breakfast**

| Food item | Serving Size | Calories | Carbohydrates (gr) | Fat (gr) | Protein (gr) |
|---|---|---|---|---|---|
| 6. | | | | | |
| 7. | | | | | |
| 8. | | | | | |

**Lunch**

| Food item | Serving Size | Calories | Carbohydrates (gr) | Fat (gr) | Protein (gr) |
|---|---|---|---|---|---|
| 1. | | | | | |
| 2. | | | | | |
| 3. | | | | | |
| 4. | | | | | |
| 5. | | | | | |
| 6. | | | | | |
| 7. | | | | | |
| 8. | | | | | |

**Snack**

| Food item | Serving Size | Calories | Carbohydrates (gr) | Fat (gr) | Protein (gr) |
|---|---|---|---|---|---|
| 1. | | | | | |

**Dinner**

| Food item | Serving Size | Calories | Carbohydrates (gr) | Fat (gr) | Protein (gr) |
|---|---|---|---|---|---|
| 1. | | | | | |
| 2. | | | | | |
| 3. | | | | | |
| 4. | | | | | |
| 5. | | | | | |
| 6. | | | | | |
| 7. | | | | | |
| 8. | | | | | |
| Totals: | | | | | |

## IV. Percent of Macronutrients

Determine the percent of total calories that are derived from carbohydrates, fat, and protein.

A. Total calories = [        ]

B. Grams of carbohydrates [        ] $\times 4 \div$ [        ] (total calories) = [        ] %

C. Grams of fat [        ] $\times 9 \div$ [        ] (total calories) = [        ] %

D. Grams of protein [        ] $\times 4 \div$ [        ] (total calories) = [        ] %

E. Body weight (BW) in kilograms (BW in pounds divided by 2.2046) = [        ] kg

F. Grams of protein per kilogram of body weight [        ] (grams of protein) $\div$ [        ] (BW in kg) = [        ] gr/kg

G. Please summarize your diet and protein intake to either maintain or gain weight.

_____

_____

# LAB 5E: Weight Management: Measuring Progress

Name _____     Date _____     Grade _____

Instructor _____     Course _____     Section _____

### Necessary Lab Equipment
None.

### Lab Preparation
Read Chapters 2, 3, 4, and 5 prior to this lab.

### Objective
To prepare and monitor behavioral changes for weight management.

## I. Please answer all of the following:

1. State your own feelings regarding your current body weight, your target body composition, and a completion date for this goal.

_____

_____

_____

_____

Completion date: _____

2. Do you have an eating disorder? If so, express your feelings about it. Can your instructor help you find professional advice so that you can work toward resolving this problem?

_____

_____

_____

_____

_____

3. Is your present diet adequate according to the nutrient analysis?   Yes _____   No _____

4. State dietary changes necessary to achieve a balanced diet and/or to lose weight (increase or decrease caloric intake, decrease fat intake, increase intake of complex carbohydrates, etc.). List specific foods that will help you improve in areas where you may have deficiencies and food items to avoid or consume in moderation to help you achieve better nutrition.

Changes to make: _____

_____

Foods that will help: _____

_____

Foods to avoid: _____

_____

## II. Behavior Modification Progress Form

**Instructions:** Read the section on tips for behavior modification and adherence to a weight management program (pages 176–177). On a weekly or bi-weekly basis, go through the list of strategies and provide a "Yes" or "No" answer to each statement. If you are able to answer "Yes" to most questions, you have been successful in implementing positive weight management behaviors. (Make additional copies of this page as needed.)

| Strategy                                                              Date | | | | | | |
|----------------------------------------------------------------------------|--|--|--|--|--|--|
| 1. I have made a commitment to change. | | | | | | |
| 2. I set realistic goals. | | | | | | |
| 3. I exercise regularly. | | | | | | |
| 4. I have healthy eating patterns. | | | | | | |
| 5. I exercise control over my appetite. | | | | | | |
| 6. I am consuming less fat in my diet. | | | | | | |
| 7. I pay attention to the number of calories in food. | | | | | | |
| 8. I have eliminated unnecessary food items from my diet. | | | | | | |
| 9. I use craving-reducing foods in my diet. | | | | | | |
| 10. I avoid automatic eating. | | | | | | |
| 11. I stay busy. | | | | | | |
| 12. I plan meals ahead of time. | | | | | | |
| 13. I cook wisely. | | | | | | |
| 14. I do not serve more food than I should eat. | | | | | | |
| 15. I use portion control in my diet. | | | | | | |
| 16. I eat slowly and at the table only. | | | | | | |
| 17. I avoid social binges. | | | | | | |
| 18. I avoid food raids. | | | | | | |
| 19. I do not eat out more than once per week. When I do, I eat low-fat meals. | | | | | | |
| 20. I practice stress management. | | | | | | |
| 21. I have a strong support group. | | | | | | |
| 22. I monitor behavior changes. | | | | | | |
| 23. I prepare for lapses/relapses. | | | | | | |
| 24. I reward my accomplishments. | | | | | | |
| 25. I think positive. | | | | | | |

# Cardiorespiratory Endurance

**6**

© Fitness & Wellness, Inc.

Exercise is the closest thing we'll ever get to the miracle pill that people seek. It brings weight loss, appetite control, improved mood and self-esteem, an energy kick, and longer life by decreasing the risk of heart disease, diabetes, stroke, osteoporosis, and chronic disabilities.[1]

## Objectives

- Define cardiorespiratory endurance and describe the benefits of cardiorespiratory endurance training in maintaining health and well-being
- Define aerobic and anaerobic exercise, and give examples
- Be able to assess cardiorespiratory fitness through five different test protocols: 1.5-Mile Run Test, 1.0-Mile Walk Test, Step Test, Astrand-Rhyming Test, and 12-Minute Swim Test
- Be able to interpret the results of cardiorespiratory endurance assessments according to health fitness and physical fitness standards

- Be able to estimate oxygen uptake and caloric expenditure from walking and jogging
- Determine your readiness to start an exercise program
- Explain the principles that govern cardiorespiratory exercise prescription: intensity, mode, duration, and frequency
- Learn some ways to foster adherence to exercise

CENGAGENOW™

Assess your cardiorespiratory endurance. Maintain a log of all your fitness activities.

Check your understanding of the chapter contents by logging on to CengageNOW and accessing the pre-test, personalized learning plan, and post-test for this chapter.

# FAQ

## Does aerobic exercise make a person immune to heart and blood vessel disease?

Although aerobically fit individuals as a whole have a lower incidence of cardiovascular disease, a regular aerobic exercise program by itself does not offer an absolute guarantee against cardiovascular disease. The best way to minimize the risk for cardiovascular disease is to manage the risk factors. Many factors, including a genetic predisposition, can increase the risk. Data, however, indicate that a regular aerobic exercise program will delay the onset of cardiovascular problems and also will improve the chances of surviving a heart attack.

Even moderate increases in aerobic fitness significantly lower the incidence of premature cardiovascular deaths. Data from the research study on death rates by physical fitness groups (illustrated in Figure 1.10, page 15) indicate that the decrease in cardiovascular mortality is greatest between the unfit and the moderately fit groups. A further decrease in cardiovascular mortality is observed between the moderately fit and the highly fit groups, although the difference is not as pronounced as that between the unfit and moderately fit groups.

## Is low-intensity aerobic exercise more effective in burning fat for weight loss purposes?

Without question, vigorous-intensity aerobic exercise is more effective. True, during low-intensity exercise a greater percentage of the energy is derived from fat. It is also true that an even greater percentage of the energy comes from fat when doing absolutely nothing (resting/sleeping). And when one does nothing, as in a sedentary lifestyle, one doesn't burn many calories.

Let's examine this issue. During resting conditions, the human body is a very efficient "fat-burning machine." That is, most of the energy, approximately 70 percent, is derived from fat and only 30 percent from carbohydrates. But we burn few calories at rest, about 1.5 calories per minute compared with 3 to 4 calories during low-intensity exercise and 8 to 10 calories per minute during vigorous-intensity exercise. As we begin to exercise and subsequently increase its intensity, we progressively rely more on carbohydrates and less on fat for energy, until we reach maximal intensity, when 100 percent of the energy is derived from carbohydrates. Even though a lower percentage of the energy is derived from fat during vigorous-intensity exercise, the total caloric expenditure is so much greater (twice as

---

**Cardiorespiratory endurance** is the single most important component of health-related physical fitness. The exception occurs among older adults, for whom muscular strength is particularly important. In any case, people can get by without high levels of strength and flexibility, but we cannot do without a good cardiorespiratory system, facilitated by aerobic exercise.

Aerobic exercise is especially important in preventing cardiovascular disease. A poorly conditioned heart, which has to pump more often just to keep a person alive, is sub-

ject to more wear and tear than a well-conditioned heart. In situations that place strenuous demands on the heart, such as doing yard work, lifting heavy objects or weights, or running to catch a bus, the unconditioned heart may not be able to sustain the strain. Regular participation in cardiorespiratory endurance activities also helps a person achieve and maintain recommended body weight—the fourth component of health-related physical fitness.

Physical activity, unfortunately, is no longer a natural part of our existence. Technological developments have driven most people in developed countries into sedentary lifestyles. For instance, when many people go to a store only a couple of blocks away, they drive their automobiles and then spend a couple of minutes driving around the parking lot to find a spot 20 yards closer to the store's entrance. They do not even have to carry the groceries to the car, as an employee working at the store usually offers to do this for them.

---

**Cardiorespiratory endurance** The ability of the lungs, heart, and blood vessels to deliver adequate amounts of oxygen to the cells to meet the demands of prolonged physical activity.

**Hypokinetic diseases** "Hypo" denotes "lack of" and kinetic denotes "motion"; therefore, lack of physical activity.

high or more) that overall the total fat burned is still higher than during moderate intensity.

A word of caution, nonetheless; do not start vigorous-intensity exercise without several weeks of proper and gradual conditioning. Even worse is if such exercise is a weight-bearing activity. If you do such exercise from the outset, you increase the risk of injury and may have to stop exercising altogether.

### Do energy drinks enhance performance?

People tend to associate energy with work. If an energy drink can enhance work capacity, the benefits of such drinks would surpass plain thirst-quenching drinks. Energy drinks typically contain sugar, herbal extracts, large amounts of caffeine, and water-soluble vitamins. Consumers are led to believe that these ingredients increase energy metabolism, provide an energy boost, improve endurance, and aid in weight loss. These purported benefits are yet to be proven through scientific research.

The energy content of many of these drinks is around 60 grams of sugar and 240 calories in a 16-ounce drink, with little additional nutritive value. If you are going to participate in an intense and lengthy workout, the carbohydrate content can boost performance and help you get through the workout. If, however, you are concerned with weight management, 240 calories is an extraordinarily large amount of calories in a two-cup drink. Weight gain may be the end result if you drink a few of these throughout the day to give you a boost while studying or while at work. Sugar-free energy drinks, available for the weight-conscious consumer, provide little or no energy (calories), although they are packed with nervous system stimulants.

The high caffeine content can also have adverse health effects. Caffeine intake above 400 mg can precipitate cardiac arrhythmias, nervousness, irritability, and gastrointestinal discomfort. Many of the popular energy drinks (Red Bull, Sobe Adrenaline Rush, Full Throttle, Rip It Energy Fuel) contain about 80 mg of caffeine per 8 ounce cup. If you drink two 16-ounce cans, you'll end up with upward of 300 mg of caffeine through these drinks alone. You may also have to consider additional caffeine intake from other beverages that you routinely consume during the day (coffee, tea, sodas). As with most addictive substances, invariably a sugar and caffeine rush is likely to end up in a physiologic crash, requiring a subsequent larger intake to obtain a similar "physical high."

Similarly, during a visit to a multilevel shopping mall, almost everyone chooses to take the escalator instead of the stairs (which tend to be inaccessible). Automobiles, elevators, escalators, telephones, intercoms, remote controls, electric garage door openers—all are modern-day commodities that minimize the amount of movement and effort required of the human body.

One of the most harmful effects of modern-day technology is an increase in chronic conditions related to a lack of physical activity. These **hypokinetic diseases** include hypertension, heart disease, chronic low back pain, and obesity. (The term "hypo" means low or little, and "kinetic" implies motion.) Lack of adequate physical activity is a fact of modern life that most people can avoid no longer. To enjoy modern-day conveniences and still expect to live life to its fullest, however, one has to make a personalized lifetime exercise program a part of daily living.

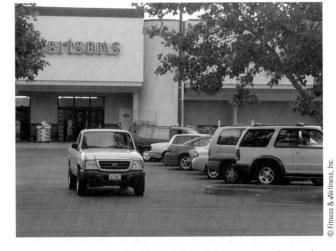

The epitome of physical inactivity: driving around a parking lot for several minutes in search of a parking spot 20 yards closer to the store's entrance.

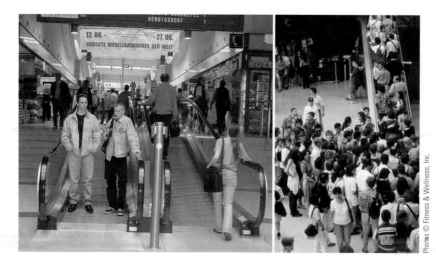

Advances in modern technology have almost completely eliminated the need for physical activity, significantly enhancing the deterioration rate of the human body.

# Basic Cardiorespiratory Physiology: A Quick Survey

Before we begin to overhaul our bodies with an exercise program, we should understand the mechanisms that we propose to alter and survey the ways by which to measure how well we perform them. Cardiorespiratory endurance is a measure of how the pulmonary (lungs), cardiovascular (heart and blood vessels), and muscular systems work together during aerobic activities. As a person breathes, part of the oxygen in the air is taken up by the **alveoli** in the lungs. As blood passes through the alveoli, oxygen is picked up by **hemoglobin** and transported in the blood to the heart. The heart then is responsible for pumping the oxygenated blood through the circulatory system to all organs and tissues of the body.

At the cellular level, oxygen is used to convert food substrates (primarily carbohydrates and fats) through aerobic metabolism into **adenosine triphosphate (ATP)**. This compound provides the energy for physical activity, body functions, and maintenance of a constant internal equilibrium. During physical exertion, more ATP is needed to perform the activity. As a result, the lungs, heart, and blood vessels have to deliver more oxygen to the muscle cells to supply the required energy.

During prolonged exercise, an individual with a high level of cardiorespiratory endurance is able to deliver the required amount of oxygen to the tissues with relative ease. In contrast, the cardiorespiratory system of a person with a low level of endurance has to work much harder, the heart has to work at a higher rate, less oxygen is delivered to the tissues, and consequently, the individual fatigues faster. Hence, a higher capacity to deliver and utilize oxygen—called **oxygen uptake**, or

VO₂—indicates a more efficient cardiorespiratory system. Measuring oxygen uptake, therefore, is an important way by which to evaluate our cardiorespiratory health.

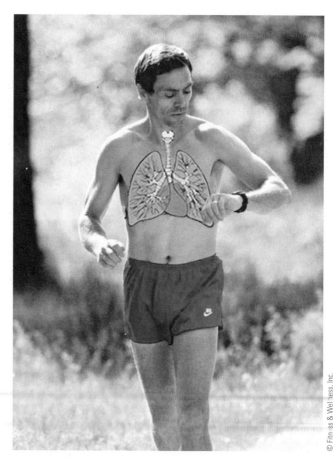

Cardiorespiratory endurance refers to the ability of the lungs, heart, and blood vessels to deliver adequate amounts of oxygen to the cells to meet the demands of prolonged physical activity.

# Aerobic and Anaerobic Exercise

Cardiorespiratory endurance activities often are called **aerobic** exercises. Examples are walking, jogging, swimming, cycling, cross-country skiing, water aerobics, rope skipping, and aerobics. By contrast, the intensity of **anaerobic** exercise is so high that oxygen cannot be delivered and utilized to produce energy. Because energy production is limited in the absence of oxygen, anaerobic activities can be carried out for only short periods—2 to 3 minutes. The higher the intensity of the activity, the shorter the duration.

Good examples of anaerobic activities are track and field (the 100, 200, and 400 meters), swimming (the 100 meters),

gymnastics routines, and strength training. Anaerobic activities do not contribute much to developing the cardiorespiratory system. Only aerobic activities will increase cardiorespiratory endurance. The basic guidelines for cardiorespiratory exercise prescription are set forth later in this chapter.

## Critical Thinking

Your friend Joe is not physically active and doesn't exercise. He manages to keep his weight down by dieting and tells you that because he feels and looks good, he doesn't need to exercise. How do you respond to your friend?

**Benefits of Aerobic Training** Everyone who participates in a cardiorespiratory or aerobic exercise program can expect a number of beneficial physiological adaptations from training. Among them are the following:

1. A higher **maximal oxygen uptake.** The amount of oxygen the body is able to use during exercise increases significantly. This allows the individual to exercise longer and more intensely before becoming fatigued. Depending on the initial fitness level, the increases in maximal oxygen uptake ($VO_{2max}$) average 15 to 20 percent, although increases greater than 50 percent have been reported in people who have very low initial levels of fitness or who were significantly overweight prior to starting the aerobic exercise program.

2. An increase in the oxygen-carrying capacity of the blood. As a result of training, the red blood cell count goes up. Red blood cells contain hemoglobin, which transports oxygen in the blood.

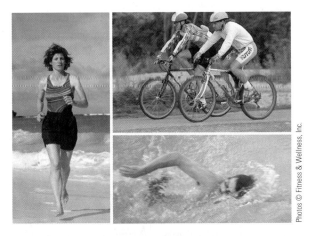

Aerobic activities.

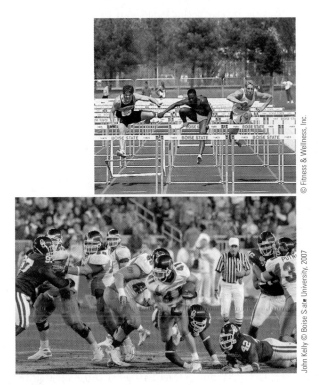

Anaerobic activities.

**Alveoli** Air sacs in the lungs where oxygen is taken up and carbon dioxide (produced by the body) is released from the blood.

**Hemoglobin** Iron-containing compound, found in red blood cells, that transports oxygen.

**Adenosine triphosphate (ATP)** A high-energy chemical compound that the body uses for immediate energy.

**Oxygen uptake ($VO_2$)** The amount of oxygen the human body uses.

**Aerobic** Describes exercise that requires oxygen to produce the necessary energy (ATP) to carry out the activity.

**Anaerobic** Describes exercise that does not require oxygen to produce the necessary energy (ATP) to carry out the activity.

**Maximal oxygen uptake ($VO_{2max}$)** Maximum amount of oxygen the body is able to utilize per minute of physical activity, commonly expressed in mL/kg/min; the best indicator of cardiorespiratory or aerobic fitness.

**TABLE 6.1** Average Resting and Maximal Cardiac Output, Stroke Volume, and Heart Rate for Sedentary, Trained, and Highly Trained Males*

| | Resting | | | Maximal | | |
|---|---|---|---|---|---|---|
| | Cardiac Output (l/min) | Stroke Volume (ml) | Heart Rate (bpm) | Cardiac Output (l/min) | Stroke Volume (ml) | Heart Rate (bpm) |
| Sedentary | 5–6 | 68 | 74 | 20 | 100 | 200 |
| Trained | 5–6 | 90 | 56 | 30 | 150 | 200 |
| Highly Trained | 5–6 | 110 | 45 | 35 | 175 | 200 |

* Cardiac output and stroke volume in women are about 25 percent lower than in men.

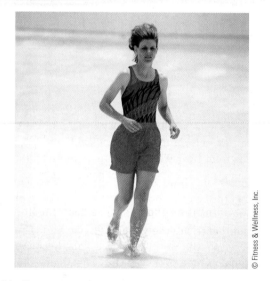

Aerobic fitness leads to better health and a higher quality of life.

© Fitness & Wellness, Inc.

3. A decrease in heart rate at rest and an increase in cardiac muscle strength. The **resting heart rate** ejects between 5 and 6 liters of blood per minute (a liter is slightly larger than a quart). This amount of blood, also referred to as **cardiac output,** meets the body's energy demands in the resting state. Like any other muscle, the heart responds to training by increasing in strength and size. As the heart gets stronger, the muscle can produce a more forceful contraction, which helps the heart to eject more blood with each beat. This **stroke volume** yields a lower heart rate. The lower heart rate also allows the heart to rest longer between beats. Average resting and maximal cardiac outputs, stroke volumes, and heart rates for sedentary, trained, and highly trained (elite) males are shown in Table 6.1. Resting heart rates frequently decrease by 10 to 20 beats per minute (bpm) after only 6 to 8 weeks of training. A reduction of 20 bpm saves the heart about 10,483,200 beats per year. The average heart beats between 70 and 80 bpm. As seen in Table 6.1, resting heart rates in highly trained athletes are often around 45 bpm.

4. A lower heart rate at given **workloads.** When compared with untrained individuals, a trained person has a lower heart rate response to a given task because of greater efficiency of the cardiorespiratory system. Individuals are surprised to find that following several weeks of training, a given workload (let's say a 10-minute mile) elicits a much lower heart rate response than that when they first started training.

5. An increase in the number and size of the **mitochondria.** All energy necessary for cell function is produced in the mitochondria. As their size and numbers increase, so does their potential to produce energy for muscular work.

6. An increase in the number of functional **capillaries.** Capillaries allow for the exchange of oxygen and carbon dioxide between the blood and the cells. As more vessels open up, more gas exchange can take place, delaying the onset of fatigue during prolonged exercise. This increase in capillaries also speeds the rate at which waste products of cell metabolism can be removed. This increased capillarization also occurs in the heart, which enhances the oxygen delivery capacity to the heart muscle itself.

7. Ability to recover rapidly. Trained individuals have a faster **recovery time** after exercising. A fit system is able to more quickly restore any internal equilibrium disrupted during exercise.

8. Lower blood pressure and blood lipids. A regular aerobic exercise program leads to lower blood pressure (thereby reducing a major risk factor for stroke) and lower levels of fats (such as cholesterol and triglycerides), all of which have been linked to the formation of atherosclerotic plaque, which obstructs the arteries. This decreases the risk for coronary heart disease (see Chapter 11).

9. An increase in fat-burning enzymes. These enzymes are significant because fat is lost primarily by burning it in muscle. As the concentration of the enzymes increases, so does the ability to burn fat.

## Behavior Modification Planning

### TIPS TO INCREASE DAILY PHYSICAL ACTIVITY

Adults need recess, too! There are 1440 minutes in every day. Schedule a minimum of 30 of these minutes for physical activity. With a little creativity and planning, even the person with the busiest schedule can make room for physical activity. For many folks, before or after work or meals is often an available time to cycle, walk, or play. Think about your weekly or daily schedule and look for or make opportunities to be more active. Every little bit helps. Consider the following suggestions:

☐ I PLAN TO
☐ I DID IT

☐ ☐ Walk, cycle, jog, skate, etc., to school, work, the store, or place of worship.
☐ ☐ Use a pedometer to count your daily steps.
☐ ☐ Walk while doing errands.
☐ ☐ Get on or off the bus several blocks away.
☐ ☐ Park the car farther away from your destination.
☐ ☐ At work, walk to nearby offices instead of sending e-mails or using the phone.
☐ ☐ Walk or stretch a few minutes every hour that you are at your desk.
☐ ☐ Take fitness breaks—walking or doing desk exercises—instead of taking cigarette breaks or coffee breaks.
☐ ☐ Incorporate activity into your lunch break (walk to the restaurant).
☐ ☐ Take the stairs instead of the elevator or escalator.

☐ ☐ Play with children, grandchildren, or pets. Everybody wins. If you find it too difficult to be active after work, try it before work.
☐ ☐ Do household tasks.
☐ ☐ Work in the yard or garden.
☐ ☐ Avoid labor-saving devices. Turn off the self-propelled option on your lawnmower or vacuum cleaner.
☐ ☐ Use leg power. Take small trips on foot to get your body moving.
☐ ☐ Exercise while watching TV (for example, use hand weights, stationary bicycle/treadmill/stairclimber, or stretch).
☐ ☐ Spend more time playing sports than sitting in front of the TV or the computer.
☐ ☐ Dance to music.
☐ ☐ Keep a pair of comfortable walking or running shoes in your car and office. You'll be ready for activity wherever you go!
☐ ☐ Make a Saturday morning walk a group habit.
☐ ☐ Learn a new sport or join a sports team.
☐ ☐ Avoid carts when golfing.
☐ ☐ When out of town, stay in hotels with fitness centers.

***Source:*** Adapted from Centers for Disease Control and Prevention, Atlanta, 2005.

## Try It

Keep a three-day log of all your activities. List the activities performed, time of day, and how long you were engaged in these activities. You may be surprised by your findings.

# Physical Fitness Assessment

Assessment of physical fitness serves several purposes:

- To educate participants regarding their present fitness levels and compare them with health fitness and physical fitness standards
- To motivate individuals to participate in exercise programs

**Resting heart rate (RHR)** Heart rate after a person has been sitting quietly for 15–20 minutes.

**Cardiac output** Amount of blood pumped by the heart in one minute.

**Stroke volume** Amount of blood pumped by the heart in one beat.

**Workload** Load (or intensity) placed on the body during physical activity.

**Mitochondria** Structures within the cells where energy transformations take place.

**Capillaries** Smallest blood vessels carrying oxygenated blood to the tissues in the body.

**Recovery time** Amount of time the body takes to return to resting levels after exercise.

- To provide a starting point for individualized exercise prescription
- To evaluate improvements in fitness achieved through exercise programs and adjust exercise prescription accordingly
- To monitor changes in fitness throughout the years

**Responders Versus Nonresponders** Individuals who follow similar training programs show a wide variation in physiologic responses. Heredity plays a crucial role in how each person responds to and improves after beginning an exercise program. Several studies have documented that following exercise training, most individuals, called **responders**, readily show improvements, but a few, **nonresponders**, exhibit small or no improvements at all. This concept is referred to as the **principle of individuality.**

After several months of aerobic training, increases in $VO_{2max}$ are between 15 and 20 percent, on the average, although individual responses can range from 0 percent (in a few selected cases) to more than 50 percent improvement, even when all participants follow exactly the same training program. Nonfitness and low-fitness participants, however, should not label themselves as nonresponders based on the previous discussion. Nonresponders constitute less than 5 percent of exercise participants. Although additional research is necessary, lack of improvement in cardiorespiratory endurance among nonresponders might be related to low levels of leg strength. A lower-body strength-training program has been shown to help these individuals improve $VO_{2max}$ through aerobic exercise.[2]

Following your self-assessment of cardiorespiratory fitness, if your fitness level is less than adequate, do not let that discourage you, but do set a priority to be physically active every day. In addition to regular exercise, lifestyle behaviors—walking, taking stairs, cycling to work, parking farther from the office, doing household tasks, gardening and doing yard work, for example—provide substantial benefits. In this regard, daily **physical activity** and **exercise** habits should be monitored in conjunction with fitness testing to evaluate adherence among nonresponders. After all, it is through increased daily activity that we reap the health benefits that improve our quality of life.

# Assessment of Cardiorespiratory Endurance

Cardiorespiratory endurance, cardiorespiratory fitness, or aerobic capacity is determined by the maximal amount of oxygen the human body is able to utilize (the oxygen uptake) per minute of physical activity ($VO_{2max}$). This value can be expressed in liters per minute (L/min) or milliliters per kilogram per minute (mL/kg/min). The relative value in mL/kg/min is used most often because it considers total body mass (weight) in kilograms. When comparing two individuals with the same absolute value, the one with the lesser body mass will have a higher relative value, indicating that more oxygen is available to each kilogram (2.2 pounds) of body weight. Because all tissues and organs of the body need oxygen to function, higher oxygen consumption indicates a more efficient cardiorespiratory system.

**Components of Oxygen Uptake ($VO_2$)** The amount of oxygen the body actually uses at rest or during submaximal ($VO_2$) or maximal ($VO_{2max}$) exercise is determined by the heart rate, the stroke volume, and the amount of oxygen removed from the vascular system (for use by all organs and tissues of the body, including the muscular system).

**Heart Rate** Normal heart rate ranges from about 40 bpm during resting conditions in trained athletes to 200 bpm or higher during maximal exercise. The **maximal heart rate (MHR)** that a person can achieve starts to drop by about one beat per year beginning at about 12 years of age. Maximal heart rate in trained endurance athletes is sometimes slightly lower than in untrained individuals. This adaptation to training is thought to allow the heart more time to effectively fill with blood so as to produce a greater stroke volume.

**Stroke Volume** Stroke volume ranges from 50 mL per beat (stroke) during resting conditions in untrained individuals to 200 mL at maximum in endurance-trained athletes (see Table 6.1). Following endurance training, stroke volume increases significantly. Some of the increase is the result of a stronger heart muscle, but it also is related to an increase in total blood volume and a greater filling capacity of the ventricles during the resting phase (diastole) of the cardiac cycle. As more blood enters the heart, more blood can be ejected with each heartbeat (systole). The increase in stroke volume is primarily responsible for the increase in $VO_{2max}$ with endurance training.

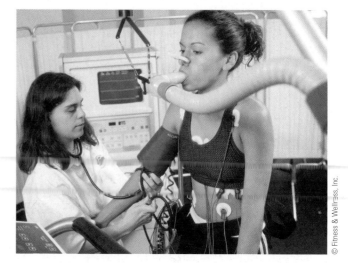

Oxygen uptake ($VO_2$), as determined through direct gas analysis.

## Amount of Oxygen Removed from Blood

The amount of oxygen removed from the vascular system is known as the **arterial–venous oxygen difference (a-v̄O2$_{diff}$).** The oxygen content in the arteries at sea level is typically 20 mL of oxygen per 100 cc of blood. (This value decreases at higher altitudes because of the drop in barometric pressure, which affects the amount of oxygen picked up by hemoglobin.) The oxygen content in the veins during a resting state is about 15 mL per 100 cc. Thus, the a-v̄O2$_{diff}$—the amount of oxygen in the arteries minus the amount in the veins—at rest is 5 mL per 100 cc. The arterial value remains constant during both resting and exercise conditions, but during maximal exercise the venous oxygen content drops to about 5 mL per 100 cc, yielding an a-v̄O2$_{diff}$ of 15 mL per 100 cc. The latter value may be slightly higher in endurance athletes.

These three factors are used to compute VO$_2$ using the following equation:

$$VO_2 \text{ in L/min} = (HR \times SV \times \text{a-v̄O2}_{diff}) \div 100,000,$$

where

HR = heart rate and SV = stroke volume.

For example, the resting VO$_2$ (also known as the resting metabolic rate) of an individual with a resting heart rate of 76 bpm and a stroke volume of 79 mL would be:

$$VO_2 \text{ in L/min} = (76 \times 79 \times 5) \div 100,000 = 0.3 \text{ L/min.}$$

Likewise, the VO$_{2max}$ of a person exercising maximally who achieves a heart rate of 190 bpm and a maximal stroke volume of 120 mL would be:

$$VO_{2max} \text{ in L/min} = (190 \times 120 \times 15) \div 100,000 = 3.42 \text{ L/min.}$$

To convert L/min to mL/kg/min, multiply the L/min value by 1,000 and divide by body weight in kilograms. In the above example, if the person weighs 70 kilograms, the VO$_{2max}$ in mL/kg/min is 48.9 ($3.42 \times 1000 \div 70$).

## Critical Thinking

You can improve your relative VO$_{2max}$ without engaging in an aerobic exercise program. How do you accomplish this? Would you benefit from doing so?

Because the actual measurement of the stroke volume and the a-v̄O2$_{diff}$ is impractical in the fitness setting, VO$_2$ also is determined through gas (air) analysis. The person being tested breathes into a metabolic cart that measures the difference in oxygen content between the person's exhaled air and the atmosphere. The air we breathe contains 21 percent oxygen; thus, VO$_2$ can be assessed by establishing the difference between 21 percent and the percent of oxygen left in the air the person exhales, according to the total amount of air taken into the lungs. This type of equipment, however, is expensive. Consequently, several alternative methods of estimating VO$_{2max}$ using limited equipment have been developed. These methods are discussed next.

VO$_{2max}$ is affected by genetics, training, gender, age, and body composition. Although aerobic training can help people attain good or excellent cardiorespiratory fitness, only those with a strong genetic component are able to reach an "elite" level of aerobic capacity (60 to 80 mL/kg/min). Further, VO$_{2max}$ is 15 to 30 percent higher in men. This is related to a greater hemoglobin content, lower body fat (see "Essential and Storage Fat" in Chapter 4, page 123), and larger heart size in men (a larger heart pumps more blood, and thus produces a greater stroke volume). VO$_{2max}$ also decreases by about 1 percent per year starting at age 25. This decrease, however, is only 0.5 percent per year in physically active individuals.

# Tests to Estimate VO$_{2max}$

Even though most cardiorespiratory endurance tests probably are safe to administer to apparently healthy individuals (those with no major coronary risk factors or symptoms), a health history questionnaire, such as found in Lab 1C in Chapter 1, should be used as a minimum screening tool prior to exercise testing or participation. The American College of Sports Medicine (ACSM) also recommends that a physician be present for all maximal exercise tests on apparently healthy men 45 or older and women 55 or older.[3] A maximal test is any test that requires the participant's all-out or nearly all-out effort. For submaximal exercise tests, a physician should be present

**Responders** Individuals who exhibit improvements in fitness as a result of exercise training.

**Nonresponders** Individuals who exhibit small or no improvements in fitness as compared with others who undergo the same training program.

**Principle of individuality** Training concept holding that genetics plays a major role in individual responses to exercise training and that these differences must be considered when designing exercise programs for different people.

**Physical activity** Bodily movement produced by skeletal muscles; requires expenditure of energy and produces progressive health benefits. Examples include walking, taking the stairs, dancing, gardening, yard work, house cleaning, snow shoveling, washing the car, and all forms of structured exercise.

**Exercise** A type of physical activity that requires planned, structured, and repetitive bodily movement with the intent of improving or maintaining one or more components of physical fitness.

**Maximal heart rate (MHR)** Highest heart rate for a person, related primarily to age.

**Arterial–venous oxygen difference (a-v̄O$_2$diff)** The amount of oxygen removed from the blood as determined by the difference in oxygen content between arterial and venous blood.

**FIGURE 6.1** Procedure for the 1.5-Mile Run Test.

1. Make sure you qualify for this test. This test is contraindicated for unconditioned beginners, individuals with symptoms of heart disease, and those with known heart disease or risk factors.
2. Select the testing site. Find a school track (each lap is one-fourth of a mile) or a premeasured 1.5-mile course.
3. Have a stopwatch available to determine your time.
4. Conduct a few warm-up exercises prior to the test. Do some stretching exercises, some walking, and slow jogging.
5. Initiate the test and try to cover the distance in the fastest time possible (walking or jogging). Time yourself during the run to see how fast you have covered the distance. If any unusual symptoms arise during the test, do not continue. Stop

immediately and retake the test after another 6 weeks of aerobic training.
6. At the end of the test, cool down by walking or jogging slowly for another 3 to 5 minutes. Do not sit or lie down after the test.
7. According to your performance time, look up your estimated maximal oxygen uptake ($VO_{2max}$) in Table 6.2.

**Example:** A 20-year-old female runs the 1.5-mile course in 12 minutes and 40 seconds. Table 6.2 shows a $VO_{2max}$ of 39.8 ml/kg/min for a time of 12:40. According to Table 6.8, this $VO_{2max}$ would place her in the "good" cardiorespiratory fitness category.

when testing higher-risk/symptomatic individuals or diseased people, regardless of the participants' current age.

Five exercise tests used to assess cardiorespiratory fitness are introduced in this chapter: the 1.5-Mile Run Test, the 1.0-Mile Walk Test, the Step Test, the Astrand-Rhyming Test, and the 12-Minute Swim Test. The procedures for each test are explained in detail in Figures 6.1, 6.2, 6.3, 6.4, and 6.5, respectively.

Several tests are provided in this chapter, so you may choose one depending on time, equipment, and individual physical limitations. For example, people who can't jog or walk can take the Astrand-Rhyming (bicycle) or swim test. You may perform more than one test, but because they are different and they estimate $VO_{2max}$, they will not necessarily yield the same results. Therefore, to make valid comparisons, you should take the same test when doing pre- and post-assessments. You may record the results of your test(s) in Lab 6A.

## 1.5-Mile Run Test
The 1.5-Mile Run Test is used most frequently to predict $VO_{2max}$ according to the time the person takes to run or walk a 1.5-mile course (Figure 6.1). $VO_{2max}$ is estimated based on the time the person takes to cover the distance (Table 6.2).

The only equipment necessary to conduct this test is a stopwatch and a track or premeasured 1.5-mile course. This perhaps is the easiest test to administer, but a note of caution is in order when conducting the test: Given that the objective is to cover the distance in the shortest time, it is considered a maximal exercise test. The 1.5-Mile Run Test should be limited to conditioned individuals who have been cleared for exercise. The test is not recommended for unconditioned beginners, men over age 45 and women over age 55 without proper medical clearance, symptomatic individuals, and those with known disease or risk factors for coronary heart disease. A program of at least 6 weeks of aerobic training is recommended before unconditioned individuals take this test.

## 1.0-Mile Walk Test
The 1.0-Mile Walk Test can be used by individuals who are unable to run because of low fitness levels or injuries. All that is required is a brisk 1.0-mile walk that will elicit an exercise heart rate of at least 120 bpm at the end of the test.

You will need to know how to take your heart rate by counting your pulse. You can do this by gently placing the middle and index fingers over the radial artery on the inside of the wrist on the side of the thumb or over the carotid artery in the neck just below the jaw next to the voice box. You should not use the thumb to check the pulse because it has a strong pulse of its own, which can make you miscount. When checking the carotid pulse, do not press too hard, because it may cause a reflex action that slows the heart. For checking the pulse over the carotid artery, some exercise experts recommend that the hand on the same side of the neck (left hand over left carotid artery) be used to avoid excessive pressure on the artery. With minimum experience, however, you can be accurate using either hand as long as you apply only gentle pressure. If available, heart rate monitors can be used to increase the accuracy of heart rate assessment.

$VO_{2max}$ is estimated according to a prediction equation that requires the following data: 1.0-mile walk time, exercise heart rate at the end of the walk, gender, and body weight in pounds. The procedure for this test and the equation are given in Figure 6.2.

## Step Test
The Step Test requires little time and equipment and can be administered to almost anyone, because a submaximal workload is used to estimate $VO_{2max}$. Symptomatic and diseased individuals should not take this test. Significantly overweight individuals and those with joint

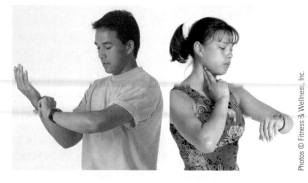

Pulse taken at the radial artery.

Pulse taken at the carotid artery.

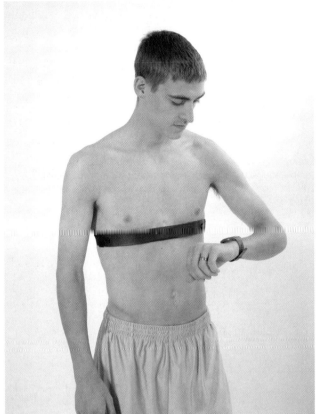

Heart rate monitors increase the accuracy of heart rate assessment.

problems in the lower extremities may have difficulty performing the test.

The actual test takes only 3 minutes. A 15-second recovery heart rate is taken between 5 and 20 seconds following the test (Figure 6.3 and Table 6.3). The required equipment consists of a bench or gymnasium bleacher 16¼ inches high, a stopwatch, and a metronome.

You also will need to know how to take your heart rate by counting your pulse, as we have just discussed. Once people learn to take their own heart rate, a large group of people can be tested at once, using gymnasium bleachers for the steps.

Astrand-Rhyming Test  Because of its simplicity and practicality, the Astrand-Rhyming Test is one of the most popular tests used to estimate $VO_{2max}$ in the laboratory setting. The test is conducted on a bicycle ergometer and, similar to the Step Test, requires only submaximal workloads and little time to administer.

The cautions given for the Step Test also apply to the Astrand-Rhyming Test. Nevertheless, because the participant does not have to support his or her own body weight while riding the bicycle, overweight individuals and those with limited joint problems in the lower extremities can take this test.

The bicycle ergometer to be used for this test should allow for the regulation of workloads (see the test procedure in Figure 6.4). Besides the bicycle ergometer, a stop-

**TABLE 6.2**  Estimated Maximal Oxygen Uptake ($VO_{2max}$) for the 1.5-Mile Run Test

| Time | $VO_{2max}$ (ml/kg/min) | Time | $VO_{2max}$ (ml/kg/min) |
|------|------|------|------|
| 6:10 | 80.0 | 12:40 | 39.8 |
| 6:20 | 79.0 | 12:50 | 39.2 |
| 6:30 | 77.9 | 13:00 | 38.6 |
| 6:40 | 76.7 | 13:10 | 38.1 |
| 6:50 | 75.5 | 13:20 | 37.8 |
| 7:00 | 74.0 | 13:30 | 37.2 |
| 7:10 | 72.6 | 13:40 | 36.8 |
| 7:20 | 71.3 | 13:50 | 36.3 |
| 7:30 | 69.9 | 14:00 | 35.9 |
| 7:40 | 68.3 | 14:10 | 35.5 |
| 7:50 | 66.8 | 14:20 | 35.1 |
| 8:00 | 65.2 | 14:30 | 34.7 |
| 8:10 | 63.9 | 14:40 | 34.3 |
| 8:20 | 62.5 | 14:50 | 34.0 |
| 8:30 | 61.2 | 15:00 | 33.6 |
| 8:40 | 60.2 | 15:10 | 33.1 |
| 8:50 | 59.1 | 15:20 | 32.7 |
| 9:00 | 58.1 | 15:30 | 32.2 |
| 9:10 | 56.9 | 15:40 | 31.8 |
| 9:20 | 55.9 | 15:50 | 31.4 |
| 9:30 | 54.7 | 16:00 | 30.9 |
| 9:40 | 53.5 | 16:10 | 30.5 |
| 9:50 | 52.3 | 16:20 | 30.2 |
| 10:00 | 51.1 | 16:30 | 29.8 |
| 10:10 | 50.4 | 16:40 | 29.5 |
| 10:20 | 49.5 | 16:50 | 29.1 |
| 10:30 | 48.6 | 17:00 | 28.9 |
| 10:40 | 48.0 | 17:10 | 28.5 |
| 10:50 | 47.4 | 17:20 | 28.3 |
| 11:00 | 46.6 | 17:30 | 28.0 |
| 11:10 | 45.8 | 17:40 | 27.7 |
| 11:20 | 45.1 | 17:50 | 27.4 |
| 11:30 | 44.4 | 18:00 | 27.1 |
| 11:40 | 43.7 | 18:10 | 26.8 |
| 11:50 | 43.2 | 18:20 | 26.6 |
| 12:00 | 42.3 | 18:30 | 26.3 |
| 12:10 | 41.7 | 18:40 | 26.0 |
| 12:20 | 41.0 | 18:50 | 25.7 |
| 12:30 | 40.4 | 19:00 | 25.4 |

***Source:*** Adapted from K. H. Cooper, "A Means of Assessing Maximal Oxygen Intake," in *Journal of the American Medical Association,* 203 (1968): 201–204; M. L. Pollock, J. H. Wilmore, and S. M. Fox III, *Health and Fitness Through Physical Activity,* (New York: John Wiley & Sons, 1978); and J. H. Wilmore and D. L. Costill, *Training for Sport and Activity* (Dubuque, IA: Wm. C. Brown Publishers, 1988).

© Fitness & Wellness, Inc.

**FIGURE 6.2  Procedure for the 1.0-Mile Walk Test.**

1. Select the testing site. Use a 440-yard track (4 laps to a mile) or a premeasured 1.0-mile course.
2. Determine your body weight in pounds prior to the test.
3. Have a stopwatch available to determine total walking time and exercise heart rate.
4. Walk the 1.0-mile course at a brisk pace (the exercise heart rate at the end of the test should be above 120 beats per minute).
5. At the end of the 1.0-mile walk, check your walking time and immediately count your pulse for 10 seconds. Multiply the 10-second pulse count by 6 to obtain the exercise heart rate in beats per minute.
6. Convert the walking time from minutes and seconds to minute units. Because each minute has 60 seconds, divide the seconds by 60 to obtain the fraction of a minute. For instance, a walking time of 12 minutes and 15 seconds would equal 12 + (15 ÷ 60), or 12.25 minutes.
7. To obtain the estimated maximal oxygen uptake ($VO_{2max}$) in mL/kg/min, plug your values in the following equation:
   $VO_{2max} = 88.768 - (0.0957 \times W) + (8.892 \times G) - (1.4537 \times T) - (0.1194 \times HR)$

**Where:**

$W$ = Weight in pounds
$G$ = Gender (use 0 for women and 1 for men)
$T$ = Total time for the one-mile walk in minutes (see item 6)
$HR$ = Exercise heart rate in beats per minute at the end of the 1.0-mile walk

**Example:** A 19-year-old female who weighs 140 pounds completed the 1.0-mile walk in 14 minutes 39 seconds with an exercise heart rate of 148 beats per minute. Her estimated $VO_{2max}$ would be:

$W$ = 140 lbs
$G$ = 0 (female gender = 0)
$T$ = 14:39 = 14 + (39 ÷ 60) = 14.65 min
$HR$ = 148 bpm
$VO_{2max} = 88.768 - (0.0957 \times 140) + (8.892 \times 0) - (1.4537 \times 14.65) - (0.1194 \times 148)$
$VO_{2max}$ = 36.4 mL/kg/min

*Source:* F. A. Dolgener, L. D. Hensley, J. J. Marsh, and J. K. Fjelstul, "Validation of the Rockport Fitness Walking Test in college males and females," *Research Quarterly for Exercise and Sport* 65 (1994): 152–158.

**FIGURE 6.3  Procedure for the Step Test.**

1. Conduct the test with a bench or gymnasium bleacher 16¼ inches high.
2. Perform the stepping cycle to a four-step cadence (up-up-down-down). Men should perform 24 complete step-ups per minute, regulated with a metronome set at 96 beats per minute. Women perform 22 step-ups per minute, or 88 beats per minute on the metronome.
3. Allow a brief practice period of 5 to 10 seconds to familiarize yourself with the stepping cadence.
4. Begin the test and perform the step-ups for exactly 3 minutes.
5. Upon completing the 3 minutes, remain standing and take your heart rate for a 15-second interval from 5 to 20 seconds into recovery. Convert recovery heart rate to beats per minute (multiply 15-second heart rate by 4).
6. Maximal oxygen uptake ($VO_{2max}$) in mL/kg/min is estimated

according to the following equations:
Men:
$VO_{2max} = 111.33 - (0.42 \times$ recovery heart rate in bpm)
Women:
$VO_{2max} = 65.81 - (0.1847 \times$ recovery heart rate in bpm)

**Example:** The recovery 15-second heart rate for a male following the 3-minute step test is found to be 39 beats. His $VO_{2max}$ is estimated as follows:
15-second heart rate = 39 beats
Minute heart rate = 39 × 4 = 156 bpm
$VO_{2max} = 111.33 - (0.42 \times 156) = 45.81$ mL/kg/min
$VO_{2max}$ also can be obtained according to recovery heart rates in Table 6.3.

*Source:* From W. D. McArdle et al., *Exercise Physiology: Energy, Nutrition, and Human Performance* (Philadelphia: Lea & Febiger, 1986).

watch and an additional technician to monitor the heart rate are needed to conduct the test.

The heart rate is taken every minute for 6 minutes. At the end of the test, the heart rate should be in the range given for each workload in Table 6.5 (generally between 120 and 170 bpm).

When administering the test to older people, good judgment is essential. Low workloads should be used, because if the higher heart rates (around 150 to 170 bpm) are reached, these individuals could be working near or at their maximal capacity, making this an unsafe test without adequate medical supervision. When testing older people, choose workloads so that the final exercise heart rates do not exceed 130 to 140 bpm.

**12-Minute Swim Test** Similar to the 1.5-Mile Run Test, the 12-Minute Swim Test is considered a maximal exercise test, and the same precautions apply. The objective is to swim as far as possible during the 12-Minute Swim Test (Figure 6.5).

Unlike land-based tests, predicting $VO_{2max}$ through a swimming test is difficult. A swimming test is practical only for those who are planning to take part in a swimming program or who cannot perform any of the other tests. Differences in skill level, swimming conditioning, and body composition greatly affect the energy requirements (oxygen uptake) of swimming.

Unskilled and unconditioned swimmers can expect lower cardiorespiratory fitness ratings than those ob-

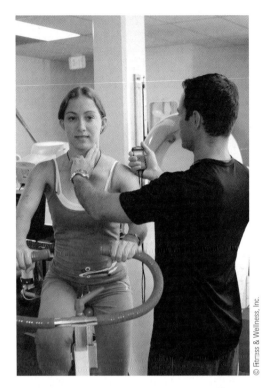

Monitoring heart rate on the carotid artery during the Astrand-Rhyming Test.

**TABLE 6.3** Predicted Maximal Oxygen Uptake for the Step Test

| 15-Sec Heart Rate | Heart Rate (bpm) | $VO_{2max}$ (mL/kg/min) Men | $VO_{2max}$ (mL/kg/min) Women |
|---|---|---|---|
| 30 | 120 | 60.9 | 43.6 |
| 31 | 124 | 59.3 | 42.9 |
| 32 | 128 | 57.6 | 42.2 |
| 33 | 132 | 55.9 | 41.4 |
| 34 | 136 | 54.2 | 40.7 |
| 35 | 140 | 52.5 | 40.0 |
| 36 | 144 | 50.9 | 39.2 |
| 37 | 148 | 49.2 | 38.5 |
| 38 | 152 | 47.5 | 37.7 |
| 39 | 156 | 45.8 | 37.0 |
| 40 | 160 | 44.1 | 36.3 |
| 41 | 164 | 42.5 | 35.5 |
| 42 | 168 | 40.8 | 34.8 |
| 43 | 172 | 39.1 | 34.0 |
| 44 | 176 | 37.4 | 33.3 |
| 45 | 180 | 35.7 | 32.6 |
| 46 | 184 | 34.1 | 31.8 |
| 47 | 188 | 32.4 | 31.1 |
| 48 | 192 | 30.7 | 30.3 |
| 49 | 196 | 29.0 | 29.6 |
| 50 | 200 | 27.3 | 28.9 |

tained with a land-based test. A skilled swimmer is able to swim more efficiently and expend much less energy than an unskilled swimmer. Improper breathing patterns cause premature fatigue. Overweight individuals are more buoyant in the water, and the larger surface area (body size) produces more friction against movement in the water medium.

**FIGURE 6.4** Procedure for the Astrand-Rhyming Test.

1. Adjust the bike seat so the knees are almost completely extended as the foot goes through the bottom of the pedaling cycle.
2. During the test, keep the speed constant at 50 revolutions per minute. Test duration is 6 minutes.
3. Select the appropriate workload for the bike based on gender, age, weight, health, and estimated fitness level. For unconditioned individuals: women, use 300 kpm (kilopounds per meter) or 450 kpm; men, 300 kpm or 600 kpm. Conditioned adults: women, 450 kpm or 600 kpm; men, 600 kpm or 900 kpm.*
4. Ride the bike for 6 minutes and check the heart rate every minute, during the last 15 seconds of each minute. Determine heart rate by recording the time it takes to count 30 pulse beats and then converting to beats per minute using Table 6.4.
5. Average the final two heart rates (5th and 6th minutes). If these two heart rates are not within 5 beats per minute of each other, continue the test for another few minutes until this is accomplished. If the heart rate continues to climb significantly after the 6th minute, stop the test and rest for 15 to 20 minutes. You may then retest, preferably at a lower workload. The final average

heart rate should also fall between the ranges given for each workload in Table 6.5 (men: 300 kpm = 120 to 140 beats per minute; 600 kpm = 120 to 170 beats per minute).
6. Based on the average heart rate of the final 2 minutes and your workload, look up the maximal oxygen uptake ($VO_{2max}$) in Table 6.5 (for example: men: 600 kpm and average heart rate = 145, $VO_{2max}$ = 2.4 L/min).
7. Correct $VO_{2max}$ using the correction factors found in Table 6.6 (if $VO_{2max}$ = 2.4 and age 35, correction factor = .870. Multiply 2.4 × .870 and final corrected $VO_{2max}$ = 2.09 L/min).
8. To obtain $VO_{2max}$ in mL/kg/min, multiply the $VO_{2max}$ by 1,000 (to convert liters to milliliters) and divide by body weight in kilograms (to obtain kilograms, divide your body weight in pounds by 2.2046).

**Example:** Corrected $VO_{2max}$ = 2.09 L/min
Body weight = 132 pounds ÷ 2.2046 = 60 kilograms

$$VO_{2max} \text{ in mL/kg/min} = \frac{2.09 \times 1,000}{60} = 34.8 \text{ mL/kg/min}$$

*On the Monarch bicycle ergometer, at a speed of 50 revolutions per minute, a load of 1 kp = 300 kpm, 1.5 kp = 450 kpm, 2 kp = 600 kpm, and so forth, with increases of 150 kpm to each half kp.

**TABLE 6.4** Conversion of the Time for 30 Pulse Beats to Pulse Rate per Minute

| Sec. | bpm | Sec. | bpm | Sec. | bpm | Sec. | bpm | Sec. | bpm | Sec. | bpm |
|------|-----|------|-----|------|-----|------|-----|------|-----|------|-----|
| 22.0 | 82 | 19.6 | 92 | 17.2 | 105 | 14.8 | 122 | 12.4 | 145 | 10.0 | 180 |
| 21.9 | 82 | 19.5 | 92 | 17.1 | 105 | 14.7 | 122 | 12.3 | 146 | 9.9 | 182 |
| 21.8 | 83 | 19.4 | 93 | 17.0 | 106 | 14.6 | 123 | 12.2 | 148 | 9.8 | 184 |
| 21.7 | 83 | 19.3 | 93 | 16.9 | 107 | 14.5 | 124 | 12.1 | 149 | 9.7 | 186 |
| 21.6 | 83 | 19.2 | 94 | 16.8 | 107 | 14.4 | 125 | 12.0 | 150 | 9.6 | 188 |
| 21.5 | 84 | 19.1 | 94 | 16.7 | 108 | 14.3 | 126 | 11.9 | 151 | 9.5 | 189 |
| 21.4 | 84 | 19.0 | 95 | 16.6 | 108 | 14.2 | 127 | 11.8 | 153 | 9.4 | 191 |
| 21.3 | 85 | 18.9 | 95 | 16.5 | 109 | 14.1 | 128 | 11.7 | 154 | 9.3 | 194 |
| 21.2 | 85 | 18.8 | 96 | 16.4 | 110 | 14.0 | 129 | 11.6 | 155 | 9.2 | 196 |
| 21.1 | 85 | 18.7 | 96 | 16.3 | 110 | 13.9 | 129 | 11.5 | 157 | 9.1 | 198 |
| 21.0 | 86 | 18.6 | 97 | 16.2 | 111 | 13.8 | 130 | 11.4 | 158 | 9.0 | 200 |
| 20.9 | 86 | 18.5 | 97 | 16.1 | 112 | 13.7 | 131 | 11.3 | 159 | 8.9 | 202 |
| 20.8 | 87 | 18.4 | 98 | 16.0 | 113 | 13.6 | 132 | 11.2 | 161 | 8.8 | 205 |
| 20.7 | 87 | 18.3 | 98 | 15.9 | 113 | 13.5 | 133 | 11.1 | 162 | 8.7 | 207 |
| 20.6 | 87 | 18.2 | 99 | 15.8 | 114 | 13.4 | 134 | 11.0 | 164 | 8.6 | 209 |
| 20.5 | 88 | 18.1 | 99 | 15.7 | 115 | 13.3 | 135 | 10.9 | 165 | 8.5 | 212 |
| 20.4 | 88 | 18.0 | 100 | 15.6 | 115 | 13.2 | 136 | 10.8 | 167 | 8.4 | 214 |
| 20.3 | 89 | 17.9 | 101 | 15.5 | 116 | 13.1 | 137 | 10.7 | 168 | 8.3 | 217 |
| 20.2 | 89 | 17.8 | 101 | 15.4 | 117 | 13.0 | 138 | 10.6 | 170 | 8.2 | 220 |
| 20.1 | 90 | 17.7 | 102 | 15.3 | 118 | 12.9 | 140 | 10.5 | 171 | 8.1 | 222 |
| 20.0 | 90 | 17.6 | 102 | 15.2 | 118 | 12.8 | 141 | 10.4 | 173 | 8.0 | 225 |
| 19.9 | 90 | 17.5 | 103 | 15.1 | 119 | 12.7 | 142 | 10.3 | 175 | | |
| 19.8 | 91 | 17.4 | 103 | 15.0 | 120 | 12.6 | 143 | 10.2 | 176 | | |
| 19.7 | 91 | 17.3 | 104 | 14.9 | 121 | 12.5 | 144 | 10.1 | 178 | | |

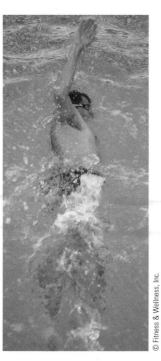

Only those with swimming skill and proper conditioning should take the 12-minute swimming test.

Lack of conditioning affects swimming test results as well. An unconditioned skilled swimmer who is in good cardiorespiratory shape because of a regular jogging program will not perform as effectively in a swimming test. Swimming conditioning is important for adequate performance on this test.

Because of these limitations, $VO_{2max}$ cannot be estimated for a swimming test, and the fitness categories given in Table 6.7 are only estimated ratings.

## Critical Thinking

Should fitness testing be a part of a fitness program? Why or why not? Does preparticipation fitness testing have benefits, or should fitness testing be done at a later date?

**TABLE 6.5** Maximal Oxygen Uptake (VO$_{2max}$) Estimates in L/min for the Astrand-Rhyming Test

| Heart Rate | Men Workload 300 | 600 | 900 | 1200 | 1500 | Women Workload 300 | 450 | 600 | 750 | 900 |
|---|---|---|---|---|---|---|---|---|---|---|
| 120 | 2.2 | 3.4 | 4.8 | | | 2.6 | 3.4 | 4.1 | 4.8 | |
| 121 | 2.2 | 3.4 | 4.7 | | | 2.5 | 3.3 | 4.0 | 4.8 | |
| 122 | 2.2 | 3.4 | 4.6 | | | 2.5 | 3.2 | 3.9 | 4.7 | |
| 123 | 2.1 | 3.4 | 4.6 | | | 2.4 | 3.1 | 3.9 | 4.6 | |
| 124 | 2.1 | 3.3 | 4.5 | 6.0 | | 2.4 | 3.1 | 3.8 | 4.5 | |
| 125 | 2.0 | 3.2 | 4.4 | 6.0 | | 2.3 | 3.0 | 3.7 | 4.4 | |
| 126 | 2.0 | 3.2 | 4.4 | 5.8 | | 2.3 | 3.0 | 3.6 | 4.3 | |
| 127 | 2.0 | 3.1 | 4.3 | 5.7 | | 2.2 | 2.9 | 3.5 | 4.2 | |
| 128 | 2.0 | 3.1 | 4.2 | 5.6 | | 2.2 | 2.8 | 3.5 | 4.2 | 4.8 |
| 129 | 1.9 | 3.0 | 4.2 | 5.6 | | 2.2 | 2.8 | 3.4 | 4.1 | 4.8 |
| 130 | 1.9 | 3.0 | 4.1 | 5.5 | | 2.1 | 2.7 | 3.4 | 4.0 | 4.7 |
| 131 | 1.9 | 2.9 | 4.0 | 5.4 | | 2.1 | 2.7 | 3.4 | 4.0 | 4.6 |
| 132 | 1.8 | 2.9 | 4.0 | 5.3 | | 2.0 | 2.7 | 3.3 | 3.9 | 4.5 |
| 133 | 1.8 | 2.8 | 3.9 | 5.3 | | 2.0 | 2.6 | 3.2 | 3.8 | 4.4 |
| 134 | 1.8 | 2.8 | 3.9 | 5.2 | | 2.0 | 2.6 | 3.2 | 3.8 | 4.4 |
| 135 | 1.7 | 2.8 | 3.8 | 5.1 | | 2.0 | 2.6 | 3.1 | 3.7 | 4.3 |
| 136 | 1.7 | 2.7 | 3.8 | 5.0 | | 1.9 | 2.5 | 3.1 | 3.6 | 4.2 |
| 137 | 1.7 | 2.7 | 3.7 | 5.0 | | 1.9 | 2.5 | 3.0 | 3.6 | 4.2 |
| 138 | 1.6 | 2.7 | 3.7 | 4.9 | | 1.8 | 2.4 | 3.0 | 3.5 | 4.1 |
| 139 | 1.6 | 2.6 | 3.6 | 4.8 | | 1.8 | 2.4 | 2.9 | 3.5 | 4.0 |
| 140 | 1.6 | 2.6 | 3.6 | 4.8 | 6.0 | 1.8 | 2.4 | 2.8 | 3.4 | 4.0 |
| 141 | | 2.6 | 3.5 | 4.7 | 5.9 | 1.8 | 2.3 | 2.8 | 3.4 | 3.9 |
| 142 | | 2.5 | 3.5 | 4.6 | 5.8 | 1.7 | 2.3 | 2.8 | 3.3 | 3.9 |
| 143 | | 2.5 | 3.4 | 4.6 | 5.7 | 1.7 | 2.2 | 2.7 | 3.3 | 3.8 |
| 144 | | 2.5 | 3.4 | 4.5 | 5.7 | 1.7 | 2.2 | 2.7 | 3.2 | 3.8 |
| 145 | | 2.4 | 3.4 | 4.5 | 5.6 | 1.6 | 2.2 | 2.7 | 3.2 | 3.7 |
| 146 | 2.4 | 3.3 | 4.4 | 5.6 | | 1.6 | 2.2 | 2.6 | 3.2 | 3.7 |
| 147 | 2.4 | 3.3 | 4.4 | 5.5 | | 1.6 | 2.1 | 2.6 | 3.1 | 3.6 |
| 148 | 2.4 | 3.2 | 4.3 | 5.4 | | 1.6 | 2.1 | 2.6 | 3.1 | 3.6 |
| 149 | 2.3 | 3.2 | 4.3 | 5.4 | | | 2.1 | 2.6 | 3.0 | 3.5 |
| 150 | 2.3 | 3.2 | 4.2 | 5.3 | | | 2.0 | 2.5 | 3.0 | 3.5 |
| 151 | 2.3 | 3.1 | 4.2 | 5.2 | | | 2.0 | 2.5 | 3.0 | 3.4 |
| 152 | 2.3 | 3.1 | 4.1 | 5.2 | | | 2.0 | 2.5 | 2.9 | 3.4 |
| 153 | 2.2 | 3.0 | 4.1 | 5.1 | | | 2.0 | 2.4 | 2.9 | 3.3 |
| 154 | 2.2 | 3.0 | 4.0 | 5.1 | | | 2.0 | 2.4 | 2.8 | 3.3 |
| 155 | 2.2 | 3.0 | 4.0 | 5.0 | | | 1.9 | 2.4 | 2.8 | 3.2 |
| 156 | 2.2 | 2.9 | 4.0 | 5.0 | | | 1.9 | 2.3 | 2.8 | 3.2 |
| 157 | 2.1 | 2.9 | 3.9 | 4.9 | | | 1.9 | 2.3 | 2.7 | 3.2 |
| 158 | 2.1 | 2.9 | 3.9 | 4.9 | | | 1.8 | 2.3 | 2.7 | 3.1 |
| 159 | 2.1 | 2.8 | 3.8 | 4.8 | | | 1.8 | 2.2 | 2.7 | 3.1 |
| 160 | 2.1 | 2.8 | 3.8 | 4.8 | | | 1.8 | 2.2 | 2.6 | 3.0 |
| 161 | 2.0 | 2.8 | 3.7 | 4.7 | | | 1.8 | 2.2 | 2.6 | 3.0 |
| 162 | 2.0 | 2.8 | 3.7 | 4.6 | | | 1.8 | 2.2 | 2.6 | 3.0 |
| 163 | 2.0 | 2.8 | 3.7 | 4.6 | | | 1.7 | 2.2 | 2.6 | 2.9 |
| 164 | 2.0 | 2.7 | 3.6 | 4.5 | | | 1.7 | 2.1 | 2.5 | 2.9 |
| 165 | 2.0 | 2.7 | 3.6 | 4.5 | | | 1.7 | 2.1 | 2.5 | 2.9 |
| 166 | 1.9 | 2.7 | 3.6 | 4.5 | | | 1.7 | 2.1 | 2.5 | 2.8 |
| 167 | 1.9 | 2.6 | 3.5 | 4.4 | | | 1.6 | 2.1 | 2.4 | 2.8 |
| 168 | 1.9 | 2.6 | 3.5 | 4.4 | | | 1.6 | 2.0 | 2.4 | 2.8 |
| 169 | 1.9 | 2.6 | 3.5 | 4.3 | | | 1.6 | 2.0 | 2.4 | 2.8 |
| 170 | 1.8 | 2.6 | 3.4 | 4.3 | | | 1.6 | 2.0 | 2.4 | 2.7 |

From Astrand, I. *Acta Physiologica Scandinavica* 49 (1960). Supplementum 169: 45–60.

## Interpreting the Results of Your Maximal Oxygen Uptake

After obtaining your VO$_{2max}$, you can determine your current level of cardiorespiratory fitness by consulting Table 6.8. Locate the VO$_{2max}$ in your age category, and on the top row you will find your present level of cardiorespiratory fitness. For example, a 19-year-old male with a VO$_{2max}$ of 35 mL/kg/min would be classified in the "average" cardiorespiratory fitness category. After you initiate your personal cardiorespiratory exercise program (see Lab 6D), you may wish to retest yourself periodically to evaluate your progress.

## Predicting Oxygen Uptake and Caloric Expenditure from Walking and Jogging

As indicated earlier in the chapter, oxygen uptake can be expressed in liters per minute (L/min) or milliliters per kilogram per minute (mL/kg/min). The latter is used to classify individuals into the various cardiorespiratory fitness categories (see Table 6.8).

Oxygen uptake expressed in L/min is valuable in determining the caloric expenditure of physical activity. The human body burns about 5 calories for each liter of oxygen consumed. During aerobic exercise the average

**TABLE 6.6** Age-Based Correction Factors for Maximal Oxygen Uptake

| Age | Correction Factor | Age | Correction Factor | Age | Correction Factor |
|---|---|---|---|---|---|
| 14 | 1.11 | 32 | .909 | 50 | .750 |
| 15 | 1.10 | 33 | .896 | 51 | .742 |
| 16 | 1.09 | 34 | .883 | 52 | .734 |
| 17 | 1.08 | 35 | .870 | 53 | .726 |
| 18 | 1.07 | 36 | .862 | 54 | .718 |
| 19 | 1.06 | 37 | .854 | 55 | .710 |
| 20 | 1.05 | 38 | .846 | 56 | .704 |
| 21 | 1.04 | 39 | .838 | 57 | .698 |
| 22 | 1.03 | 40 | .830 | 58 | .692 |
| 23 | 1.02 | 41 | .820 | 59 | .686 |
| 24 | 1.01 | 42 | .810 | 60 | .680 |
| 25 | 1.00 | 43 | .800 | 61 | .674 |
| 26 | .987 | 44 | .790 | 62 | .668 |
| 27 | .974 | 45 | .780 | 63 | .662 |
| 28 | .961 | 46 | .774 | 64 | .656 |
| 29 | .948 | 47 | .768 | 65 | .650 |
| 30 | .935 | 48 | .762 | | |
| 31 | .922 | 49 | .756 | | |

Adapted from Astrand, I. *Acta Physiologica Scandinavica* 49 (1960). Supplementum 169: 45–60.

**FIGURE 6.5** Procedure for the 12-Minute Swim Test.

1. Enlist a friend to time the test. The only other requisites are a stopwatch and a swimming pool. Do not attempt to do this test in an unsupervised pool.
2. Warm up by swimming slowly and doing a few stretching exercises before taking the test.
3. Start the test and swim as many laps as possible in 12 minutes. Pace yourself throughout the test and do not swim to the point of complete exhaustion.
4. After completing the test, cool down by swimming another 2 or 3 minutes at a slower pace.
5. Determine the total distance you swam during the test and look up your fitness category in Table 6.7.

**TABLE 6.7** 12-Minute Swim Test Fitness Categories

| Distance (yards) | Fitness Category |
|---|---|
| ≥700 | Excellent |
| 500–700 | Good |
| 400–500 | Average |
| 200–400 | Fair |
| ≤200 | Poor |

Adapted from K. H. Cooper, *The Aerobics Program for Total Well-Being* (New York: Bantam Books, 1982).

**TABLE 6.8** Cardiorespiratory Fitness Classification According to Maximal Oxygen Uptake (VO$_{2max}$)

| Gender | Age | FITNESS CLASSIFICATION (based on VO$_{2max}$ in mL/kg/min) | | | | |
|---|---|---|---|---|---|---|
| | | Poor | Fair | Average | Good | Excellent |
| Men | <29 | <24.9 | 25–33.9 | 34–43.9 | 44–52.9 | >53 |
| | 30–39 | <22.9 | 23–30.9 | 31–41.9 | 42–49.9 | >50 |
| | 40–49 | <19.9 | 20–26.9 | 27–38.9 | 39–44.9 | >45 |
| | 50–59 | <17.9 | 18–24.9 | 25–37.9 | 38–42.9 | >43 |
| | 60–69 | <15.9 | 16–22.9 | 23–35.9 | 36–40.9 | >41 |
| | ≥70 | ≤12.9 | 13–20.9 | 21–32.9 | 33–37.9 | ≥38 |
| Women | <29 | <23.9 | 24–30.9 | 31–38.9 | 39–48.9 | >49 |
| | 30–39 | <19.9 | 20–27.9 | 28–36.9 | 37–44.9 | >45 |
| | 40–49 | <16.9 | 17–24.9 | 25–34.9 | 35–41.9 | >42 |
| | 50–59 | <14.9 | 15–21.9 | 22–33.9 | 34–39.9 | >40 |
| | 60–69 | <12.9 | 13–20.9 | 21–32.9 | 33–36.9 | >37 |
| | ≥70 | ≤11.9 | 12–19.9 | 20–30.9 | 31–34.9 | ≥35 |

Health fitness standard ▨ High physical fitness standard
See the Chapter 1 discussion on health fitness versus physical fitness.

person trains between 50 and 75 percent of maximal oxygen uptake.

A person with a maximal oxygen uptake of 3.5 L/min who trains at 60 percent of maximum uses 2.1 (3.5 × .60) liters of oxygen per minute of physical activity. This indicates that 10.5 calories are burned each minute of exercise (2.1 × 5). If the activity is carried out for 30 minutes, 315 calories (10.5 × 30) have been burned.

For individuals concerned about weight management, these computations are valuable in determining energy expenditure. Because a pound of body fat represents 3,500 calories, this individual would have to exercise for a total of 333 minutes (3,500 ÷ 10.5) to burn the equivalent of a pound of body fat. At 30 minutes per exercise session, approximately 11 sessions would be required to expend the 3,500 calories.

Applying the principle of 5 calories burned per liter of oxygen consumed, you can determine with reasonable accuracy your own caloric output for walking and jogging. Table 6.9 contains the oxygen requirement (uptake) for walking speeds between 50 and 100 meters per minute and for jogging speeds in excess of 80 meters per minute.

There is a transition period from walking to jogging for speeds in the range of 80 to 134 meters per minute. Consequently, the person must be truly jogging at these lower speeds to use the estimated oxygen uptakes for jogging in Table 6.9. Because these uptakes are expressed in mL/kg/min, you will need to convert this figure to L/min to predict caloric output. This is done by multiplying the oxygen uptake in mL/kg/min by your body weight in kilograms (kg) and then dividing by 1,000.

For example, let's estimate the caloric cost for an individual who weighs 145.5 pounds and runs 3 miles in 21 minutes. Each mile is about 1,600 meters, or four laps around a 400-meter (440-yard) track. Three miles then would be 4,800 meters (1,600 × 3). Therefore, 3 miles (4,800 meters) in 21 minutes represents a pace of 228.6 meters per minute (4,800 ÷ 21).

Table 6.9 indicates an oxygen requirement (uptake) of about 49.5 mL/kg/min for a speed of 228.6 meters per minute. A weight of 145.5 pounds equals 66 kilograms (145.5 ÷ 2.2046). The oxygen uptake in L/min now can be calculated by multiplying the value in mL/kg/min by body weight in kg and dividing by 1,000. In our example, it is (49.5 × 66) ÷ 1,000 = 3.3 L/min. This oxygen uptake in 21 minutes represents a total of 347 calories (3.3 × 5 × 21).

In Lab 6B you have an opportunity to determine your own oxygen uptake and caloric expenditure for walking and jogging. Using your oxygen uptake information in conjunction with exercise heart rates allows you to estimate your caloric expenditure for almost any activity, as long as the heart rate ranges from 110 to 180 beats per minute.

To make an accurate estimate, you have to be skilled in assessing exercise heart rate. Also, as your level of fitness improves, you will need to reassess your exercise heart rate because it will drop (given the same workload) with improved physical condition.

**TABLE 6.9** Oxygen Requirement Estimates for Selected Walking and Jogging Speeds

| Walking | | Jogging | | | |
|---|---|---|---|---|---|
| Speed (m/min) | VO₂ (mL/kg/min) | Speed (m/min) | VO₂ (mL/kg/min) | Speed (m/min) | VO₂ (mL/kg/min) |
| 50 | 8.5 | 80 | 19.5 | 210 | 45.5 |
| 52 | 8.7 | 85 | 20.5 | 215 | 46.5 |
| 54 | 8.9 | 90 | 21.5 | 220 | 47.5 |
| 56 | 9.1 | 95 | 22.5 | 225 | 48.5 |
| 58 | 9.3 | 100 | 23.5 | 230 | 49.5 |
| 60 | 9.5 | 105 | 24.5 | 235 | 50.5 |
| 62 | 9.7 | 110 | 25.5 | 240 | 51.5 |
| 64 | 9.9 | 115 | 26.5 | 245 | 52.5 |
| 66 | 10.1 | 120 | 27.5 | 250 | 53.5 |
| 68 | 10.3 | 125 | 28.5 | 255 | 54.5 |
| 70 | 10.5 | 130 | 29.5 | 260 | 55.5 |
| 72 | 10.7 | 135 | 30.5 | 265 | 56.5 |
| 74 | 10.9 | 140 | 31.5 | 270 | 57.5 |
| 76 | 11.1 | 145 | 32.5 | 275 | 58.5 |
| 78 | 11.3 | 150 | 33.5 | 280 | 59.5 |
| 80 | 11.5 | 155 | 34.5 | | |
| 82 | 11.7 | 160 | 35.5 | | |
| 84 | 11.9 | 165 | 36.5 | | |
| 86 | 12.1 | 170 | 37.5 | | |
| 88 | 12.3 | 175 | 38.5 | | |
| 90 | 12.5 | 180 | 39.5 | | |
| 92 | 12.7 | 185 | 40.5 | | |
| 94 | 12.9 | 190 | 41.5 | | |
| 96 | 13.1 | 195 | 42.5 | | |
| 98 | 13.3 | 200 | 43.5 | | |
| 100 | 13.5 | 205 | 44.5 | | |

m/min = meters per minute
mL/kg/min = milliliters per kilogram per minute

Table developed using the metabolic calculations contained in *Guidelines for Exercise Testing and Exercise Prescription,* by the American College of Sports Medicine (Baltimore: Williams & Wilkins, 2006).

# Principles of Cardiorespiratory Exercise Prescription

Before proceeding with the principles of exercise prescription, you should ask yourself if you are willing to give exercise a try. A low percentage of the U.S. population is truly committed to exercise. Further, more than half of the people who start exercising drop out during the first 3 to 6 months of the program. Sports psychologists are trying to find out why some people exercise habitually and many do not. None of the benefits of exercise can help unless people commit to a lifetime program of physical activity. Lab 6D allows you to look at the implications of your results on your future health and well-being.

### Readiness for Exercise

The first step is to ask yourself: Am I ready to start an exercise program? The information provided in Lab 6C can help you answer this question. You are evaluated in four categories: mastery (self-control), attitude, health, and commitment. The higher you score in any category—mastery, for example—the more important that reason is for you to exercise.

Scores can vary from 4 to 16. A score of 12 or above is a strong indicator that the factor is important to you, whereas 8 or below is low. If you score 12 or more points in each category, your chances of initiating and sticking to an exercise program are good. If you do not score at least 12 points in each of any three categories, your chances of succeeding at exercise may be slim. You need to be better informed about the benefits of exercise, and a retraining process might be helpful to change core values regarding exercise. More tips on how you can become committed to exercise are provided in "Getting Started and Adhering to a Lifetime Exercise Program" (page 218).

Next you will have to decide positively that you will try. Using Lab 6C, you can list the advantages and disadvantages of incorporating exercise into your lifestyle. Your list might include advantages such as:

- It will make me feel better.
- I will lose weight.
- I will have more energy.
- It will lower my risk for chronic diseases.

Your list of disadvantages might include the following:

- I don't want to take the time.
- I'm too out of shape.
- There's no good place to exercise.
- I don't have the willpower to do it.

When your reasons for exercising outweigh your reasons for not exercising, you will find it easier to try. In Lab 6C you will also determine your stage of change for aerobic exercise. Using the information learned in Chapter 2, you can outline specific processes and techniques for change (also see the example in Chapter 9, page 343).

# Guidelines for Cardiorespiratory Exercise Prescription

In spite of the release of the U.S. Surgeon General's statement on physical activity and health more than a decade ago and the overwhelming evidence validating the benefits of exercise on health and longevity, only about 19 percent of adults in the United States meet minimum recommendations of the ACSM for the improvement and maintenance of cardiorespiratory fitness.[4]

Most people are not familiar with the basic principles of cardiorespiratory exercise prescription. Thus, although they exercise regularly, they do not reap significant improvements in cardiorespiratory endurance.

To develop the cardiorespiratory system, the heart muscle has to be overloaded like any other muscle in the human body. Just as the biceps muscle in the upper arm is developed through strength-training exercises, the heart muscle has to be exercised to increase in size, strength, and efficiency. To better understand how the cardiorespiratory system can be developed, you have to be familiar with the four **FITT** variables that govern exercise prescription: *f*requency, *i*ntensity, *t*ype (mode), and *t*ime (duration).[5]

First, however, you should be aware that the ACSM recommends that apparently healthy men over age 45 and women over age 55 get a diagnostic exercise stress test prior to **vigorous exercise**.[6] The ACSM has defined vigorous exercise as an exercise **intensity** above 60 percent of maximal capacity. For individuals initiating an exercise program, this intensity is the equivalent of exercise that provides a "substantial challenge" to the participant or one that cannot be maintained for 20 continuous minutes.

### Intensity of Exercise

When trying to develop the cardiorespiratory system, many people ignore intensity of exercise. For muscles to develop, they have to be overloaded to a given point. The training stimulus to develop the biceps muscle, for example, can be accomplished with arm curl-up exercises with increasing weights. Likewise, the cardiorespiratory system is stimulated by making the heart pump faster for a specified period.

Health and cardiorespiratory fitness benefits result when the person is working between 40 and 85 percent of **heart rate reserve (HRR)** combined with an appropriate duration and frequency of training (see how to calculate intensity, below).[7] Health benefits are achieved when training at a lower exercise intensity (40 to 60 percent) for a longer time. However, new research indicates that greater cardioprotective benefits and higher and faster improvements in cardiorespiratory fitness ($VO_{2max}$) are achieved primarily through vigorous-intensity programs.[8]

Most people who initiate exercise programs have a difficult time adhering to vigorous-intensity exercise. Thus, unconditioned individuals and older adults should start at a 40 to 50 percent training intensity (TI). Active and fit people can train at higher intensities. Increases in $VO_{2max}$ are accelerated when the heart is working closer to 85 percent of HRR. For this reason, after several weeks of progressive training at lower (40 to 50 percent) to moderate (50 to 60 percent) intensities, exercise can be performed between 60 and 85 percent TI.

Exercise training above 85 percent is recommended only for healthy, performance-oriented individuals and

**FIGURE 6.6** Recommended cardiorespiratory or aerobic training pattern.

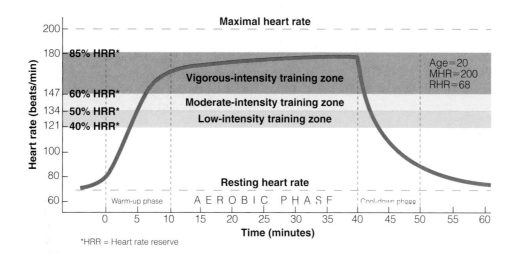

*HRR = Heart rate reserve

competitive athletes. For most people, training above 85 percent is discouraged to avoid potential cardiovascular problems associated with high-intensity exercise. As intensity increases, exercise adherence decreases and the risk of orthopedic injuries increases.

Intensity of exercise can be calculated easily, and training can be monitored by checking your pulse. To determine the intensity of exercise, or the **cardiorespiratory training zone**, according to HRR, follow these steps:

1. Estimate your maximal heart rate (MHR) using the following formula:

    MHR = 220 minus age (220 – age).

2. Check your resting heart rate (RHR) some time after you have been sitting quietly for 15 to 20 minutes. You may take your pulse for 30 seconds and multiply by 2, or take it for a full minute. As explained on page 202, you can check your pulse on the wrist by placing two or three fingers over the radial artery, or on the neck using the carotid artery.

3. Determine the HRR by subtracting the RHR from the MHR or:

    HRR = MHR – RHR.

4. Calculate the TI at 40, 50, 60, and 85 percent by multiplying HRR by .40, .50, .60, and .85, respectively, and then adding the RHR to each of these four figures (for example, 85% TI = HRR × .85 + RHR).

    Example. The 40, 50, 60, and 85 percent TIs for a 20-year-old with RHR of 68 bpm would be as follows:

MHR: 220 – 20 = 200 bpm

RHR: = 68 bpm

HRR: 200 – 68 = 132 bpm

40% TI = (132 × .40) + 68 = 121 bpm

50% TI = (132 × .50) + 68 = 134 bpm

60% TI = (132 × .60) + 68 = 147 bpm

85% TI = (132 × .85) + 68 = 180 bpm

Low-intensity cardiorespiratory training zone: 121 to 134 bpm

Moderate-intensity cardiorespiratory training zone: 134 to 147 bpm

Vigorous-intensity cardiorespiratory training zone: 147 to 180 bpm

To accelerate cardiorespiratory development, maintain your exercise heart rate between the 60 and 85 percent TIs (Figure 6.6). If you have been physically inactive, start at 40 to 50 percent intensity and gradually increase to 60 percent during the first 6 to 8 weeks of the exercise program. After that, you may exercise between 60 and 85 percent TI.

Following a few weeks of training, you may have a considerably lower resting heart rate (10 to 20 beats fewer in 8 to 12 weeks). Therefore, you should recompute your target zone periodically. You can compute your own cardiorespiratory training zone using Lab 6D, or you can use the

**FITT** An acronym used to describe the four cardiorespiratory exercise prescription variables: *f*requency, *i*ntensity, *t*ype (mode), and *t*ime (duration).

**Vigorous exercise** Cardiorespiratory exercise that requires an intensity level of approximately 70 percent of capacity.

**Intensity** In cardiorespiratory exercise, how hard a person has to exercise to improve or maintain fitness.

**Heart rate reserve (HRR)** The difference between maximal heart rate and resting heart rate.

**Cardiorespiratory training zone** Recommended training intensity range, in terms of exercise heart rate, to obtain adequate cardiorespiratory endurance development.

CengageNOW online resources available with this book to obtain a printout of your personalized cardiorespiratory exercise prescription (see Chapter 9, Figure 9.5). You also can use CengageNOW to create and regularly update an exercise log to keep a record of your activity program (see Chapter 9, Figure 9.6). Once you have reached an ideal level of cardiorespiratory endurance, frequent training in the 60 to 85 percent range will allow you to maintain your fitness level.

## Moderate- Versus Vigorous-Intensity Exercise

As fitness programs became popular in the 1970s, vigorous-intensity exercise (70 percent TI or above) was routinely prescribed for all fitness participants. Following extensive research in the late 1980s and 1990s, we learned that moderate-intensity physical activity (about 50 percent TI) provided many health benefits, including decreased risk for cardiovascular mortality—a statement endorsed by the U.S. Surgeon General in 1996.[9] Thus, the emphasis switched from vigorous- to moderate-intensity training in the late 1990s. In the 1996 report, the Surgeon General also stated that vigorous-intensity exercise would provide even greater benefits. Limited attention, however, has been paid to this recommendation since the publication of the report.

Vigorous-intensity programs yield higher improvements in $VO_{2max}$ than do moderate-intensity programs. And higher levels of aerobic fitness are associated with lower cardiovascular mortality, even when the duration of moderate-intensity activity is prolonged to match the energy expenditure performed during a shorter vigorous-intensity effort.[10] A recent review of several clinical studies substantiated that vigorous-intensity compared with moderate-intensity exercise leads to better improvements in coronary heart disease risk factors, including aerobic endurance, blood pressure, and blood glucose control.[11] As a result, the pendulum is again swinging toward vigorous intensity because of the added aerobic benefits, greater protection against disease, and larger energy expenditure that helps with weight management.

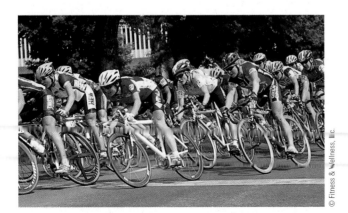

High-intensity exercise is required to achieve the high physical fitness standard ("excellent" category) for cardiorespiratory endurance.

**Monitoring Exercise Heart Rate** During the first few weeks of an exercise program, you should monitor your exercise heart rate regularly to make sure you are training in the proper zone. Wait until you are about 5 minutes into the aerobic phase of your exercise session before taking your first reading. When you check your heart rate, count your pulse for 10 seconds, then multiply by 6 to get the per minute pulse rate. The exercise heart rate will remain at the same level for about 15 seconds after you stop aerobic exercise, then drop rapidly. Do not hesitate to stop during your exercise bout to check your pulse. If the rate is too low, increase the intensity of exercise. If the rate is too high, slow down.

When determining the training intensity for your own program, you need to consider your personal fitness goals and possible cardiovascular risk factors. Individuals who exercise at around the 50 percent TI still reap significant health benefits—in particular, improvements in the metabolic profile (see "Health Fitness Standards" in Chapter 1, page 17). Training at this lower percentage, however, may place you in only the "average" (moderate fitness) category (see Table 6.8). Exercising at this lower intensity will not allow you to achieve a "good" or "excellent" cardiorespiratory endurance fitness rating (the physical fitness standard). The latter ratings are obtained by exercising closer to the 85 percent threshold.

**Rate of Perceived Exertion** Because many people do not check their heart rate during exercise, an alternative method of prescribing intensity of exercise has been devised using the **physical activity perceived exertion (H-PAPE) scale.** Using the scale in Figure 6.7, a person subjectively rates the perceived exertion or dif-

**FIGURE 6.7** Physical activity perceived exertion (H-PAPE) scale.

The H-PAPE (Hoeger-Physical Activity Perceived Exertion) Scale provides a subjective rating of the perceived exertion or difficulty of physical activity and exercise when training at a given intensity level. The intensity level is associated with the corresponding perceived exertion phrase provided. These phases are based on common terminology used in physical activity and exercise prescription guidelines.

| Perceived Exertion | Training Intensity |
| --- | --- |
| Low | 40% |
| Moderate | 50% |
| Somewhat hard | 60% |
| Vigorous | 70% |
| Hard | 80% |
| Very hard | 90% |
| All-out effort (10) | 100% |

***Source:*** Adapted from Werner W. K. Hoeger, "Training for a walkathon," *Diabetes Self-Management* 24(4) (2007): 56–68.

ficulty of exercise when training at different intensity levels. The exercise heart rate then is associated with the corresponding perceived exertion phrase.

For example, if training between 147 (60% TI) and 160 (70% TI) bpm, the person may associate this with training between "somewhat hard" and "vigorous." Some individuals perceive less exertion than others when training at a certain intensity level. Therefore, you have to associate your own inner perception of the task with the phrases given on the scale. You then may proceed to exercise at that rate of perceived exertion.

You must be sure to cross-check your target zone with your perceived exertion during the first weeks of your exercise program. To help you develop this association, you should regularly keep a record of your activities, using the form provided in Figure 6.10. After several weeks of training, you should be able to predict your exercise heart rate just by your own perceived exertion of the intensity of exercise.

Whether you monitor the intensity of exercise by checking your pulse or through the H-PAPE scale, you should be aware that changes in normal exercise conditions will affect the training intensity. For example, exercising on a hot, humid day or at high altitude increases the heart rate response to a given task, requiring adjustments in the intensity of your exercise.

## Mode of Exercise
The **mode,** or type, of exercise that develops the cardiorespiratory system has to be aerobic in nature. Once you have established your cardiorespiratory training zone, any activity or combination of activities that will get your heart rate up to that training zone and keep it there for as long as you exercise will give you adequate development. Examples of these activities are walking, jogging, stair climbing, elliptical activity, aerobics, swimming, water aerobics, cross-country skiing, rope skipping, cycling, racquetball, stair climbing, and stationary running or cycling.

Aerobic exercise has to involve the major muscle groups of the body, and it has to be rhythmic and continuous. As the amount of muscle mass involved during exercise increases, so do the demands on the cardiorespiratory system. The activity you choose should be based on your personal preferences, what you most enjoy doing, and your physical limitations. Low-impact activities greatly reduce the risk for injuries. Most injuries to beginners result from high-impact activities. Also, general strength conditioning (see Chapter 7) is also recommended prior to initiating an aerobic exercise program for individuals who have been inactive. Strength conditioning can significantly reduce the incidence of injuries.

The amount of strength or flexibility you develop through various activities differs. In terms of cardiorespiratory development, though, the heart doesn't know whether you are walking, swimming, or cycling. All the heart knows is that it has to pump at a certain rate, and as long as that rate is in the desired range, your cardiorespiratory fitness will improve. From a health fitness point

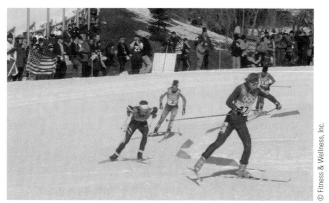

Cross-country skiing requires more oxygen and energy than most other aerobic activities.

of view, training in the lower end of the cardiorespiratory zone will yield optimal health benefits. The closer the heart rate is to the higher end of the cardiorespiratory training zone, however, the greater will be the improvements in $VO_{2max}$ (high physical fitness).

Because of the specificity of training, to ascertain changes in fitness, it is recommended that you use the same mode of exercise for training and testing. If your primary mode of training is cycling, it is recommended that you assess $VO_{2max}$ using a bicycle test. For joggers, a field or treadmill running test is best. Swimmers should use a swim test.

## Duration of Exercise
The general recommendation is that a person exercise between 20 and 60 minutes per session. For people who have been successful at losing a large amount of weight, however, up to 90 minutes of moderate-intensity activity daily may be required to prevent weight regain.

The duration of exercise is based on how intensely a person trains. The variables are inversely related. If the training is done at around 85 percent, a session of 20 to 30 minutes is sufficient. At about 50 percent intensity, the person should train between 30 and 60 minutes. As mentioned under "Intensity of Exercise" on page 210, unconditioned people and older adults should train at lower percentages, and therefore the activity should be carried out over a longer time.

Although the recommended guideline is 20 to 60 minutes of aerobic exercise per session, in the early stages of conditioning and for individuals who are pressed for time, accumulating 30 minutes or more of moderate-intensity aerobic physical activity throughout the day, in activity bouts of at least 10 minutes each, does provide health benefits. Three 10-minute exercise sessions per day (sepa-

---

**Physical Activity Perceived Exertion Scale (H-PAPE)** A perception scale to monitor or interpret the intensity of aerobic exercise.

**Mode** Form or type of exercise.

rated by at least 4 hours), at approximately 70 percent of maximal heart rate, have been shown to produce training benefits.[12] Although the increases in $VO_{2max}$ with the latter program were not as large (57 percent) as those found in a group performing a continuous 30-minute bout of exercise per day, the researchers concluded that moderate-intensity physical activity, conducted for 10 minutes three times per day, benefits the cardiorespiratory system significantly.

Results of this study are meaningful because people often mention lack of time as the reason they do not take part in an exercise program. Many think they have to exercise at least 20 continuous minutes to get any benefits at all. A duration of 20 to 30 vigorous-intensity minutes is ideal, but short, intermittent exercise bouts are beneficial to the cardiorespiratory system.

From a weight management point of view, the recommendation to prevent weight gain is for people to accumulate 60 minutes of moderate-intensity physical activity most days of the week,[13] whereas 60 to 90 minutes of daily moderate-intensity activity is necessary to prevent weight regain.[14] These recommendations are based on evidence that people who maintain healthy weight typically accumulate between 1 and 1½ hours of physical activity daily. The duration of exercise should be increased gradually to avoid undue fatigue and exercise-related injuries.

If lack of time is a concern, you should exercise at a vigorous intensity for 30 minutes, which can burn as many calories as 60 minutes of moderate intensity (also see "Low-Intensity Versus Vigorous-Intensity Exercise for Weight Loss" in Chapter 5, page 167), but only 19 percent of adults in the United States typically exercise at a high intensity level. Novice and overweight exercisers also need proper conditioning prior to vigorous-intensity exercise to avoid injuries or cardiovascular-related problems.

Exercise sessions always should be preceded by a 5- to 10-minute **warm-up** and be followed by a 10-minute **cool-down** period (see Figure 6.6). The purpose of the warm-up is to aid in the transition from rest to exercise. A good warm-up increases extensibility of the muscles and connective tissue, extends joint range of motion, and enhances muscular activity. A warm-up consists of general calisthenics, mild stretching exercises, and walking/jogging/cycling for a few minutes at a lower intensity than the actual target zone. The concluding phase of the warm-up is a gradual increase in exercise intensity to the lower end of the target training zone.

In the cool-down, the intensity of exercise is decreased gradually to help the body return to near resting levels, followed by stretching and relaxation activities. Stopping abruptly causes blood to pool in the exercised body parts, diminishing the return of blood to the heart. Less blood return can cause a sudden drop in blood pressure, with dizziness and faintness, or it can bring on cardiac abnormalities. The cool-down phase also helps dissipate body heat and aids in removing the lactic acid produced during high-intensity exercise.

## Behavior Modification Planning

### TIPS FOR PEOPLE WHO HAVE BEEN PHYSICALLY INACTIVE

❑ I PLAN TO  ❑ I DID IT

❑ ❑ Take the sensible approach by starting slowly.

❑ ❑ Begin by choosing moderate-intensity activities you enjoy the most. By choosing activities you enjoy, you'll be more likely to stick with them.

❑ ❑ Gradually build up the time spent exercising by adding a few minutes every few days or so until you can comfortably perform a minimum recommended amount of exercise (20 minutes per day).

❑ ❑ As the minimum amount becomes easier, gradually increase either the length of time exercising or increase the intensity of the activity, or both.

❑ ❑ Vary your activities, both for interest and to broaden the range of benefits.

❑ ❑ Explore new physical activities.

❑ ❑ Reward and acknowledge your efforts.

*Source:* Adapted from: Centers for Disease Control and Prevention, Atlanta, 2008.

### Try It

Fill out the cardiorespiratory exercise prescription in Lab 6D either in your text or online. In your Online Journal or class notebook, describe how well you implement the above suggestions.

**Frequency of Exercise** The recommended **frequency** for aerobic exercise is three to five days per week. Initially, only three weekly training sessions of 15 to 20 minutes are recommended, to avoid musculoskeletal injuries. You may then increase the frequency so that by the third week you are exercising four to five times per week for 20 minutes per session in the appropriate heart rate target zone (see Lab 6D and Figure 9.5 in Chapter 9). Thereafter, progressively continue to increase frequency, duration, and intensity of exercise until you have accomplished your goals.

When exercising at 60 to 85 percent of HRR, three 20- to 30-minute exercise sessions per week, on nonconsecutive days, are sufficient to improve (in the early stages) or maintain $VO_{2max}$. When training at lower intensities, exercising 30 to 60 minutes more than three days per week is required. If training is conducted more than five days a week, further improvements in $VO_{2max}$ are minimal. Although endurance athletes often train six or seven days per week (often twice per day), their training programs are designed to increase training mileage to endure long-distance races (6 to 100 miles) at a high percentage of $VO_{2max}$. These athletes often train at or above maximal steady state, also known as **anaerobic threshold**.

For individuals on a weight loss program, the recommendation is 60 to 90 minutes of low-intensity to moderate-intensity activity on most days of the week. Longer exercise sessions increase caloric expenditure for faster weight reduction (see Chapter 5, "Exercise: The Key to Weight Management," page 165).

Although three exercise sessions per week will maintain cardiorespiratory fitness, the importance of regular physical activity in preventing disease and enhancing quality of life has been pointed out clearly by the ACSM, the U.S. Centers for Disease Control and Prevention, and the President's Council on Physical Fitness and Sports.[15] These organizations, along with the U.S. Surgeon General, advocate at least 30 minutes of moderate-intensity physical activity at least five days per week. This routine has been promoted as an effective way to improve health and quality of life. Further, the Surgeon General states that no one, including older adults, is too old to enjoy the benefits of regular physical activity.

If you want to enjoy better health and fitness, physical activity must be pursued regularly. According to Dr. William Haskell of Stanford University: "Most of the health-related benefits of exercise are relatively short-term, so people should think of exercise as medication and take it on a daily basis."[16] Many of the benefits of exercise and activity diminish within 2 weeks of substantially decreased physical activity. These benefits are completely lost within 2 to 8 months of inactivity.[17]

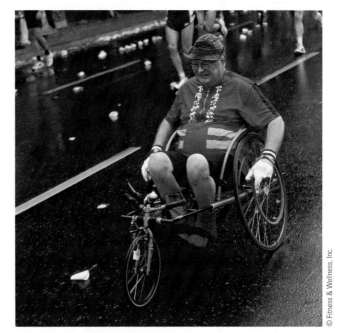

Physically challenged people can participate in and derive health and fitness benefits from a high-intensity exercise program.

To sum up: Ideally, a person should engage in physical activity six or seven times per week. Based on the previous discussion, to reap both the high fitness and health fitness benefits of exercise, a person should do vigorous exercise a minimum of three times per week for high fitness maintenance, and three or four additional times per week in moderate-intensity activities to maintain good health. Depending on the intensity of the activity and the health/fitness goals, all exercise sessions should last between 20 and 60 minutes. For adequate weight management purposes, additional daily physical activity, up to 90 minutes, may be necessary. A summary of the cardiorespiratory exercise prescription guidelines according to the ACSM is provided in Figure 6.8. Comprehensive guidelines for weekly physical activity are also provided in Figure 6.9.

---

**FIGURE 6.8** Cardiorespiratory exercise prescription guidelines.

| | |
|---|---|
| **Activity:** | Aerobic (examples: walking, jogging, cycling, swimming, aerobics, racquetball, soccer, stair climbing) |
| **Intensity:** | 40/50%–85% of heart rate reserve |
| **Duration:** | 20–60 minutes of continuous aerobic activity |
| **Frequency:** | 3 to 5 days per week |

*Source:* American College of Sports Medicine, *ACSM's Guidelines for Exercise Testing and Prescription* (Philadelphia: Lippincott Williams & Wilkins, 2006).

**Warm-up** Starting a workout slowly.

**Cool-down** Tapering off an exercise session slowly.

**Frequency** Number of times per week a person engages in exercise.

**Anaerobic threshold** The highest percentage of the $VO_{2max}$ at which an individual can exercise (maximal steady state) for an extended time without accumulating significant amounts of lactic acid (accumulation of lactic acid forces an individual to slow down the exercise intensity or stop altogether).

**FIGURE 6.9** The Physical Activity Pyramid

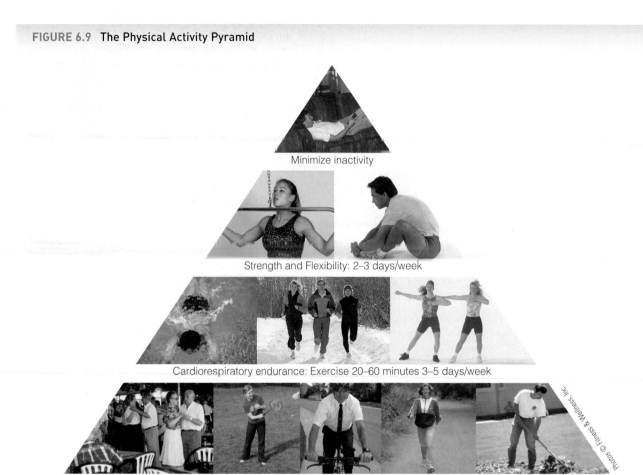

Minimize inactivity

Strength and Flexibility: 2–3 days/week

Cardiorespiratory endurance: Exercise 20–60 minutes 3–5 days/week

Physical activity: Accumulate 60 to 90 minutes of moderate-intensity activity nearly every day.

# Fitness Benefits of Aerobic Activities

The contributions of different aerobic activities to the health-related components of fitness vary. Although an accurate assessment of the contributions to each fitness component is difficult to establish, a summary of likely benefits of several activities is provided in Table 6.10. Instead of a single rating or number, ranges are given for some of the categories. The benefits derived are based on the person's effort while participating in the activity.

The nature of the activity often dictates the potential aerobic development. For example, jogging is much more strenuous than walking. The effort during exercise also affects the amount of physiological development. During a low-impact aerobics routine, accentuating all movements (instead of just going through the motions) increases training benefits by orders of magnitude.

Table 6.10 indicates a starting fitness level for each aerobic activity. Attempting to participate in high-intensity activities without proper conditioning often leads to injuries, not to mention discouragement. Beginners should start with low-intensity activities that carry a minimum risk for injuries.

In some cases, such as high-impact aerobics and rope skipping, the risk for orthopedic injuries remains high even if the participants are adequately conditioned. These activities should be supplemental only and are not recommended as the sole mode of exercise. Most exercise-related injuries occur as a result of high-impact activities, not high intensity of exercise.

Physicians who work with cardiac patients frequently use metabolic equivalents (**METs**) as an alternative method of prescribing exercise intensity. One MET represents the rate of energy expenditure at rest, that is, 3.5 mL/kg/min. METs are used to measure the intensity of physical activity and exercise in multiples of the resting metabolic rate. At an intensity level of 10 METs, the activity requires a tenfold increase in the resting energy requirement (or approximately 35 mL/kg/min). MET levels for a given activity vary according to the effort expended. The MET range for various activities is included in Table 6.10. The harder a person exercises, the higher is the MET level.

The effectiveness of various aerobic activities in weight management is charted in Table 6.10. As a general rule, the greater the muscle mass involved in exercise, the better the results. Rhythmic and continuous activities that involve large amounts of muscle mass are most effective in burning calories.

Higher-intensity activities increase caloric expenditure as well. Exercising longer, however, compensates for lower

**TABLE 6.10** Ratings for Selected Aerobic Activities

| Activity | Recommended Starting Fitness Level[1] | Injury Risk[2] | Potential Cardiorespiratory Endurance Development ($VO_{2max}$)[3.5] | Upper Body Strength Development[3] | Lower Body Strength Development[3] | Upper Body Flexibility Development[3] | Lower Body Flexibility Development[3] | Weight Control[3] | MET Level[4,5,6] | Caloric Expenditure (cal/hour)[5,6] |
|---|---|---|---|---|---|---|---|---|---|---|
| Aerobics | | | | | | | | | | |
| High-Impact Aerobics | A | H | 3–4 | 2 | 4 | 3 | 2 | 4 | 6–12 | 450–900 |
| Moderate-Impact Aerobics | I | M | 2–4 | 2 | 3 | 3 | 2 | 3 | 6–12 | 450–900 |
| Low-Impact Aerobics | B | L | 2–4 | 2 | 3 | 3 | 2 | 3 | 5–10 | 375–750 |
| Step Aerobics | I | M | 2–4 | 2 | 3–4 | 3 | 2 | 3–4 | 5–12 | 375–900 |
| Cross-Country Skiing | B | M | 4–5 | 4 | 4 | 2 | 2 | 4–5 | 10–16 | 750–1,200 |
| Cross-Training | I | M | 3–5 | 2–3 | 3–4 | 2–3 | 1–2 | 3–5 | 6–15 | 450–1,125 |
| Cycling | | | | | | | | | | |
| Road | I | M | 2–5 | 1 | 4 | 1 | 1 | 3 | 6–12 | 450–900 |
| Stationary | B | L | 2–4 | 1 | 4 | 1 | 1 | 3 | 6–10 | 450–750 |
| Hiking | B | L | 2–4 | 1 | 3 | 1 | 1 | 3 | 6–10 | 450–750 |
| In-Line Skating | I | M | 1–4 | 2 | 4 | 2 | 2 | 3 | 6–10 | 450–750 |
| Jogging | I | M | 3–5 | 1 | 3 | 1 | 1 | 5 | 6–15 | 450–1,125 |
| Jogging, Deep Water | A | L | 3–5 | 2 | 2 | 1 | 1 | 5 | 8–15 | 600–1,125 |
| Racquet Sports | I | M | 2–4 | 3 | 3 | 3 | 2 | 3 | 6–10 | 450–750 |
| Rope Skipping | I | H | 3–5 | 2 | 4 | 1 | 2 | 3–5 | 8–15 | 600–1,125 |
| Rowing | B | L | 3–5 | 4 | 2 | 3 | 1 | 4 | 8–14 | 600–1,050 |
| Spinning | I | L | 4–5 | 1 | 4 | 1 | 1 | 4 | 8–15 | 600–1,125 |
| Stair Climbing | B | L | 3–5 | 1 | 4 | 1 | 1 | 4–5 | 8–15 | 600–1,125 |
| Swimming (front crawl) | B | L | 3–5 | 4 | 2 | 3 | 1 | 3 | 6–12 | 450–900 |
| Walking | B | L | 1–2 | 1 | 2 | 1 | 1 | 3 | 4–6 | 300–450 |
| Walking, Water, Chest-Deep | I | L | 2–4 | 2 | 3 | 1 | 1 | 3 | 6–10 | 450–750 |
| Water Aerobics | B | L | 2–4 | 3 | 3 | 3 | 2 | 3 | 6–12 | 450–900 |

[1]B = Beginner, I = Intermediate, A = Advanced
[2]L = Low, M = Moderate, H = High
[3]1 = Low, 2 = Fair, 3 = Average, 4 = Good, 5 = Excellent
[4]One MET represents the rate of energy expenditure at rest (3.5 ml/kg/min). Each additional MET is a multiple of the resting value. For example, 5 METs represents an energy expenditure equivalent to five times the resting value, or about 17.5 ml/kg/min.
[5]Varies according to the person's effort (intensity) during exercise.
[6]Varies according to body weight.

intensities. If carried out long enough (45 to 60 minutes five or six times per week), even walking is a good exercise mode for weight management. Additional information on a comprehensive weight management program is given in Chapter 5.

**MET** Short for metabolic equivalent, the rate of energy expenditure at rest; 1 MET is the equivalent of a $VO_2$ of 3.5 mL/kg/min.

## Behavior Modification Planning

### TIPS TO ENHANCE EXERCISE COMPLIANCE

☐ I PLAN TO ☐ I DID IT

☐ ☐ 1. Set aside a regular time for exercise. If you don't plan ahead, it is a lot easier to skip. On a weekly basis, using red ink, schedule your exercise time into your day planner. Next, hold your exercise hour "sacred." Give exercise priority equal to the most important school or business activity of the day.

If you are too busy, attempt to accumulate 30 to 60 minutes of daily activity by doing separate 10-minute sessions throughout the day. Try reading the mail while you walk, taking stairs instead of elevators, walking the dog, or riding the stationary bike as you watch the evening news.

☐ ☐ 2. Exercise early in the day, when you will be less tired and the chances of something interfering with your workout are minimal; thus, you will be less likely to skip your exercise session.

☐ ☐ 3. Select aerobic activities you enjoy. Exercise should be as much fun as your favorite hobby. If you pick an activity you don't enjoy, you will be unmotivated and less likely to keep exercising. Don't be afraid to try out a new activity, even if that means learning new skills.

☐ ☐ 4. Combine different activities. You can train by doing two or three different activities the same week. This cross-training may reduce the monotony of repeating the same activity every day. Try lifetime sports. Many endurance sports, such as racquetball, basketball, soccer, badminton, roller skating, cross-country skiing, and body surfing (paddling the board), provide a nice break from regular workouts.

☐ ☐ 5. Use the proper clothing and equipment for exercise. A poor pair of shoes, for example, can make you more prone to injury, discouraging you from the beginning.

☐ ☐ 6. Find a friend or group of friends to exercise with. Social interaction will make exercise more fulfilling. Besides, exercise is harder to skip if someone is waiting to go with you.

☐ ☐ 7. Set goals and share them with others. Quitting is tougher when someone else knows what you are trying to accom-

### Critical Thinking

Mary started an exercise program last year as a means to lose weight and enhance her body image. She now runs more than 6 miles every day, works out regularly on stairclimbers and elliptical machines, strength trains daily, participates in step aerobics three times per week, and plays tennis or racquetball twice a week. Evaluate her program and make suggestions for improvements.

# Getting Started and Adhering to a Lifetime Exercise Program

Following the guidelines provided in Lab 6D, you may proceed to initiate your own cardiorespiratory endurance program. If you have not been exercising regularly, you might begin by attempting to train five or six times a week for 30 minutes at a time. You might find this discouraging, however, and drop out before getting too far, because you will probably develop some muscle soreness and stiffness and possibly incur minor injuries. Muscle plish. When you reach a targeted goal, reward yourself with a new pair of shoes or a jogging suit.

❑ ❑ 8. Purchase a pedometer (step counter) and build up to 10,000 steps per day. These 10,000 steps may include all forms of daily physical activity combined. Pedometers motivate people toward activity because they track daily activity, provide feedback on activity level, and remind the participant to enhance daily activity.

❑ ❑ 9. Don't become a chronic exerciser. Over-exercising can lead to chronic fatigue and injuries. Exercise should be enjoyable, and in the process you should stop and smell the roses.

❑ ❑ 10. Exercise in different places and facilities. This will add variety to your workouts.

❑ ❑ 11. Exercise to music. People who listen to fast-tempo music tend to exercise more vigorously and longer. Using headphones when exercising outdoors, however, can be dangerous. Even indoors, it is preferable not to use headphones so you still can be aware of your surroundings.

❑ ❑ 12. Keep a regular record of your activities. Keeping a record allows you to monitor your progress and compare it against previous months and years (see Figure 6.10, page 220).

❑ ❑ 13. Conduct periodic assessments. Improving to a higher fitness category is often a reward in itself, and creating your own rewards is even more motivating.

❑ ❑ 14. Listen to your body. If you experience pain or unusual discomfort, stop exercising. Pain and aches are an indication of potential injury. If you do suffer an injury, don't return to your regular workouts until you are fully recovered. You may cross train using activities that don't aggravate your injury (for instance, swimming instead of jogging).

❑ ❑ 15. If a health problem arises, see a physician. When in doubt, it's better to be safe than sorry.

## Try It

The most difficult challenge about exercise is to keep going once you start. The above behavioral change tips will enhance your chances for exercise adherence. In your Online Journal or class notebook, describe which suggestions were most useful

soreness and stiffness and the risk for injuries can be lessened or eliminated by increasing the intensity, duration, and frequency of exercise progressively, as outlined in Lab 6D.

Once you have determined your exercise prescription, the difficult part begins: starting and sticking to a lifetime exercise program. Although you may be motivated after reading about the benefits to be gained from physical activity, lifelong dedication and perseverance are necessary to reap and maintain good fitness.

The first few weeks probably will be the most difficult for you, but where there's a will, there's a way. Once you begin to see positive changes, it won't be as hard. Soon you will develop a habit of exercising that will be deeply satisfying and will bring about a sense of self-accomplishment.

The suggestions provided in the accompanying Behavior Modification Planning box have been used successfully to help change behavior and adhere to a lifetime exercise program.

**A Lifetime Commitment to Fitness** The benefits of fitness can be maintained only through a regular lifetime program. Exercise is not like putting money in the bank. It doesn't help much to exercise 4 or 5 hours on Saturday and not do anything else the rest of the week. If anything, exercising only once a week is not safe for unconditioned adults.

The time involved in losing the benefits of exercise varies among the different components of physical fitness and also depends on the person's condition before the interrup-

**FIGURE 6.10** Cardiorespiratory exercise record form.

Name: _____   Date: _____   Course: _____   Section: _____   Gender: _____   Age: _____

Month [ ]

| Date | Body Weight | Exercise Heart Rate | Type of Activity | Distance in Miles | Time Minutes | H-PAPE* | Daily Steps |
|------|-------------|---------------------|------------------|-------------------|--------------|---------|-------------|
| 1 | | | | | | | |
| 2 | | | | | | | |
| 3 | | | | | | | |
| 4 | | | | | | | |
| 5 | | | | | | | |
| 6 | | | | | | | |
| 7 | | | | | | | |
| 8 | | | | | | | |
| 9 | | | | | | | |
| 10 | | | | | | | |
| 11 | | | | | | | |
| 12 | | | | | | | |
| 13 | | | | | | | |
| 14 | | | | | | | |
| 15 | | | | | | | |
| 16 | | | | | | | |
| 17 | | | | | | | |
| 18 | | | | | | | |
| 19 | | | | | | | |
| 20 | | | | | | | |
| 21 | | | | | | | |
| 22 | | | | | | | |
| 23 | | | | | | | |
| 24 | | | | | | | |
| 25 | | | | | | | |
| 26 | | | | | | | |
| 27 | | | | | | | |
| 28 | | | | | | | |
| 29 | | | | | | | |
| 30 | | | | | | | |
| 31 | | | | | | | |
| Total | | | | | | | |

*Physical activity perceived exertion.

Month [ ]

| Date | Body Weight | Exercise Heart Rate | Type of Activity | Distance in Miles | Time Minutes | H-PAPE* | Daily Steps |
|------|-------------|---------------------|------------------|-------------------|--------------|---------|-------------|
| 1 | | | | | | | |
| 2 | | | | | | | |
| 3 | | | | | | | |
| 4 | | | | | | | |
| 5 | | | | | | | |
| 6 | | | | | | | |
| 7 | | | | | | | |
| 8 | | | | | | | |
| 9 | | | | | | | |
| 10 | | | | | | | |
| 11 | | | | | | | |
| 12 | | | | | | | |
| 13 | | | | | | | |
| 14 | | | | | | | |
| 15 | | | | | | | |
| 16 | | | | | | | |
| 17 | | | | | | | |
| 18 | | | | | | | |
| 19 | | | | | | | |
| 20 | | | | | | | |
| 21 | | | | | | | |
| 22 | | | | | | | |
| 23 | | | | | | | |
| 24 | | | | | | | |
| 25 | | | | | | | |
| 26 | | | | | | | |
| 27 | | | | | | | |
| 28 | | | | | | | |
| 29 | | | | | | | |
| 30 | | | | | | | |
| 31 | | | | | | | |
| Total | | | | | | | |

*Rate of perceived exertion.

tion. In regard to cardiorespiratory endurance, it has been estimated that 4 weeks of aerobic training are completely reversed in 2 consecutive weeks of physical inactivity. But if you have been exercising regularly for months or years, 2 weeks of inactivity won't hurt you as much as it will someone who has exercised only a few weeks. As a rule, after 48 to 72 hours of aerobic inactivity, the cardiorespiratory system starts to lose some of its capacity.

To maintain fitness, you should keep up a regular exercise program, even during vacations. If you have to inter-rupt your program for reasons beyond your control, you should not attempt to resume training at the same level you left off but, rather, build up gradually again.

Even the greatest athletes on earth, if they were to stop exercising, would be, after just a few years, at about the same risk for disease as someone who has never done any physical activity. Staying with a physical fitness program long enough brings about positive physiological and psychological changes. Once you are there, you will not want to have it any other way.

## ASSESS YOUR BEHAVIOR

 Log on to http://www.cengage.com/sso/ to update your exercise log to include all your physical activity (climbing stairs, walking around campus, etc.). Be sure to update your pedometer log as well.

1. Do you consciously attempt to incorporate as much physical activity as possible in your daily living (walk, take stairs, cycle, participate in sports and recreational activities)?

2. Are you accumulating at least 30 minutes of moderate-intensity physical activity a minimum of five days per week?

3. Is aerobic exercise in the appropriate target zone a priority in your life a minimum of three times per week for at least 20 minutes per exercise session?

4. Do you own a pedometer and do you accumulate 10,000 or more steps on most days of the week?

5. Have you evaluated your aerobic fitness and do you meet at least the health fitness category?

## ASSESS YOUR KNOWLEDGE

 Log on to http://www.cengage.com/sso/ to assess your understanding of this chapter's topics by taking the Student Practice Test and exploring the modules recommended in your Personalized Study Plan.

1. Cardiorespiratory endurance is determined by
   a. the amount of oxygen the body is able to utilize per minute of physical activity.
   b. the length of time it takes the heart rate to return to 120 bpm following the 1.5-Mile Run Test.
   c. the difference between the maximal heart rate and the resting heart rate.
   d. the product of the heart rate and blood pressure at rest versus exercise.
   e. the time it takes a person to reach a heart rate between 120 and 170 bpm during the Astrand-Rhyming test.

2. Which of the following is *not* a benefit of aerobic training?
   a. A higher $VO_{2max}$
   b. An increase in red blood cell count
   c. A decrease in resting heart rate
   d. An increase in heart rate at a given workload
   e. An increase in functional capillaries

3. The oxygen uptake for a person with an exercise heart rate of 130, a stroke volume of 100, and an a-vO2$_{diff}$ of 10 is
   a. 130,000 mL/kg/min.
   b. 1,300 L/min.
   c. 1.3 L/min.
   d. 130 mL/kg/min.
   e. 13 mL/kg/min.

4. The oxygen uptake, in mL/kg/min, for a person with a $VO_2$ of 2.0 L/min who weighs 60 kilograms is
   a. 120.
   b. 26.5.
   c. 33.3.
   d. 30.
   e. 120,000.

5. The Step Test estimates $VO_{2max}$ according to
   a. how long a person is able to sustain the proper Step Test cadence.
   b. the lowest heart rate achieved during the test.
   c. the recovery heart rate following the test.
   d. the difference between the maximal heart rate achieved and the resting heart rate.
   e. the exercise heart rate and the total stepping time.

6. An "excellent" cardiorespiratory fitness rating, in mL/kg/min, for young male adults is about
   a. 10.
   b. 20.
   c. 30.
   d. 40.
   e. 50.

7. How many minutes would a person training at 2 L/min have to exercise to burn the equivalent of one pound of fat?
   a. 700
   b. 350
   c. 120
   d. 60
   e. 20

8. The high-intensity cardiorespiratory training zone for a 22-year-old individual with a resting heart rate of 68 bpm is
   a. 120 to 148.
   b. 132 to 156.
   c. 138 to 164.
   d. 146 to 179.
   e. 154 to 188.

9. Which of the following activities does *not* contribute to the development of cardiorespiratory endurance?
   a. Low-impact aerobics
   b. Jogging
   c. 400-yard dash
   d. Racquetball
   e. All of these activities contribute to its development.

10. The recommended duration for each cardiorespiratory training session is
    a. 10 to 20 minutes.
    b. 15 to 30 minutes.
    c. 20 to 60 minutes.
    d. 45 to 70 minutes.
    e. 60 to 120 minutes.

Correct answers can be found at the back of the book.

# MEDIA MENU

You can find the links below at the book companion site: www.cengage.com/health/hoeger/plfw10e

- Chronicle your daily activities using the exercise log.
- Determine your readiness to exercise.
- Check how well you understand the chapter's concepts.

## Internet Connections

- FitFacts. This site features information about a variety of cardiovascular forms of exercise, including walking, running, jumping rope, swimming, spinning, cross-training, interval training, and others. *http://www.acefitness.org/default.aspx*

- Fitness Fundamentals: Guidelines for Personal Exercise Programs. This site, developed by the President's Council on Physical Fitness and Sports, features information about starting an exercise program, including tips on how to select the right kinds of exercise to improve cardiovascular health, flexibility, and muscle strength and endurance. *http://www.hoptechno.com/book11.htm*

- Exercise Physiology: The Methods and Mechanisms Underlying Performance. This site features information on the principles of training, gender differences in performance and training, cardiovascular benefits, and much more. *http://home.hia.no/~stephens/exphys.htm*

- Check Your Physical Activity and Heart IQ. This site, sponsored by the National Heart, Lung, and Blood Institute, provides a true/false quiz to allow you to assess what you know about how physical activity affects your heart. The answers provided will uncover exercise myths and give you information on ways to improve your heart health. *http://www.nhlbi.nih.gov/health/public/heart/obesity/pa_iq_ab.htm*

# NOTES

1. H. Atkinson, "Exercise for Longer Life: The Physician's Perspective," *HealthNews* 7:3 (1997), 3.

2. R. B. O'Hara, et al., "Increased Volume Resistance Training: Effects upon Predicted Aerobic Fitness in a Select Group of Air Force Men," *ACSM's Health & Fitness Journal* 8, no. 4 (2004): 16–25.

3. American College of Sports Medicine, *ACSM's Guidelines for Exercise Testing and Prescription* (Philadelphia: Lippincott Williams & Wilkins, 2006).

4. U.S. Department of Health and Human Services, Centers for Disease Control and Prevention, National Center for Health Statistics, *Physical Activity Among Adults: United States, 2000*, no. 15 (May 14, 2003).

5. American College of Sports Medicine, "Position Stand: The Recommended Quantity and Quality of Exercise for Developing and Maintaining Cardiorespiratory, Muscular Fitness, and Flexibility in Healthy Adults," *Medicine and Science in Sports and Exercise* 30 (1998): 975–991.

6. See note 3.

7. See note 3.

8. S. E. Gormley, et al., "Effect of Intensity of Aerobic Training on $VO_{2max}$," *Medicine and Science in Sports and Exercise* 40 (2008): 1336–1343.

9. U.S. Department of Health and Human Services, *Physical Activity and Health: A Report of the Surgeon General* (Atlanta: Centers for Disease Control and Prevention, National Center for Chronic Disease Prevention and Health Promotion, 1996).

10. D. P. Swain, "Moderate- or Vigorous-Intensity Exercise: What Should We Prescribe?" *ACSM's Health & Fitness Journal* 10, no. 5 (2006): 7–11.

11. D. P. Swain and B. A. Franklin, "Comparative Cardioprotective Benefits of Vigorous vs. Moderate Intensity Aerobic Exercise," *American Journal of Cardiology* 97, no. 1 (2006): 141–147.

12. R. F. DeBusk, U. Stenestrand, M. Sheehan, and W. L. Haskell, "Training Effects of Long Versus Short Bouts of Exercise in Healthy Subjects," *American Journal of Cardiology* 65 (1990): 1010–1013.

13. National Academy of Sciences, Institute of Medicine, *Dietary Reference Intakes for Energy, Carbohydrates, Fiber, Fat, Protein and Amino Acids (Macronutrients).* (Washington, DC: National Academy Press, 2002).

14. U.S. Department of Health and Human Services, Department of Agriculture, *Dietary Guidelines for Americans 2005* (Washington, DC: DHHS, 2005).

15. "Summary Statement: Workshop on Physical Activity and Public Health," *Sports Medicine Bulletin* 28 (1993): 7.

16. "Scanning Sports," *Physician and Sportsmedicine* 21, no. 11 (1993): 34.

17. See note 3.

# SUGGESTED READINGS

*ACSM's Guidelines for Exercise Testing and Prescription* (Philadelphia: Lippincott Williams & Wilkins, 2006).

*ACSM's Resource Manual for Guidelines for Exercise Testing and Prescription* (Philadelphia: Lippincott Williams & Wilkins, 2006).

Akalan, C., L. Kravitz, and R. Robergs. "VO$_{2max}$: Essentials of the Most Widely Used Test in Exercise Physiology." *ACSM's Health & Fitness Journal* 8, no. 3 (2004): 5–9.

Hoeger, W. W. K., and S. A. Hoeger. *Lifetime Fitness & Wellness: A Personalized Program* (Belmont, CA: Wadsworth/Thomson Learning, 2009).

Karvonen, M. J., E. Kentala, and O. Mustala. "The Effects of Training on the Heart Rate, a Longitudinal Study." *Annales Medicinae Experimetalis et Biologiae Fenniae* 35 (1957): 307–315.

McArdle, W. D., F. I. Katch, and V. L. Katch. *Exercise Physiology: Energy, Nutrition, and Human Performance* (Philadelphia: Lippincott Williams & Wilkins, 2007).

Nieman, D. C. *Exercise Testing and Prescription: A Health-Related Approach* (Boston: McGraw-Hill, 2003).

Wilmore, J. H., and D. L. Costill. *Physiology of Sport and Exercise* (Champaign, IL: Human Kinetics, 2008).

# LAB 6A: Cardiorespiratory Endurance Assessment

Name _____  Date _____  Grade _____

Instructor _____  Course _____  Section _____

### Necessary Lab Equipment

**1.5-Mile Run:** School track or premeasured course and a stopwatch.

**1.0-Mile Walk Test:** School track or premeasured course and a stopwatch.

Step Test: A bench or gymnasium bleachers 16¼ inches high, a metronome, and a stopwatch.

Astrand–Rhyming Test: A bicycle ergometer that allows for regulation of workloads in kilopounds per meter (or watts) and a stopwatch.

12-Minute Swim Test: Swimming pool and a stopwatch.

### Objective

To estimate maximal oxygen uptake ($VO_{2max}$) and cardiorespiratory endurance classification.

### Lab Preparation

Wear appropriate exercise clothing including jogging shoes and a swimsuit if required. Be prepared to take the 1.0-Mile Walk Test, the Step Test, the Astrand–Rhyming Test, the 1.5-Mile Run Test, and/or the 12-Minute Swim Test. If more than one test will be conducted, perform them in the order just listed and allow at least 15 minutes between tests. Avoid vigorous physical activity 24 hours prior to this lab.

I. **1.5-Mile Run Test**

1.5-Mile Run Time: _____ min and _____ sec    $VO_{2max}$ (see Table 6.2, page 203): _____ mL/kg/min

Cardiorespiratory Fitness Category (Table 6.8, page 208): _____

II. **1.0-Mile Walk Test**

Weight (W) = _____ lbs    Gender (G) = _____ (female = 0, male = 1)    Time = _____ min and _____ sec

Heart Rate (HR) = _____ bpm

Time in minutes (T) = min + (sec ÷ 60) or T = _____ + (_____ ÷ 60) = _____ min

$VO_{2max}$ = 88.768 − (0.0957 × W) + (8.892 × G) − (1.4537 × T) − (0.1194 × HR)

$VO_{2max}$ = 88.768 − (0.0957 × _____) + (8.892 × _____) − (1.4537 × _____) − (0.1194 × _____)

$VO_{2max}$ = 88.768 − (_____) + (_____) − (_____) − (_____) = _____ mL/kg/min

Cardiorespiratory Fitness Category (Table 6.8, page 208): _____

III. **Step Test**

15-second recovery heart rate: _____ beats    $VO_{2max}$ (Table 6.3, page 205): _____ mL/kg/min

Cardiorespiratory Fitness Category (Table 6.8, page 208): _____

## IV. Astrand–Rhyming Test

Weight (W) = _____ lbs    Weight (BW) in kilograms = (W ÷ 2.2046) = _____ kg    Workload = _____ kpm

| Exercise Heart Rates | Time to count 30 beats | Heart Rate (bpm) (from Table 6.4, page 206) | | Time to count 30 beats | Heart Rate (bpm) (from Table 6.4, page 206) |
|---|---|---|---|---|---|
| First minute: | | | Fourth minute: | | |
| Second minute: | | | Fifth minute: | | |
| Third minute: | | | Sixth minute: | | |

Average heart rate for the fifth and sixth minutes = _____ bpm

$VO_{2max}$ in L/min (Table 6.5, page 207) = _____ L min    Correction factor (from Table 6.6, page 208) = _____

Corrected $VO_{2max}$ = $VO_{2max}$ in L/min × correction factor = _____ × _____ – _____ L/min

$VO_{2max}$ in mL/kg/min = corrected $VO_{2max}$ in L/min × 1000 ÷ BW in kg = \_\_\_\_ × 1000 ÷ \_\_\_\_ = \_\_\_\_ mL/kg/min

Cardiorespiratory Fitness Category (Table 6.8, page 208): _____

## V. 12-Minute Swim Test

Distance swum in 12 minutes: _____ yards

Cardiorespiratory Fitness Category (Table 6.7, page 208): _____

## VI. What I Learned and Where I Go From Here:

1. Interpret the results of your cardiorespiratory endurance test(s). Indicate the cardiorespiratory fitness classification you would like to achieve by the end of the term and explain how you are planning to achieve this goal.

_____

_____

_____

_____

_____

_____

_____

2. Briefly discuss the advantages and disadvantages of the cardiorespiratory endurance tests used in this lab.

_____

_____

_____

_____

_____

_____

_____

# LAB 6B: Caloric Expenditure and Exercise Heart Rate

Name _____  Date _____  Grade _____

Instructor _____  Course _____  Section _____

### Necessary Lab Equipment

A school track (or premeasured course) and a stopwatch. Each student also should bring a watch with a second hand.

### Objective

To monitor exercise heart rate and determine the caloric cost of physical activity based on exercise heart rate.

### Lab Preparation

Wear exercise clothing, including jogging shoes. Do not engage in vigorous physical activity prior to this lab. Read the information on predicting oxygen uptake and caloric expenditure in this chapter, pages 207–209.

### Procedure

1. **Cardiorespiratory Training Zone.** Look up your cardiovascular training zone at 60 percent and 85 percent of heart rate reserve in Lab 6D. Record this information in beats per minute (bpm) and in 10-second pulse counts in the blank spaces provided below.

|  | | **Beats/minute** | **10-sec count** |
|---|---|---|---|
| 60% intensity | = | | |
| 85% intensity | = | | |

2. **Resting Heart Rate (HR) and Body Weight (BW).** Determine your resting HR prior to exercise and your body weight in kilograms (divide pounds by 2.2046).

   Resting HR: _____ bpm

   BW: _____ lbs ÷ 2.2046 = _____ kg

3. **Walking HR, Oxygen Uptake (VO$_2$), and Caloric Expenditure.** Walk two laps around a 400-meter (440-yard) track at an average speed of 75 to 100 meters per minute. Try to maintain a constant speed around the track. You can monitor your speed by starting the walk at the beginning of the 100-meter straightway and making sure you have walked at least 75 meters and no more than 100 meters in one minute. As soon as you complete the two laps (800 meters), notice the time required to walk this distance and immediately check your exercise HR by taking a 10-second pulse count. Record this information in the spaces provided below. Do not record the time until after you have checked your pulse. Exercise HR will remain at the same rate for about 15 seconds following cessation of exercise. Therefore, you need to check your pulse as soon as you finish the walk, after noticing the 800-meter walk time.

   10-sec. pulse count: _____ beats (from question 1 above)

   800-meter time: _____ min _____ sec

   HR in bpm = 10-sec pulse count × 6

   HR in bpm = _____ × 6 = _____ bpm

   800-meter time in minutes = min + (sec ÷ 60)

   800-meter time in minutes = _____ + (_____ ÷ 60) = _____ min

   Speed in meters per minute (mts/min) = 800 ÷ 800-meter time in min

   Speed in mts/min = 800 ÷ _____ = _____ mts/min

$VO_2$ in mL/kg/min at this walking speed (Use Table 6.9, page 209) = _____ mL/kg/min

$VO_2$ in L/min = $VO_2$ in mL/kg/min × BW in kg ÷ 1,000

$VO_2$ in L/min = _____ × _____ ÷ 1,000 = _____ L/min

Caloric expenditure for 800-meter walk = $VO_2$ in L/min × 5 × 800-meter time in min

Caloric expenditure for 800-meter walk = _____ × 5 × _____ = _____ calories

4. **Slow-Jogging HR, $VO_2$, and Caloric Expenditure.** Slowly jog 800 meters (two laps) around the track. Try to maintain the same slow-jogging pace throughout the two laps. Do NOT jog fast or sprint. This is not a speed test and is intended to be a slow jog only. As soon as you complete the 800 meters, notice the time required to complete the distance and check your exercise HR immediately by taking another 10-second pulse count. Record this information below.

10-sec pulse count: _____ beats

800-meter time: _____ min _____ sec.

HR in bpm = 10-sec pulse count × 6

HR in bpm = _____ × 6 = _____ bpm

800-meter time in minutes = min + (sec ÷ 60)

800-meter time in minutes = _____ + (_____ ÷ 60) = _____ min

Speed in mts/min = 800 ÷ 800-meter time in min

Speed in mts/min = 800 ÷ _____ = _____ mts/min.

$VO_2$ in mL/kg/min at this slow-jogging speed (Use Table 6.9, page 209) = _____ mL/kg/min

$VO_2$ in L/min = $VO_2$ in mL/kg/min × BW in kg ÷ 1,000

$VO_2$ in L/min = _____ × _____ ÷ 1,000 = _____ L/min

Caloric expenditure for 800-meter slow jog = $VO_2$ in L/min × 5 × 800-meter time in min

Caloric expenditure for 800-meter slow jog = _____ × 5 × _____ = _____ calories

5. **Fast-Jogging HR, VO2, Caloric Expenditure, and Recovery HR.** Jog another 800 meters at a faster speed around the track. Again try to maintain the same jogging pace throughout the two laps. Do NOT sprint. Your HR should not exceed 180 bpm on this test. As soon as you complete the 800 meters, notice your time for the two laps and check your 10-second pulse count. Record this information below. You also should check your 2- and 5-minute recovery HRs after the run and record these rates below.

10-sec pulse count: _____ beats

800-meter time: _____ min _____ sec

HR in bpm = 10-sec pulse count × 6

HR in bpm = _____ × 6 = _____ bpm

800-meter time in minutes = min + (sec ÷ 60)

800-meter time in minutes = _____ + (_____ ÷ 60) = _____ min

Speed in mts/min = 800 ÷ 800-meter time in min

Speed in mts/min = 800 ÷ _____ = _____ mts/min

$VO_2$ in mL/kg/min at this fast-jogging speed (Use Table 6.9, page 209) = _____ mL/kg/min

$VO_2$ in L/min = $VO_2$ in mL/kg/min × BW in kg ÷ 1,000

$\text{VO}_2 \text{ in L/min} = \underline{\hspace{2cm}} \times \underline{\hspace{2cm}} \div 1{,}000 = \underline{\hspace{2cm}} \text{ L/min}$

Caloric expenditure for 800-meter fast jog = $\text{VO}_2$ in L/min × 5 × 800-meter time in min

Caloric expenditure for 800-meter fast jog = $\underline{\hspace{2cm}}$ × 5 × $\underline{\hspace{2cm}}$ = $\underline{\hspace{2cm}}$ calories

**Recovery HRs**

|  | 10-sec count | bpm |
|---|---|---|
| 2 minutes |  |  |
| 5 minutes* |  |  |

6. **Resting, Exercise, and Recovery HRs.** Plot your resting, exercise, and recovery HRs on the graph provided below.

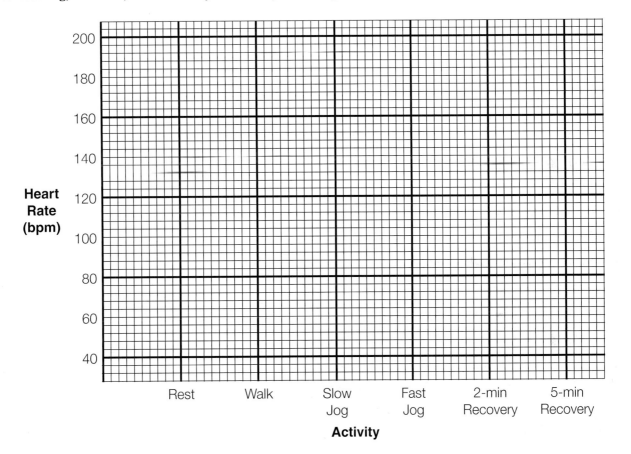

7. **Training Exercise HR and Equivalent Caloric Expenditure.** This part of the lab should be completed outside your regular lab time, during the next 2 or 3 days prior to turning in the assignment. According to the previous exercise HRs (items 3, 4, and 5), try to select a walking or jogging speed that will allow you to maintain your exercise HR in the appropriate cardiorespiratory training zone. Using a 400-meter track, walk or jog for 20 minutes at the selected speed and again try to maintain a constant speed throughout the exercise time. At the end of the 20 minutes, check your 10-second pulse count and estimate the distance covered in meters. Record this information below and estimate the $\text{VO}_2$ and caloric expenditure.

10-sec pulse count: $\underline{\hspace{2cm}}$ beats

HR in bpm = 10-sec pulse count × 6

HR in bpm = $\underline{\hspace{2cm}}$ × 6 = $\underline{\hspace{1cm}}$ bpm

Approximate distance covered in 20 minutes: $\underline{\hspace{2cm}}$ meters

---

*Your 5-minute recovery HR should be below 120 bpm. If it is above 120, you most likely have overexerted yourself and, therefore, need to decrease the intensity of exercise (and/or duration when exercising for long periods of time). If your 5-minute recovery HR is still above 120 after decreasing the intensity of exercise, you should consult a physician regarding this condition.

Speed in mts/min = distance in meters ÷ 20 minutes

Speed in mts/min = _____ ÷ 20 = _____ mts/min

$VO_2$ at this speed (see Table 6.9, page 209) = _____ mL/kg/min

$VO_2$ in L/min = $VO_2$ in mL/kg/min × BW in kg ÷ 1,000

$VO_2$ in L/min = _____ × _____ ÷ 1,000 = _____ L/min

Caloric expenditure for 20-min walk/jog = $VO_2$ in L/min × 5 × 20 min

Caloric expenditure for 20-min walk/jog = _____ × 5 × 20 = _____ calories

Using the previous information, how many calories would you have burned if you had maintained this pace for:

10 minutes ($VO_2$ in L/min × 5 × 10) = _____ × 5 × 10 = _____ calories

30 minutes ($VO_2$ in L/min × 5 × 30) = _____ × 5 × 30 = _____ calories

60 minutes ($VO_2$ in L/min × 5 × 60) = _____ × 5 × 60 = _____ calories

### Predicting Caloric Expenditure According to Exercise HR

Research indicates that there is a linear relationship between HR and $VO_2$, as long as the HR ranges from about 110 to 180 bpm. If you obtain two exercise HRs in this range and the equivalent oxygen uptakes (in L/min), you can easily predict your $VO_2$ and caloric expenditure for any given HR in the specified range. Plot your two exercise HRs and the corresponding $VO_2$ values on the graph provided below. Next, draw a line between these two points on the graph and extend the line to 110 and 180 bpm. You now may look up the $VO_2$ for any HR by finding the desired HR on the Y axis, then going across to the reference line and straight down to the X axis, where you will find the corresponding $VO_2$ in L/min. To obtain the caloric expenditure in calories per minute, simply multiply the $VO_2$ by 5. You also may predict your maximal $VO_2$ (in L/min) by extending the line up to your estimated maximal HR. The maximal HR is estimated by subtracting your age from 220. To convert the maximal VO2 to mL/kg/min, multiply the L/min value by 1,000 and divide by body weight in kilograms.

Using the results from your lab and the graph below, indicate the $VO_2$ in L/min and the caloric expenditure at the following HRs:

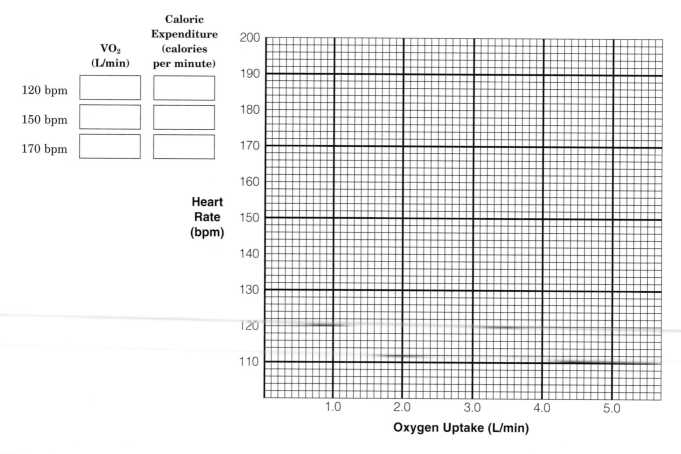

# LAB 6C: Exercise Readiness Questionnaire

Name _____ Date _____ Grade _____

Instructor _____ Course _____ Section _____

**Necessary Lab Equipment**
None required.

**Objective**
To determine your preparedness to start an exercise program.

**Instructions**
Read each statement carefully and circle the number that best describes your feelings in each statement. Please be completely honest with your answers. Interpret the results of this questionnaire using the guidelines provided on the next page.

| I. | Strongly Agree | Mildly Agree | Mildly Disagree | Strongly Disagree |
|---|---|---|---|---|
| 1. I can walk, ride a bike (or use a wheelchair), swim, or walk in a shallow pool. | 4 | 3 | 2 | 1 |
| 2. I enjoy exercise. | 4 | 3 | 2 | 1 |
| 3. I believe exercise can help decrease the risk for disease and premature mortality. | 4 | 3 | 2 | 1 |
| 4. I believe exercise contributes to better health. | 4 | 3 | 2 | 1 |
| 5. I have previously participated in an exercise program. | 4 | 3 | 2 | 1 |
| 6. I have experienced the feeling of being physically fit. | 4 | 3 | 2 | 1 |
| 7. I can envision myself exercising. | 4 | 3 | 2 | 1 |
| 8. I am contemplating an exercise program. | 4 | 3 | 2 | 1 |
| 9. I am willing to stop contemplating and give exercise a try for a few weeks. | 4 | 3 | 2 | 1 |
| 10. I am willing to set aside time at least three times a week for exercise. | 4 | 3 | 2 | 1 |
| 11. I can find a place to exercise (the streets, a park, a YMCA, a health club). | 4 | 3 | 2 | 1 |
| 12. I can find other people who would like to exercise with me. | 4 | 3 | 2 | 1 |
| 13. I will exercise when I am moody, fatigued, and even when the weather is bad. | 4 | 3 | 2 | 1 |
| 14. I am willing to spend a small amount of money for adequate exercise clothing (shoes, shorts, leotards, swimsuit). | 4 | 3 | 2 | 1 |
| 15. If I have any doubts about my present state of health, I will see a physician before beginning an exercise program. | 4 | 3 | 2 | 1 |
| 16. Exercise will make me feel better and improve my quality of life. | 4 | 3 | 2 | 1 |

Scoring Your Test:

This questionnaire allows you to examine your readiness for exercise. You have been evaluated in four categories: mastery (self-control), attitude, health, and commitment. Mastery indicates that you can be in control of your exercise program. Attitude examines your mental disposition toward exercise. Health measures the strength of your convictions about the wellness benefits of exercise. Commitment shows dedication and resolution to carry out the exercise program. Write the number you circled after each statement in the corresponding spaces below. Add the scores on each line to get your totals. Scores can vary from 4 to 16. A score of 12 and above is a strong indicator that that factor is important to you, and 8 and below is low. If you score 12 or more points in each category, your chances of initiating and adhering to an exercise program are good. If you fail to score at least 12 points in three categories, your chances of succeeding at exercise may be slim. You need to be better informed about the benefits of exercise, and a retraining process may be required.

Mastery:  1. [ ]  +  5. [ ]  +  6. [ ]  +  9. [ ]  =  [ ]

Attitude:  2. [ ]  +  7. [ ]  +  8. [ ]  +  13. [ ]  =  [ ]

Health:  3. [ ]  +  4. [ ]  +  15. [ ]  +  16. [ ]  =  [ ]

Commitment:  10. [ ]  +  11. [ ]  +  12. [ ]  +  14. [ ]  =  [ ]

## II. Stage of Change for Cardiorespiratory Endurance Exercise

Using Figure 2.5 (page 57) and Table 2.3 (page 57), identify your current stage of change in regard to participation in a cardiorespiratory endurance exercise program:

[ ]

## III. Advantages and Disadvantages for Adding Aerobic Exercise to Your Lifestyle

Advantages: _____

_____

_____

_____

_____

_____

_____

Disdvantages: _____

_____

_____

_____

_____

_____

_____

# LAB 6D: Cardiorespiratory Exercise Prescription

Name _____    Date _____    Grade _____

Instructor _____    Course _____    Section _____

**Necessary Lab Equipment**
None required.

**Objective**
To write your own cardiorespiratory exercise prescription.

## I. Intensity of Exercise

1. Estimate your own maximal heart rate (MHR)

    MHR = 220 minus age (220 − age)

    MHR = 220 − [          ] = [          ] bpm

2. Resting Heart Rate (RHR) = [          ] bpm

3. Heart Rate Reserve (HRR) = MHR − RHR

    HRR = [          ] − [          ] = [          ] beats

4. Training Intensities (TI) = HRR × TI + RHR

    40 Percent TI = [          ] × .40 + [          ] = [          ] bpm

    50 Percent TI = [          ] × .50 + [          ] = [          ] bpm

    60 percent TI = [          ] × .60 + [          ] = [          ] bpm

    85 Percent TI = [          ] × .85 + [          ] = [          ] bpm

5. Cardiorespiratory Training Zone. The optimum cardiorespiratory training zone is found between the 60 percent and 85 percent training intensities. Older adults, individuals who have been physically inactive or are in the poor or fair cardiorespiratory fitness categories, however, should follow a 40 percent to 50 percent training intensity during the first few weeks of the exercise program.

    Cardiorespiratory Training Zone: [          ] (60% TI) to [          ] (85% TI)

    Physical Activity Perceived Exertion (see Figure 6.7, page 212): [          ] to [          ]

## II. Mode of Exercise

Select any activity or combination of activities that you enjoy doing. The activity has to be continuous in nature and must get your heart rate up to the cardiorespiratory training zone and keep it there for as long as you exercise. Indicate your preferred mode(s) of exercise:

1. [          ]    2. [          ]    3. [          ]

4. [          ]    5. [          ]    6. [          ]

## III. Cardiorespiratory Exercise Program

The following is your weekly program for development of cardiorespiratory endurance. If you are in the average, good, or excellent fitness category, you may start at week 5. After completing this 12-week program, for you to maintain your fitness level, you should exercise in the 60 percent to 85 percent training zone for about 20 to 30 minutes, a minimum of three times per week, on nonconsecutive days. You should also recompute your target zone periodically because you will experience a significant reduction in resting heart rate with aerobic training (approximately 10 to 20 beats in about 8 to 12 weeks).

| Week | Duration (min) | Frequency | Training Intensity | Heart Rate (bpm) | 10-Sec Pulse Count* |
|------|---------------|-----------|--------------------|------------------|---------------------|
| 1 | 15 | 3 | Between 40% and 50% | ☐ to ☐ | ☐ to ☐ beats |
| 2 | 15 | 4 | Between 40% and 50% | | |
| 3 | 20 | 4 | Between 40% and 50% | | |
| 4 | 20 | 5 | Between 40% and 50% | | |
| 5 | 20 | 4 | Between 50% and 60% | ☐ to ☐ | ☐ to ☐ beats |
| 6 | 20 | 5 | Between 50% and 60% | | |
| 7 | 30 | 4 | Between 50% and 60% | | |
| 8 | 30 | 5 | Between 50% and 60% | | |
| 9 | 30 | 4 | Between 60% and 85% | ☐ to ☐ | ☐ to ☐ beats |
| 10 | 30 | 5 | Between 60% and 85% | | |
| 11 | 30–40 | 5 | Between 60% and 85% | | |
| 12 | 30–40 | 5 | Between 60% and 85% | | |

*Fill out your own 10-second pulse count under this column.

## IV. Briefly State Your Experiences and Feelings Regarding Aerobic Exercise:

_____

_____

_____

_____

_____

_____

_____

_____

_____

## V. Monitoring Daily Physical Activity

What is your average total number of daily steps (use a 7-day average): ☐

What is your current activity category (use Table 1.2, page 10): ☐

Do you accumulate 10,000 steps on most days of the week (at least five days)? ☐ Yes ☐ No

# Muscular Strength and Endurance

**7**

## Objectives

- Explain the importance of adequate strength levels in maintaining good health and well-being
- Clarify misconceptions about strength fitness
- Define muscular strength and muscular endurance
- Be able to assess muscular strength and endurance and learn to interpret test results according to health fitness and physical fitness standards
- Identify the factors that affect strength
- Understand the principles of overload and specificity of training for strength development
- Become acquainted with two distinct strength-training programs—with weights and without weights
- Chart your achievements for strength tests.

Check your understanding of the chapter contents by logging on to CengageNOW and accessing the pre-test, personalized learning plan, and post-test for this chapter.

© Fitness & Wellness, Inc.

# FAQ

### What is more important for good health: aerobic fitness or muscular strength?

They are both important. During the initial fitness boom in the 1970s and 1980s, the emphasis was almost exclusively on aerobic fitness. We now know that they both contribute to health, fitness, work capacity, and overall quality of life. Aerobic fitness is important in the prevention of cardiovascular diseases and some types of cancer, whereas muscular fitness will build strong muscles and bones, increase functional capacity, prevent osteoporosis, and decrease the risk for low back pain and other musculoskeletal injuries.

### Should I do aerobic exercise or strength training first?

Ideally, allow some recovery hours between the two types of training. If you can't afford the time, the training order should be based on your fitness goals and preferences. Unless extremely exhausting, aerobics provides a good lead into strength training. Excessive fatigue can lead to bad form while lifting and may result in injury. If your primary goal is strength development, lift first, as you'll be less fatigued and will end up with a more productive workout. On the other hand, if you are trying to develop the cardiorespiratory system or enhance caloric expenditure for weight loss purposes, heavy lower body lifting will make it very difficult to sustain a good cardio workout thereafter. Thus, evaluate your goals, and select the training order accordingly.

### Do big muscles turn into fat when the person stops training?

Muscle and fat tissue are two completely different types of tissue. Just as an apple will not turn into an orange, muscle tissue cannot turn into fat or vice versa. Muscle cells increase and decrease in size according to your training program. If you train quite hard, muscle cells increase in size. This increase is limited in women due to hormonal differences compared with men. When one stops training, muscle cells again decrease in size. If the person maintains a high caloric intake without physical training, however, fat cells will increase in size as weight (fat) is gained.

### What strength-training exercises are best to get an abdominal "six-pack"?

Most men tend to store body fat around the waist, while women do so around the hips. There are, however, no "miracle" exercises to spot-reduce. Multiple sets of abdominal curl-ups, crunches, reverse crunches, or sit-ups performed three to five times per week will strengthen the abdominal musculature but will not be sufficient to allow the muscles to appear through the layer of fat between the skin and the muscles. The total energy (caloric) expenditure of a few sets of abdominal exercises will not be sufficient to lose a significant amount of weight (fat). If you want to get a "washboard stomach" (or, for women, achieve shapely hips), you need to engage in a moderate to vigorous aerobic and strength-training program combined with a moderate reduction in daily caloric intake (diet).

The need for strength fitness is not confined to highly trained athletes, fitness enthusiasts, and individuals who have jobs that require heavy muscular work. In fact, a well-planned **strength-training** program leads to increased muscle strength and endurance, muscle tone, tendon and ligament strength, and bone density—all of which help to improve and maintain everyday functional physical capacity. The benefits of strength training or resistance training on health and well-being are well documented.

# Benefits of Strength Training

Strength is a basic health-related fitness component and is an important wellness component for optimal performance in daily activities such as sitting, walking, running, lifting and carrying objects, doing housework, and enjoying recreational activities. Strength also is of great value in improving posture, personal appearance, and self-image; in developing sports skills; in promoting stability of joints; and in meeting certain emergencies in life.

From a health standpoint, increasing strength helps to increase or maintain muscle and a higher resting metabolic rate, encourages weight loss and maintenance, lessens the risk for injury, prevents osteoporosis, reduces chronic low back pain, alleviates arthritic pain, aids in childbearing, improves cholesterol levels, promotes psychological well-being, and may help to lower the risk of high blood pressure and diabetes.

Furthermore, with time, the heart rate and blood pressure response to lifting a heavy resistance (a weight) decreases. This adaptation reduces the demands on the cardiovascular system when you perform activities such as carrying a child, the groceries, or a suitcase.

Regular strength training can also help control blood sugar. Much of the blood glucose from food consumption goes to the muscles, where it is stored as glycogen. When muscles are not used, muscle cells may become insulin resistant, and glucose cannot enter the cells, thereby increasing the risk for diabetes. Following 16 weeks of strength training, a group of diabetic men and women improved their blood sugar control, gained strength, increased lean body mass, lost body fat, and lowered blood pressure.[1]

## Muscular Strength and Aging

In the older adult population, muscular strength may be the most important health-related component of physical fitness. Though proper cardiorespiratory endurance is necessary to help maintain a healthy heart, good strength contributes more to independent living than any other fitness component. Older adults with good strength levels can successfully perform most **activities of daily living.**

A common occurrence as people age is **sarcopenia,** the loss of lean body mass, strength, and function. How much of this loss is related to the aging process itself or to actual physical inactivity and faulty nutrition is unknown. And whereas thinning of the bones from osteoporosis renders them prone to fractures, the gradual loss of muscle mass and ensuing frailty are what lead to falls and subsequent loss of function in older adults. Strength training helps to slow the age-related loss of muscle function. Protein deficiency, seen in some older adults, also contributes to loss of lean tissue.

More than anything else, older adults want to enjoy good health and to function independently. Many of them, however, are confined to nursing homes because they lack sufficient strength to move about. They cannot walk very far, and many have to be helped in and out of beds, chairs, and tubs.

A strength-training program can enhance quality of life tremendously, and nearly everyone can benefit from it. Only people with advanced heart disease are advised to refrain from strength training. Inactive adults between the ages of 56 and 86 who participated in a 12-week strength-training program increased their lean body mass by about 3 pounds, lost about 4 pounds of fat, and increased their resting metabolic rate by almost 7 percent.[2] In other research, leg strength improved by as much as 200 percent in previously inactive adults over age 90.[3] As strength improves, so does the ability to move about, the capacity for independent living, and enjoyment of life during the "golden years." More specifically, good strength enhances quality of life in that it

- improves balance and restores mobility,
- makes lifting and reaching easier,
- decreases the risk for injuries and falls, and
- stresses the bones and preserves bone mineral density, thereby decreasing the risk for osteoporosis.

Another benefit of maintaining a good strength level is its relationship to human **metabolism.** A primary outcome of a strength-training program is an increase in muscle mass or size (lean body mass), known as muscle **hypertrophy.**

Muscle tissue uses more energy than fatty tissue. That is, your body expends more calories to maintain muscle than to maintain fat. All other factors being equal, if two individuals both weigh 150 pounds but have different amounts of muscle mass, the one with more muscle mass will have a higher **resting metabolism** (also see "Exercise: The Key to Weight Management," pages 165–169). Even small increases in muscle mass have a long-term positive effect on metabolism.

Loss of lean tissue also is thought to be a primary reason for the decrease in metabolism as people grow older. Contrary to some beliefs, metabolism does not have to slow down significantly with aging. It is not so much that metabolism slows down. It's that we slow down. Lean body mass decreases with sedentary living, which in turn slows down the resting metabolic rate. Thus, if people continue eating at the same rate as they age, body fat increases.

Daily energy requirements decrease an average of 360 calories between age 26 and age 60.[4] Participating in

---

**Strength training** A program designed to improve muscular strength and/or endurance through a series of progressive resistance (weight) training exercises that overload the muscle system and cause physiologic development.

**Activities of daily living** Everyday behaviors that people normally do to function in life (cross the street, carry groceries, lift objects, do laundry, sweep floors).

**Sarcopenia** Age-related loss of lean body mass, strength, and function.

**Metabolism** All energy and material transformations that occur within living cells; necessary to sustain life.

**Hypertrophy** An increase in the size of the cell, as in muscle hypertrophy.

**Resting metabolism** Amount of energy (expressed in milliliters of oxygen per minute or total calories per day) an individual requires during resting conditions to sustain proper body function.

a strength-training program can offset much of the decline and prevent and reduce excess body fat. One research study found an increase in resting metabolic rate of 35 calories per pound of muscle mass in older adults who participated in a strength-training program.[5]

**Gender Differences** A common misconception about physical fitness concerns women in strength training. Because of the increase in muscle mass typically seen in men, some women think that a strength-training program will result in their developing large musculature.

Even though the quality of muscle in men and women is the same, endocrinological differences do not allow women to achieve the same amount of muscle hypertrophy (size) as men. Men also have more muscle fibers, and because of the sex-specific male hormones, each individual fiber has more potential for hypertrophy. On the average, following 6 months of training, women can achieve up to a 50 percent increase in strength but only a 10 percent increase in muscle size.

The idea that strength training allows women to develop muscle hypertrophy to the same extent as men is as false as the notion that playing basketball will turn women into giants. Masculinity and femininity are established by genetic inheritance, not by the amount of physical activity. Variations in the extent of masculinity and femininity are determined by individual differences in hormonal secretions of androgen, testosterone, estrogen, and progesterone. Women with a bigger-than-average build often are inclined to participate in sports because of their natural physical advantage. As a result, many people have associated women's participation in sports and strength training with large muscle size.

As the number of females who participate in sports has increased steadily during the last few years, the myth of

## Selected Detrimental Effects from Using Anabolic Steroids

- Liver tumors
- Hepatitis
- Hypertension
- Reduction of high-density lipoprotein (HDL) cholesterol
- Elevation of low-density lipoprotein (LDL) cholesterol
- Hyperinsulinism
- Impaired pituitary function
- Impaired thyroid function
- Mood swings
- Aggressive behavior
- Increased irritability
- Acne
- Fluid retention
- Decreased libido
- HIV infection (via injectable steroids)
- Prostate problems (men)
- Testicular atrophy (men)
- Reduced sperm count (men)
- Clitoral enlargement (women)
- Decreased breast size (women)
- Increased body and facial hair (nonreversible in women)
- Deepening of the voice (nonreversible in women)

strength training in women leading to large increases in muscle size has abated somewhat. For example, per pound of body weight, female gymnasts are among the strongest athletes in the world. These athletes engage regularly in vigorous strength-training programs. Yet, female gymnasts have some of the most well-toned and graceful figures of all women.

In recent years, improved body appearance has become the rule rather than the exception for women who participate in strength-training programs. Some of the most attractive female movie stars also train with weights to further improve their personal image.

Nonetheless, you may ask, "If weight training does not masculinize women, why do so many women body builders develop such heavy musculature?" In the sport of body building, the athletes follow intense training routines consisting two or more hours of constant weight lifting with short rest intervals between sets. Many body-building training routines call for back-to-back exercises using the

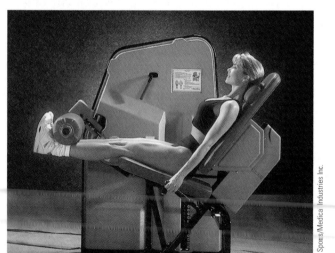

Improved body appearance has become the rule rather than the exception for women who participate in strength-training exercises.

© Nautilus Sports/Medica Industries Inc.

**FIGURE 7.1** Changes in body composition as a result of a combined aerobic and strength-training program.

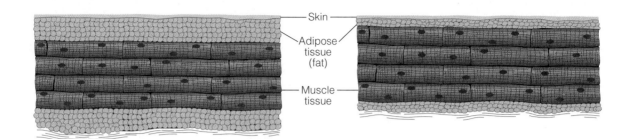

same muscle groups. The objective of this type of training is to pump extra blood into the muscles. This additional fluid makes the muscles appear much bigger than they do in a resting condition. Based on the intensity and the length of the training session, the muscles can remain filled with blood, appearing measurably larger for several hours after completing the training session. Performing such routines is a common practice before competitions. Therefore, in real life, these women are not as muscular as they seem when they are participating in a contest.

In the sport of body building (among others), a big point of controversy is the use of **anabolic steroids** and human growth hormones. These hormones produce detrimental and undesirable side effects in women (such as hypertension, fluid retention, decreased breast size, deepening of the voice, and whiskers and other atypical body hair growth), which some women deem tolerable. Anabolic steroid use in general—except for medical reasons and when carefully monitored by a physician—can lead to serious health consequences.

## Critical Thinking

What role should strength training have in a fitness program? Should people be motivated for the health fitness benefits, or should they participate to enhance their body image? What are your feelings about individuals (male or female) with large body musculature?

Use of anabolic steroids by female body builders and female track-and-field athletes around the world is widespread. These athletes use anabolic steroids to remain competitive at the highest level. During the 2004 Olympic Games In Athens, Greece, two women shot putters, including the gold medal winner (later stripped of the medal), were expelled from the games for using steroids. Women who take steroids undoubtedly will build heavy musculature, and if they take them long enough, the steroids will produce masculinizing effects.

To prevent steroid use, the International Federation of Body Building instituted a mandatory steroid-testing program for women participating in the Miss Olympia contest. When drugs are not used to promote development, improved body image is the rule rather than the exception among women who participate in body building, strength training, and sports in general.

## Changes in Body Composition

A benefit of strength training, accentuated even more when combined with aerobic exercise, is a decrease in adipose or fatty tissue around muscle fibers themselves. This decrease is often greater than the amount of muscle hypertrophy (see Figure 7.1). Therefore, losing inches but not body weight is common.

Because muscle tissue is more dense than fatty tissue (and despite the fact that inches are lost during a combined strength-training and aerobic program), people, especially women, often become discouraged because they cannot see the results readily on the scale. They can offset this discouragement by determining body composition regularly to monitor their changes in percent body fat rather than simply measuring changes in total body weight (see Chapter 4).

## Assessment of Muscular Strength and Endurance

Although muscular strength and endurance are interrelated, they do differ. **Muscular strength** is the ability to exert maximum force against resistance. **Muscular endurance** is the ability of a muscle to exert submaximal force repeatedly over time.

**Anabolic steroids** Synthetic versions of the male sex hormone testosterone, which promotes muscle development and hypertrophy.

**Muscular strength** The ability of a muscle to exert maximum force against resistance (for example, 1 repetition maximum [or 1 RM] on the bench press exercise).

**Muscular endurance** The ability of a muscle to exert submaximal force repeatedly over time.

Muscular endurance (also referred to as "localized muscular endurance") depends to a large extent on muscular strength. Weak muscles cannot repeat an action several times or sustain it. Based upon these principles, strength tests and training programs have been designed to measure and develop absolute muscular strength, muscular endurance, or a combination of the two.

Muscular strength is usually determined by the maximal amount of resistance (weight)—**one repetition maximum**, or 1 RM—an individual is able to lift in a single effort. Although this assessment yields a good measure of absolute strength, it does require considerable time, because the 1 RM is determined through trial and error. For example, strength of the chest muscles is frequently measured through the bench press exercise. If an individual has not trained with weights, he may try 100 pounds and lift this resistance easily. After adding 50 pounds, he fails to lift the resistance. Then he decreases resistance by 20 or 30 pounds. Finally, after several trials, the 1 RM is established.

Using this method, a true 1 RM might be difficult to obtain the first time an individual is tested, because fatigue becomes a factor. By the time the 1 RM is established, the person already has made several maximal or near-maximal attempts.

In contrast, muscular endurance typically is established by the number of repetitions an individual can

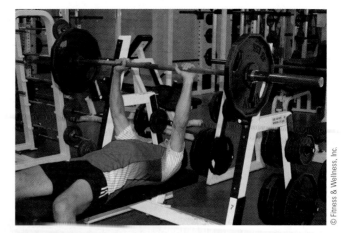

The maximal amount of resistance that an individual is able to lift in one single effort (1 repetition maximum or 1 RM) is a measure of absolute strength.

perform against a submaximal resistance or by the length of time a given contraction can be sustained. For example: How many push-ups can an individual do? Or how many times can a 30-pound resistance be lifted? Or how long can a person hold a chin-up?

If time is a factor and only one test item can be done, the Hand Grip Strength Test, described in Figure 7.2, is commonly used to assess strength. This test, though, provides only a weak correlation with overall body strength. Two additional strength tests are provided in Figures 7.3 and 7.4. Lab 7A also offers you the opportunity to assess your own level of muscular strength or endurance with all three tests. You may take one or more of these tests, according to your time and the facilities available.

In strength testing, several body sites should be assessed, because muscular strength and muscular endurance are both highly specific. A high degree of strength or endurance in one body part does not necessarily indicate similarity in other parts, so no single strength test provides a good assessment of overall body strength. Accordingly, exercises for the strength tests were selected to include the upper body, lower body, and abdominal regions.

---

**FIGURE 7.2** Procedure for the Hand Grip Strength Test.

1. Adjust the width of the dynamometer* so the middle bones of your fingers rest on the distant end of the dynamometer grip.
2. Use your dominant hand for this test. Place your elbow at a 90° angle and about 2 inches away from the body.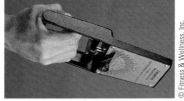
3. Now grip as hard as you can for a few seconds. Do not move any other body part as you perform the test (do not flex or extend the elbow, do not move the elbow away or toward the body, and do not lean forward or backward during the test).
4. Record the dynamometer reading in pounds (if reading is in kilograms, multiply by 2.2046).
5. Three trials are allowed for this test. Use the highest reading for your final test score. Look up your percentile rank for this test in Table 7.1.
6. Based on your percentile rank, obtain the hand grip strength fitness category according to the following guidelines:

| Percentile Rank | Fitness Category |
| --- | --- |
| ≥90 | Excellent |
| 70–80 | Good |
| 50–60 | Average |
| 30–40 | Fair |
| ≤20 | Poor |

*A Lafayette 78010 dynamometer is recommended for this test (Lafayette Instruments Co., Sagamore and North 9th Street, Lafayette, IN 47903).

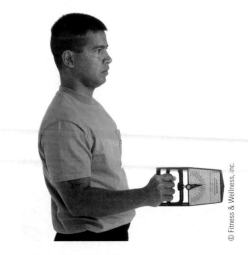

The hand grip tests strength.

Before strength testing, you should become familiar with the procedures for the respective tests. For safety reasons, always take at least one friend with you whenever you train with weights or undertake any type of strength assessment. Also, these are different tests, so to make valid comparisons, you should use the same test for pre- and post-assessments. The following are your options.

## Muscular Strength: Hand Grip Strength Test

As indicated previously, when time is a factor, the Hand Grip Test can be used to provide a rough estimate of strength. Unlike the next two tests, this one is isometric (involving static contraction, discussed later in the chapter). If the proper grip is used, no finger motion or body movement is visible during the test. The test procedure is given in Figure 7.2, and percentile ranks based on your results are provided in Table 7.1. You can record the results of this test in Lab 7A.

Changes in strength may be more difficult to evaluate with the Hand Grip Strength Test. Most strength-training programs are dynamic in nature (body segments are moved through a range of motion, discussed later in the chapter), whereas this test provides an isometric assessment. Further, grip-strength exercises seldom are used in strength training, and increases in strength are specific to the body parts exercised. This test, however, can be used to supplement the following strength tests.

## Muscular Endurance Test

Three exercises were selected to assess the endurance of the upper body, lower body, and midbody muscle groups (see Figure 7.3). The advantage of the Muscular Endurance Test is that it does not require strength-training equipment—only a stop-watch, a metronome, a bench or gymnasium bleacher 16¼ inches high, a cardboard strip 3½ inches wide by 30 inches long, and a partner. A percentile rank is given for each exercise according to the number of repetitions performed (see Table 7.2). An overall endurance rating can be obtained by totaling the number of points obtained on each exercise. Record the results of this test in Lab 7A.

## Muscular Strength and Endurance Test

In the Muscular Strength and Endurance Test, you will lift a submaximal resistance as many times as possible using the six strength-training exercises listed in Figure 7.4. The resistance for each lift is determined according to selected percentages of body weight shown in Figure 7.1 and Lab 7A.

With this test, if an individual does only a few repetitions, the test will measure primarily absolute strength. For those who are able to do a lot of repetitions, the test will be an indicator of muscular endurance. If you are not familiar with the different lifts, illustrations are provided at the end of this chapter.

A strength/endurance rating is determined according to the maximum number of repetitions you are able to perform on each exercise. Fixed-resistance strength units are necessary to administer all but the abdominal exercises in this test (see "Dynamic Training" on pages 246–247 for an explanation of fixed-resistance equipment).

A percentile rank for each exercise is given based on the number of repetitions performed (see Table 7.3). As with the Muscular Endurance Test, an overall muscular strength/endurance rating is obtained by totaling the number of points obtained on each exercise.

If no fixed-resistance equipment is available, you can still perform the test using different equipment. In that case, though, the percentile rankings and strength fitness categories may not be completely accurate because a certain resistance (for example, 50 pounds) is seldom the same on two different weight machines (for example, Universal Gym versus Nautilus). The industry has no standard calibration procedure for strength equipment. Consequently, if you lift a certain resistance for a specific exercise (for example, bench press) on one machine, you may or may not be able to lift the same amount for this exercise on a different machine.

Even though the percentile ranks may not be valid across different equipment, test results can be used to evaluate changes in fitness. For example, you may be able to do 7 repetitions during the initial test, but if you can perform 14 repetitions after 12 weeks of training, that's a measure of improvement. Results of the Muscular Strength and Endurance Test can be recorded in Lab 7A.

**TABLE 7.1** Scoring Table for Hand Grip Strength Test

| Percentile Rank | Men | Women |
|---|---|---|
| 99 | 153 | 101 |
| 95 | 145 | 94 |
| 90 | 141 | 91 |
| 80 | 139 | 86 |
| 70 | 132 | 80 |
| 60 | 124 | 78 |
| 50 | 122 | 74 |
| 40 | 114 | 71 |
| 30 | 110 | 66 |
| 20 | 100 | 64 |
| 10 | 91 | 60 |
| 5 | 76 | 58 |

High physical fitness standard

Health fitness standard

**One repetition maximum (1 RM)** The maximum amount of resistance an individual is able to lift in a single effort.

**FIGURE 7.3** Muscular Endurance Test.

Three exercises are conducted on this test: bench jumps, modified dips (men) or modified push-ups (women), and bent-leg curl-ups or abdominal crunches. All exercises should be conducted with the aid of a partner. The correct procedure for performing each exercise is as follows:

**Bench-jump.** Using a bench or gymnasium bleacher 16¼" high, attempt to jump up onto and down off of the bench as many times as possible in 1 minute. If you cannot jump the full minute, you may step up and down. A repetition is counted each time both feet return to the floor.

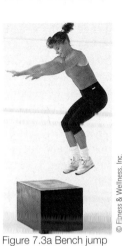

Figure 7.3a Bench jump

**Modified dip.** Men only: Using a bench or gymnasium bleacher, place the hands on the bench with the fingers pointing forward. Have a partner hold your feet in front of you. Bend the hips at approximately 90° (you also may use three sturdy chairs: Put your hands on two chairs placed by the sides of your body and place your feet on the third chair in front of you). Lower your body by flexing the elbows until they reach a 90° angle, then return to the starting position (also see Exercise 6, page 263). Perform the repetitions to a two-step cadence (down-up) regulated with a metronome set at 56 beats per minute. Perform as many continuous repetitions as possible. Do not count any more repetitions if you fail to follow the metronome cadence.

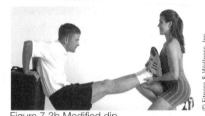

Figure 7.3b Modified dip

**Modified push-up.** Women: Lie down on the floor (face down), bend the knees (feet up in the air), and place the hands on the floor by the shoulders with the fingers pointing forward. The lower body will be supported at the knees (as opposed to the feet) throughout the test (see Figure 7.3c). The chest must touch the floor on each repetition. As with the modified-dip exercise (above), perform the repetitions to a two-step cadence (up-down) regulated with a metronome set at 56 beats per minute. Perform as many continuous repetitions as possible. Do not count any more repetitions if you fail to follow the metronome cadence.

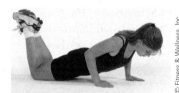

Figure 7.3c Modified push-up

**Bent-leg curl-up.** Lie down on the floor (face up) and bend both legs at the knees at approximately 100°. The feet should be on the floor, and you must hold them in place yourself throughout the test. Cross the arms in front of the chest, each hand on the opposite shoulder. Now raise the head off the floor, placing the chin against the chest. This is the starting and finishing position for each curl-up (see Figure 7.3d). **The back of the head may not come in contact with the floor, the hands cannot be removed from the shoulders, nor may the feet or hips be raised off the floor at any time during the test. The test is terminated if any of these four conditions occur.**

When you curl up, the upper body must come to an upright position before going back down (see Figure 7.3e). The repetitions are performed to a two-step cadence (up-down)

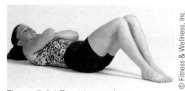

Figure 7.3d Bent-leg curl-up

regulated with the metronome set at 40 beats per minute. For this exercise, you should allow a brief practice period of 5 to 10 seconds to familiarize yourself with the cadence (the *up* movement is initiated with the first beat, then you must wait for the next beat to initiate the *down* movement; one repetition is accomplished every two beats of the metronome). Count as many repetitions as you are able to perform following the proper cadence. The test is also terminated if you fail to maintain the appropriate cadence or if you accomplish 100 repetitions. Have your partner check the angle at the knees throughout the test to make sure to maintain the 100° angle as close as possible.

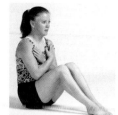

Figure 7.3e Bent-leg curl-up

**Abdominal crunch.** This test is recommended only for individuals who are unable to perform the bent-leg curl-up test because of susceptibility to low-back injury. Exercise form must be carefully monitored during the test. Several authors and researchers have indicated that proper form during this test is extremely difficult to control. Subjects often slide their bodies, bend their elbows, or shrug their shoulders during the test. Such actions facilitate the performance of the test and misrepresent the actual test results. Biomechanical factors also limit the ability to perform this test. Further, lack of spinal flexibility keeps some individuals from being able to move the full 3½" range of motion. Others are unable to keep their heels on the floor during the test. The validity of this test as an effective measure of abdominal strength or abdominal endurance has also been questioned through research.

Tape a 3½" × 30" strip of cardboard onto the floor. Lie down on the floor in a supine position (face up) with the knees bent at approximately 100° and the legs slightly apart. The feet should be on the floor, and you must hold them in place yourself throughout the test. Straighten out your arms and place them on the floor alongside the trunk with the palms down and the fingers fully extended. The fingertips of both hands should barely touch the closest edge of the cardboard (see Figure 7.3f). Bring the head off the floor until the chin is 1" to 2" away from your chest. Keep the head in this position during the entire test (do not move the head by flexing or extending the neck). You are now ready to begin the test.

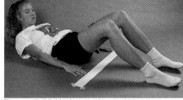

Figure 7.3f Abdominal crunch test

Perform the repetitions to a two-step cadence (up-down) regulated with a metronome set at 60 beats per minute. As you curl up, slide the fingers over the cardboard until the fingertips reach the far edge (3½") of the board (see Figure 7.3g), then return to the starting position.

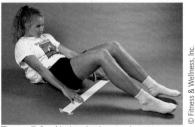

Figure 7.3g Abdominal crunch test

Allow a brief practice period of 5 to 10 seconds to familiarize yourself with the cadence. Initiate the *up* movement with the first beat and the *down* movement with the next beat. Accomplish one repetition every two beats of the metronome. Count as many repetitions as you are able to perform following the proper cadence. You may not count a repetition if the fingertips fail to reach the distant edge of the cardboard.

Terminate the test if you (a) fail to maintain the appropriate cadence, (b) bend the elbows, (c) shrug the shoulders, (d) slide

**FIGURE 7.3** Muscular Endurance Test. *(continued)*

the body, (e) lift heels off the floor, (f) raise the chin off the chest, (g) accomplish 100 repetitions, or (h) no longer can perform the test. Have your partner check the angle at the knees throughout the test to make sure that the 100° angle is maintained as closely as possible.

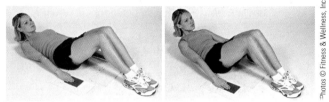

Figure 7.3h      Figure 7.3i
Abdominal crunch test performed with a Crunch-Ster Curl-Up Tester.

For this test you may also use a Crunch-Ster Curl-Up Tester, available from Novel Products.* An illustration of the test performed with this equipment is provided in Figures 7.3h and 7.3i.

According to the results, look up your percentile rank for each exercise in the far left column of Table 7.2 and determine your

muscular endurance fitness category according to the following classification:

| Average Score | Fitness Category | Points |
|---|---|---|
| ≥90 | Excellent | 5 |
| 70–80 | Good | 4 |
| 50–60 | Average | 3 |
| 30–40 | Fair | 2 |
| ≤20 | Poor | 1 |

Look up the number of points assigned for each fitness category above. Total the number of points and determine your overall strength endurance fitness category according to the following ratings:

| Total Points | Strength Endurance Category |
|---|---|
| ≥13 | Excellent |
| 10–12 | Good |
| 7–9 | Average |
| 4–6 | Fair |
| ≤3 | Poor |

*Novel Products, Inc. Figure Finder Collection, P.O. Box 408, Rockton, IL, 61072-0408. 1-800-323-5143, Fax 815-624-4866.

**TABLE 7.2** Muscular Endurance Scoring Table

| Percentile Rank | Men | | | | Women | | | |
|---|---|---|---|---|---|---|---|---|
| | Bench Jumps | Modified Dips | Bent-Leg Curl-Ups | Abdominal Crunches | Bench Jumps | Modified Push-Ups | Bent-Leg Curl-Ups | Abdominal Crunches |
| 99 | 66 | 54 | 100 | 100 | 58 | 95 | 100 | 100 |
| 95 | 63 | 50 | 81 | 100 | 54 | 70 | 100 | 100 |
| 90 | 62 | 38 | 65 | 100 | 52 | 50 | 97 | 69 |
| 80 | 58 | 32 | 51 | 66 | 48 | 41 | 77 | 49 |
| 70 | 57 | 30 | 44 | 45 | 44 | 38 | 57 | 37 |
| 60 | 56 | 27 | 31 | 38 | 42 | 33 | 45 | 34 |
| 50 | 54 | 26 | 28 | 33 | 39 | 30 | 37 | 31 |
| 40 | 51 | 23 | 25 | 29 | 38 | 28 | 28 | 27 |
| 30 | 48 | 20 | 22 | 26 | 36 | 25 | 22 | 24 |
| 20 | 47 | 17 | 17 | 22 | 32 | 21 | 17 | 21 |
| 10 | 40 | 11 | 10 | 18 | 28 | 18 | 9 | 15 |
| 5 | 34 | 7 | 3 | 16 | 26 | 15 | 4 | 0 |

▢ High physical fitness standard      ▢ Health fitness standard

# Strength-Training Prescription

The capacity of muscle cells to exert force increases and decreases according to the demands placed upon the muscular system. If muscle cells are overloaded beyond their normal use, such as in strength-training programs, the cells increase in size (hypertrophy) and strength. If the demands placed on the muscle cells decrease, such as in sedentary living or required rest because of illness or injury, the cells **atrophy** and lose strength. A good level of

**Atrophy** Decrease in the size of a cell.

244

PRINCIPLES AND LABS

## FIGURE 7.4  Muscular Strength and Endurance Test.

1. Familiarize yourself with the six lifts used for this test: lat pull-down, leg extension, bench press, bent-leg curl-up or abdominal crunch,* leg curl, and arm curl. Graphic illustrations for each lift are given on pages 271, 273, 266, 262, 268, and 264, respectively. For the leg curl exercise, the knees should be flexed to 90°. A description and illustration of the bent-leg curl-up and the abdominal crunch exercises are provided in Figure 7.3. On the leg extension lift, maintain the trunk in an upright position.
2. Determine your body weight in pounds.
3. Determine the amount of resistance to be used on each lift. To obtain this number, multiply your body weight by the percent given below for each lift.

| Lift | Percent of Body Weight | |
|---|---|---|
| | Men | Women |
| Lat Pull-Down | .70 | .45 |
| Leg Extension | .65 | .50 |
| Bench Press | .75 | .45 |
| Bent-Leg Curl-Up or Abdominal Crunch* | NA** | NA** |
| Leg Curl | .32 | .25 |
| Arm Curl | .35 | .18 |

*The abdominal crunch exercise should be used only by individuals who suffer or are susceptible to low-back pain.
**NA = not applicable—see Figure 7.3

4. Perform the maximum continuous number of repetitions possible.
5. Based on the number of repetitions performed, look up the percentile rank for each lift in the left column of Table 7.3.
6. The individual strength fitness category is determined according to the following classification:

| Percentile Rank | Fitness Category | Points |
|---|---|---|
| ≥90 | Excellent | 5 |
| 70–80 | Good | 4 |
| 50–60 | Average | 3 |
| 30–40 | Fair | 2 |
| ≤20 | Poor | 1 |

7. Look up the number of points assigned for each fitness category under item 6 above. Total the number of points and determine your overall strength fitness category according to the following ratings:

| Total Points | Strength Category |
|---|---|
| ≥25 | Excellent |
| 19–24 | Good |
| 13–18 | Average |
| 7–12 | Fair |
| ≤6 | Poor |

8. Record your results in Lab 7A.

## TABLE 7.3  Muscular Strength and Endurance Scoring Table

| | Men | | | | | | | Women | | | | | | |
|---|---|---|---|---|---|---|---|---|---|---|---|---|---|---|
| Percentile Rank | Lat Pull-Down | Leg Extension | Bench Press | Bent-Leg Curl-Up | Abdominal Crunch | Leg Curl | Arm Curl | Lat Pull-Down | Leg Extension | Bench Press | Bent-Leg Curl-Up | Abdominal Crunch | Leg Curl | Arm Curl |
| 99 | 30 | 25 | 26 | 100 | 100 | 24 | 25 | 30 | 25 | 27 | 100 | 100 | 20 | 25 |
| 95 | 25 | 20 | 21 | 81 | 100 | 20 | 21 | 25 | 20 | 21 | 100 | 100 | 17 | 21 |
| 90 | 19 | 19 | 19 | 65 | 100 | 19 | 19 | 21 | 18 | 20 | 97 | 69 | 12 | 20 |
| 80 | 16 | 15 | 16 | 51 | 66 | 15 | 15 | 16 | 13 | 16 | 77 | 49 | 10 | 16 |
| 70 | 13 | 14 | 13 | 44 | 45 | 13 | 12 | 13 | 11 | 13 | 57 | 37 | 9 | 14 |
| 60 | 11 | 13 | 11 | 31 | 38 | 11 | 10 | 11 | 10 | 11 | 45 | 34 | 7 | 12 |
| 50 | 10 | 12 | 10 | 28 | 33 | 10 | 9 | 10 | 9 | 10 | 37 | 31 | 6 | 10 |
| 40 | 9 | 10 | 7 | 25 | 29 | 8 | 8 | 9 | 8 | 5 | 28 | 27 | 5 | 8 |
| 30 | 7 | 9 | 5 | 22 | 26 | 6 | 7 | 7 | 7 | 3 | 22 | 24 | 4 | 7 |
| 20 | 6 | 7 | 3 | 17 | 22 | 4 | 5 | 6 | 5 | 1 | 17 | 21 | 3 | 6 |
| 10 | 4 | 5 | 1 | 10 | 18 | 3 | 3 | 3 | 3 | 0 | 9 | 15 | 1 | 3 |
| 5 | 3 | 3 | 0 | 3 | 16 | 1 | 2 | 2 | 1 | 0 | 4 | 0 | 0 | 2 |

☐ High physical fitness standard   ▨ Health fitness standard

muscular strength is important to develop and maintain fitness, health, and total well-being.

## Factors That Affect Strength
Several physiological factors combine to create muscle contraction and subsequent strength gains: neural stimulation, type of muscle fiber, overload, and specificity of training. Basic knowledge of these concepts is important to understand the principles involved in strength training.

**Neural Stimulation** Within the neuromuscular system, single **motor neurons** branch and attach to multiple muscle fibers. The motor neuron and the fibers it innervates (supplies with nerves) form a **motor unit.** The number of fibers a motor neuron can innervate varies from just a few in muscles that require precise control (eye muscles, for example) to as many as 1,000 or more in large muscles that do not perform refined or precise movements.

Stimulation of a motor neuron causes the muscle fibers to contract maximally or not at all. Variations in the number of fibers innervated and the frequency of their stimulation determine the strength of the muscle contraction. As the number of fibers innervated and frequency of stimulation increase, so does the strength of the muscular contraction.

**Types of Muscle Fiber** The human body has two basic types of muscle fibers: (a) slow-twitch or red fibers and (b) fast-twitch or white fibers. **Slow-twitch fibers** have a greater capacity for aerobic work. **Fast-twitch fibers** have a greater capacity for anaerobic work and produce more overall force. The latter are important for quick and powerful movements commonly used in strength-training activities.

The proportion of slow- and fast-twitch fibers is determined genetically and consequently varies from one person to another. Nevertheless, training increases the functional capacity of both types of fiber, and more specifically, strength training increases their ability to exert force.

During muscular contraction, slow-twitch fibers always are recruited first. As the force and speed of muscle contraction increase, the relative importance of the fast-twitch fibers increases. To activate the fast-twitch fibers, an activity must be intense and powerful.

**Overload** Strength gains are achieved in two ways:

1. Through increased ability of individual muscle fibers to generate a stronger contraction

2. By recruiting a greater proportion of the total available fibers for each contraction

These two factors combine in the **overload principle.** The demands placed on the muscle must be increased systematically and progressively over time, and the resistance must be of a magnitude significant enough to cause physiological adaptation. In simpler terms, just like all other organs and systems of the human body, to increase in physical capacity, muscles have to be taxed repeatedly beyond their accustomed loads. Because of this principle, strength training also is called progressive resistance training.

Several procedures can be used to overload in strength training:[6]

1. Increasing the resistance

2. Increasing the number of repetitions

3. Increasing or decreasing the speed of the normal repetition

4. Decreasing the rest interval for endurance improvements (with lighter resistances) or lengthening the rest interval for strength gains (with higher resistances)

5. Increasing the volume (sum of the repetitions performed multiplied by the resistance used)

6. Using any combination of the above

**Specificity of Training** The principle of **specificity of training** holds that for a muscle to increase in strength or endurance, the training program must be specific to obtain the desired effects (see also the discussion on resistance on pages 248–249).

The principle of specificity also applies to activity or sport-specific development and is commonly referred to as SAID training (**specific adaptation to imposed demand**). The SAID principle implies that if an individual is attempting to improve specific sport skills, the strength-training exercises performed should resemble as closely as possible the movement patterns encountered in that particular activity or sport.

For example, a soccer player who wishes to become stronger and faster would emphasize exercises that will develop leg strength and power. In contrast, an individual recovering from a lower-limb fracture initially exercises to increase strength and stability, and subsequently muscle endurance. Additional information on the principle of specificity is provided in Chapter 9, the section "Sport-Specific Conditioning," pages 340–341. Understanding all four concepts discussed thus far (neural stimulation, muscle fiber types, overload, and specificity) is required to design an effective strength-training program.

## Principles Involved in Strength Training

Because muscular strength and endurance are important in developing and maintaining overall fitness and well-being, the principles necessary to develop a strength-training program have to be understood, just as in the prescription for cardiorespiratory endurance. These principles are mode, resistance, sets, frequency, and volume of

---

**Motor neurons** Nerves connecting the central nervous system to the muscle.

**Motor unit** The combination of a motor neuron and the muscle fibers that neuron innervates.

**Slow-twitch fibers** Muscle fibers with greater aerobic potential and slow speed of contraction.

**Fast-twitch fibers** Muscle fibers with greater anaerobic potential and fast speed of contraction.

**Overload principle** Training concept that the demands placed on a system (cardiorespiratory or muscular) must be increased systematically and progressively over time to cause physiologic adaptation (development or improvement).

**Specificity of training** Principle that training must be done with the specific muscle the person is attempting to improve.

**Specific adaptation to imposed demand (SAID) training** Training principle stating that, for improvements to occur in a specific activity, the exercises performed during a strength-training program should resemble as closely as possible the movement patterns encountered in that particular activity.

training. The key factor in successful muscular strength development, however, is the individualization of the program according to these principles and the person's goals, as well as the magnitude of the individual's effort during training itself.[7]

**Mode of Training** Two types of training methods are used to improve strength, isometric (static) and dynamic (previously called "isotonic"). In **isometric training**, muscle contractions produce little or no movement, such as pushing or pulling against an immovable object. In dynamic training, the muscle contractions produce movement, such as extending the knees with resistance on the ankles (leg extension). The specificity of training principle applies here, too. To increase isometric versus dynamic strength, an individual must use static instead of dynamic training to achieve the desired results.

**Isometric Training** Isometric training does not require much equipment, and its popularity of several years ago has waned. Because strength gains with isometric training are specific to the angle of muscle contraction, this type of training is beneficial in a sport such as gymnastics, which requires regular static contractions during routines. As presented in Chapter 8, however, isometric training is a critical component of health conditioning programs for the back (see "Preventing and Rehabilitating Low-Back Pain," pages 299–303).

## Dynamic Training

Dynamic training is the most popular mode for strength training. The primary advantage is that strength is gained through the full **range of motion.** Most daily activities are dynamic in nature. We are constantly lifting, pushing, and pulling objects, and strength is needed through a complete range of motions. Another advantage is that improvements are measured easily by the amount lifted.

**Dynamic training** consists of two action phases when an exercise is performed: (1) **concentric** or **positive resistance** and (2) **eccentric** or **negative resistance.** In the concentric phase, the muscle shortens as it contracts to overcome the resistance. In the eccentric phase, the muscle lengthens to overcome the resistance. For example, during a bench press exercise, when the person lifts the resistance from the chest to full-arm extension, the triceps muscle on the back of the upper arm shortens to extend (straighten) the elbow. During the eccentric phase, the same triceps muscle is used to lower the weight during elbow flexion, but the muscle lengthens slowly to avoid dropping the resistance. Both motions work the same muscle against the same resistance.

Eccentric muscle contractions allow us to lower weights in a smooth, gradual, and controlled manner. Without eccentric contractions, weights would be suddenly dropped on the way down. Because the same muscles work when you lift and lower a resistance, always be sure to execute both actions in a controlled manner. Failure to do so diminishes the benefits of the training program and increases the risk for injuries. Eccentric contractions seem to be more effective in producing muscle hypertrophy but result in greater muscle soreness.[8]

Dynamic training programs can be conducted without weights; using exercise bands; and with **free weights,** **fixed-resistance** machines, **variable-resistance** machines, or isokinetic equipment. When you perform dynamic exercises without weights (for example, pull-ups and push-ups), with free weights, or with fixed-resistance machines, you move a constant resistance through a joint's full range of motion. The greatest resistance that can be lifted equals the maximum weight that can be moved at the weakest angle of the joint. This is because of changes in length of muscle and angle of pull as the joint moves through its range of motion. This type of training is also referred to as **dynamic constant external resistance,** or DCER.

As strength training became more popular, new strength-training machines were developed. This technology brought about **isokinetic training** and variable-resistance training programs, which require special ma-

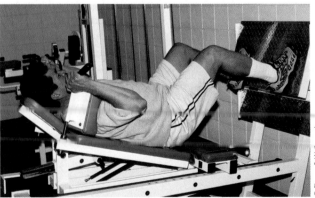

In isometric training, muscle contraction produces little or no movement.

In dynamic training, muscle contraction produces movement in the respective joint.

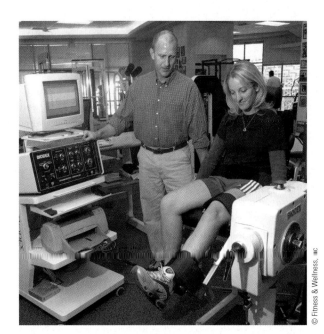

In isokinetic training, the speed of muscle contraction is constant.

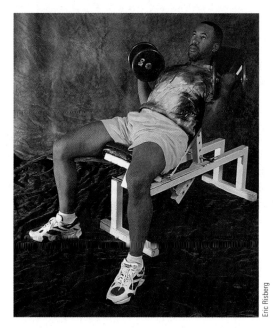

Strength training can be done using free weights.

chines equipped with mechanical devices that provide differing amounts of resistance, with the intent of over-loading the muscle group maximally through the entire range of motion. A distinction of isokinetic training is that the speed of the muscle contraction is kept constant because the machine provides resistance to match the user's force through the range of motion. The mode of training that an individual selects depends mainly on the type of equipment available and the specific objective the training program is attempting to accomplish.

The benefits of isokinetic and variable-resistance training are similar to those of the other dynamic training methods. Theoretically, strength gains should be better because maximum resistance is applied at all angles. Research, however, has not shown this type of training to be more effective than other modes of dynamic training.

## Free Weights Versus Machines in Dynamic Training

The most popular weight-training devices available during the first half of the 20th century were plate-loaded barbells (free weights). Strength-training machines were developed in the middle of the century but did not become popular until the 1970s. With subsequent technological improvements to these machines, a debate arose over which of the two training modalities was better.

Free weights require that the individual balance the resistance through the entire lifting motion. Thus, one could logically assume that free weights are a better training modality because additional stabilizing muscles are needed to balance the resistance as it is moved through the range of motion. Research, however, has not shown any differences in strength development between the two exercise modalities.[9]

Although each modality has pros and cons, muscles do not know whether the source of a resistance is a barbell, a dumbbell, a Universal Gym machine, a Nautilus machine, or a simple cinder block. What determines the extent of a

**Isometric training** Strength-training method referring to a muscle contraction that produces little or no movement, such as pushing or pulling against an immovable object.

**Range of motion** Entire arc of movement of a given joint.

**Dynamic training** Strength-training method referring to a muscle contraction with movement.

**Concentric** Describes shortening of a muscle during muscle contraction.

**Positive resistance** The lifting, pushing, or concentric phase of a repetition during a strength-training exercise.

**Eccentric** Describes lengthening of a muscle during muscle contraction.

**Negative resistance** The lowering or eccentric phase of a repetition during a strength-training exercise.

**Free weights** Barbells and dumbbells.

**Fixed resistance** Type of exercise in which a constant resistance is moved through a joint's full range of motion (dumbbells, barbells, machines using a constant resistance).

**Variable resistance** Training using special machines equipped with mechanical devices that provide differing amounts of resistance through the range of motion.

**Dynamic constant external resistance (DCER)** See fixed resistance.

**Isokinetic training** Strength-training method in which the speed of the muscle contraction is kept constant because the equipment (machine) provides an accommodating resistance to match the user's force (maximal) through the range of motion.

person's strength development is the quality of the program and the individual's effort during the training program itself—not the type of equipment used.

**Advantages of Free Weights.** Following are the advantages of using free weights instead of machines in a strength-training program:

- Cost: Free weights are much less expensive than most exercise machines. On a limited budget, free weights are a better option.
- Variety: A bar and a few plates can be used to perform many exercises to strengthen most muscles in the body.
- Portability: Free weights can be easily moved from one area or station to another.
- Balance: Free weights require that a person balance the weight through the entire range of motion. This feature involves additional stabilizing muscles to keep the weight moving properly.
- One size fits all: People of almost all ages can use free weights. A drawback of machines is that individuals who are at the extremes in terms of height or limb length often do not fit into the machines. In particular, small women and adolescents are at a disadvantage.

**Advantages of Machines.** Strength-training machines have the following advantages over free weights:

- Safety: Machines are safer because spotters are rarely needed to monitor exercises.
- Selection: A few exercises—such as hip flexion, hip abduction, leg curls, lat pull-downs, and neck exercises—can be performed only with machines.
- Variable resistance: Most machines provide variable resistance. Free weights provide only fixed resistance.
- Isolation: Individual muscles are better isolated with machines because stabilizing muscles are not used to balance the weight during the exercise.
- Time: Exercising with machines requires less time because you can set the resistance quickly by using a selector pin instead of having to manually change dumbbells or weight plates on both sides of a barbell.
- Flexibility: Most machines can provide resistance over a greater range of movement during the exercise, thereby contributing to more flexibility in the joints. For example, a barbell pullover exercise provides resistance over a range of 100 degrees, whereas a weight machine may allow for as much as 260 degrees.
- Rehabilitation: Machines are more useful during injury rehabilitation. A knee injury, for instance, is practically impossible to rehab using free weights, whereas, with a weight machine, small loads can be easily selected through a limited range of motion.
- Skill acquisition: Learning a new exercise movement—and performing it correctly—is faster because the machine controls the direction of the movement.

## Resistance

**Resistance** in strength training is the equivalent of intensity in cardiorespiratory exercise prescription. To stimulate strength development, the general recommendation has been to use a resistance of approximately 80 percent of the maximum capacity (1 RM). For example, a person with a 1 RM of 150 pounds should work with about 120 pounds ($150 \times .80$).

The number of repetitions that one can perform at 80 percent of the 1 RM varies among exercises (i.e., bench press, lat pull-down, leg curl; see Table 7.4). Data indicate that the total number of repetitions performed at a certain percentage of the 1 RM depends on the amount of muscle mass involved (bench press versus triceps extension) and whether it is a single or multi-joint exercise (leg press versus leg curl). In trained and untrained subjects alike, the number of repetitions is greater with larger muscle mass involvement and multi-joint exercises.[10]

Because of the time factor involved in constantly determining the 1 RM on each lift to ensure that the person is indeed working around 80 percent, the accepted rule for many years has been that individuals perform between 3 and 12 repetitions maximum (or 3 to 12 RM zone) for adequate strength gains. For example, if a person is training with a resistance of 120 pounds and cannot lift it more than 12 times—that is, the person reaches volitional fatigue at or before 12 repetitions—the training stimulus (weight used) is adequate for strength development. Once the person can lift the resistance more than 12 times, the resistance is increased by 5 to 10 pounds and the person again should build up to 12 repetitions. This is referred to as **progressive resistance training.**

Strength development, however, also can occur when working with less than 80 percent of the 1 RM. Although the 3 to 12 RM zone is the most commonly prescribed resistance training zone, benefits do accrue when working below 3 RM or above 12 RM.

At least in the health fitness area, little evidence supports the notion that working with a given number of repeti-

**TABLE 7.4  Number of Repetitions Performed at 80 Percent of the One Repetition Maximum (1 RM)**

|  | Trained | | Untrained | |
|---|---|---|---|---|
| Exercise | Men | Women | Men | Women |
| Leg press | 19 | 22 | 15 | 12 |
| Lat pulldown | 12 | 10 | 10 | 10 |
| Bench press | 12 | 14 | 10 | 10 |
| Leg extension | 12 | 10 | 9 | 8 |
| Sit-up* | 12 | 12 | 8 | 7 |
| Arm curl | 11 | 7 | 8 | 6 |
| Leg curl | 7 | 5 | 6 | 6 |

*Sit-up exercise performed with weighted plates on the chest and feet held in place with an ankle strap.
***Source:*** W. W. K. Hoeger, D. R. Hopkins, S. L. Barette, and D. F. Hale, "Relationship Between Repetitions and Selected Percentages of One Repetition Maximum: A Comparison Between Untrained and Trained Males and Females," *Journal of Applied Sport Science Research* 4, no. 2 (1990): 47–51.

tions elicits specific or greater strength, endurance, or hypertrophy.[11] Although not precisely to the same extent, muscular strength and endurance are both increased when training within a reasonable amount of repetitions. Thus, the American College of Sports Medicine recommends a range between 3 RM and 20 RM. The individual may choose the number of repetitions based on personal preference.

Elite strength athletes typically work between 1 and 6 RM, but they often shuffle training with a different number of repetitions for selected periods (weeks) of time (see "Training Volume" on next page). Body builders tend to work with moderate resistance levels (60 to 85 percent of the 1 RM) and perform 8 to 20 repetitions to near fatigue. A foremost objective of body building is to increase muscle size. Moderate resistance promotes blood flow to the muscles, "pumping up the muscles" (also known as "the pump"), which makes them look much larger than they do in a resting state.

From a general fitness point of view, working near a 10-repetition threshold seems to improve overall performance most effectively. We live in a dynamic world in which muscular strength and endurance are both required to lead an enjoyable life. Working around 10 RM produces good results in terms of strength, endurance, and hypertrophy.

## Sets

In strength training, a **set** is the number of repetitions performed for a given exercise. For example, a person lifting 120 pounds eight times has performed one set of eight repetitions ($1 \times 8 \times 120$). For general fitness, the recommendation is one to three sets per exercise. Some evidence suggests greater strength gains using multiple sets rather than a single set for a given exercise. Other research, however, concludes that similar increases in strength, endurance, and hypertrophy are derived between single- and multiple-set strength training, as long as the single set, or at least one of the multiple sets, is a heavy (maximum) set performed to volitional exhaustion using an RM zone (for example, 9 RM using an 8 to 12 RM zone).[12]

Because of the characteristics of muscle fiber, the number of sets the exerciser can do is limited. As the number of sets increases, so does the amount of muscle fatigue and subsequent recovery time. Therefore, strength gains may be lessened by performing too many sets. When time is a factor, single-set programs are preferable because they require less time and can enhance compliance with exercise. You may also choose to do multiple sets for multijoint exercises (bench press, leg press, lat pull-down) and a single RM-zone set for single joint exercises (arm curl, triceps extension, knee extension).

A recommended program for beginners in their first year of training is one or two light warm-up sets per exercise, using about 50 percent of the 1 RM (no warm-up sets are necessary for subsequent exercises that use the same muscle group), followed by one to three sets to near fatigue per exercise. Maintaining a resistance and effort that will temporarily fatigue the muscle (volitional exhaustion) from the number of repetitions selected in at least one of the sets is crucial to achieve optimal progress. Because of the lower resistances used in body building, four to eight sets can be done for each exercise.

To avoid muscle soreness and stiffness, new participants ought to build up gradually to three sets of maximal repetitions. They can do this by performing only one set of each exercise with a lighter resistance on the first day, two sets of each exercise on the second day—the first light and the second with the required resistance to volitional exhaustion. If you choose to do so, you can increase to three sets on the third day—one light and two heavy. After that, a person should be able to perform all three heavy sets.

The time necessary to recover between sets depends mainly on the resistance used during each set. In strength training, the energy to lift heavy weights is derived primarily from the system involving adenosine triphosphate (ATP) and creatine phosphate (CP) or phosphagen (see Chapter 3, the section "Energy (ATP) Production," pages 101–102). Ten seconds of maximal exercise nearly depletes the CP stores in the exercised muscle(s). These stores are replenished in about 3 to 5 minutes of recovery.

Based on this principle, rest intervals between sets vary in length depending on the program goals and are dictated by the amount of resistance used in training. Short rest intervals of less than 2 minutes are commonly used when one is trying to develop local muscular endurance. Moderate rest intervals of two to four minutes are used for strength development. Long intervals of more than 4 minutes are used when one is training for power development.[13] Using these guidelines, individuals training for health fitness purposes might allow 2 minutes of rest between sets. Body builders, who use lower resistances, should rest no more than 1 minute to maximize the "pumping" effect.

For individuals who are trying to maximize strength gains, the exercise program will be more time-effective if two or three exercises are alternated that require different muscle groups, called **circuit training.** In this way, an individual will not have to wait 2 to 4 minutes before proceeding to a new set on a different exercise. For example, the bench press, leg extension, and abdominal curl-up exercises may be combined so that the person can go almost directly from one exercise set to the next.

Men and women alike should observe the guidelines given previously. Many women do not follow them. They erroneously believe that training with low resistances and many repetitions is best to enhance body composition and maximize energy expenditure. Unless a person is seeking

---

**Resistance** Amount of weight lifted.

**Progressive resistance training** A gradual increase of resistance over a period of time.

**Set** A fixed number of repetitions; one set of bench presses might be 10 repetitions.

**Circuit training** Alternating exercises by performing them in a sequence of three to six or more.

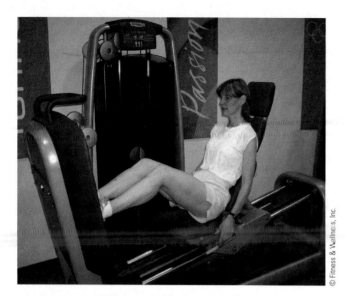

From a health-fitness standpoint, one strength-training session per week is sufficient to maintain strength.

to increase muscular endurance for a specific sport-related activity, the use of low resistances and high repetitions is not recommended to achieve optimal strength-fitness goals and maximize long-term energy expenditure (also see Chapter 5, the section "Exercise: The Key to Weight Management," pages 165–169).

## Frequency

Strength training can be done through a total body workout two or three times a week or more frequently if using a split-body routine (upper body one day, lower body the next). After a maximum strength workout, the muscles should be rested for about 2 to 3 days to allow adequate recovery. If not completely recovered in 2 to 3 days, the person most likely is overtraining and therefore not reaping the full benefits of the program. In that case, the person should do fewer sets of exercises than in the previous workout. A summary of strength-training guidelines for health fitness purposes is provided in Figure 7.5.

To achieve significant strength gains, a minimum of 8 weeks of consecutive training is necessary. After an individual has achieved a recommended strength level, from a health fitness standpoint, one training session per week

will be sufficient to maintain it. Highly trained athletes will have to train twice a week to maintain their strength levels.

Frequency of strength training for body builders varies from person to person. Because they use moderate resistance, daily or even two-a-day workouts are common. The frequency depends on the amount of resistance, number of sets performed per session, and the person's ability to recover from the previous exercise bout (see Table 7.5). The latter often is dictated by level of conditioning.

## Training Volume

**Volume** is the sum of all the repetitions performed multiplied by the resistances used during a strength-training session.[14] Volume frequently is used to quantify the amount of work performed in a given training session. For example, an individual who does three sets of six repetitions with 150 pounds has performed a training volume of 2,700 ($3 \times 6 \times 150$) for this exercise. The total training volume can be obtained by totaling the volume of all exercises performed.

The volume of training done in a strength-training session can be modified by changing the total number of exercises performed—either by changing the number of sets done per exercise or the number of repetitions performed per set. Athletes typically use high training volumes and low intensities to achieve muscle hypertrophy, and low volumes and high intensities to increase strength and power.

Altering training volume and intensity is known as **periodization**, a training approach that athletes frequently use to achieve peak fitness and prevent **overtraining**. Periodization means cycling one's training objectives (hypertrophy, strength, and endurance), with each phase of the program lasting anywhere from 2 to 12 weeks. To prevent overtraining during periodization, the volume should not increase by more than 5 percent from one phase to the next.

Periodization now is becoming popular among fitness participants who want to achieve higher levels of fitness. A more thorough discussion on periodization is provided in Chapter 9 (pages 342–343).

---

**FIGURE 7.5 Strength-training guidelines.**

| | |
|---|---|
| **Mode:** | 8 to 10 dynamic strength-training exercises involving the body's major muscle groups |
| **Resistance:** | 8 to 12 repetitions per set to complete or near-complete fatigue. A range of 3 to 20 repetitions to complete or near complete fatigue, however, may also be used and appears to be just as effective. The number of repetitions is optional; you may use 3 to 6, 8 to 12, 12 to 15, or 16 to 20 repetitions. |
| **Sets:** | A minimum of 1 set |
| **Frequency:** | 2 to 3 days per week on nonconsecutive days |

Adapted from American College of Sports Medicine, *Guidelines for Exercise Testing and Prescription* (Baltimore: Lippincott Williams & Wilkins, 2006).

---

**TABLE 7.5 Guidelines for Various Strength-Training Programs**

| Strength-Training Program | Resistance | Sets | Rest Between Sets* | Frequency (workouts per week)** |
|---|---|---|---|---|
| General fitness | 8–20 reps max | 1–3 | 2 min | 2–3 |
| Strength athletes | 1–6 reps max | 3–6 | 3 min | 2–3 |
| Body building | 8–20 reps near max | 3–8 | up to 1 min | 4–12 |

*Recovery between sets can be decreased by alternating exercises that use different muscle groups.
**Weekly training sessions can be increased by using a split-body routine.

Plyometrics Strength, speed, and explosiveness are all crucial for success in athletics. All three of these factors are enhanced with a progressive resistance training program, but greater increases in speed and explosiveness are thought to be possible with **plyometric exercise.** The objective is to generate the greatest amount of force in the shortest time. A solid strength base is necessary before attempting plyometric exercises.

Plyometric training is popular in sports that require powerful movements, such as basketball, volleyball, sprinting, jumping, and gymnastics. A typical plyometric exercise involves jumping off and back onto a box, attempting to rebound as quickly as possible on each jump. Box heights are increased progressively from about 12 to 22 inches.

The bounding action attempts to take advantage of the stretch-recoil and stretch reflex characteristics of muscle. The rapid stretch applied to the muscle during contact with the ground is thought to augment muscle contraction, leading to more explosiveness. Plyometrics can be used, too, for strengthening upper body muscles. An example is doing push-ups so the extension of the arms is forceful enough to drive the hands (and body) completely off the floor during each repetition.

A drawback of plyometric training is its higher risk for injuries compared with conventional modes of progressive resistance training. For instance, the potential for injury in rebound exercise escalates with the increase in box height or the number of repetitions.

# Strength Gains

A common question by many strength-training participants is: How quickly can strength gains be observed? Strength-training studies have revealed that most of the strength gains are seen in the first 8 weeks of training. The amount of improvement, however, is related to previous training status. Increases of 40 percent are seen in individuals with no previous strength-training experience, 16 percent in previously strength-trained people, and 10 percent in advanced individuals.[15] Adhering to a periodized strength-training program can yield further improvements (see "Periodization," Chapter 9).

# Strength-Training Exercises

The strength-training programs introduced on pages 261–278 provide a complete body workout. The major muscles of the human body referred to in the exercises are pointed out in Figure 7.7 and with the exercises themselves at the end of the chapter.

Only a minimum of equipment is required for the first program, Strength-Training Exercises without Weights (Exercises 1 through 14). You can conduct this program in your own home. Your body weight is used as the primary resistance for most exercises. A few exercises call for a friend's help or some basic implements from around your house to provide greater resistance.

Strength-Training Exercises with Weights (Exercises 15 through 37) require machines (shown in the accompanying photographs). These exercises can be conducted on either fixed-resistance or variable-resistance equipment. Many of these exercises also can be performed with free weights. The first 13 of these exercises (15 to 27) are recommended to get a complete workout. You can do these exercises as circuit training. If time is a factor, as a minimum perform the first nine (15 through 23) exercises. Exercises 28 to 37 are supplemental or can replace some of the basic 13 (for instance, substitute Exercise 29 or 30 for 15; 31 for 16; 33 for 19; 34 for 24; 35 for 26; 32 for 27). Exercises 38 to 46 are stability ball exercises that can be used to complement your workout. Some of these exercises can also take the place of others that you use to strengthen similar muscle groups.

Selecting different exercises for a given muscle group is recommended between training sessions (for example, chest press for bench press). No evidence indicates that a given exercise is best for a given muscle group. Changing exercises works the specific muscle group through a different range of motion and may change the difficulty of the exercise. Alternating exercises is also beneficial to avoid the monotony of repeating the same training program each training session.

## Critical Thinking

Your roommate started a strength-training program last year and has seen good results. He is now strength training on a nearly daily basis and taking performance-enhancing supplements hoping to accelerate results. What are your feelings about his program? What would you say (and not say) to him?

**Volume (in strength training)** The sum of all the repetitions performed multiplied by the resistances used during a strength-training session.

**Periodization** A training approach that divides the season into cycles using a systematic variation in intensity and volume of training to enhance fitness and performance.

**Overtraining** An emotional, behavioral, and physical condition marked by increased fatigue, decreased performance, persistent muscle soreness, mood disturbances, and feelings of "staleness" or "burnout" as a result of excessive physical training.

**Plyometric exercise** Explosive jump training, incorporating speed and strength training to enhance explosiveness.

# Dietary Guidelines for Strength Development

Individuals who wish to enhance muscle growth and strength during periods of intense strength training should increase protein intake from 0.8 gram per kilogram of body weight per day to about 1.5 grams per kilogram of body weight per day. An additional 500 daily calories are also recommended to optimize muscle mass gain. If protein intake is already at 1.5 grams per kilogram of body weight, the additional 500 calories should come primarily from complex carbohydrates to provide extra nutrients to the body and glucose for the working muscles.

The time of day when carbohydrates and protein are consumed in relation to the strength-training workout also plays a role in promoting muscle growth. Studies suggest that consuming a pre-exercise snack consisting of a combination of carbohydrates and protein is beneficial to muscle development. The carbohydrates supply energy for training, and the availability of amino acids (the building blocks of protein) in the blood during training enhances muscle building. A peanut butter, turkey, or tuna sandwich, milk or yogurt and fruit, or nuts and fruit consumed 30 to 60 minutes before training are excellent choices for a pre-workout snack.

Consuming a carbohydrate/protein snack immediately following strength training and a second snack an hour thereafter further promotes muscle growth and strength development. Post-exercise carbohydrates help restore muscle glycogen depleted during training and, in combination with protein, induce an increase in blood insulin and growth hormone levels. These hormones are essential to the muscle-building process.

Muscle fibers also absorb a greater amount of amino acids up to 48 hours following strength training. The first hour, nonetheless, seems to be the most critical. A higher level of circulating amino acids in the bloodstream immediately after training is believed to increase protein synthesis to a greater extent than amino acids made available later in the day. A ratio of 4 to 1 grams of carbohydrates to protein is recommended for a post-exercise snack—for example, a snack containing 40 grams of carbohydrates (160 calories) and 10 grams of protein (40 calories).

# Core Strength Training

The trunk (spine) and pelvis are referred to as the "core" of the body. Core muscles include the abdominal muscles (rectus, transversus, and internal and external obliques), hip muscles (front and back), and spinal muscles (lower and upper back muscles). These muscle groups are responsible for maintaining the stability of the spine and pelvis.

Many of the major muscle groups of the legs, shoulders, and arms attach to the core. A strong core allows a person to perform activities of daily living with greater ease, improve sports performance through a more effective energy transfer from large to small body parts, and decrease the incidence of low back pain. Core strength training also contributes to better posture and balance.

Interest in **core strength training** programs has increased recently. A major objective of core training is to exercise the abdominal and lower back muscles in unison. Furthermore, individuals should spend as much time training the back muscles as they do the abdominal muscles. Besides enhancing stability, core training improves dynamic balance, which is often required during physical activity and participation in sports.

Key core training exercises include the abdominal crunch and bent-leg curl-up, reverse crunch, pelvic tilt, lateral bridge, prone bridge, leg press, seated back, lat pull-down, back extension, lateral trunk flexion, supine bridge, and pelvic clock (Exercises 4, 11, 12, 13, 14, 16, 20, 24, 36, and 37 in this chapter and Exercises 26 and 27 in Chapter 8, respectively). Stability ball exercises 38 through 46 are also used to strengthen the core.

When core training is used in athletic conditioning programs, athletes attempt to mimic the dynamic skills they use in their sport. To do so, they use special equipment such as balance boards, stability balls, and foam pads. Using this equipment allows the athletes to train the core while seeking balance and stability in a sport-specific manner.[16]

### Pilates Exercise System

**Pilates** exercises have become increasingly popular in recent years. Previously, Pilates training was used primarily by dancers, but now this exercise modality is embraced by a large number of fitness participants, rehab patients, models, actors, and even professional athletes. Pilates studios, college courses, and classes at health clubs are available nationwide.

The Pilates training system was originally developed in the 1920s by German physical therapist Joseph Pilates. He designed the exercises to help strengthen the body's core by developing pelvic stability and abdominal control, coupled with focused breathing patterns.

Pilates exercises are performed either on a mat (floor) or with specialized equipment to help increase strength and flexibility of deep postural muscles. The intent is to improve muscle tone and length (a limber body), instead of increasing muscle size (hypertrophy). Pilates mat classes focus on body stability and proper body mechanics. The exercises are performed in a slow, controlled, precise manner. When performed properly, these exercises require intense concentration. Initially, Pilates training should be conducted under the supervision of certified instructors with extensive Pilates teaching experience.

Fitness goals of Pilates programs include better flexibility, muscle tone, posture, spinal support, body balance, low back health, sports performance, and mind–body awareness. Individuals with loose or unstable joints benefit from Pilates because the exercises are designed to enhance joint stability. The Pilates program is also used to help lose weight, increase lean tissue, and manage stress. Although Pilates programs are quite popular, more re-

## Behavior Modification Planning

### HEALTHY STRENGTH TRAINING

☐ ☐ Make a progressive resistance strength-training program a priority in your weekly schedule.

☐ ☐ Strength train at least once a week; even better, twice a week.

☐ ☐ Find a facility where you feel comfortable training and where you can get good professional guidance.

☐ ☐ Learn the proper technique for each exercise.

☐ ☐ Train with a friend or group of friends.

☐ ☐ Consume a pre-exercise snack consisting of a combination of carbohydrates and some protein about 30 to 60 minutes before each strength-training session.

☐ ☐ Use a minimum of 8 to 10 exercises that involve all major muscle groups of your body.

☐ ☐ Perform at least one set of each exercise to near muscular fatigue.

☐ ☐ To enhance protein synthesis, consume one post-exercise snack with a 4-to-l gram ratio of carbohydrates to protein immediately following strength training; and a second snack one hour thereafter.

☐ ☐ Allow at least 48 hours between strength-training sessions that involve the same muscle groups.

### Try It

Attend the school's fitness or recreation center and have an instructor or fitness trainer help you design a progressive resistance strength-training program. Train twice a week for the next 4 weeks. Thereafter, evaluate the results and write down your feelings about the program.

search is required to corroborate the benefits attributed to this training system.

### Stability Exercise Balls

A stability exercise ball is a large, flexible, and inflatable ball used for exercises that combine the principles of Pilates with core strength training. Stability exercises are specifically designed to develop abdominal, hip, chest, and spinal muscles by addressing core stabilization while the exerciser maintains a balanced position over the ball. Particular emphasis is placed on correct movement and maintenance of proper body alignment to involve as much of the core as possible. Although the primary objective is core strength and stability, many stability exercises can be performed to strengthen other body areas as well.

Stability exercises are thought to be more effective than similar exercises on the ground. For example, just sitting on the ball requires the use of stabilizing core muscles (including the rectus abdominis and the external and internal obliques) to keep the body from falling off the ball. Traditional strength-training exercises are primarily for strength and power development and do not contribute as much to body balance.

When performing stability exercises, choose a ball size based on your height. Your thighs should be parallel to the floor when you sit on the ball. A slightly larger ball may be used if you suffer from back problems. Several stability ball exercises are provided on pages 279–282. For best results, have a trained specialist teach you the proper technique and watch your form while you learn the exercises. Individuals who have a weak muscular system or poor balance or who are over the age of 65 should perform stability exercises under the supervision of a qualified trainer.

### Elastic-Band Resistive Exercise

Elastic bands and tubing can also be used for strength training. This type of constant-resistance training has increased in popularity and has been shown to help increase strength, mobility, functional ability (particularly in older adults), and aid in the rehab of many types of injuries. Some of the advantages to using this type of training include low cost, versatility (you can create resistance in almost all angles and directions of the range of motion), use of a large number of exercises to work all joints of the body, and they provide a great way to workout while traveling (exercise bands can be easily packed in a suitcase). Use of elastic-band resistive exercises can also add variety to your routine workout.

Due to the constant resistance provided by the bands or tubing, the training may appear more difficult to some individuals, because the resistance is used both during the eccentric and concentric phases of the repetition. Workouts, however, can be just as challenging as with free weights or machines. Additionally, the bands can be used

**Core strength training** A program designed to strengthen the abdominal, hip, and spinal muscles (the core of the body).

**Pilates** A training program that uses exercises designed to help strengthen the body's core by developing pelvic stability and abdominal control; exercises are coupled with focused breathing patterns.

**FIGURE 7.6** Sample elastic-band resistive exercises

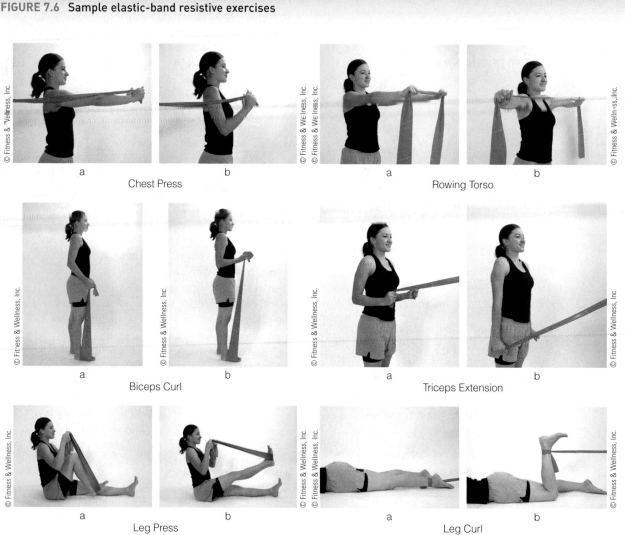

Chest Press

Rowing Torso

Biceps Curl

Triceps Extension

Leg Press

Leg Curl

by beginners and strength-trained individuals. That is because several different tension cords (up to eight bands) are available and all participants can progress through various resistance levels.

At the beginning, it may be a little confusing trying to determine how to use the bands and create the proper loops to grip the bands. The assistance of a training video, an instructor, or a personal trainer is helpful. The bands can be wrapped around a post, a door knob, or you can stand on them as well for some of the exercises. A few sample exercises with elastic-band resistive exercises are provided in Figure 7.6. Instructional booklets are available to purchase with your elastic band or tubing.

# Exercise Safety Guidelines

As you prepare to design your strength-training program, keep the following guidelines in mind:

- Select exercises that will involve all major muscle groups: chest, shoulders, back, legs, arms, hip, and trunk.
- Select exercises that will strengthen the core. Use controlled movements and start with light-to-moderate resistances (later, athletes may use explosive movements with heavier resistances).
- Never lift weights alone. Always have someone work out with you in case you need a spotter or help with an injury. When you use free weights, one to two spotters are recommended for certain exercises (for example, bench press, squats, overhead press).
- Prior to lifting weights, warm up properly by performing a light- to moderate-intensity aerobic activity (5 to 7 minutes) and some gentle stretches for a few minutes.
- Use proper lifting technique for each exercise. The correct lifting technique will involve only those muscles and joints intended for a specific exercise. Involving other muscles and joints to "cheat" during the exercise to complete a repetition or to be able to lift a greater resistance decreases the long-term effectiveness of the exercise and can lead to injury (such as arching the

back during the push-up, squat, or bench press exercises). Proper lifting technique also implies performing the exercises in a controlled manner and throughout the entire range of motion. Perform each repetition in a rhythmic manner and at a moderate speed. Avoid fast and jerky movements, and do not throw the entire body into the lifting motion. Do not arch the back when lifting a weight.

- Maintain proper body balance while lifting. Proper balance involves good posture, a stable body position, and correct seat and arm/leg settings on exercise machines. Loss of balance places undue strain on smaller muscles and leads to injuries because of the heavy resistances suddenly placed on them. In the early stages of a program, first-time lifters often struggle with bar control and balance when using free weights. This problem is overcome quickly with practice following a few training sessions.

- Exercise larger muscle groups (such as those in the chest, back, and legs) before exercising smaller muscle groups (arms, abdominals, ankles, neck). For example, the bench press exercise works the chest, shoulders, and back of the upper arms (triceps), whereas the triceps extension works the back of the upper arms only.

- Exercise opposing muscle groups for a balanced workout. When you work the chest (bench press), also work the back (rowing torso). If you work the biceps (arm curl), also work the triceps (triceps extension).

- Breathe naturally. Inhale during the eccentric phase (bringing the weight down), and exhale during the concentric phase (lifting or pushing the weight up). Practice proper breathing with lighter weights when you are learning a new exercise.

- Avoid holding your breath while straining to lift a weight. Holding your breath increases the pressure inside the chest and abdominal cavity greatly, making it nearly impossible for the blood in the veins to return to the heart. Although rare, a sudden high intrathoracic pressure may lead to dizziness, a blackout, a stroke, a heart attack, or a hernia.

- Based on the program selected, allow adequate recovery time between sets of exercises (see Table 7.5).

- If you experience unusual discomfort or pain, discontinue training. The high tension loads used in strength training can exacerbate potential injuries. Discomfort and pain are signals to stop and determine what's wrong. Be sure to evaluate your condition properly before you continue training.

- Use common sense on days when you feel fatigued or when you are performing sets to complete fatigue. Excessive fatigue affects lifting technique, body balance, muscles involved, and range of motion—all of which increase the risk for injury. A spotter is recommended when sets are performed to complete fatigue. The spotter's help through the most difficult part of the repetition will relieve undue stress on muscles, ligaments, and tendons—and help ensure that you perform the exercise correctly.

- At the end of each strength-training workout, stretch out for a few minutes to help your muscles return to their normal resting length and to minimize muscle soreness and risk for injury.

# Setting Up Your Own Strength-Training Program

The same pre-exercise guidelines outlined for cardiorespiratory endurance training apply to strength training (see Lab 1C, "Health History Questionnaire," on page 35). If you have any concerns about your present health status or ability to participate safely in strength training, consult a physician before you start. Strength training is not advised for people with advanced heart disease.

Before you proceed to write your strength-training program, you should determine your stage of change for this fitness component in Lab 7B at the end of the chapter. Next, if you are prepared to do so, and depending on the facilities available, you can choose one of the training programs outlined in this chapter (use Lab 7B). Once you begin your strength-training program, you may use the form provided in Figure 7.8 to keep a record of your training sessions.

You should base the resistance, number of repetitions, and sets you use with your program on your current strength-fitness level and the amount of time that you have for your strength workout. If you are training for reasons other than general health fitness, review Table 7.5 for a summary of the guidelines.

**FIGURE 7.7** Major muscles of the human body.

**THE MUSCULAR SYSTEM**

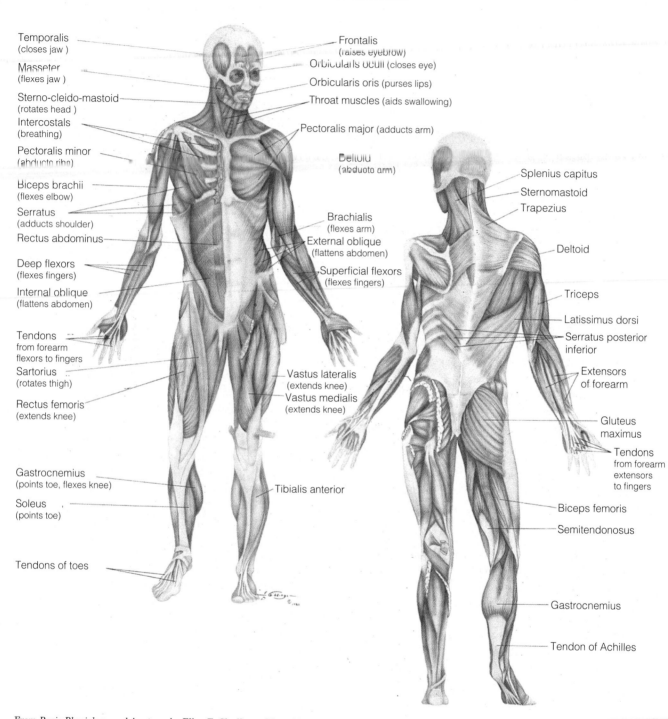

Temporalis (closes jaw )

Masseter (flexes jaw )

Sterno-cleido-mastoid (rotates head )

Intercostals (breathing)

Pectoralis minor (abducts ribs)

Biceps brachii (flexes elbow)

Serratus (adducts shoulder)

Rectus abdominus

Deep flexors (flexes fingers)

Internal oblique (flattens abdomen)

Tendons from forearm flexors to fingers

Sartorius (rotates thigh)

Rectus femoris (extends knee)

Gastrocnemius (points toe, flexes knee)

Soleus (points toe)

Tendons of toes

Frontalis (raises eyebrow)

Orbicularis oculi (closes eye)

Orbicularis oris (purses lips)

Throat muscles (aids swallowing)

Pectoralis major (adducts arm)

Deltoid (abducts arm)

Brachialis (flexes arm)

External oblique (flattens abdomen)

Superficial flexors (flexes fingers)

Vastus lateralis (extends knee)

Vastus medialis (extends knee)

Tibialis anterior

Splenius capitus

Sternomastoid

Trapezius

Deltoid

Triceps

Latissimus dorsi

Serratus posterior inferior

Extensors of forearm

Gluteus maximus

Tendons from forearm extensors to fingers

Biceps femoris

Semitendonosus

Gastrocnemius

Tendon of Achilles

From *Basic Physiology and Anatomy* by Ellen E. Chaffee and Ivan M. Lytle. Reprinted by permission of J. B. Lippincott.

FIGURE 7.8  Strength training record form.

Name

| Date | | | | | | | | | | |
|------|---|---|---|---|---|---|---|---|---|---|
| Exercise | St/Reps/Res* | St/Reps/Res* | St/Reps/Res* | St/Reps/Res* | St/Reps/Res* | St/Reps/Res* | St/Reps/Res* | St/Reps/Res* | St/Reps/Res* | St/Reps/Res* |
| | | | | | | | | | | |
| | | | | | | | | | | |
| | | | | | | | | | | |
| | | | | | | | | | | |
| | | | | | | | | | | |
| | | | | | | | | | | |
| | | | | | | | | | | |
| | | | | | | | | | | |
| | | | | | | | | | | |
| | | | | | | | | | | |
| | | | | | | | | | | |
| | | | | | | | | | | |
| | | | | | | | | | | |
| | | | | | | | | | | |
| | | | | | | | | | | |

*Sets, Repetitions, and Resistance (e.g., 1/6/125 = 1 set of 6 repetitions with 125 pounds)

# ASSESS YOUR BEHAVIOR

Log on to http://www.cengage.com/sso/ to assess your muscular strength and endurance and to track your strength activities.

1. Are your strength levels sufficient to perform tasks of daily living (climbing stairs, carrying a backpack, opening jars, doing housework, mowing the yard) without requiring additional assistance or feeling unusually fatigued?

2. Do you regularly participate in a strength-training program that includes all major muscle groups of the body, and do you perform at least one set of each exercise to near fatigue?

# ASSESS YOUR KNOWLEDGE

Log on to http://www.cengage.com/sso/ to assess your understanding of this chapter's topics by taking the Student Practice Test and exploring the modules recommended in your Personalized Study Plan.

1. The ability of a muscle to exert submaximal force repeatedly over time is known as
   a. muscular strength.
   b. plyometric training.
   c. muscular endurance.
   d. isokinetic training.
   e. isometric training.

2. In older adults, each additional pound of muscle tissue increases resting metabolism by
   a. 10 calories.
   b. 17 calories.
   c. 23 calories.
   d. 35 calories.
   e. 50 calories.

3. The Hand Grip Strength Test is an example of
   a. an isometric test.
   b. an isotonic test.
   c. a dynamic test.
   d. an isokinetic test.
   e. a plyometric test.

4. A 70th percentile rank places an individual in the _____ fitness category.
   a. excellent
   b. good
   c. average
   d. fair
   e. poor

5. During an eccentric muscle contraction,
   a. the muscle shortens as it overcomes the resistance.
   b. there is little or no movement during the contraction.
   c. a joint has to move through the entire range of motion.
   d. the muscle lengthens as it contracts.
   e. the speed is kept constant throughout the range of motion.

6. The training concept stating that the demands placed on a system must be increased systematically and progressively over time to cause physiologic adaptation is referred to as
   a. the overload principle.
   b. positive-resistance training.
   c. specificity of training.
   d. variable-resistance training.
   e. progressive resistance.

7. A set in strength training refers to
   a. the starting position for an exercise.
   b. the recovery time required between exercises.
   c. a given number of repetitions.
   d. the starting resistance used in an exercise.
   e. the sequence in which exercises are performed.

8. For health fitness, the recommendation of the American College of Sports Medicine is that a person should perform a maximum of between
   a. 1 and 6 reps.
   b. 4 and 10 reps.
   c. 8 and 12 reps.
   d. 10 and 25 reps.
   e. 20 and 30 reps.

9. Plyometric training frequently is used to help with performance in
   a. gymnastics.
   b. basketball.
   c. volleyball.
   d. sprinting.
   e. all of these sports.

10. The posterior deltoid, rhomboid, and trapezius muscles can be developed with the
    a. bench press.
    b. lat pull-down.
    c. rotary torso.
    d. squat.
    e. rowing torso.

Correct answers can be found at the back of the book.

# MEDIA MENU

You can find the links below at the book companion site: www.cengage.com/health/hoeger/plfw10e

- Chart your achievements for strength tests.
- Check how well you understand the chapter's concepts.

## Internet Connections

**Muscle and Fitness.** This comprehensive site features information on intermediate and advanced training techniques, with photographs and informative articles on the use of dietary supplements as well as the importance of mind–body activities to enhance your workout. *http://www.muscleandfitness.com/training/29*

**Strength Training Muscle Map & Explanation.** This site provides an anatomical map of the body's muscles. Click on the muscle for exercises designed to specifically strengthen that muscle, complete with a video and safety information. *http://www.global-fitness.com/strength/s_musclemap.html*

**SportSpecific.com.** Inside SportSpecific.com, you'll find more than 5,370 pages jam-packed with sports training programs, exercises, interviews, forums, and much more. The site includes sport-specific training programs, a sports nutrition section, animated sports training exercises, exercise spreadsheets for sets and reps, case studies, and a variety of articles. *http://www.sportspecific.com*

# NOTES

1. C. Castaneda, et al., "A Randomized Controlled Trial of Resistance Exercise Training to Improve Glycemic Control in Older Adults with Type 2 Diabetes," *Diabetes Care* 25 (2002): 2335–2341.

2. W. W. Campbell, M. C. Crim, V. R. Young, and W. J. Evans, "Increased Energy Requirements and Changes in Body Composition with Resistance Training in Older Adults," *American Journal of Clinical Nutrition* 60 (1994): 167–175.

3. W. J. Evans, "Exercise, Nutrition and Aging," *Journal of Nutrition* 122 (1992): 796–801.

4. P. E. Allsen, *Strength Training: Beginners, Body Builders and Athletes* (Dubuque, IA: Kendall/Hunt, 2003).

5. See note 2.

6. American College of Sports Medicine, "Progression Models in Resistance Training for Healthy Adults," *Medicine and Science in Sports and Exercise* 34 (2002): 364–380.

7. J. K. Kraemer and N. A. Ratamess, "Fundamentals of Resistance Training: Progression and Exercise Prescription," *Medicine and Science in Sports and Exercise* 36 (2004): 674–688.

8. B. M. Hather, P. A. Tesch, P. Buchanan, and G. A. Dudley, "Influence of Eccentric Actions on Skeletal Muscle Adaptations to Resistance Training," *Acta Physiologica Scandinavica* 143 (1991): 177–185; C. B. Ebbeling and P. M. Clarkson, "Exercise-Induced Muscle Damage and Adaptation," *Sports Medicine* 7 (1989): 207–234.

9. S. P. Messier and M. Dill, "Alterations in Strength and Maximal Oxygen Uptake Consequent to Nautilus Circuit Weight Training," *Research Quarterly for Exercise and Sport* 56 (1985): 345–351; T. V. Pipes, "Variable Resistance Versus Constant Resistance Strength Training in Adult Males," *European Journal of Applied Physiology* 39 (1978): 27–35.

10. W. W. K. Hoeger, D. R. Hopkins, S. L. Barette, and D. F. Hale, "Relationship Between Repetitions and Selected Percentages of One Repetition Maximum: A Comparison Between Untrained and Trained Males and Females," *Journal of Applied Sport Science Research* 4, no. 2 (1990): 47–51.

11. American College of Sports Medicine, *ACSM's Guidelines for Exercise Testing and Prescription* (Baltimore: Williams & Wilkins, 2006).

12. See note 11.

13. W. J. Kraemer and M. S. Fragala, "Personalize It: Program Design in Resistance Training," *ACSM's Health and Fitness Journal* 10, no. 4 (2006): 7–17.

14. See note 6.

15. See note 6.

16. Gatorade Sports Science Institute, "Core Strength Training," *Sports Science Exchange Roundtable* 13, no. 1 (2002): 1–4.

# SUGGESTED READINGS

American College of Sports Medicine. "Progression Models in Resistance Training for Healthy Adults." *Medicine and Science in Sports and Exercise* 34 (2002): 364–380.

Hesson, J. L. *Weight Training for Life*. Belmont, CA: Wadsworth/Cengage, 2007.

Heyward, V. H. *Advanced Fitness Assessment and Exercise Prescription*. Champaign, IL: Human Kinetics Press, 2006.

Hoeger, W. W. K., and S. A. Hoeger. *Lifetime Physical Fitness and Wellness: A Personalized Program*. Belmont, CA: Thomson/Wadsworth, 2009.

Kraemer, J. K., and N. A. Ratamess. "Fundamentals of Resistance Training: Progression and Exercise Prescription." *Medicine and Science in Sports and Exercise* 36 (2004): 674–688.

Kraemer, W. J., and S. J. Fleck. *Optimizing Strength Training*. Champaign, IL: Human Kinetic Press, 2007.

Liemohn, W., and G. Pariser. "Core Strength: Implications for Fitness and Low Back Pain." *ACSM's Health and Fitness Journal* 6, no. 5 (2002): 10–16.

Volek, J. "Influence of Nutrition on Responses to Resistance Training." *Medicine and Science in Sports and Exercise* 36 (2004): 689–696.

# Strength-Training Exercises without Weights

## EXERCISE 1   Step Up

ACTION Step up and down using a box or chair approximately 12 to 15 inches high (a). Conduct one set using the same leg each time you step up, and then conduct a second set using the other leg. You also could alternate legs on each step-up cycle. You may increase the resistance by holding an object in your arms (b). Hold the object close to the body to avoid increased strain in the lower back.

MUSCLES DEVELOPED Gluteal muscles, quadriceps, gastrocnemius, and soleus

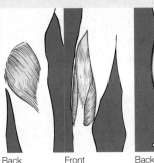

Back    Front    Back

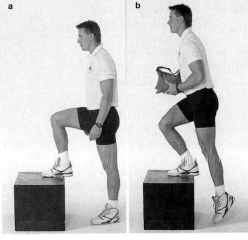

a    b

Photos © Fitness & Wellness, Inc.

## EXERCISE 2   Rowing Torso

ACTION Raise your arms laterally (abduction) to a horizontal position and bend your elbows to 90°. Have a partner apply enough pressure on your elbows to gradually force your arms forward (horizontal flexion) while you try to resist the pressure. Next, reverse the action, horizontally forcing the arms backward as your partner applies sufficient forward pressure to create resistance.

MUSCLES DEVELOPED Posterior deltoid, rhomboids, and trapezius

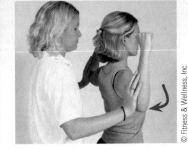

Back

© Fitness & Wellness, Inc.

## EXERCISE 3   Push Up

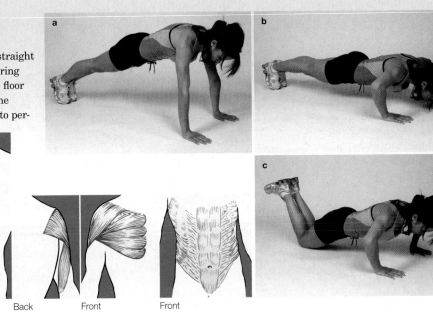

a    b    c

ACTION Maintaining your body as straight as possible (a), flex the elbows, lowering the body until you almost touch the floor (b), then raise yourself back up to the starting position. If you are unable to perform the push-up as indicated, decrease the resistance by supporting the lower body with the knees rather than the feet (c).

MUSCLES DEVELOPED Triceps, deltoid, pectoralis major, abdominals, and erector spinae

Back    Back    Front    Front

Photos © Fitness & Wellness, Inc.

# EXERCISE 4  Abdominal Crunch and Bent-Leg Curl-Up

**ACTION** Start with your head and shoulders off the floor, arms crossed on your chest, and knees slightly bent (a). The greater the flexion of the knee, the more difficult the curl-up. Now curl up to about 30° (abdominal crunch—illustration b) or curl up all the way (abdominal curl-up—illustration c), then return to the starting position without letting the head or shoulders touch the floor or allowing the hips to come off the floor. If you allow the hips to raise off the floor and the head and shoulders to touch the floor, you most likely will "swing up" on the next crunch or curl-up, which minimizes the work of the abdominal muscles. If you cannot curl up with the arms on the chest, place the hands by the side of the hips or even help yourself up by holding on to your thighs (d and e). Do not perform the sit-up exercise with your legs completely extended, because this will strain the lower back. For additional resistance during the abdominal crunch, have a partner add slight resistance to your shoulders as you "crunch up" (f).

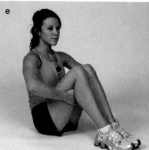

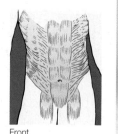

**MUSCLES DEVELOPED**
Abdominal muscles and hip flexors

Front

**NOTE:** The abdominal curl-up exercise should be used only by individuals of at least average fitness without a history of lower back problems. New participants and those with a history of lower-back problems should use the abdominal crunch exercise in its place.

Photos © Fitness & Wellness, Inc.

# EXERCISE 5  Leg Curl

**ACTION** Lie on the floor face down. Cross the right ankle over the left heel (a). Apply resistance with your right foot while you bring the left foot up to 90° at the knee joint (b). Apply enough resistance so the left foot can only be brought up slowly. Repeat the exercise, crossing the left ankle over the right heel.

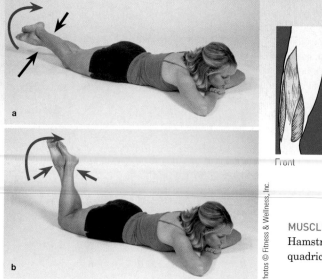

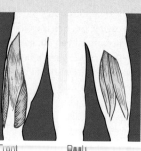

Front   Back

Photos © Fitness & Wellness, Inc.

**MUSCLES DEVELOPED**
Hamstrings (and quadriceps)

# EXERCISE 6 Modified Dip

ACTION Using a gymnasium bleacher or box and with the help of a partner, dip down at least to a 90° angle at the elbow joint and then return to the initial position.

MUSCLES DEVELOPED Triceps, deltoid, and pectoralis major

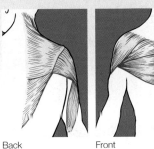

Back        Front

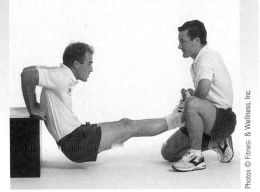

# EXERCISE 7 Pull-Up

ACTION Suspend yourself from a bar with a pronated (thumbs-in) grip (a). Pull your body up until your chin is above the bar (b), then lower the body slowly to the starting position. If you are unable to perform the pull-up as described, either have a partner hold your feet to push off and facilitate the movement upward (c and d).

MUSCLES DEVELOPED
Biceps, brachioradialis, brachialis, trapezius, and latissimus dorsi

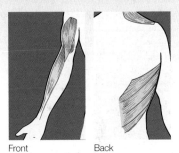

Front        Back

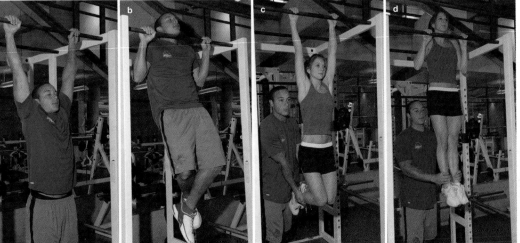

# EXERCISE 8    Arm Curl

**ACTION** Using a palms-up grip, start with the arm completely extended and, with the aid of a sandbag or bucket filled (as needed) with sand or rocks (a), curl up as far as possible (b), then return to the initial position. Repeat the exercise with the other arm.

**MUSCLES DEVELOPED** Biceps, brachioradialis, and brachialis

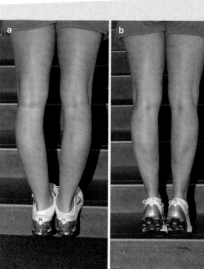

Front

# EXERCISE 9    Heel Raise

**ACTION** From a standing position with feet flat on the floor or at the edge of a step (a), raise and lower your body weight by moving at the ankle joint only (b). For added resistance, have someone else hold your shoulders down as you perform the exercise.

**MUSCLES DEVELOPED** Gastrocnemius and soleus

Back

# EXERCISE 10    Leg Abduction and Adduction

**ACTION** Both participants sit on the floor. The person on the left places the feet on the inside of the other person's feet. Simultaneously, the person on the left presses the legs laterally (to the outside—abduction), while the person on the right presses the legs medially (adduction). Hold the contraction for 5 to 10 seconds. Repeat the exercise at all three angles, and then reverse the pressing sequence: The person on the left places the feet on the outside and presses inward while the person on the right presses outward.

**MUSCLES DEVELOPED** Hip abductors (rectus femoris, sartori, gluteus medius and minimus) and adductors (pectineus, gracilis, adductor magnus, adductor longus, and adductor brevis)

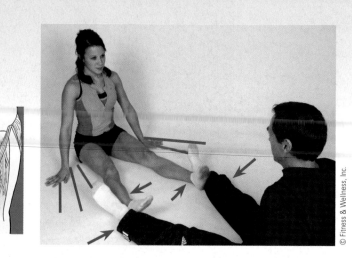

Back

## EXERCISE 11    Reverse Crunch

**ACTION** Lie on your back with arms to the sides and knees and hips flexed at 90° (a). Now attempt to raise the pelvis off the floor by lifting vertically from the knees and lower legs (b). This is a challenging exercise that may be difficult for beginners to perform.

**MUSCLES DEVELOPED** Abdominals

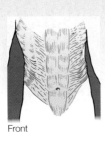

Front

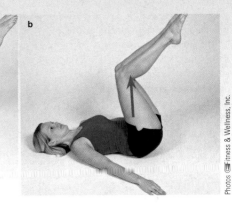

## EXERCISE 12    Pelvic Tilt

**ACTION** Lie flat on the floor with the knees bent at about a 90° angle (a). Tilt the pelvis by tightening the abdominal muscles, flattening your back against the floor, and raising the lower gluteal area ever so slightly off the floor (b). Hold the final position for several seconds.

**AREAS STRETCHED** Low back muscles and ligaments

**AREAS STRENGTHENED** Abdominal and gluteal muscles

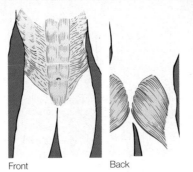

Front        Back

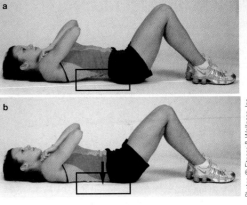

## EXERCISE 13    Lateral Bridge

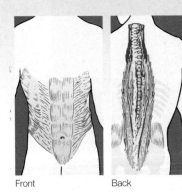

Front        Back

**MUSCLES DEVELOPED** Abdominals (obliques and transversus abdominus) and quadratus lumborum (lower back)

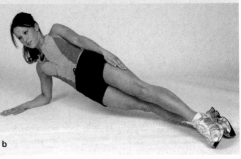

**ACTION** Lie on your side with legs bent (a: easier version) or straight (b: harder version) and support the upper body with your arm. Straighten your body by raising the hip off the floor and hold the position for several seconds. Repeat the exercise with the other side of the body.

## EXERCISE 14  Prone Bridge

**ACTION** Starting in a prone position on a floor mat, balance yourself on the tips of your toes and elbows while attempting to maintain a straight body from heels to shoulders (do not arch the lower back). You can increase the difficulty of this exercise by placing your hands in front of you and straightening the arms (elbows off the floor).

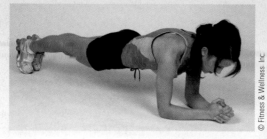

**MUSCLES DEVELOPED** Anterior and posterior muscle groups of the trunk and pelvis

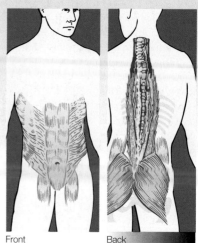

© Fitness & Wellness, Inc

Front          Back

# Strength-Training Exercises with Weights

## EXERCISE 15  Bench (Chest) Press

**MUSCLES DEVELOPED** Pectoralis major, triceps, and deltoid

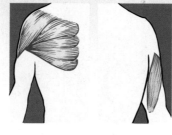

**MACHINE** From a seated position, grasp the bar handles (a) and press forward until the arms are completely extended (b), then return to the original position. Do not arch the back during this exercise.

**FREE WEIGHTS** Lie on the bench with arms extended and have one or two spotters help you place the barbell directly over your shoulders (a). Lower the weight to your chest (b) and then push it back up until you achieve full extension of the arms. Do not arch the back during this exercise.

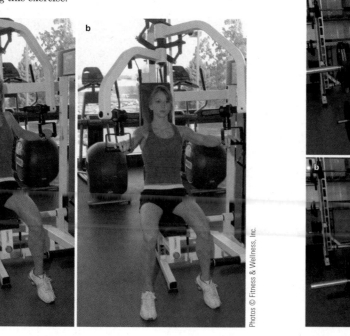

a          b

Photos © Fitness & Wellness, Inc.

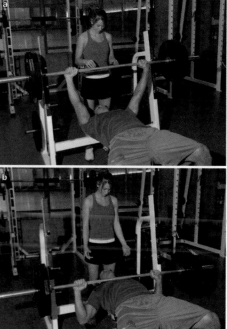

Photos © Fitness & Wellness, Inc.

## EXERCISE 16  Leg Press

**ACTION** From a sitting position with the knees flexed at about 90° and both feet on the footrest (a), extend the legs fully (b), then return slowly to the starting position.

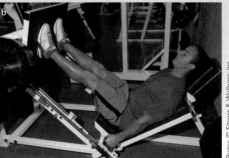

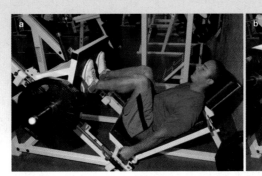

MUSCLES DEVELOPED
Quadriceps and gluteal muscles

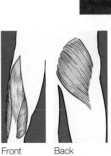

Front    Back

Photos © Fitness & Wellness, Inc.

## EXERCISE 17  Abdominal Crunch

**ACTION** Sit in an upright position. Grasp the handles in front of you and crunch forward. Return slowly to the original position.

MUSCLES DEVELOPED  Abdominals

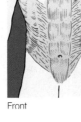

Front

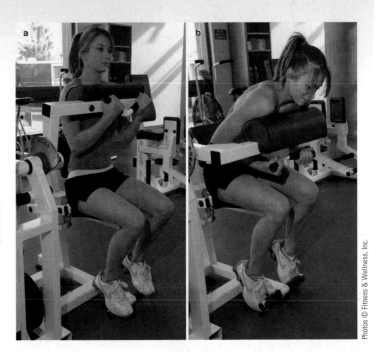

Photos © Fitness & Wellness, Inc.

# EXERCISE 18   Rowing Torso

**ACTION** Sit in the machine and grasp the handles in front of you (a). Press back as far as possible, drawing the shoulder blades together (b). Return to the original position.

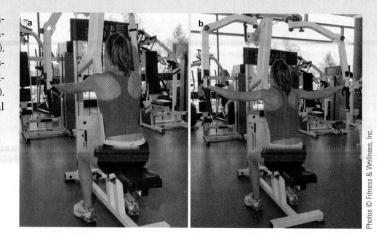

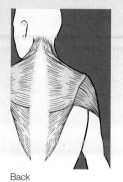

Back

**MUSCLES DEVELOPED**
Posterior deltoid, rhomboids, and trapezius

## Bent-Over Lateral Raise

**ACTION** Bend over with your back straight and knees bent at about 5 to 10° (a). Hold one dumbbell in each hand. Raise the dumbbells laterally to about shoulder level (b) and then slowly return them to the starting position.

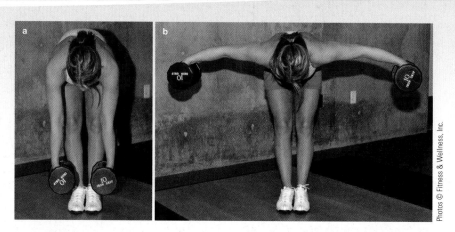

# EXERCISE 19   Leg Curl

**ACTION** Lie face down on the bench, legs straight, and place the back of the feet under the padded bar (a). Curl up to at least 90° (b), and return to the original position.

**MUSCLES DEVELOPED**
Hamstrings

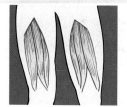

Back

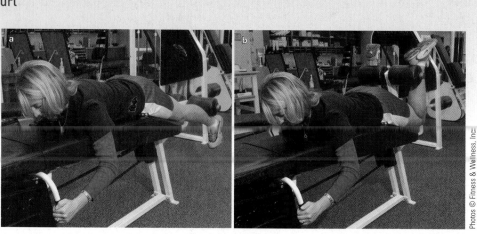

Photos © Fitness & Wellness, Inc.

## EXERCISE 20  Seated Back

ACTION Sit in the machine with your trunk flexed and the upper back against the shoulder pad. Place the feet under the padded bar and hold on with your hands to the bars on the sides (a). Start the exercise by pressing backward, simultaneously extending the trunk and hip joints (b). Slowly return to the original position.

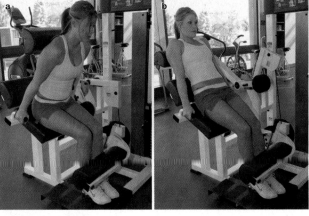

MUSCLES DEVELOPED Erector spinae and gluteus maximus

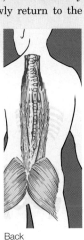

Back

## EXERCISE 21  Calf Press

FREE WEIGHTS In a standing position, place a barbell across the shoulders and upper back. Grip the bar by the shoulders (a). Raise your heels off the floor or step box as far as possible (b) and then slowly return them to the starting position.

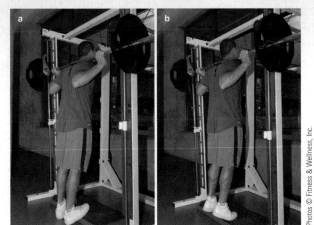

MACHINE Start with your feet flat on the plate (a). Now extend the ankles by pressing on the plate with the balls of your feet (b).

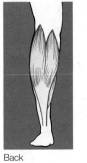

Back

MUSCLES DEVELOPED
Gastrocnemius, soleus

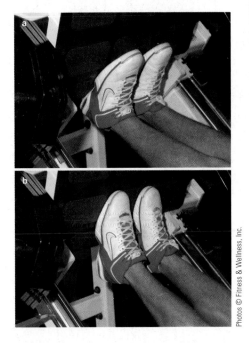

## EXERCISE 22    Leg (Hip) Adduction

ACTION Adjust the pads on the inside of the thighs as far out as the desired range of motion to be accomplished during the exercise (a). Press the legs together until both pads meet at the center (b). Slowly return to the starting position.

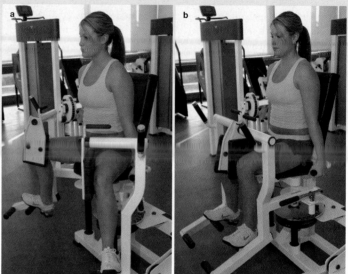

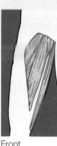

MUSCLES DEVELOPED Hip adductors (pectineus, gracilis, adductor magnus, adductor longus, and adductor brevis)

Front

Photos © Fitness & Wellness, Inc.

## EXERCISE 23    Leg (Hip) Abduction

ACTION Place your knees together with the pads directly outside the knees (a). Press the legs laterally out as far as possible (b). Slowly return to the starting position.

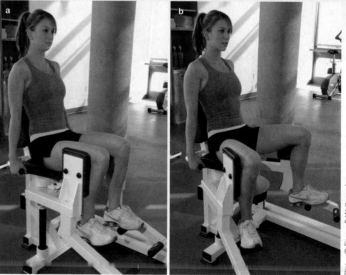

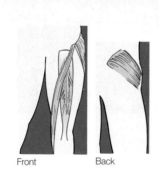

MUSCLES DEVELOPED
Hip abductors (rectus femoris, sartori, gluteus medius and minimus)

Front          Back

Photos © Fitness & Wellness, Inc.

## EXERCISE 24    Lat Pull-Down

ACTION Starting from a sitting position, hold the exercise bar with a wide grip (a). Pull the bar down in front of you until it reaches the upper chest (b), then return to the starting position.

MUSCLES DEVELOPED Latissimus dorsi, pectoralis major, and biceps

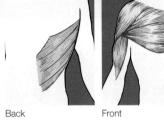

Back          Front

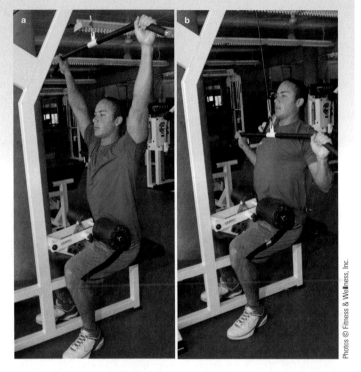

Photos © Fitness & Wellness, Inc.

## EXERCISE 25    Rotary Torso

MACHINE Sit upright in the machine and place the elbows behind the padded bars. Rotate the torso as far as possible to one side and then return slowly to the starting position. Repeat the exercise to the opposite side.

MUSCLES DEVELOPED Internal and external obliques (abdominal muscles)

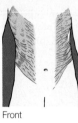

Front

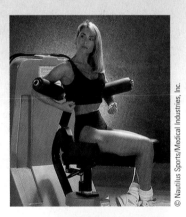

© Nautilus Sports/Medical Industries, Inc.

FREE WEIGHTS Stand with your feet slightly apart. Place a barbell across your shoulders and upper back, holding on to the sides of the barbell. Now gently, and in a controlled manner, twist your torso to one side as far as possible and then do so in the opposite direction.

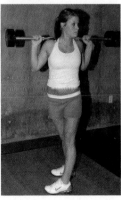

© Fitness & Wellness, Inc.

## EXERCISE 26  Triceps Extension

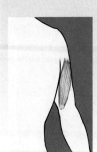

**MUSCLES DEVELOPED** Triceps

Back

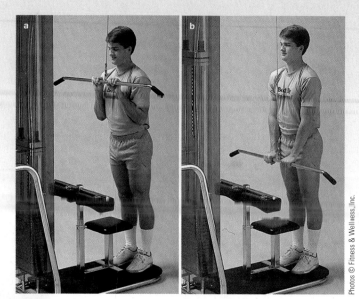

Photos © Fitness & Wellness, Inc.

**MACHINE** Sit in an upright position and grasp the bar behind the shoulders (a). Fully extend the arms (b) and then return to the original position.

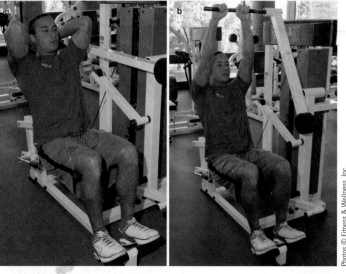

Photos © Fitness & Wellness, Inc.

**MACHINE** Using a palms-down grip, grasp the bar slightly closer than shoulder-width and start with the elbows almost completely bent (a). Extend the arms fully (b), then return to starting position.

**FREE WEIGHTS** In a standing position, hold a barbell with both hands overhead and with the arms in full extension (a). Slowly lower the barbell behind your head (b) and then return it to the starting position.

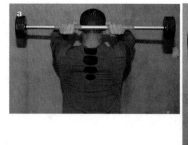

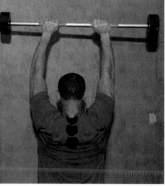

Photos © Fitness & Wellness, Inc.

## EXERCISE 27 Arm Curl

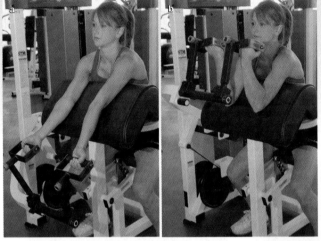

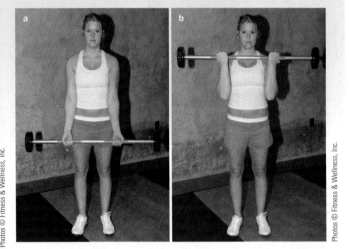

Photos © Fitness & Wellness, Inc.

**MACHINE** Using a supinated (palms-up) grip, start with the arms almost completely extended (a). Curl up as far as possible (b), then return to the starting position.

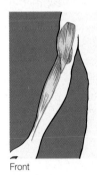

Front

**MUSCLES DEVELOPED** Biceps, brachioradialis, and brachialis

**FREE WEIGHTS** Standing upright, hold a barbell in front of you at about shoulder width with arms extended and the hands in a thumbs-out position (supinated grip) (a). Raise the barbell to your shoulders (b) and slowly return it to the starting position.

## EXERCISE 28 Leg Extension

**ACTION** Sit in an upright position with the feet under the padded bar and grasp the handles at the sides (a). Extend the legs until they are completely straight (b), then return to the starting position.

**MUSCLES DEVELOPED** Quadriceps

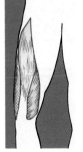

Front

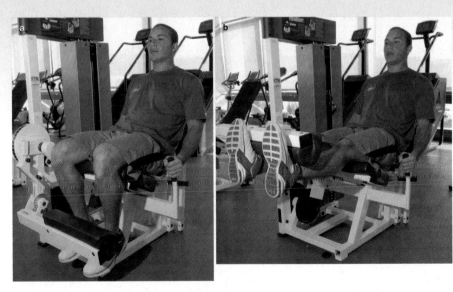

Photos © Fitness & Wellness, Inc.

## EXERCISE 29 Shoulder Press

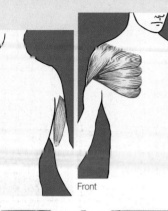

Front

Back

MUSCLES DEVELOPED Triceps, deltoid, and pectoralis major

MACHINE Sit in an upright position and grasp the bar wider than shoulder width (a). Press the bar all the way up until the arms are fully extended (b), then return to the initial position.

FREE WEIGHTS Place a barbell on your shoulders in front of the body (a) and press the weight overhead until complete extension of the arms is achieved (b). Return the weight to the original position. Be sure not to arch the back or lean back during this exercise.

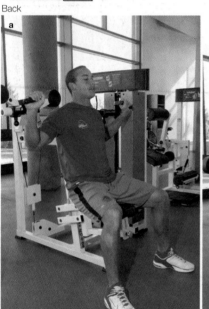

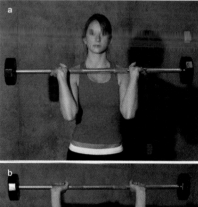

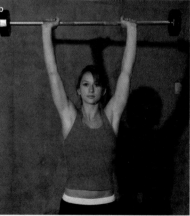

Photos © Fitness & Wellness, Inc.

## EXERCISE 30  Chest Press

ACTION Start with the arms out to the side, and grasp the handle bars with the arms straight (a). Press the movement arms forward until they are completely in front of you (b). Slowly return to the starting position.

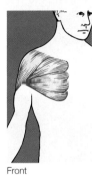

**MUSCLES DEVELOPED**
Pectoralis major and deltoid

Front

**Bent-Arm Flyes**

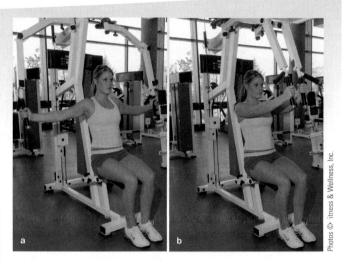

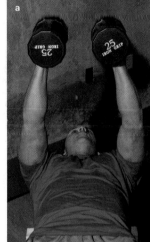

ACTION Lie down on your back on a bench and hold a dumbbell in each hand directly overhead (a). Keeping your elbows slightly bent, lower the weights laterally to a horizontal position (b) and then bring them back up to the starting position.

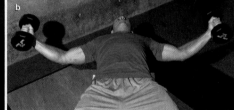

*Photos © Fitness & Wellness, Inc.*

## EXERCISE 31  Squat

**MUSCLES DEVELOPED**
Quadriceps, gluteus maximus, erector spinae

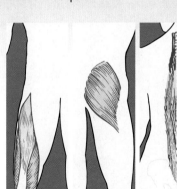

Front     Back     Back

FREE WEIGHTS From a standing position, and with a spotter to each side, support a barbell over your shoulders and upper back (a). Keeping your head up and back straight, bend at the knees and the hips until you achieve an approximate 120° angle at the knees (b). Return to the starting position. *Do not perform this exercise alone.* If no spotters are available, use a squat rack to ensure that you will not get trapped under a heavy weight.

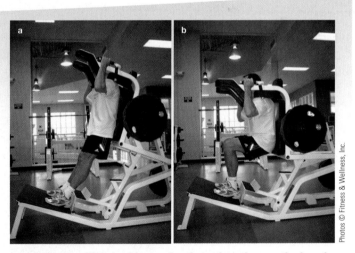

MACHINE Place the shoulders under the pads and grasp the bars by the sides of the shoulders (a). Slowly bend the knees to between 90° and 120° (b). Return to the starting position.

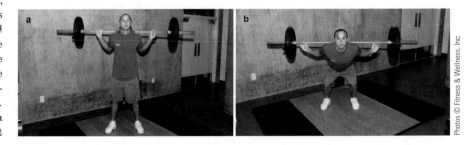

*Photos © Fitness & Wellness, Inc.*

# EXERCISE 32  Upright Rowing

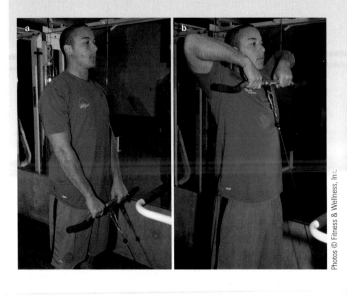

**FREE WEIGHTS** Hold a barbell in front of you, with the arms fully extended and hands in a thumbs-in (pronated) grip less than shoulder-width apart (a). Pull the barbell up until it reaches shoulder level (b) and then slowly return it to the starting position.

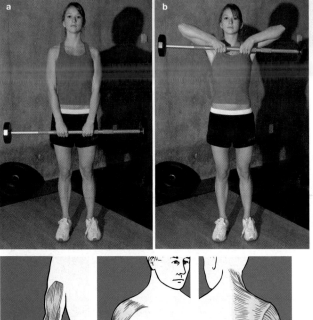

Photos © Fitness & Wellness, Inc.

**MACHINE** Start with the arms extended and grip the handles with the palms down (a). Pull all the way up to the chin (b), then return to the starting position.

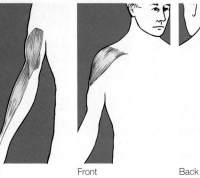

Front    Front    Back

**MUSCLES DEVELOPED** Biceps, brachioradialis, brachialis, deltoid, and trapezius

# EXERCISE 33  Seated Leg Curl

**ACTION** Sit in the unit and place the strap over the upper thighs. With legs extended, place the back of the feet over the padded rollers (a). Flex the knees until you reach a 90° to 100° angle (b). Slowly return to the starting position.

**MUSCLES DEVELOPED** Hamstrings

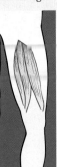

Back

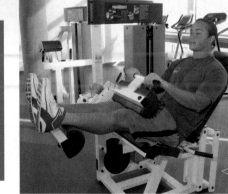

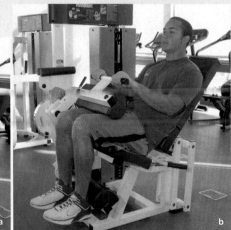

Photos © Fitness & Wellness, Inc.

## EXERCISE 34   Bent-Arm Pullover

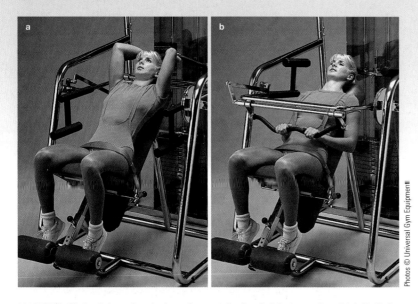

**FREE WEIGHTS** Lie on your back on an exercise bench with your head over the edge of the bench. Hold a barbell over your chest with the hands less than shoulder-width apart (a). Keeping the elbows shoulder-width apart, lower the weight over your head until your shoulders are completely extended (b). Slowly return the weight to the starting position.

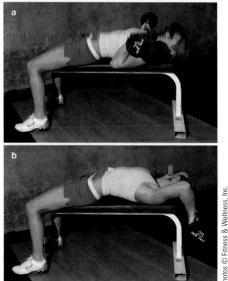

Photos © Universal Gym Equipment

**MACHINE** Sit back into the chair and grasp the bar behind your head (a). Pull the bar over your head all the way down to your abdomen (b) and slowly return to the original position.

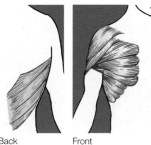

Back          Front

**MUSCLES DEVELOPED** Latissimus dorsi, pectoral muscles, deltoid, and serratus anterior

Photos © Fitness & Wellness, Inc.

## EXERCISE 35   Dip

**ACTION** Start with the elbows flexed (a), then extend the arms fully (b), and return slowly to the initial position.

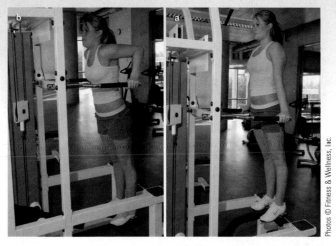

Photos © Fitness & Wellness, Inc.

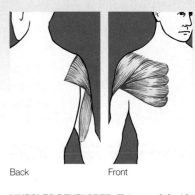

Back          Front

**MUSCLES DEVELOPED** Triceps, deltoid, and pectoralis major

## EXERCISE 36   Back Extension

ACTION Place your feet under the ankle rollers and the hips over the padded seat. Start with the trunk in a flexed position and the arms crossed over the chest (a). Slowly extend the trunk to a horizontal position (b), hold the extension for 2 to 5 seconds, then slowly flex (lower) the trunk to the original position.

MUSCLES DEVELOPED Erector spinae, gluteus maximus, and quadratus lumborum (lower back)

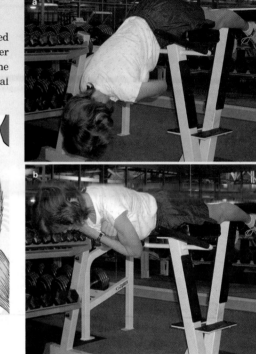

Back

Photos © Fitness & Wellness, Inc.

## EXERCISE 37   Lateral Trunk Flexion

ACTION Lie sideways on the padded seat with the right foot under the right side of the padded ankle pad (right knee slightly bent) and the left foot stabilized on the vertical bar. Cross the arms over the abdomen or chest and start with the body in a straight line. Raise (flex) your upper body about 30 to 40° and then slowly return to the starting position.

MUSCLES DEVELOPED Erector spinae, rectus abdominus, internal and external abdominal obliques, quadratus lumborum, gluteal muscles

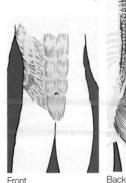

Front                Back

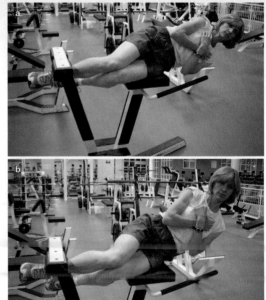

Photos © Fitness & Wellness, Inc.

# Stability Ball Exercises

## EXERCISE 38   The Plank

ACTION  Place your knees or feet (increased difficulty) on the ball and raise your body off the floor to a horizontal position. Pull the abdominal muscles in and hold the body in a straight line for 5 to 10 seconds. Repeat the exercise 3 to 5 times.

MUSCLES INVOLVED  Abdominals, erector spinae, lower back, hip flexors, gluteal, quadriceps, hamstrings, chest, shoulder, and triceps

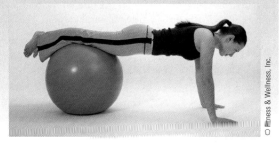

## EXERCISE 39   Abdominal Crunches

ACTION  On your back and with the feet slightly separated, lie with the ball under your back and shoulder blades. Cross the arms over your chest (a). Press your lower back into the ball and crunch up 20 to 30°. Keep your neck and shoulders in line with your trunk (b). Repeat the exercise 10 to 20 times (you may also do an oblique crunch by rotating the ribcage to the opposite hip at the end of the crunch [c]).

MUSCLES INVOLVED  Rectus abdominus, internal and external abdominal obliques

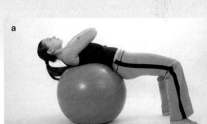

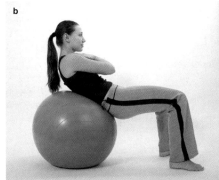

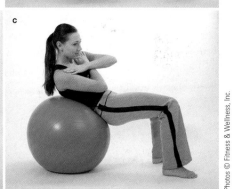

## EXERCISE 40   Supine Bridge

ACTION  With the feet slightly separated and knees bent, lie with your neck and upper back on the ball; hands placed on the abdomen. Gently squeeze the gluteal muscles while raising your hips off the floor until the upper legs and trunk reach a straight line. Hold this position for 5 to 10 seconds. Repeat the exercise 3 to 5 times.

MUSCLES INVOLVED  Gluteal, abdominals, lower back, hip flexors, quadriceps, and hamstrings

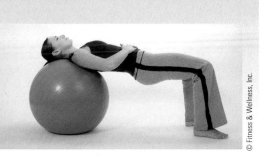

# EXERCISE 41  Reverse Supine Bridge

ACTION Lie face up on the floor with the heels on the ball. Keeping the abdominal muscles tight, slowly lift the hips off the floor and squeeze the gluteal muscles until the body reaches a straight line. Hold the position for 5 to 10 seconds. Repeat the exercise 3 to 5 times.

MUSCLES INVOLVED Gluteal, abdominals, lower back, erector spinae, hip flexors, quadriceps, and hamstrings

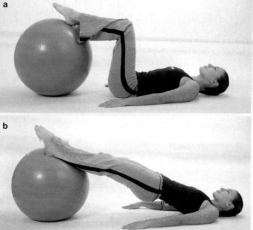

Photos © Fitness & Wellness, Inc.

# EXERCISE 42  Push-Ups

ACTION Place the front of your thighs (knees or feet–more difficult) over the ball with the body straight, the arms extended, and the hands under your shoulders. Now bend the elbows and lower the upper body as far as possible. Return to the original position. Repeat the exercise 10 times.

MUSCLES INVOLVED Triceps, chest, shoulder, abdominals, erector spinae, lower back, hip flexors, quadriceps, and hamstrings

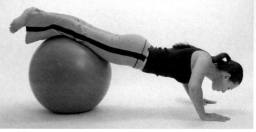

© Fitness & Wellness, Inc.

## EXERCISE 43   Back Extension

ACTION Lie face down with the hips over the ball. Keep the legs straight with the toes on the floor and slightly separated (a). Keep your arms to the sides and extend the trunk until the body reaches a straight position (b). Repeat the exercise 10 times.

MUSCLES INVOLVED Erector spinae, abdominals, and lower back

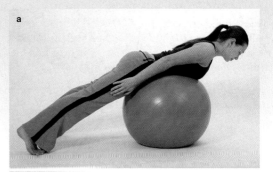
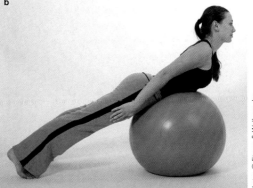

Photos © Fitness & Wellness, Inc.

## EXERCISE 44   Wall Squat

ACTION Stand upright and position the ball between your lower back and a wall. Place your feet slightly in front of you, about a foot apart (a). Lean into the ball and lower your body by bending the knees until the thighs are parallel to the ground (b) (to avoid excessive strain on the knees, it is not recommended that you go beyond this point). Return to the starting position. Repeat the exercise 10 to 20 times.

MUSCLES INVOLVED Quadriceps, hip flexors, hamstrings, abdominals, erector spinae, lower back, gastrocnemius, and soleus

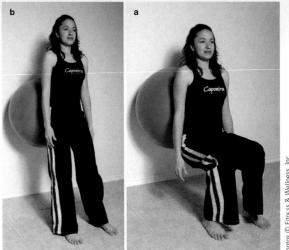

Photos © Fitness & Wellness, Inc.

## EXERCISE 45    Jackknives

ACTION  Lie face down with the hips on the ball and walk forward with your hands until the thighs are over the ball. Keep the arms fully extended, hands on floor, and the body straight (a). Now, pull the ball forward with your legs by bending at the knees and raising your hips while keeping the abdominal muscles tight (b). Repeat the exercise 10 times.

MUSCLES INVOLVED  Hip flexors, abdominals, erector spinae, lower back, quadriceps, hamstrings, chest, and shoulder

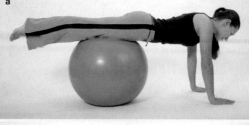

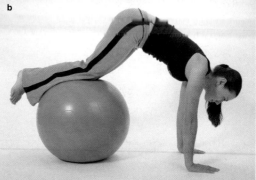

## EXERCISE 46    Hamstring Roll

ACTION  Lie on your back with your knees bent and the heels on the ball. Raise your hips off the floor, while keeping the knees bent (a). Tighten the abdominal muscles and roll the ball out with your feet to extend the legs (b). Now roll the ball back into the original position. Repeat the exercise 10 times.

MUSCLES INVOLVED  Hamstrings, abdominals, erector spinae, lower back, hip flexors, quadriceps, and chest

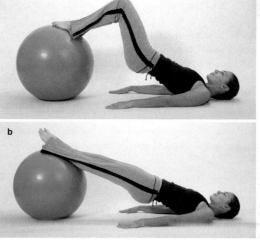

Photos © Fitness & Wellness, Inc.

# LAB 7A: Muscular Strength and Endurance Assessment

Name _____  Date _____  Grade _____

Instructor _____  Course _____  Section _____

### Necessary Lab Equipment
A Lafayette hand grip dynamometer model 78010 is recommended for the Hand Grip Test. A metronome, gymnasium bleachers, and a stopwatch are needed for the Muscular Endurance Test. A metronome is also needed for the Muscular Strength and Endurance Test.

### Objective
To determine muscular strength and/or endurance and the respective fitness classification.

### Lab Preparation
Wear exercise clothing and avoid strenuous strength training 48 hours prior to this lab.

### I. Hand Grip Strength Test
The instructions for the Hand Grip Strength Test are provided in Figure 7.2, page 240. Perform the test according to the instructions and look up your results in Table 7.1, page 241.

Hand used: _____ Right _____ Left

Reading: _____ lbs.

Fitness category (see Figure 7.2, page 240): _____

### II. Muscular Endurance Test
Conduct this test using the guidelines provided in Figure 7.3 and Table 7.2, pages 242–243. Record your repetitions, fitness category, and points in the spaces provided below.

| Exercise | Metronome Cadence | Repetitions | Fitness Category | Points |
|---|---|---|---|---|
| Bench jumps | none | | | |
| Modified dips — men only | 56 bpm | | | |
| Modified push-ups — women only | 56 bpm | | | |
| Bent-leg curl-ups | 40 bpm | | | |
| Abdominal crunches | 60 bpm | | | |
| | | | Total Points: | |

Overall muscular endurance fitness category (see Figure 7.3, pages 242–243): _____

## III. Muscular Strength and Endurance Test

Perform the Muscular Strength and Endurance Test according to the procedure outlined in Figure 7.4, page 244. Record the results, fitness category, and points in the appropriate blanks provided below.

Body weight: _____ lbs.

| Lift | Percent of Body Weight (pounds) | | Resistance | Repetitions |
|------|------|------|------|------|
| | Men | Women | | |
| Lat pull-down | .70 | .45 | | |
| Leg extension | .65 | .50 | | |
| Bench press | .75 | .45 | | |
| Bent-leg curl-up or abdominal crunch | NA* | NA* | | |
| Leg curl | .32 | .25 | | |
| Arm curl | .35 | .18 | | |

*Not applicable—no resistance required. Use test described in Figure 7.3, pages 242–243.

## IV. Muscular Strength and Endurance Goals

Indicate the muscular strength/endurance category that you would like to achieve by the end of the term: [          ]

Briefly state your feelings about your current strength level and indicate how you are planning to achieve your strength objective:

_____

_____

_____

_____

_____

_____

_____

_____

_____

_____

_____

_____

_____

_____

# LAB 7B: Strength-Training Program

Name _____ Date _____ Grade _____

Instructor _____ Course _____ Section _____

## Necessary Lab Equipment

Free weights, strength-training machines, or no equipment if the "Strength-Training Exercises without Weights" program is selected.

## Objective

To develop your personal strength-training exercise program.

## Lab Preparation

Wear exercise clothing and prepare to participate in a sample strength-training exercise session. All of the strength-training exercises are illustrated on pages 261–278.

## I. Stage of Change for Muscular Strength or Endurance

Using Figure 2.5 (page 57) and Table 2.3 (page 57), identify your current stage of change for participation in a muscular strength or muscular endurance program:

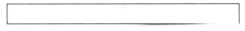

## II. Instructions

Select one of the two strength-training exercise programs. Perform all of the recommended exercises and, with the exception of the abdominal curl-up exercises, determine the resistance required to do approximately 10 repetitions maximum. For "Strength-Training Exercises without Weights," simply indicate the total number of repetitions performed. For the abdominal crunches or curl-up exercises, perform or build up to about 20 repetitions.

**1. Strength-Training Exercises without Weights**

| Exercise | Repetitions |
|---|---|
| Step-up | |
| Rowing torso | |
| Push-up | |
| Abdominal curl-up or abdominal crunch | |
| Leg curl | |
| Modified dip | |
| Pull-up or arm curl | |
| Heel raise | |
| Leg abduction and adduction | |
| Reverse crunch | |
| Pelvic tilt | |
| Lateral bridge | |
| Prone bridge | |

**2. Strength-Training Exercises with Weights**

| Exercise | Repetitions | Resistance |
|---|---|---|
| Bench press, shoulder press, or chest press (select and circle one) | | |
| Leg press or squat (select one) | | |
| Abdominal curl-up or abdominal crunch (select one) | | N/A |
| Rowing torso | | |
| Arm curl or upright rowing (select one) | | |
| Leg curl or seated leg curl (select one) | | |
| Seated back or back extension (select one) | | |
| Calf press | | |
| Hip adduction | | |
| Hip abduction | | |
| Lat pull-down or bent-arm pullover (select one) | | |
| Rotary torso | | |
| Triceps extension or dip (select one) | | |
| Leg extension | | |
| Lateral trunk flexion | | |

### 3. Stability Ball Exercises

| Exercise | Length of Hold (if applicable) | Reptitions |
|---|---|---|
| The plank | | |
| Abdominal crunches | | |
| Supine bridge or reverse supine bridge | | N/A |
| Push-ups | | |
| Back extension | | |
| Wall squats | | |
| Jackknives | | |
| Hamstring roll | | |
| Lateral trunk flexion | | |

## III. Your Personalized Strength-Training Program

Once you have performed the strength-training exercises in this lab, and depending on your personal preference (strength versus endurance), design your strength-training program selecting a minimum of 8 to 10 exercises. Indicate the number of sets, repetitions, and approximate resistance that you will use. Also state the days of the week, time, and facility that will be used for this program.

Strength-training days: M ☐ T ☐ W ☐ Th ☐ F ☐ Sa ☐ Su ☐ Time of day: ☐ Facility: ☐

| | Exercise | Sets / Reps / Resistance | | Exercise | Sets / Reps / Resistance |
|---|---|---|---|---|---|
| 1. | | | 9. | | |
| 2. | | | 10. | | |
| 3. | | | 11. | | |
| 4. | | | 12. | | |
| 5. | | | 13. | | |
| 6. | | | 14. | | |
| 7. | | | 15. | | |
| 8. | | | 16. | | |

# Muscular Flexibility

# 8

© Fitness & Wellness, Inc.

## Objectives

- Explain the importance of muscular flexibility to adequate fitness and preventive health care
- Identify the factors that affect muscular flexibility
- Explain the health-fitness benefits of stretching
- Become familiar with a battery of tests to assess overall body flexibility (Modified Sit-and-Reach Test, Total Body Rotation Test, Shoulder Rotation Test)
- Be able to interpret flexibility test results according to health-fitness and physical-fitness standards
- Learn the principles that govern development of muscular flexibility
- List some exercises that may cause injury
- Become familiar with a program for preventing and rehabilitating low-back pain
- Create your own personal flexibility profile.

Check your understanding of the chapter contents by logging on to CengageNOW and accessing the pre-test, personalized learning plan, and post-test for this chapter.

# FAQ

### Will stretching before exercise prevent injuries?

The research on this subject is limited and controversial. Some data suggest that extensive stretching prior to physical activity actually increases the risk for injuries. A temporary decrease in strength and power is also seen with intense stretching before exercise. The most important factor prior to vigorous exercise is to gradually increase the exercise intensity through mild calisthenics and low- to moderate-intensity aerobic exercise. Until more definite data are available, you may be better off performing your flexibility program following the aerobic and/or strength-training phase of your training.

### Does strength training limit flexibility?

A popular myth is that individuals with large musculature, frequently referred to as "muscle-bound," are inflexible. Data show that strength-training exercises, when performed through a full range of motion, do not limit flexibility. With few exceptions, most strength-training exercises can be performed from complete extension to complete flexion. Body builders and gymnasts, who train heavily with weights, have better than average flexibility.

### Will stretching exercises help me lose weight?

The energy (caloric) expenditure of stretching exercises is extremely low. In 30 minutes of aerobic exercise you can easily burn an additional 250–300 calories compared with 30 minutes of stretching. Flexibility exercises help develop overall health-related fitness but do not contribute much to weight loss or weight maintenance.

### How much should stretching "hurt" to gain flexibility?

Proper stretching should not hurt. Stretch to the point of only mild tension. Pain is an indication that you are stretching too aggressively. It is best to decrease the degree of stretch and hold the final position for a longer period of time.

---

Very few people who exercise take the time to stretch, and only a few of those who stretch do so properly. When joints are not regularly moved through their entire range of motion, muscles and ligaments shorten in time, and flexibility decreases. Repetitive movement through regular/structured exercise, such as with running, cycling, or aerobics, without proper stretching, also causes muscles and ligaments to tighten. Most fitness participants underestimate and overlook the contribution of good muscular flexibility to overall fitness and preventive health care.

**Flexibility** refers to the achievable range of motion at a joint or group of joints without causing injury. Some muscular/skeletal problems and injuries are related to a lack of flexibility. In daily life, we often have to make rapid or strenuous movements we are not accustomed to making. Abruptly forcing a tight muscle beyond its achievable range of motion may lead to injury.

A decline in flexibility can cause poor posture and subsequent aches and pains that lead to limited and painful joint movement. Inordinate tightness is uncomfortable and debilitating. Approximately 80 percent of all low-back problems in the United States stem from improper alignment of the vertebral column and pelvic girdle, a direct result of inflexible and weak muscles. This backache syndrome costs U.S. industry billions of dollars each year in lost productivity, health services, and worker compensation.

# Benefits of Good Flexibility

Improving and maintaining good range of motion in the joints enhances the quality of life. Good flexibility promotes healthy muscles and joints. Improving elasticity of muscles and connective tissue around joints enables greater freedom of movement and the individual's ability to participate in many types of sports and recreational activities. Adequate flexibility also makes activities of daily living such as turning, lifting, and bending much easier to perform. A person must take care, however, not to overstretch joints. Too much flexibility leads to unstable and loose joints, which may increase injury rate, including joint **subluxation** and dislocation.

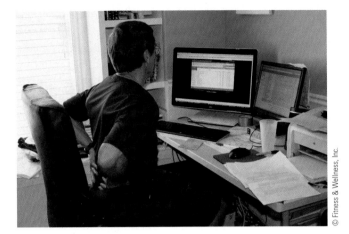

Excessive sitting and lack of physical activity lead to chronic back pain.

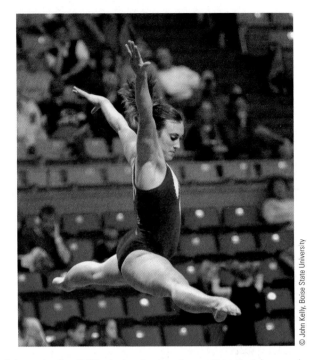

Adequate flexibility helps to develop and maintain sports skill throughout life.

Taking part in a regular **stretching** program increases circulation to the muscle(s) being stretched, prevents low-back and other spinal column problems, improves and maintains good postural alignment, promotes proper and graceful body movement, improves personal appearance and self-image, and helps to develop and maintain motor skills throughout life.

Flexibility exercises have been prescribed successfully to treat **dysmenorrhea**[1] (painful menstruation), general neuromuscular tension (stress), and knots (trigger points) in muscles and fascia. Regular stretching helps decrease the aches and pains caused by psychological stress and contributes to a decrease in anxiety, blood pressure, and breathing rate.[2] Stretching also helps relieve muscle cramps encountered at rest or during participation in exercise.

Mild stretching exercises in conjunction with calisthenics are helpful in warm-up routines to prepare for more vigorous aerobic or strength-training exercises, and in cool-down routines following exercise to facilitate the return to a normal resting state. Fatigued muscles tend to contract to a shorter-than-average resting length, and stretching exercises help fatigued muscles reestablish their normal resting length.

Flexibility in Older Adults Similar to muscular strength, good range of motion is critical in older life (see discussion in Chapter 9). Because of decreased flexibility, older adults lose mobility and may be unable to perform simple daily tasks such as bending forward or turning. Many older adults cannot turn their heads or rotate their trunks to look over their shoulders but, rather, must step around 90° to 180° to see behind them. Adequate flexibility is also important in driving. Individuals who lose range of motion with age are unable to look over their shoulders to switch lanes or to parallel-park, which increases the risk for automobile accidents.

Physical activity and exercise can be hampered severely by lack of good range of motion. Because of the pain during activity, older people who have tight hip flexors

(muscles) cannot jog or walk very far. A vicious circle ensues, because the condition usually worsens with further inactivity. Lack of flexibility also may be a cause of falls and subsequent injury in older adults. A simple stretching program can alleviate or prevent this problem and help people return to an exercise program.

# Factors Affecting Flexibility

The total range of motion around a joint is highly specific and varies from one joint to another (hip, trunk, shoulder), as well as from one individual to the next. Muscular flexibility relates primarily to genetic factors and to physical activity. Joint structure (shape of the bones), joint cartilage, ligaments, tendons, muscles, skin, tissue injury, and adipose tissue (fat)—all influence range of motion about a joint. Body temperature, age, and gender also affect flexibility.

The range of motion about a given joint depends mostly on the structure of that joint. Greater range of motion, however, can be attained through plastic and elastic elon-

**Flexibility** The achievable range of motion at a joint or group of joints without causing injury.

**Subluxation** Partial dislocation of a joint.

**Stretching** Moving the joints beyond the accustomed range of motion.

**Dysmenorrhea** Painful menstruation.

gation. **Plastic elongation** is the permanent lengthening of soft tissue. Even though joint capsules, ligaments, and tendons are basically nonelastic, they can undergo plastic elongation. This permanent lengthening, accompanied by increased range of motion, is best attained through slow-sustained stretching exercises.

**Elastic elongation** is the temporary lengthening of soft tissue. Muscle tissue has elastic properties and responds to stretching exercises by undergoing elastic or temporary lengthening. Elastic elongation increases extensibility, the ability to stretch the muscles.

Changes in muscle temperature can increase or decrease flexibility by as much as 20 percent. Individuals who warm up properly have better flexibility than people who do not. Cool temperatures have the opposite effect, impeding range of motion. Because of the effects of temperature on muscular flexibility, many people prefer to do their stretching exercises after the aerobic phase of their workout. Aerobic activities raise body temperature, facilitating plastic elongation.

Another factor that influences flexibility is the amount of adipose (fat) tissue in and around joints and muscle tissue. Excess adipose tissue will increase resistance to movement, and the added bulk also hampers joint mobility because of the contact between body surfaces.

On the average, women have better flexibility than men, and they seem to retain this advantage throughout life. Aging does decrease the extensibility of soft tissue, though, resulting in less flexibility in both sexes.

The most significant contributor to lower flexibility is sedentary living. With less physical activity, muscles lose their elasticity and tendons and ligaments tighten and shorten. Inactivity also tends to be accompanied by an increase in adipose tissue, which further decreases the range of motion around a joint. Finally, injury to muscle tissue and tight skin from excessive scar tissue have negative effects on range of motion.

# Assessment of Flexibility

Many flexibility tests developed over the years were specific to certain sports or not practical for the general population. Their application in health and fitness programs was limited. For example, the Front-to-Rear Splits Test and the Bridge-Up Test had applications in sports such as gymnastics and several track-and-field events, but they did not represent actions that most people encounter in daily life.

Because of the lack of practical flexibility tests, most health and fitness centers rely strictly on the Sit and Reach Test as an indicator of flexibility. This test measures flexibility of the hamstring muscles (back of the thigh) and, to a lesser extent, the lower back muscles.

Flexibility is joint specific. This means that a lot of flexibility in one joint does not necessarily indicate that other joints are just as flexible. Therefore, the Total Body Rotation Test and the Shoulder Rotation Test—indicators of the ability to perform everyday movements such as reach-ing, bending, and turning—are included to determine your flexibility profile.

The Sit-and-Reach Test has been modified from the traditional test to take length of arms and legs into consideration in determining the score (see Figure 8.1). In the original Sit-and-Reach Test, the 15-inch mark of the yard-stick used to measure flexibility is always set at the edge of the box where the feet are placed. This does not take into consideration an individual with long arms and/or short legs or one with short arms and/or long legs.[3] All other factors being equal, an individual with longer arms or shorter legs, or both, receives a better rating because of the structural advantage.

The procedures and norms for the flexibility tests are described in Figures 8.1 through 8.3 and Tables 8.1 through 8.3. The flexibility test results in these three tables are provided in both inches and centimeters (cm). Be sure to use the proper column to read your percentile score based on your test results. For the flexibility profile, you should take all three tests. You will be able to assess your flexibility profile in Lab 8A. Because of the specificity of flexibility, pinpointing an "ideal" level of flexibility is difficult. Nevertheless, flexibility is important to health and independent living, so an assessment will give an indication of your current level of flexibility.

**Interpreting Flexibility Test Results** After obtaining your scores and fitness ratings for each test, you can determine the fitness category for each flexibility test using the guidelines given in Table 8.4. You also should look up the number of points assigned for each fitness category in this table. The overall flexibility fitness category is obtained by totaling the number of points from all three tests and using the ratings given in Table 8.5. Record your results in Lab 8A.

# Evaluating Body Posture

Good posture enhances personal appearance, self-image, confidence, and your overall sense of well-being; improves balance and endurance; protects against misalignment-related pains and aches; and prevents falls.[4] The relationship between different body parts is the essence of posture.

Poor posture is a risk factor for musculoskeletal problems of the neck, shoulders, and lower back. Incorrect posture also strains hips and knees. Faulty posture and weak and inelastic muscles are a leading cause of chronic low-back problems. Evaluating these areas is crucial to prevent and rehabilitate low-back pain. The results of these tests can be used to prescribe corrective exercises.

Adequate body mechanics also aid in reducing chronic low-back pain. Proper body mechanics means using correct positions in all the activities of daily life, including sleeping, sitting, standing, walking, driving, working, and exercising. Because of the high incidence of low-back pain, illustrations of proper body mechanics and a series of corrective and preventive exercises are shown in Figure 8.7 on pages 301–302.

FIGURE 8.1  Procedure for the Modified Sit-and-Reach Test.

To perform this test, you will need the Acuflex I* Sit-and-Reach Flexibility Tester, or you may simply place a yardstick on top of a box 12" high.

1. Warm up properly before the first trial.
2. Remove your shoes for the test. Sit on the floor with the hips, back, and head against a wall, the legs fully extended, and the bottom of the feet against the Acuflex I or sit-and-reach box.
3. Place the hands one on top of the other and reach forward as far as possible without letting the head and back come off the wall (the shoulders may be rounded as much as possible, but neither the head nor the back should come off the wall at this time). The technician then can slide the reach indicator on the Acuflex I (or yardstick) along the top of the box until the end of the indicator touches the participant's fingers. The indicator then must be held firmly in place throughout the rest of the test.

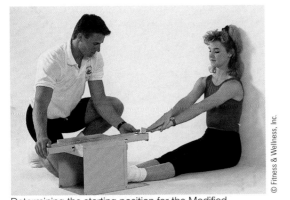

Determining the starting position for the Modified Sit-and-Reach Test.

4. Now your head and back can come off the wall. Gradually reach forward three times, the third time stretching forward as far as possible on the indicator (or yardstick) and holding the final position for at least 2 seconds. Be sure that during the test you keep the backs of the knees flat against the floor.
5. Record the final number of inches reached to the nearest ½".

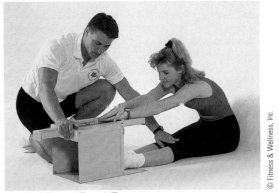

Modified Sit-and-Reach Test.

You are allowed two trials, and an average of the two scores is used as the final test score. The respective percentile ranks and fitness categories for this test are given in Tables 8.1 and 8.4.

*The Acuflex I Flexibility Tester for the Modified Sit-and-Reach Test can be obtained from Figure Finder Collection, Novel Products, P. O. Box 408, Rockton, IL 61072-0480. Phone: 800-323-5143, Fax 815-624-4866.

Most people are unaware of how faulty their posture is until they see themselves in a photograph. This can be quite a shock and is often enough to motivate change.

Besides engaging in the recommended exercises to elicit changes in postural alignment, people need to be continually aware of the corrections they are trying to make. As posture improves, you frequently become motivated to change other aspects, such as improving muscular strength and flexibility and decreasing body fat.

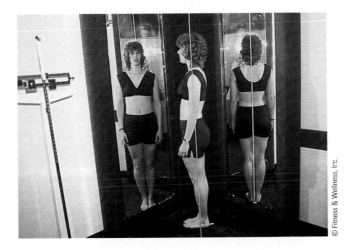

Photographic technique used for posture evaluation.

Posture tests are used to detect deviations from normal body alignment and prescribe corrective exercises or procedures to improve alignment. These analyses are best conducted early in life, because certain postural deviations are more difficult to correct in older people. If deviations are allowed to go uncorrected, they usually become more serious as the person grows older. Consequently, corrective exercises or other medical procedures should be used to stop or slow down postural degeneration.

Proper body alignment has been difficult to evaluate because most experts still don't know exactly what constitutes good posture. To objectively analyze a person's posture, an observer either must be adequately trained or must have some guidelines to identify abnormalities and assign ratings according to the amount of deviation from "normal" posture.

A posture rating chart, such as that in Lab 8B, provides simple guidelines for evaluating posture. Assuming the drawings in the left column to be proper alignment and the drawings in the right column to be extreme deviations

**Plastic elongation**  Permanent lengthening of soft tissue.
**Elastic elongation**  Temporary lengthening of soft tissue.

**FIGURE 8.2 Procedure for the Total Body Rotation Test.**

An Acuflex II* Total Body Rotation Flexibility Tester or a measuring scale with a sliding panel is needed to administer this test. The Acuflex II or scale is placed on the wall at shoulder height and should be adjustable to accommodate individual differences in height. If you need to build your own scale, use two measuring tapes and glue them above and below the sliding panel centered at the 15" mark. Each tape should be at least 30" long. If no sliding panel is available, simply tape the measuring tapes onto a wall oriented in opposite directions as shown below. A line also must be drawn on the floor and centered with the 15" mark.

1. Warm up properly before beginning this test.
2. Stand with one side toward the wall, an arm's length away from the wall, with the foot straight ahead, slightly separated, and the toes touching the center line drawn on the floor. Hold out the arm away from the wall horizontally from the body, making a fist with the hand. The Acuflex II measuring scale (or tapes) should be shoulder height at this time.
3. Rotate the trunk, the extended arm going backward (always maintaining a horizontal plane) and making contact with the panel, gradually sliding it forward as far as possible. If no panel is available, slide the fist alongside the tapes as far as possible. Hold the final position at least 2 seconds. Position the hand with the little finger side forward during the entire sliding movement. **Proper hand position is crucial. Many people attempt to open the hand, or push with extended fingers, or slide the panel with the knuckles—none of which is acceptable.** During the test the knees can be bent slightly, but **the feet cannot be moved or rotated**—they must point forward. The body must be kept as straight (vertical) as possible.

4. Conduct the test on either the right or the left side of the body. Perform two trials on the selected side. Record the farthest point reached, measured to the nearest half inch and held for at least 2 seconds. Use the average of the two trials as the final test score. Refer to Tables 8.2 and 8.4 to determine the percentile rank and flexibility fitness category for this test.

*The Acuflex II Flexibility Tester for the Total Body Rotation Test can be obtained from Figure Finder Collection, Novel Products, P.O. Box 408, Rockton, IL 61072-0408. Phone: 800-323-5143, Fax 815-624-4866.

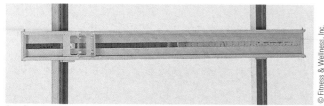

Acuflex II measuring device for the Total Body Rotation Test.

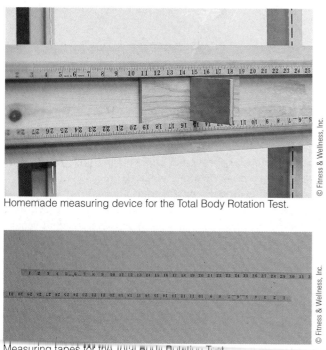

Homemade measuring device for the Total Body Rotation Test.

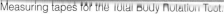

Measuring tapes for the Total Body Rotation Test.

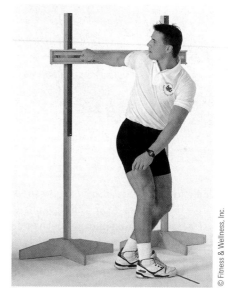

Total Body Rotation Test.

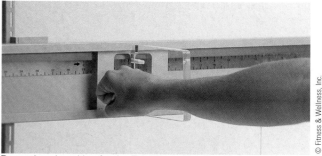

Proper hand position for the Total Body Rotation Test.

from normal, an observer is able to rate each body segment on a scale from 1 to 5.

Postural analysis can be done with more precision with the aid of a plumb line, two mirrors, and a camera. The mirrors are placed at an 80° to 85° angle, and the plumb line is centered in front of the mirrors. Another line is drawn down the center of the mirror on the right. The person should stand with the left side to the plumb line. The plumb line is used as a reference to divide the body into front and back halves (try to center the line with the hip joint and the shoulder). The line on the back (right) mirror should divide the body into right and left halves. A

**FIGURE 8.3** Procedure for the Shoulder Rotation Test.

This test can be done using the Acuflex III* Flexibility Tester, which consists of a shoulder caliper and a measuring device for shoulder rotation. If this equipment is unavailable, you can construct your own device quite easily. The caliper can be built with three regular yardsticks. Nail and glue two of the yardsticks at one end at a 90° angle, and use the third one as the sliding end of the caliper. Construct the rotation device by placing a 60" measuring tape on an aluminum or wood stick, starting at about 6" or 7" from the end of the stick.

1. Warm up before the test.
2. Using the shoulder caliper, measure the biacromial width to the nearest ¼" (use the top scale on the Acuflex III). Measure biacromial width between the lateral edges of the acromion processes of the shoulders.
3. Place the Acuflex III or homemade device behind the back and use a reverse grip (thumbs out) to hold on to the device. Place the index finger of the right hand next to the zero point of the scale or tape (lower scale on the Acuflex III) and hold it firmly in place throughout the test. Place the left hand on the other end of the measuring device wherever comfortable.

4. Standing straight up and extending both arms to full length, with elbows locked, slowly bring the measuring device over the head until it reaches about forehead level. For subsequent trials, depending on the resistance encountered when rotating the shoulders, move the left grip in ½" to 1" at a time, and repeat the task until you no longer can rotate the shoulders without undue strain or starting to bend the elbows. Always keep the right-hand grip against the zero point of the scale. Measure the last successful trial to the nearest ½". Take this measurement at the inner edge of the left hand on the side of the little finger.
5. Determine the final score for this test by subtracting the biacromial width from the best score (shortest distance) between both hands on the rotation test. For example, if the best score is 35" and the biacromial width is 15", the final score is 20" (35 − 15 = 20). Using Tables 8.3 and 8.4, determine the percentile rank and flexibility fitness category for this test.

*The Acuflex III Flexibility Tester for the Shoulder Rotation Test can be obtained from Figure Finder Collection, Novel Products, Inc., P. O. Box 408, Rockton, IL 61072-0408. Phone: (800) 323-5143, Fax 815-624-4866.

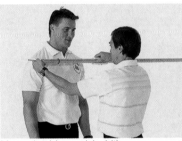

Measuring biacromial width.

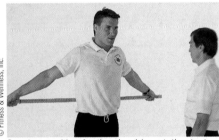

Starting position for the shoulder rotation test (note the reverse grip used for this test).

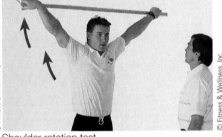

Shoulder rotation test.

© Fitness & Wellness, Inc.

**TABLE 8.1** Percentile Ranks for the Modified Sit-and-Reach Test

| Percentile Rank | Age Category—Men | | | | | | | | Percentile Rank | Age Category—Women | | | | | | | |
|---|---|---|---|---|---|---|---|---|---|---|---|---|---|---|---|---|---|
| | ≤18 | | 19–35 | | 36–49 | | ≥50 | | | ≤18 | | 19–35 | | 36–49 | | ≥50 | |
| | in. | cm | in. | cm | in. | cm | in. | cm | | in. | cm | in. | cm | in. | cm | in. | cm |
| 99 | 20.8 | 52.8 | 20.1 | 51.1 | 18.9 | 48.0 | 16.2 | 41.1 | 99 | 22.6 | 57.4 | 21.0 | 53.3 | 19.8 | 50.3 | 17.2 | 43.7 |
| 95 | 19.6 | 49.8 | 18.9 | 48.0 | 18.2 | 46.2 | 15.8 | 40.1 | 95 | 19.5 | 49.5 | 19.3 | 49.0 | 19.2 | 48.8 | 15.7 | 39.9 |
| 90 | 18.2 | 46.2 | 17.2 | 43.7 | 16.1 | 40.9 | 15.0 | 38.1 | 90 | 18.7 | 47.5 | 17.9 | 45.5 | 17.4 | 44.2 | 15.0 | 38.1 |
| 80 | 17.8 | 45.2 | 17.0 | 43.2 | 14.6 | 37.1 | 13.3 | 33.8 | 80 | 17.8 | 45.2 | 16.7 | 42.4 | 16.2 | 41.1 | 14.2 | 36.1 |
| 70 | 16.0 | 40.6 | 15.8 | 40.1 | 13.9 | 35.3 | 12.3 | 31.2 | 70 | 16.5 | 41.9 | 16.2 | 41.1 | 15.2 | 38.6 | 13.6 | 34.5 |
| 60 | 15.2 | 38.6 | 15.0 | 38.1 | 13.4 | 34.0 | 11.5 | 29.2 | 60 | 16.0 | 40.6 | 15.8 | 40.1 | 14.5 | 36.8 | 12.3 | 31.2 |
| 50 | 14.5 | 36.8 | 14.4 | 36.6 | 12.6 | 32.0 | 10.2 | 25.9 | 50 | 15.2 | 38.6 | 14.8 | 37.6 | 13.5 | 34.3 | 11.1 | 28.2 |
| 40 | 14.0 | 35.6 | 13.5 | 34.3 | 11.6 | 29.5 | 9.7 | 24.6 | 40 | 14.5 | 36.8 | 14.5 | 36.8 | 12.8 | 32.5 | 10.1 | 25.7 |
| 30 | 13.4 | 34.0 | 13.0 | 33.0 | 10.8 | 27.4 | 9.3 | 23.6 | 30 | 13.7 | 34.8 | 13.7 | 34.8 | 12.2 | 31.0 | 9.2 | 23.4 |
| 20 | 11.8 | 30.0 | 11.6 | 29.5 | 9.9 | 25.1 | 8.8 | 22.4 | 20 | 12.6 | 32.0 | 12.6 | 32.0 | 11.0 | 27.9 | 8.3 | 21.1 |
| 10 | 9.5 | 24.1 | 9.2 | 23.4 | 8.3 | 21.1 | 7.8 | 19.8 | 10 | 11.4 | 29.0 | 10.1 | 25.7 | 9.7 | 24.6 | 7.5 | 19.0 |
| 05 | 8.4 | 21.3 | 7.9 | 20.1 | 7.0 | 17.8 | 7.2 | 18.3 | 05 | 9.4 | 23.9 | 8.1 | 20.6 | 8.5 | 21.6 | 3.7 | 9.4 |
| 01 | 7.2 | 18.3 | 7.0 | 17.8 | 5.1 | 13.0 | 4.0 | 10.2 | 01 | 6.5 | 16.5 | 2.6 | 6.6 | 2.0 | 5.1 | 1.5 | 3.8 |

▭ High physical fitness standard    ▭ Health fitness standard

**TABLE 8.2** Percentile Ranks for the Total Body Rotation Test

| | Percentile Rank | Age Category—Left Rotation | | | | | | | | Age Category—Right Rotation | | | | | | | |
|---|---|---|---|---|---|---|---|---|---|---|---|---|---|---|---|---|---|
| | | ≤18 | | 19–35 | | 36–49 | | ≥50 | | ≤18 | | 19–35 | | 36–49 | | ≥50 | |
| | | in. | cm | in. | cm | in. | cm | in. | cm | in. | cm | in. | cm | in. | cm | in. | cm |
| **MEN** | 99 | 29.1 | 73.9 | 28.0 | 71.1 | 26.6 | 67.6 | 21.0 | 53.3 | 28.2 | 71.6 | 27.8 | 70.6 | 25.2 | 64.0 | 22.2 | 56.4 |
| | 95 | 26.6 | 67.6 | 24.8 | 63.0 | 24.5 | 62.2 | 20.0 | 50.8 | 25.5 | 64.8 | 25.6 | 65.0 | 23.8 | 60.5 | 20.7 | 52.6 |
| | 90 | 25.0 | 63.5 | 23.6 | 59.9 | 23.0 | 58.4 | 17.7 | 45.0 | 24.3 | 61.7 | 24.1 | 61.2 | 22.5 | 57.1 | 19.3 | 49.0 |
| | 80 | 22.0 | 55.9 | 22.0 | 55.9 | 21.2 | 53.8 | 15.5 | 39.4 | 22.7 | 57.7 | 22.3 | 56.6 | 21.0 | 53.3 | 16.3 | 41.4 |
| | 70 | 20.9 | 53.1 | 20.3 | 51.6 | 20.4 | 51.8 | 14.7 | 37.3 | 21.3 | 54.1 | 20.7 | 52.6 | 18.7 | 47.5 | 15.7 | 39.9 |
| | 60 | 19.9 | 50.5 | 19.3 | 49.0 | 18.7 | 47.5 | 13.9 | 35.3 | 19.8 | 50.3 | 19.0 | 48.3 | 17.3 | 43.9 | 14.7 | 37.3 |
| | 50 | 18.6 | 47.2 | 18.0 | 45.7 | 16.7 | 42.4 | 12.7 | 32.3 | 19.0 | 48.3 | 17.2 | 43.7 | 16.3 | 41.4 | 12.3 | 31.2 |
| | 40 | 17.0 | 43.2 | 16.8 | 42.7 | 15.3 | 38.9 | 11.7 | 29.7 | 17.3 | 43.9 | 16.3 | 41.4 | 14.7 | 37.3 | 11.5 | 29.2 |
| | 30 | 14.9 | 37.8 | 15.0 | 38.1 | 14.8 | 37.6 | 10.3 | 26.2 | 15.1 | 38.4 | 15.0 | 38.1 | 13.3 | 33.8 | 10.7 | 27.2 |
| | 20 | 13.8 | 35.1 | 13.3 | 33.8 | 13.7 | 34.8 | 9.5 | 24.1 | 12.9 | 32.8 | 13.3 | 33.8 | 11.2 | 28.4 | 8.7 | 22.1 |
| | 10 | 10.8 | 27.4 | 10.5 | 26.7 | 10.8 | 27.4 | 4.3 | 10.9 | 10.8 | 27.4 | 11.3 | 28.7 | 8.0 | 20.3 | 2.7 | 6.9 |
| | 05 | 8.5 | 21.6 | 8.9 | 22.6 | 8.8 | 22.4 | 0.3 | 0.8 | 8.1 | 20.6 | 8.3 | 21.1 | 5.5 | 14.0 | 0.3 | 0.8 |
| | 01 | 3.4 | 8.6 | 1.7 | 4.3 | 5.1 | 13.0 | 0.0 | 0.0 | 6.6 | 16.8 | 2.9 | 7.4 | 2.0 | 5.1 | 0.0 | 0.0 |
| **WOMEN** | 99 | 29.3 | 74.4 | 28.6 | 72.6 | 27.1 | 68.8 | 23.0 | 58.4 | 29.6 | 75.2 | 29.4 | 74.7 | 27.1 | 68.8 | 21.7 | 55.1 |
| | 95 | 26.8 | 68.1 | 24.8 | 63.0 | 25.3 | 64.3 | 21.4 | 54.4 | 27.6 | 70.1 | 25.3 | 64.3 | 25.9 | 65.8 | 19.7 | 50.0 |
| | 90 | 25.5 | 64.8 | 23.0 | 58.4 | 23.4 | 59.4 | 20.5 | 52.1 | 25.8 | 65.5 | 23.0 | 58.4 | 21.3 | 54.1 | 19.0 | 48.3 |
| | 80 | 23.8 | 60.5 | 21.5 | 54.6 | 20.2 | 51.3 | 19.1 | 48.5 | 23.7 | 60.2 | 20.8 | 52.8 | 19.6 | 49.8 | 17.9 | 45.5 |
| | 70 | 21.8 | 55.4 | 20.5 | 52.1 | 18.6 | 47.2 | 17.3 | 43.9 | 22.0 | 55.9 | 19.3 | 49.0 | 17.3 | 43.9 | 16.8 | 42.7 |
| | 60 | 20.5 | 52.1 | 19.3 | 49.0 | 17.7 | 45.0 | 16.0 | 40.6 | 20.8 | 52.8 | 18.0 | 45.7 | 16.5 | 41.9 | 15.6 | 39.6 |
| | 50 | 19.5 | 49.5 | 18.0 | 45.7 | 16.4 | 41.7 | 14.8 | 37.6 | 19.5 | 49.5 | 17.3 | 43.9 | 14.6 | 37.1 | 14.0 | 35.6 |
| | 40 | 18.5 | 47.0 | 17.2 | 43.7 | 14.8 | 37.6 | 13.7 | 34.8 | 18.3 | 46.5 | 16.0 | 40.6 | 13.1 | 33.3 | 12.8 | 32.5 |
| | 30 | 17.1 | 43.4 | 15.7 | 39.9 | 13.6 | 34.5 | 10.0 | 25.4 | 16.3 | 41.4 | 15.2 | 38.6 | 11.7 | 29.7 | 8.5 | 21.6 |
| | 20 | 16.0 | 40.6 | 15.2 | 38.6 | 11.6 | 29.5 | 6.3 | 16.0 | 14.5 | 36.8 | 14.0 | 35.6 | 9.8 | 24.9 | 3.9 | 9.9 |
| | 10 | 12.8 | 32.5 | 13.6 | 34.5 | 8.5 | 21.6 | 3.0 | 7.6 | 12.4 | 31.5 | 11.1 | 28.2 | 6.1 | 15.5 | 2.2 | 5.6 |
| | 05 | 11.1 | 28.2 | 7.3 | 18.5 | 6.8 | 17.3 | 0.7 | 1.8 | 10.2 | 25.9 | 8.8 | 22.4 | 4.0 | 10.2 | 1.1 | 2.8 |
| | 01 | 8.9 | 22.6 | 5.3 | 13.5 | 4.3 | 10.9 | 0.0 | 0.0 | 8.9 | 22.6 | 3.2 | 8.1 | 2.8 | 7.1 | 0.0 | 0.0 |

▢ High physical fitness standard     ▢ Health fitness standard

picture then is taken (like the photo on page 291) that can be compared with the rating chart given in Lab 8B.

The photographic procedure allows for a better comparison of the different body segment alignments and a more objective analysis. If no mirrors and camera are available, the participant should stand with his or her side to the line, and then repeat with the back to the line, while the evaluator does the assessment.

A final posture score is determined according to the sum of the ratings obtained for each body segment. Table 8.6 on page 295 contains the various categories as determined by the final posture score.

# Principles of Muscular Flexibility Prescription

Even though genetics play a crucial role in body flexibility, the range of joint mobility can be increased and maintained through a regular stretching program. Because range of motion is highly specific to each body part (ankle, trunk, shoulder), a comprehensive stretching program should include all body parts and follow the basic guidelines for development of flexibility.

**TABLE 8.3  Percentile Ranks for the Shoulder Rotation Test**

| Percentile Rank | Age Category—Men | | | | | | | | Percentile Rank | Age Category—Women | | | | | | | |
|---|---|---|---|---|---|---|---|---|---|---|---|---|---|---|---|---|---|
| | ≤18 | | 19–35 | | 36–49 | | ≥50 | | | ≤18 | | 19–35 | | 36–49 | | ≥50 | |
| | in. | cm | in. | cm | in. | cm | in. | cm | | in. | cm | in. | cm | in. | cm | in. | cm |
| 99 | 2.2 | 5.6 | −1.0 | −2.5 | 18.1 | 46.0 | 21.5 | 54.6 | 99 | 2.6 | 6.6 | −2.4 | −6.1 | 11.5 | 29.2 | 13.1 | 33.3 |
| 95 | 15.2 | 38.6 | 10.4 | 26.4 | 20.4 | 51.8 | 27.0 | 68.6 | 95 | 8.0 | 20.3 | 6.2 | 15.7 | 15.4 | 39.1 | 16.5 | 41.9 |
| 90 | 18.5 | 47.0 | 15.5 | 39.4 | 20.8 | 52.8 | 27.9 | 70.9 | 90 | 10.7 | 27.2 | 9.7 | 24.6 | 16.8 | 42.7 | 20.9 | 53.1 |
| 80 | 20.7 | 52.6 | 18.4 | 46.7 | 23.3 | 59.2 | 28.5 | 72.4 | 80 | 14.5 | 36.8 | 14.5 | 36.8 | 19.2 | 48.8 | 22.5 | 57.1 |
| 70 | 23.0 | 58.4 | 20.5 | 52.1 | 24.7 | 62.7 | 29.4 | 74.7 | 70 | 16.1 | 40.9 | 17.2 | 43.7 | 21.5 | 54.6 | 24.3 | 61.7 |
| 60 | 24.2 | 61.5 | 22.9 | 58.2 | 26.6 | 67.6 | 29.9 | 75.9 | 60 | 19.2 | 48.8 | 18.7 | 47.5 | 23.1 | 58.7 | 25.1 | 63.8 |
| 50 | 25.4 | 64.5 | 24.4 | 62.0 | 28.0 | 71.1 | 30.5 | 77.5 | 50 | 21.0 | 53.3 | 20.0 | 50.8 | 23.5 | 59.7 | 26.2 | 66.5 |
| 40 | 26.3 | 66.8 | 25.7 | 65.3 | 30.0 | 76.2 | 31.0 | 78.7 | 40 | 22.2 | 56.4 | 21.4 | 54.4 | 24.4 | 62.0 | 28.1 | 71.4 |
| 30 | 28.2 | 71.6 | 27.3 | 69.3 | 31.9 | 81.0 | 31.7 | 80.5 | 30 | 23.2 | 58.9 | 24.0 | 61.0 | 25.9 | 65.8 | 29.9 | 75.9 |
| 20 | 30.0 | 76.2 | 30.1 | 76.5 | 33.3 | 84.6 | 33.1 | 84.1 | 20 | 25.0 | 63.5 | 25.9 | 65.8 | 29.8 | 75.7 | 31.5 | 80.0 |
| 10 | 33.5 | 85.1 | 31.8 | 80.8 | 36.1 | 91.7 | 37.2 | 94.5 | 10 | 27.2 | 69.1 | 29.1 | 73.9 | 31.1 | 79.0 | 33.1 | 84.1 |
| 05 | 34.7 | 88.1 | 33.5 | 85.1 | 37.8 | 96.0 | 38.7 | 98.3 | 05 | 28.0 | 71.1 | 31.3 | 79.5 | 33.4 | 84.8 | 34.1 | 86.6 |
| 01 | 40.8 | 103.6 | 42.6 | 108.2 | 43.0 | 109.2 | 44.1 | 112.0 | 01 | 32.5 | 82.5 | 37.1 | 94.2 | 34.9 | 88.6 | 35.4 | 89.9 |

▨ High physical fitness standard  ▢ Health fitness standard

**TABLE 8.4  Flexibility Fitness Categories According to Percentile Ranks**

| Percentile Rank | Fitness Category | Points |
|---|---|---|
| ≥90 | Excellent | 5 |
| 70–80 | Good | 4 |
| 50–60 | Average | 3 |
| 30–40 | Fair | 2 |
| ≤20 | Poor | 1 |

**TABLE 8.6  Posture Evaluation Standards**

| Total Points | Category |
|---|---|
| ≥45 | Excellent |
| 40–44 | Good |
| 30–39 | Average |
| 20–29 | Fair |
| ≤19 | Poor |

**TABLE 8.5  Overall Flexibility Fitness Categories**

| Total Points | Flexibility Category |
|---|---|
| ≥13 | Excellent |
| 10–12 | Good |
| 7–9 | Average |
| 4–6 | Fair |
| ≤3 | Poor |

The overload and specificity of training principles (discussed in conjunction with strength development in Chapter 7) also apply to the development of muscular flexibility. To increase the total range of motion of a joint, the specific muscles surrounding that joint have to be stretched progressively beyond their accustomed length. The principles of mode, intensity, repetitions, and frequency of exercise can also be applied to flexibility programs.

## Modes of Training  Three modes of stretching exercises can increase flexibility:

1. Ballistic stretching
2. Slow-sustained stretching (static)
3. Proprioceptive neuromuscular facilitation (PNF) stretching

Although research has indicated that all three types of stretching are effective in improving flexibility, each technique has certain advantages.

**Ballistic Stretching** **Ballistic** (or **dynamic**) **stretching** exercises are done with jerky, rapid, and bouncy movements that provide the necessary force to lengthen the muscles. Although this type of stretching helps to develop flexibility, the ballistic actions may cause muscle soreness and injury from small tears to the soft tissue.

Precautions must be taken not to overstretch ligaments, because they will undergo plastic or permanent elongation. If the stretching force cannot be controlled—as often occurs in fast, jerky movements—ligaments can easily be overstretched. This, in turn, leads to excessively loose joints, increasing the risk for injuries. Slow, gentle, and **controlled ballistic stretching** (instead of jerky, rapid, and bouncy movements), however, is effective in developing flexibility, and most individuals can perform it safely.

**Slow-sustained Stretching** With the **slow-sustained stretching** technique, muscles are lengthened gradually through a joint's complete range of motion, and the final position is held for a few seconds. A slow-sustained stretch causes the muscles to relax and thereby achieve greater length. This type of stretch causes little pain and has a low risk for injury. In flexibility-development programs, slow-sustained stretching exercises are the most frequently used and recommended.

**Proprioceptive Neuromuscular Facilitation (PNF)** **Proprioceptive neuromuscular facilitation (PNF)** stretching is based on a "contract-and-relax" method and requires the assistance of another person. The procedure is as follows:

1. The person assisting with the exercise provides initial force by pushing slowly in the direction of the desired stretch. This first stretch does not cover the entire range of motion.

2. The person being stretched then applies force in the opposite direction of the stretch, against the assistant, who tries to hold the initial degree of stretch as close as possible. This results in an isometric contraction at the angle of the stretch.

3. After 4 or 5 seconds of isometric contraction, the person being stretched relaxes the target muscle completely. The assistant then increases the degree of stretch slowly to a greater angle.

4. The isometric contraction is repeated for another 4 or 5 seconds, after which the muscle is relaxed again. The assistant then can increase the degree of stretch, slowly, one more time.

Steps 1 through 4 are repeated two to five times, until the exerciser feels mild discomfort. On the last trial, the final stretched position should be held for 15 to 30 seconds.

Theoretically, with the PNF technique, the isometric contraction helps relax the muscle being stretched, which results in lengthening the muscle. Some fitness leaders believe PNF is more effective than slow-sustained stretching. Another benefit of PNF is an increase in strength of the muscle(s) being stretched. Research has shown ap-

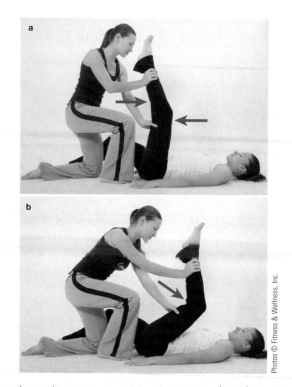

Photos © Fitness & Wellness, Inc.

Proprioceptive neuromuscular facilitation (PNF) stretching technique: (a) isometric phase, (b) stretching phase.

proximately 17 and 35 percent increases in absolute strength and muscular endurance, respectively, in the hamstring muscle group after 12 weeks of PNF stretching.[5] The results were consistent in both men and women and are attributed to the isometric contractions performed during PNF. Disadvantages of PNF are (1) more pain, (2) the need for a second person to assist, and (3) the need for more time to conduct each session.

## Intensity ☯

The **intensity,** or degree of stretch, when doing flexibility exercises should be to only a point of mild discomfort or tightness at the end of the range of motion. Pain does not have to be part of the stretching routine. All stretching should be done to slightly below the pain threshold. As participants reach this point, they should try to relax the muscle being stretched as much as possible. If you feel pain, the load is too high and may cause injury. After completing the stretch, the body part is brought back gradually to the starting point.

## Critical Thinking

Carefully consider the relevance of stretching exercises to your personal fitness program. How much importance do you place on these exercises? Have some conditions improved through your stretching program, or have certain specific exercises contributed to your health and well-being?

**FIGURE 8.4** Guidelines for flexibility development.

**Mode:** Slow-sustained, slow-controlled ballistic, slow-controlled proprioceptive neuromuscular facilitation stretching to include all major muscle groups
**Intensity:** Stretch to tightness at the end of the range of motion
**Repetitions:** Repeat each exercise 2 to 4 times and hold the final stretched position for 15 to 30 seconds
**Frequency:** Minimal, 2 or 3 days per week
Ideal, 5 to 7 days per week

*Source:* Adapted from American College of Sports Medicine, *ACSM's Guidelines for Exercise Testing and Prescription* (Baltimore: Williams & Wilkins, 2006).

**Repetitions** The time required for an exercise session for development of flexibility is based on the number of **repetitions** and the length of time each repetition is held in the final stretched position. As a general recommendation, each exercise should be done 2 to 4 times, holding the final position each time for 15 to 30 seconds.[6] Stretching for 15 to 30 seconds is better to increase range of motion than stretching for shorter periods of time and is just as effective as stretching for longer durations.[7]

As flexibility increases, a person can gradually increase the time each repetition is held, to a maximum of 1 minute. Individuals who are susceptible to flexibility injuries should limit each stretch to 20 seconds. Pilates exercises are recommended for these individuals, as they increase joint stability (also see Chapter 7, page 252).

**Frequency of Exercise** Flexibility exercises should be conducted a minimum of 2 or 3 days per week, but ideally 5 to 7 days per week. After 6 to 8 weeks of almost daily stretching, flexibility can be maintained with only 2 or 3 sessions per week, doing about three repetitions of 15 to 30 seconds each. Figure 8.4 summarizes the guidelines for flexibility development.

# When to Stretch?

Many people do not differentiate a warm-up from stretching. Warming up means starting a workout slowly with walking, cycling, or slow jogging, followed by gentle stretching (not through the entire range of motion). Stretching implies movement of joints through their full range of motion and holding the final degree of stretch according to recommended guidelines.

A warm-up that progressively increases muscle temperature and mimics movement that will occur during training enhances performance. For some activities, gentle stretching is recommended in conjunction with warm-up routines. Before steady activities (walking, jogging, cycling), a warm-up of 3 to 5 minutes is recommended. The recommendation is up to 10 minutes before stop-and-go activities (for example, racquet sports, basketball, soccer) and athletic participation in general (for example, football, gymnastics). Activities that require abrupt changes in direction are more likely to cause muscle strains if they

are performed without proper warm-up that includes mild stretching.

Sports-specific/pre-exercise stretching can improve performance in sports that require a greater-than-average range of motion, such as gymnastics, dance, swimming, and figure skating. Some evidence, however, suggests that intense stretching during warm-up can lead to a temporary short-term (up to 60 minutes) decrease in strength. Thus, extensive stretching conducted prior to participating in athletic events that rely on strength and power for peak performance is not recommended.[8]

In terms of preventing injuries, the best time to stretch is controversial. In limited studies on athletic populations, the evidence is unclear as to whether stretching before or after exercise is more beneficial in preventing injury. Additional research is necessary to clarify this issue.

In general, a good time to stretch is after aerobic workouts. Higher body temperature in itself helps to increase the joint range of motion. Muscles also are fatigued following exercise, and a fatigued muscle tends to shorten, which can lead to soreness and spasms. Stretching exercises help fatigued muscles reestablish their normal resting length and prevent unnecessary pain.

# Flexibility Exercises

To improve body flexibility, each major muscle group should be subjected to at least one stretching exercise. A complete set of exercises for developing muscular flexibility is presented on pages 307–314.

Although you may not be able to hold a final stretched position with some of these exercises (such as lateral head tilts and arm circles), you still should perform the exercise through the joint's full range of motion. Depending on the number and length of repetitions, a complete workout will last between 15 and 30 minutes.

**Contraindicated Exercises** Most strength and flexibility exercises are relatively safe to perform, but even safe exercises can be hazardous if they are performed incorrectly. Some exercises may be safe to perform occasionally but, when executed repeatedly, may cause trauma and injury. Preexisting muscle or joint conditions (old

---

**Ballistic (dynamic) stretching** Exercises done with jerky, rapid, bouncy movements or slow, short, and sustained movements.

**Controlled ballistic stretching** Exercises done with slow, short, gentle, and sustained movements.

**Slow-sustained stretching** Exercises in which the muscles are lengthened gradually through a joint's complete range of motion.

**Proprioceptive neuromuscular facilitation (PNF)** Mode of stretching that uses reflexes and neuromuscular principles to relax the muscles being stretched.

**Intensity (for flexibility exercises)** Degree of stretch when doing flexibility exercises.

**Repetitions** Number of times a given resistance is performed.

**FIGURE 8.5** Contraindicated exercises.

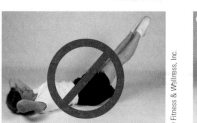

**Double-Leg Lift**

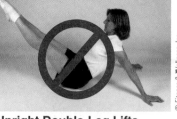

**Upright Double-Leg Lifts**

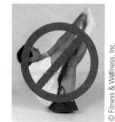

**V-Sits**

All three of these exercises cause excessive strain on the spine and may harm disks.

**Alternatives:** Strength Exercises 4 and 17, pages 262 and 267

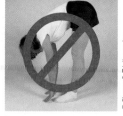

**Standing Toe Touch**

Excessive strain on the knee and lower back.

**Alternative:** Flexibility Exercise 12, page 310

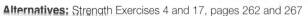

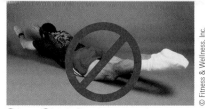

**Swan Stretch**

Excessive strain on the spine; may harm intervertebral disks.

**Alternative:** Flexibility Exercise 20, page 313

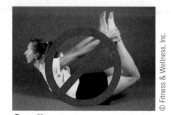

**Cradle**

Excessive strain on the spine, knees, and shoulders.

**Alternatives:** Flexibility Exercises 20, 8, and 6, pages 313, 309, and 308

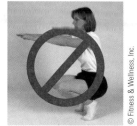

**Full Squat**

Excessive strain on the knees.

**Alternatives:**
Flexibility Exercise 8, page 309; Strength Exercises 1, 16, 27, pages 261, 267, and 273

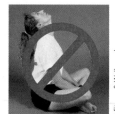

**Head Rolls**

May injure neck disks.

**Alternative:**
Flexibility Exercise 1, page 307

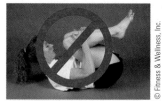

**Knee to Chest**

(with hands over the shin)
Excessive strain on the knee.

**Alternative:** Flexibility Exercises 15 and 16, pages 311 and 312

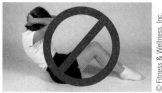

**Sit-Ups with Hands Behind the Head**

Excessive strain on the neck.

**Alternatives:** Strength Exercises 4 and 17, pages 262 and 267

**Yoga Plow**

Excessive strain on the spine, neck, and shoulders.

**Alternatives:** Flexibility Exercises 12, 15, 16, 17, and 19, pages 310, 311, and 312

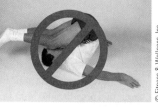

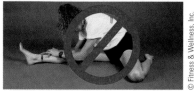

**Hurdler Stretch**

Excessive strain on the bent knee.

**Alternatives:** Flexibility Exercises 8 and 12, pages 309 and 310

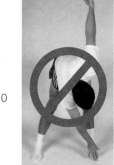

**The Hero**

Excessive strain on the knees.

**Alternatives:** Flexibility Exercises 8 and 14, pages 309 and 311

**Windmill**

Excessive strain on the spine and knees.

**Alternatives:**
Flexibility Exercises 12 and 21, pages 310 and 313

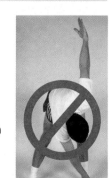

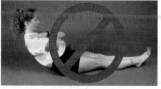

**Straight-Leg Sit-Ups**   **Alternating Bent-Leg Sit-Ups**

These exercises strain the lower back.

**Alternatives:** Strength Exercises 4 and 17, pages 262 and 267

**Donkey Kicks**

Excessive strain on the back, shoulders, and neck.

**Alternatives:**
Flexibility Exercises 20, 14, and 1, pages 313, 311, and 307

## Behavior Modification Planning

### TIPS TO PREVENT LOW-BACK PAIN

☐ I PLAN TO  ☐ I DID IT

- ☐ ☐ Be physically active.
- ☐ ☐ Stretch often using spinal exercises through a functional range of motion.
- ☐ ☐ Regularly strengthen the core of the body using sets of 10 to 12 repetitions to near fatigue with isometric contractions when applicable.
- ☐ ☐ Lift heavy objects by bending at the knees and carry them close to the body.
- ☐ ☐ Avoid sitting (over 50 minutes) or standing in one position for lengthy periods of time.
- ☐ ☐ Maintain correct posture.
- ☐ ☐ Sleep on your back with a pillow under the knees or on your side with the knees drawn up and a small pillow between the knees.
- ☐ ☐ Try out different mattresses of firm consistency before selecting a mattress.
- ☐ ☐ Warm up properly using mild stretches before engaging in physical activity.
- ☐ ☐ Practice adequate stress management techniques.

### Try It

In your class notebook, record how many of the above actions are a regular part of your healthy low-back program. If you are not using all of them, what is necessary to incorporate these behaviors into your lifestyle?

sprains or injuries) can further increase the risk of harm during certain exercises. As you develop your exercise program, you are encouraged to follow the exercise descriptions and guidelines given in this book.

A few exercises, however, are not recommended because of the potential high risk for injury. These exercises sometimes are done in videotaped workouts and some fitness classes. **Contraindicated exercises** may cause harm because of the excessive strain they place on mus-

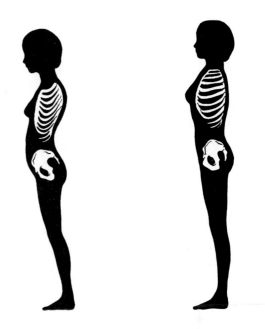

**FIGURE 8.6** Incorrect and correct pelvic alignment.

cles and joints, in particular the spine, lower back, knees, neck, or shoulders.

Illustrations of contraindicated exercises are presented in Figure 8.5. Safe alternative exercises are listed below each contraindicated exercise and are illustrated in the exercises for strength (pages 261–278) and flexibility (pages 307–314). In isolated instances, a qualified physical therapist may select one or a few of the contraindicated exercises to treat a specific injury or disability in a carefully supervised setting. Unless you are specifically instructed to use one of these exercises, it is best that you select safe exercises from this book.

## Preventing and Rehabilitating Low-Back Pain

Few people make it through life without having low-back pain at some point. An estimated 60 to 80 percent of the population has been afflicted by back pain or injury. Estimates indicate that more than 75 million Americans suffer from chronic back pain each year.

Back pain is considered chronic if it persists longer than 3 months. It has been determined that backache syndrome is preventable about 80 percent of the time, and

**Contraindicated exercises** Exercises that are not recommended because they may cause injury to a person.

is caused by (a) physical inactivity, (b) poor postural habits and body mechanics, (c) excessive body weight, and/or (d) psychological stress. Data also indicate that back injuries are more common among smokers.

More than 95 percent of all back pain is related to muscle/tendon injury, and only 1 to 5 percent is related to intervertebral disc damage.[9] Usually, back pain is the result of repeated micro injuries that occur over an extended time (sometimes years) until a certain movement, activity, or excessive overload causes a significant injury to the tissues.[10]

People tend to think of back pain as a problem with the skeleton. Actually, the spine's curvature, alignment, and movement are controlled by surrounding muscles. The most common reason for chronic low-back pain is a lack of physical activity. In particular, a major contributor to back pain is excessive sitting, which causes back muscles to shorten, stiffen, and become weaker.

Deterioration or weakening of the abdominal and gluteal muscles, along with tightening of the lower back (erector spinae) muscles, brings about an unnatural forward tilt of the pelvis (Figure 8.6). This tilt puts extra pressure on the spinal vertebrae, causing pain in the lower back. Accumulation of fat around the midsection of the body contributes to the forward tilt of the pelvis, which further aggravates the condition.

Low-back pain frequently is associated with faulty posture and improper body mechanics, or body positions in all of life's daily activities, including sleeping, sitting, standing, walking, driving, working, and exercising. Incorrect posture and poor mechanics, such as prolonged static postures, repetitive bending and pushing, twisting a loaded spine, and prolonged sitting with little movement (more than an hour) increase strain on the lower back and many other bones, joints, muscles, and ligaments. Figure 8.7 provides a summary of proper body mechanics that promote back health.

In the majority of back injuries, pain is present only with movement and physical activity. If the pain is severe and persists even at rest, the first step is to consult a physician, who can rule out any disc damage and may prescribe proper bed rest using several pillows under the knees for leg support (see Figure 8.7). This position helps release muscle spasms by stretching the muscles involved. In addition, a physician may prescribe a muscle relaxant or anti-inflammatory medication (or both) and some type of physical therapy.

In most cases of low-back pain, even with severe pain, people feel better within days or weeks without being treated by health care professionals.[11] To relieve symptoms, you may use over-the-counter pain relievers and hot or cold packs. You also should stay active to avoid further weakening of the back muscles. Low-impact activities such as walking, swimming, water aerobics, and cycling are recommended. Once you are pain-free in the resting state, you need to start correcting the muscular imbalance by stretching the tight muscles and strengthening the weak ones. Stretching exercises always are performed first.

If there is no indication of disease or injury (such as leg numbness or pain), a herniated disc, or fractures, spinal manipulation by a chiropractor or other health care professional can provide pain relief. Spinal manipulation as a treatment modality for low-back pain has been endorsed by the federal Agency for Health Care Policy and Research. The guidelines suggest that spinal manipulation may help to alleviate discomfort and pain during the first few weeks of an acute episode of low-back pain. Generally, benefits are seen in fewer than 10 treatments. People who have had chronic pain for more than 6 months should avoid spinal manipulation until they have been thoroughly examined by a physician.

Back pain can be reduced greatly through aerobic exercise, muscular flexibility exercise, and muscular strength and endurance training that includes specific exercises to strengthen the spine-stabilizing muscles. Exercise requires effort by the patient, and it may create discomfort initially, but exercise promotes circulation, healing, muscle size, and muscle strength and endurance. Many patients abstain from aggressive physical therapy because they are unwilling to commit the time required for the program.

Aerobic exercise is beneficial because it helps decrease body fat and psychological stress. During an episode of back pain, however, people often avoid activity and cope by getting more rest. Rest is recommended if the pain is associated with a herniated disc, but if your physician rules out a serious problem, exercise is a better choice of treatment. Exercise helps restore physical function, and individuals who start and maintain an aerobic exercise program have back pain less frequently. Individuals who exercise also are less likely to require surgery or other invasive treatments.

In terms of flexibility, regular stretching exercises that help the hip and trunk go through a functional range of motion, rather than increasing the range of motion, are recommended. That is, for proper back care, stretching exercises should not be performed to the extreme range of motion. Individuals with a greater spinal range of motion also have a higher incidence of back injury. Spinal stability, instead of mobility, is desirable for back health.[12]

A strengthening program for a healthy back should be conducted around the endurance threshold—10 to 12 repetitions to near fatigue. Muscular endurance of the muscles that support the spine is more important than absolute strength because these muscles perform their work during the course of an entire day.

## Critical Thinking

Consider your own low-back health. Have you ever had episodes of low-back pain? If so, how long did it take you to recover, and what helped you recover from this condition?

## FIGURE 8.7 Your back and how to care for it.

Whatever the cause of low-back pain, part of its treatment is the correction of faulty posture. But good posture is not simply a matter of "standing tall." It refers to correct use of the body at all times. In fact, for the body to function in the best of health it must be so used that no strain is put upon the muscles, joints, bones, and ligaments. To prevent low-back pain, avoiding strain must become a way of life, practiced while lying, sitting, standing, walking, working, and exercising. When body position is correct, internal organs have enough room to function normally and blood circulates more freely.

With the help of this guide, you can begin to correct the positions and movements that bring on or aggravate backache. Particular attention should be paid to the positions recommended for resting, since it is possible to strain the muscles of the back and neck even while lying in bed. By learning to live with good posture, under all circumstances, you will gradually develop the proper carriage and stronger muscles needed to protect and support your hard-working back.

### How to Stay on Your Feet Without Tiring Your Back

To prevent strain and pain in everyday activities, it is restful to change from one task to another before fatigue sets in. Housewives can lie down between chores; others should check body position frequently, drawing in the abdomen, flattening the back, bending the knees slightly.

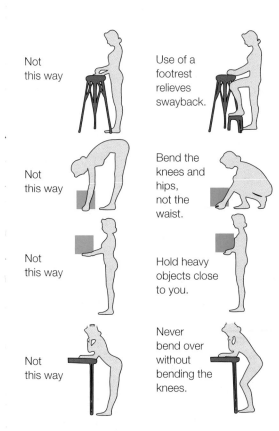

Not this way — Use of a footrest relieves swayback.

Not this way — Bend the knees and hips, not the waist.

Not this way — Hold heavy objects close to you.

Not this way — Never bend over without bending the knees.

### Check Your Carriage Here

In correct, fully erect posture, a line dropped from the ear will go through the tip of the shoulder, middle of hip, back of kneecap, and front of anklebone.

**Incorrect** — Lower back is arched or hollow.

**Incorrect** — Upper back is stooped, lower back is arched, abdomen sags.

**Incorrect** — Note how, in strained position, pelvis tilts forward, chin is out, and ribs are down, crowding internal organs.

**Correct** — In correct position, chin is in, head up, back flattened, pelvis held straight.

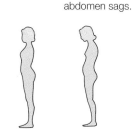

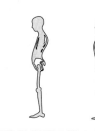

To find the correct standing position: Stand one foot away from wall. Now sit against wall, bending knees slightly. Tighten abdominal and buttock muscles.This will tilt the pelvis back and flatten the lower spine. Holding this position, inch up the wall to standing position, by straightening the legs. Now walk around the room, maintaining the same posture. Place back against wall again to see if you have held it.

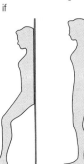

### How to Sit Correctly

A back's best friend is a straight, hard chair. If you can't get the chair you prefer, learn to sit properly on whatever chair you get. *To correct sitting position from forward slump:* Throw head well back, then bend it forward to pull in the chin. This will straighten the back. Now tighten abdominal muscles to raise the chest. Check position frequently.

Use of footrest relieves swayback. Aim is to have knees higher than hips.

Correct way to sit while driving, close to pedals. Use seat belt or hard backrest, available commercially.

TV slump leads to "dowager's hump," strains neck and shoulders.

If chair is too high, swayback is increased.

Keep neck and back in as straight a line as possible with the spine. Bend forward from hips.

Driver's seat too far from pedals emphasizes curve in lower back.

Strained reading position. Forward thrusting strains muscles of neck and head.

(continued)

**FIGURE 8.7** **Your back and how to care for it.** *(continued)*

### How to Put Your Back to Bed

For proper bed posture, a firm mattress is essential. Bedboards, sold commercially, or devised at home, may be used with soft mattresses. Bedboards, preferably, should be made of 3/4 inch plywood. Faulty sleeping positions intensify swayback and result not only in backache but in numbness, tingling, and pain in arms and legs.

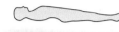

**Incorrect:**

Lying flat on back makes swayback worse.

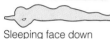

Use of high pillow strains neck, arms, shoulders.

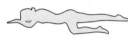

Sleeping face down exaggerates swayback, strains neck and shoulders.

Bending one hip and knee does not relieve swayback.

**Correct:**

Lying on side with knees bent effectively flattens the back. Flat pillow may be used to support neck, especially when shoulders are broad.

Sleeping on back is restful and correct when knees are properly supported.

Raise the foot of the mattress eight inches to discourage sleeping on the abdomen.

Proper arrangement of pillows for resting or reading in bed.

A straight-back chair used behind a pillow makes a serviceable backrest.

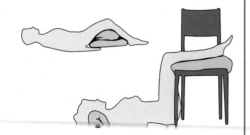

### When Doing Nothing, Do it Right

■ Rest is the first rule for the tired, painful back. The above positions relieve pain by taking all pressure and weight off the back and legs.

■ Note pillows under knees to relieve strain on spine.

■ For complete relief and relaxing effect, these positions should be maintained from 5 to 25 minutes.

### Exercise Without Getting Out of Bed

Exercises to be performed while lying in bed are aimed not so much at strengthening muscles as at teaching correct positioning. But muscles used correctly become stronger and in time are able to support the body with the least amount of effort.

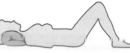

Do all exercises in this position. Legs should not be straightened.

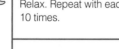

Bring knee up to chest. Lower slowly but do not straighten leg. Relax. Repeat with each leg 10 times.

Bring both knees slowly up to chest (place your hands on the lower thigh behind the knees). Tighten muscles of abdomen, press back flat against bed. Hold knees to chest 20 seconds, then lower slowly. Relax. Repeat 5 times. This exercise gently stretches the shortened muscles of the lower back, while strengthening abdominal muscles.

### Rules to Live By—From Now On

1. Never bend from the waist only; bend the hips and knees.
2. Never lift a heavy object higher than your waist.
3. Always turn and face the object you wish to lift.
4. Avoid carrying unbalanced loads; hold heavy objects close to your body.
5. Never carry anything heavier than you can manage with ease.
6. Never lift or move heavy furniture. Wait for someone to do it who knows the principles of leverage.
7. Avoid sudden movements, sudden "overloading" of muscles. Learn to move deliberately, swinging the legs from the hips.
8. Learn to keep the head in line with the spine, when standing, sitting, lying in bed.
9. Put soft chairs and deep couches on your "don't sit" list. During prolonged sitting, cross your legs to rest your back.
10. Your doctor is the only one who can determine when low-back pain is due to faulty posture and he is the best judge of when you may do general exercises for physical fitness. When you do, omit any exercise that arches

or overstrains the lower back: backward bends, or forward bends, touching the toes with the knees straight.
11. Wear shoes with moderate heels, all about the same height. Avoid changing from high to low heels.
12. Put a footrail under the desk and a footrest under the crib.
13. Diaper the baby sitting next to him or her on the bed.
14. Don't stoop and stretch to hang the wash; raise the clothesbasket and lower the washline.
15. Beg or buy a rocking chair. Rocking rests the back by changing the muscle groups used.
16. Train yourself vigorously to use your abdominal muscles to flatten your lower abdomen. In time, this muscle contraction will become habitual, making you the envied possessor of a youthful body profile!
17. Don't strain to open windows or doors.
18. For good posture, concentrate on strengthening "nature's corset"—the abdominal and buttock muscles. The pelvic roll exercise is especially recommended to correct the postural relation between the pelvis and the spine.

### Exercise Without Attracting Attention

Use these inconspicuous exercises whenever you have a spare moment during the day, both to relax tension and improve the tone of important muscle groups.

1. Rotate shoulders, forward and backward.
2. Turn head slowly side to side.
3. Watch an imaginary plane take off, just below the right shoulder. Stretch neck, follow it slowly as it moves up, around and down, disappearing below the other shoulder. Repeat, starting on left side.
4. Slowly, slowly, touch left ear to left shoulder, right ear to right shoulder. Raise both shoulders to touch ears, drop them as far down as possible.
5. At any pause in the day—waiting for an elevator to arrive, for a specific traffic light to change—pull in abdominal muscles, tighten, hold it for the count of eight without breathing. Relax slowly. Increase the count gradually after the first week, practice breathing normally with the abdomen flat and contracted. Do this sitting, standing, and walking.

Several exercises for preventing and rehabilitating the backache syndrome are given on pages 311–314. These exercises can be done twice or more daily when a person has back pain. Under normal circumstances, doing these exercises three or four times a week is enough to prevent the syndrome. Using some of the additional core exercises listed in Chapter 7 (page 252) will further enhance your low-back management program. Back pain recurs more often in people who rely solely on medication, compared with people who use both medication and exercise therapy to recover.[13]

### Effects of Stress

Psychological stress, too, may lead to back pain.[14] Excessive stress causes muscles to contract. In the case of the lower back, frequent tightening of the muscles can throw the back out of alignment and constrict blood vessels that supply oxygen and nutrients to the back. Chronic stress also increases the release of hormones that have been linked to muscle and tendon injuries. Furthermore, people under stress tend to forget proper body mechanics, placing themselves at unnecessary risk for injury. If you are undergoing excessive stress and back pain at the same time, proper stress management (see Chapter 10) should be a part of your comprehensive back-care program.

### Personal Flexibility and Low-Back Conditioning Program

Lab 8C allows you to develop your own flexibility and low-back conditioning programs. The recommendation calls for isometric contractions of 2 to 20 seconds during each repetition for some of the exercises listed for back health (see Lab 8C) to further increase spinal stability and muscular strength endurance. The length of the hold will depend on your current fitness level and the difficulty of each exercise. For most exercises, you may start with a 2- to 10-second hold. Over the course of several weeks, you can increase the length of the hold from 10 to 30 seconds.

# ASSESS YOUR BEHAVIOR

Log on to http://www.cengage.com/sso/ to create a flexibility program and track your progress in incorporating flexibility exercises in you fitness program.

1. Do you give flexibility exercises the same priority in your fitness program as you do aerobic and strength training?

2. Are stretching exercises a part of your fitness program at least two times per week?

3. Do you include exercises to strengthen and enhance body alignment in your regular strength and flexibility program?

# ASSESS YOUR KNOWLEDGE

Log on to http://www.cengage.com/sso/ to assess your understanding of this chapter's topics by taking the Student Practice Test and exploring the modules recommended in your Personalized Study Plan.

1. Muscular flexibility is defined as
   a. the capacity of joints and muscles to work in a synchronized manner.
   b. the achievable range of motion at a joint or group of joints without causing injury.
   c. the capability of muscles to stretch beyond their normal resting length without injury to the muscles.
   d. the capacity of muscles to return to their proper length following the application of a stretching force.
   e. the limitations placed on muscles as the joints move through their normal planes.

2. Good flexibility
   a. promotes healthy muscles and joints.
   b. decreases the risk of injury.
   c. improves posture.
   d. decreases the risk of chronic back pain.
   e. All are correct choices.

3. Plastic elongation is a term used in reference to
   a. permanent lengthening of soft tissue.
   b. increased flexibility achieved through dynamic stretching.
   c. temporary elongation of muscles.
   d. the ability of a muscle to achieve a complete degree of stretch.
   e. lengthening of a muscle against resistance.

4. The most significant contributors to loss of flexibility are
   a. sedentary living and lack of physical activity.
   b. weight and power training.
   c. age and injury.
   d. muscular strength and endurance.
   e. excessive body fat and low lean tissue.

5. Which of the following is *not* a mode of stretching?
   a. Proprioceptive neuromuscular facilitation
   b. Elastic elongation
   c. Ballistic stretching
   d. Slow-sustained stretching
   e. All are modes of stretching.

6. PNF can help increase
   a. muscular strength.
   b. muscular flexibility.
   c. muscular endurance.
   d. range of motion.
   e. All are correct choices.

7. When performing stretching exercises, the degree of stretch should be
   a. through the entire arc of movement.
   b. to about 80 percent of capacity.
   c. to tightness at the end of the range of motion.
   d. applied until the muscle(s) start shaking.
   e. progressively increased until the desired stretch is attained.

8. When stretching, the final stretch should be held for
   a. 1 to 10 seconds.
   b. 15 to 30 seconds.
   c. 30 to 90 seconds.
   d. 1 to 3 minutes.
   e. as long as the person is able to sustain the stretch.

9. Low-back pain is associated primarily with
   a. physical inactivity.
   b. faulty posture.
   c. excessive body weight.
   d. improper body mechanics.
   e. All are correct choices.

10. The following exercise helps stretch the lower back and hamstring muscles.
    a. Adductor stretch.
    b. Cat stretch.
    c. Back extension stretch.
    d. Single-knee-to-chest stretch.
    e. Quad stretch.

Correct answers can be found at the back of the book.

# MEDIA MENU

You can find the links below at the book companion site: www.cengage.com/health/hoeger/plfw10e

- Create your personal flexibility profile.
- Check how well you understand the chapter's concepts.

## Internet Connections

Specific Stretching Exercises, with Diagrams. Let Shape Up America show you how to develop an activity program that's right for you. Its online Fitness Center includes valuable information on improvement and assessment of, as well as barriers to, physical fitness. *http://www.shapeup.org*

Yoga and Other Stretching Exercises. This site features information on the techniques of yoga, Pilates, and other forms of stretching exercises. *http://www.yoga.com*

Stretching to Increase Flexibility. In addition to a comprehensive description of the health benefits of regular stretching, this site features a series of exercises tailored to three levels of fitness based on how often you perform stretching exercises. *http://k2.kirtland.cc.mi.us/~balbachl/flex.htm*

# NOTES

1. American College of Obstetricians and Gynecologists, *Guidelines for Exercise During Pregnancy*, 2003.

2. "Stretch Yourself Younger," *Consumer Reports on Health* 11 (August 1999): 6–7.

3. W. W. K. Hoeger and D. R. Hopkins, "A Comparison Between the Sit and Reach and the Modified Sit and Reach in the Measurement of Flexibility in Women," *Research Quarterly for Exercise and Sport* 63 (1992): 191–195; W. W. K. Hoeger, D. R. Hopkins, S. Button, and T. A. Palmer, "Comparing the Sit and Reach with the Modified Sit and Reach in Measuring Flexibility in Adolescents," *Pediatric Exercise Science* 2 (1990): 156–162; D. R. Hopkins and W. W. K. Hoeger, "A Comparison of the Sit and Reach and the Modified Sit and Reach in the Measurement of Flexibility for Males," *Journal of Applied Sports Science Research* 6 (1992): 7–10.

4. "Position Yourself to Stay Well," *Consumer Reports on Health* 18 (February 2006): 8–9.

5. J. Kokkonen and S. Lauritzen, "Isotonic Strength and Endurance Gains Through PNF Stretching," *Medicine and Science in Sports and Exercise* 27 (1995): S22, 127.

6. American College of Sports Medicine, *ACSM's Guidelines for Exercise Testing and Prescription* (Baltimore: Williams & Wilkins, 2006).

7. K. B. Fields, C. M. Burnworth, and M. Delaney, "Should Athletes Stretch before Exercise?" *Gatorade Sports Science Institute: Sports Science Exchange* 30, no. 1 (2207): 1–5.

8. S. B. Thacker, J. Gilchrist, D. F. Stroup, and C. D. Kimsey. Jr., "The Impact of Stretching on Sports Injury Risk: A Systematic Review of the Literature," *Medicine and Science in Sports and Exercise* 36 (2004): 371–378.

9. D. B. J. Andersson, L. J. Fine, and B. A. Silverstein, "Musculoskeletal Disorders," *Occupational Health: Recognizing and Preventing Work-Related Disease,* edited by B. S. Levy and D. H. Wegman (Boston: Little, Brown, 1995).

10. M. R. Bracko, "Can We Prevent Back Injuries?" *ACSM's Health & Fitness Journal* 8, no. 4 (2004): 5–11.

11. R. Deyo, "Chiropractic Care for Back Pain: The Physician's Perspective," *HealthNews* 4 (September 10, 1998).

12. See note 10.

13. J. A. Hides, G. A. Jull, and C. A. Richardson, "Long-Term Effects of Specific Stabilizing Exercises for First-Episode Low Back Pain," *Spine* 26 (2001): E243–E248.

14. "Position Yourself to Stay Well," *Consumer Reports on Health* 18 (February 2006): 8–9.

15. A. Brownstein, "Chronic Back Pain Can Be Beaten," *Bottom Line/Health* 13 (October 1999): 3–4.

# SUGGESTED READINGS

Alter, M. J. *The Science of Stretching.* Champaign, IL: Human Kinetic Press, 1996.

Alter, M. J. *Sports Stretch.* Champaign, IL: Human Kinetics, 2004.

American College of Obstetricians and Gynecologists, *Exercise During Pregnancy,* 2003.

Anderson, B. *Stretching.* Bolinas, CA: Shelter Publications, 1999.

Bracko, M. R. "Can We Prevent Back Injuries?" *ACSM's Health & Fitness Journal* 8, no. 4 (2004): 5–11.

Hoeger, W. W. K. *The Assessment of Muscular Flexibility: Test Protocols and National Flexibility Norms for the Modified Sit-and-Reach Test, Total Body Rotation Test, and Shoulder Rotation Test.* Rockton, IL: Figure Finder Collection Novel Products, Inc., 2006.

Liemohn, W., and G. Pariser. "Core Strength: Implications for Fitness and Low Back Pain." *ACSM's Health and Fitness Journal* 6, no. 5 (2002): 10–16.

McAtee, R. E., and J. Charland. *Facilitated Stretching.* Champaign, IL: Human Kinetics, 2007.

Nelson, A. G., J. Kokkonen, and J. M. McAlexander. *Stretching Anatomy.* Champaign, IL: Human Kinetics, 2006.

# Flexibility Exercises

## EXERCISE 1   Neck Stretches

ACTION Slowly and gently tilt the head laterally (a). You may increase the degree of stretch by gently pulling with one hand (b). You may also turn the head about 30° to one side and stretch the neck by raising your head toward the ceiling (see photo c—do not extend your head backward; look straight forward). Now gradually bring the head forward until you feel an adequate stretch in the muscles on the back of the neck (d). Perform the exercises on both the right and left sides. Repeat each exercise several times, and hold the final stretched position for a few seconds.

AREAS STRETCHED Neck flexors and extensors; ligaments of the cervical spine

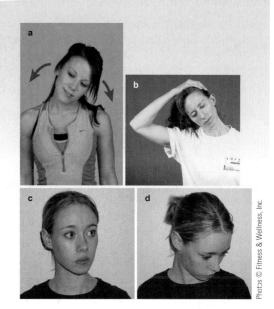

Photos © Fitness & Wellness, Inc.

## EXERCISE 2   Arm Circles

ACTION Gently circle your arms all the way around. Conduct the exercise in both directions.

AREAS STRETCHED Shoulder muscles and ligaments

© Fitness & Wellness, Inc.

## EXERCISE 3   Side Stretch

ACTION Stand straight up, feet separated to shoulder-width, and place your hands on your waist. Now move the upper body to one side and hold the final stretch for a few seconds. Repeat on the other side.

AREAS STRETCHED Muscles and ligaments in the pelvic region

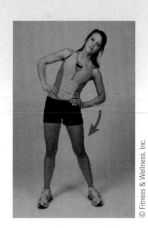

© Fitness & Wellness, Inc.

## EXERCISE 4    Body Rotation

ACTION  Place your arms slightly away from the body and rotate the trunk as far as possible, holding the final position for several seconds. Conduct the exercise for both the right and left sides of the body. You also can perform this exercise by standing about 2 feet away from the wall (back toward the wall) and then rotating the trunk, placing the hands against the wall.

AREAS STRETCHED  Hip, abdominal, chest, back, neck, and shoulder muscles; hip and spinal ligaments

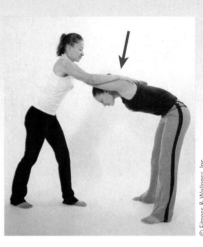

© Fitness & Wellness, Inc.

## EXERCISE 5    Chest Stretch

ACTION  Place your hands on the shoulders of your partner, who in turn will push you down by your shoulders. Hold the final position for a few seconds.

AREAS STRETCHED  Chest (pectoral) muscles and shoulder ligaments

© Fitness & Wellness, Inc.

## EXERCISE 6    Shoulder Hyperextension Stretch

ACTION  Have a partner grasp your arms from behind by the wrists and slowly push them up-ward. Hold the final position for a few seconds.

AREAS STRETCHED  Deltoid and pectoral muscles; ligaments of the shoulder joint

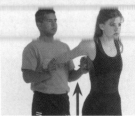

© Fitness & Wellness, Inc

## EXERCISE 7   Shoulder Rotation Stretch

ACTION  With the aid of surgical tubing or an aluminum or wood stick, place the tubing or stick behind your back and grasp the two ends using a reverse (thumbs-out) grip. Slowly bring the tubing or stick over your head, keeping the elbows straight. Repeat several times (bring the hands closer together for additional stretch).

AREAS STRETCHED  Deltoid, latissimus dorsi, and pectoral muscles; shoulder ligaments

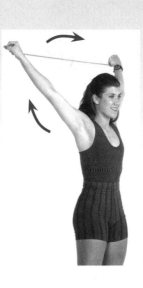
© Fitness & Wellness, Inc.

## EXERCISE 8   Quad Stretch

ACTION  Lie on your side and move one foot back by flexing the knee. Grasp the front of the lower leg and pull the ankle toward the gluteal region. Hold for several seconds. Repeat with the other leg.

AREAS STRETCHED  Quadriceps muscle; knee and ankle ligaments

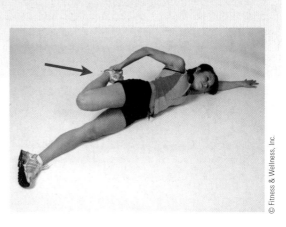
© Fitness & Wellness, Inc.

## EXERCISE 9   Heel Cord Stretch

ACTION  Stand against the wall or at the edge of a step and stretch the heel downward, alternating legs. Hold the stretched position for a few seconds.

AREAS STRETCHED  Heel cord (Achilles tendon); gastrocnemius and soleus muscles

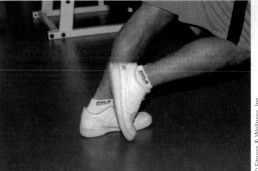
© Fitness & Wellness, Inc.

## EXERCISE 10  Adductor Stretch

**ACTION** Stand with your feet about twice shoulder-width apart and place your hands slightly above the knees. Flex one knee and slowly go down as far as possible, holding the final position for a few seconds. Repeat with the other leg.

**AREAS STRETCHED** Hip adductor muscles

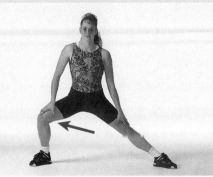

© Fitness & Wellness, Inc.

## EXERCISE 11  Sitting Adductor Stretch

**ACTION** Sit on the floor and bring your feet in close to you, allowing the soles of the feet to touch each other. Now place your forearms (or elbows) on the inner part of the thigh and push the legs downward, holding the final stretch for several seconds.

**AREAS STRETCHED** Hip adductor muscles

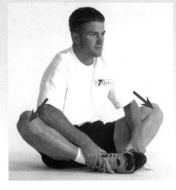

© Fitness & Wellness, Inc.

## EXERCISE 12  Sit-and-Reach Stretch

**ACTION** Sit on the floor with legs together and gradually reach forward as far as possible. Hold the final position for a few seconds. This exercise also may be performed with the legs separated, reaching to each side as well as to the middle.

**AREAS STRETCHED** Hamstrings and lower back muscles; lumbar spine ligaments

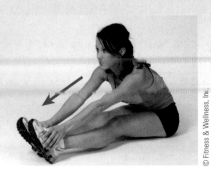

© Fitness & Wellness, Inc.

### EXERCISE 13 Triceps Stretch

ACTION Place the right hand behind your neck. Grasp the right arm above the elbow with the left hand. Gently pull the elbow backward. Repeat the exercise with the opposite arm.

AREAS STRETCHED Back of upper arm (triceps muscle); shoulder joint

NOTE Exercises 14 through 21 and 23 are also flexibility exercises and can be added to your stretching program.

© Fitness & Wellness, Inc.

# Exercises for the Prevention and Rehabilitation of Low-Back Pain

### EXERCISE 14 Hip Flexor Stretch

ACTION Kneel down on an exercise mat or a soft surface, or place a towel under your knees. Raise the right knee off the floor and place the right foot about 3 feet in front of you. Place your right hand over your right knee and the left hand over the back of the left hip. Keeping the lower back flat, slowly move forward and downward as you apply gentle pressure over the left hip. Repeat the exercise with the opposite leg forward.

AREAS STRETCHED Flexor muscles in front of the hip joint

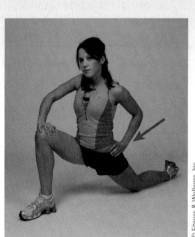

© Fitness & Wellness, Inc.

### EXERCISE 15 Single-Knee-to-Chest Stretch

ACTION Lie down flat on the floor. Bend one leg at approximately 100° and gradually pull the opposite leg toward your chest. Hold the final stretch for a few seconds. Switch legs and repeat the exercise.

AREAS STRETCHED Lower back and hamstring muscles; lumbar spine ligaments

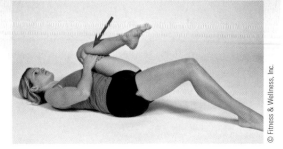

© Fitness & Wellness, Inc.

## EXERCISE 16  Double-Knee-to-Chest Stretch

ACTION Lie flat on the floor and then curl up slowly into a fetal position. Hold for a few seconds.

AREAS STRETCHED Upper and lower back and hamstring muscles; spinal ligaments

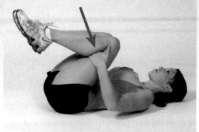

© Fitness & Wellness, Inc.

## EXERCISE 17  Upper and Lower Back Stretch

ACTION Sit on the floor and bring your feet in close to you, allowing the soles of the feet to touch each other. Holding on to your feet, bring your head and upper chest gently toward your feet.

AREAS STRETCHED Upper and lower back muscles and ligaments

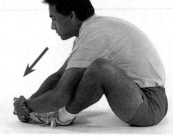

© Fitness & Wellness, Inc.

## EXERCISE 18  Sit-and-Reach Stretch

(See Exercise 12 on page 310)

## EXERCISE 19  Gluteal Stretch

ACTION Lie on the floor, bend the right leg, and place your right ankle slightly above the left knee. Grasp behind the left thigh with both hands and gently pull the leg toward the chest. Repeat the exercise with the opposite leg.

AREAS STRETCHED Buttock area (gluteal muscles)

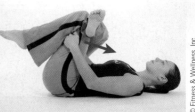

© Fitness & Wellness, Inc.

## EXERCISE 20   Back Extension Stretch

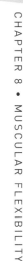

ACTION Lie face down on the floor with the elbows by the chest, forearms on the floor, and the hands beneath the chin. Gently raise the trunk by extending the elbows until you reach an approximate 90° angle at the elbow joint. Be sure the forearms remain in contact with the floor at all times. Do NOT extend the back beyond this point. Hyperextension of the lower back may lead to or aggravate an existing back problem. Hold the stretched position for about 10 seconds.

AREAS STRETCHED Abdominal region

ADDITIONAL BENEFITS Restore lower back curvature

## EXERCISE 21   Trunk Rotation and Lower Back Stretch

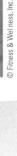

ACTION Sit on the floor and bend the left leg, placing the right foot on the outside of the left knee. Place the left elbow on the right knee and push against it. At the same time, try to rotate the trunk to the right (clockwise). Hold the final position for a few seconds. Repeat the exercise with the other side.

AREAS STRETCHED Lateral side of the hip and thigh; trunk and lower back

## EXERCISE 22   Pelvic Tilt

(See Exercise 12 in Chapter 7, page 265) This is perhaps the most important exercise for the care of the lower back. It should be included as a part of your daily exercise routine and should be performed several times throughout the day when pain in the lower back is present as a result of muscle imbalance.

## EXERCISE 23   The Cat

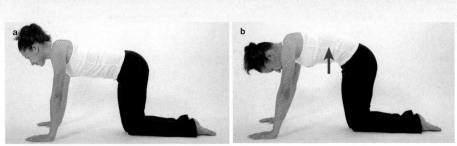

ACTION Kneel on the floor and place your hands in front of you (on the floor) about shoulder-width apart. Relax the trunk and lower back (a). Now arch the spine and pull in your abdomen as far as you can and hold this position for a few seconds (b). Repeat the exercise 4–5 times.

AREAS STRETCHED Low back muscles and ligaments

AREAS STRENGTHENED Abdominal and gluteal muscles

## EXERCISE 24   Abdominal Crunch or Abdominal Curl-Up

(See Exercise 4 in Chapter 7, page 262) It is important that you do not stabilize your feet when performing either of these exercises, because doing so decreases the work of the abdominal muscles. Also, remember not to "swing up" but, rather, to curl up as you perform these exercises.

**EXERCISE 25**  Reverse Crunch    (See Exercise 11 in Chapter 7, page 265)

**EXERCISE 26**  Supine Bridge

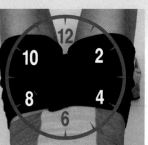

ACTION   Lie face up on the floor with the knees bent at about 120°. Do a pelvic tilt (Exercise 12 in Chapter 7, page 265) and maintain the pelvic tilt while you raise the hips off the floor until the upper body and upper legs are in a straight line. Hold this position for several seconds.

AREAS STRENGTHENED   Gluteal and abdominal flexor muscles

© Fitness & Wellness, Inc.

**EXERCISE 27**  Pelvic Clock

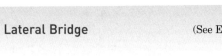

ACTION   Lie face up on the floor with the knees bent at about 120°. Fully extend the hips as in the supine bridge (Exercise 26). Now progressively rotate the hips in a clockwise manner (2 o'clock, 4 o'clock, 6 o'clock, 8 o'clock, 10 o'clock, and 12 o'clock), holding each position in an isometric contraction for about 1 second. Repeat the exercise counterclockwise.

AREAS STRENGTHENED   Gluteal, abdominal, and hip flexor muscles

© Fitness & Wellness, Inc.

**EXERCISE 28**  Lateral Bridge    (See Exercise 13 in Chapter 7, page 265)

**EXERCISE 29**  Prone Bridge    (See Exercise 14 in Chapter 7, page 266)

**EXERCISE 30**  Leg Press    (See Exercise 16 in Chapter 7, page 267)

**EXERCISE 31**  Seated Back    (See Exercise 20 in Chapter 7, page 269)

**EXERCISE 32**  Lat Pull-Down    (See Exercise 24 in Chapter 7, page 271)

**EXERCISE 33**  Back Extension    (See Exercise 36 in Chapter 7, page 278)

**EXERCISE 34**  Lateral Trunk Flexion    (See Exercise 37 in Chapter 7, page 278)

# LAB 8A: Muscular Flexibility Assessment

Name _____     Date _____     Grade _____

Instructor _____     Course _____     Section _____

### Necessary Lab Equipment
Acuflex I, Acuflex II, and Acuflex III Flexibility Testers*
or homemade flexibility testing equipment as described
in Figures 8.1, 8.2, and 8.3.

### Objective
To assess muscular flexibility and the respective fitness
categories.

### Lab Preparation
The procedures for the flexibility tests* administered in
this lab are explained in this chapter (Figures 8.1, 8.2,
and 8.3, pages 291–293. It is important that you warm
up properly before you perform any of these tests. Do
gentle stretching exercises specific to the tests that will
be administered. Wear loose exercise clothing for this lab.
Be sure to circle either inches or cm, depending on which
system you use.

## I. Modified Sit-and-Reach Test (page 291)

Trials:   1. _____ inches _____ cm   2. _____ inches _____ cm (circle either inches or cm)

Average score: _____ inches _____ cm   Percentile rank: _____   Points: _____

(Table 8.4, page 295)

Fitness category: _____

## II. Total Body Rotation Test (page 292)

Right Side     Left Side     (circle one)

Trials:   1. _____ inches _____ cm   2. _____ inches _____ cm (circle either inches or cm)

Average score: _____ inches _____ cm   Percentile rank: _____   Points: _____

(Table 8.4, page 295)

Fitness category: _____

## III. Shoulder Rotation Test (page 293)

Biacromial width: _____ inches _____ cm     Rotation score: _____ inches _____ cm

Final score = Rotation score − biacromial width

Final score = _____ − _____ = _____ inches / cm (circle one)     Percentile rank: _____

Fitness category: _____     Points: _____

(Table 8.4, page 295)

*The Acuflex I, II, and III Flexibility Testers can be obtained from Figure Finder Collection, Novel Products, Inc., P. O. Box 408, Rockton, IL 61072-0408,
Phone (800) 323-5143, Fax 815-624-4866.

IV. Overall Flexibility Rating

| Test | Points |
|------|--------|
| Modified sit-and-reach: | _____ |
| Total body rotation (right, left — circle one): | _____ |
| Shoulder rotation: | _____ |
| | Total Points: _____ |

Overall flexibility category (see Table 8.5, page 295): _____

V. Flexibility Goals

1. Indicate the flexibility category that you would like to achieve by the end of the term:

_____

2. Describe your feelings about your current body flexibility and any potential implications that your current flexibility levels may have on your health and wellness. Also, briefly state how you plan to achieve your flexibility objective by the end of the term.

_____

_____

_____

_____

_____

_____

_____

_____

_____

_____

_____

_____

_____

_____

_____

# LAB 8B: Posture Evaluation

Name _____ Date _____ Grade _____

Instructor _____ Course _____ Section _____

### Necessary Lab Equipment
A plumb line, two large mirrors set at about an 85° angle, and a Polaroid camera (the mirrors and the camera are optional—see "Evaluating Body Posture" (pages 290–294).

### Objective
To determine current body alignment.

### Lab Preparation
To conduct the posture analysis, men should wear shorts only and women, shorts and a tank top. Shoes should also be removed for this test.

### Lab Assignment
The class should be divided in groups of four students each. The group should carefully study the posture form given in this lab, then proceed to fill out the form for each member according to the instructions given under "Evaluating Body Posture" (pages 290–294). If no mirrors and camera are available, three members of the group are to rate the fourth person's posture while he/she first stands with the side of the body and then with the back to the plumb line. A final score is obtained by totaling the points given for each body segment and looking up the posture rating according to the total score found in the table provided below.

### Results

Total points: _____

Category: _____

| Posture Evaluation Standards | |
|---|---|
| Total Points | Category |
| ≥45 | Excellent |
| 40–44 | Good |
| 30–39 | Average |
| 20–29 | Fair |
| ≤19 | Poor |

### Posture Improvement
Indicate how you feel about your posture, identify areas to correct, and specify the steps you can take to make those improvements.

_____
_____
_____
_____
_____
_____
_____
_____

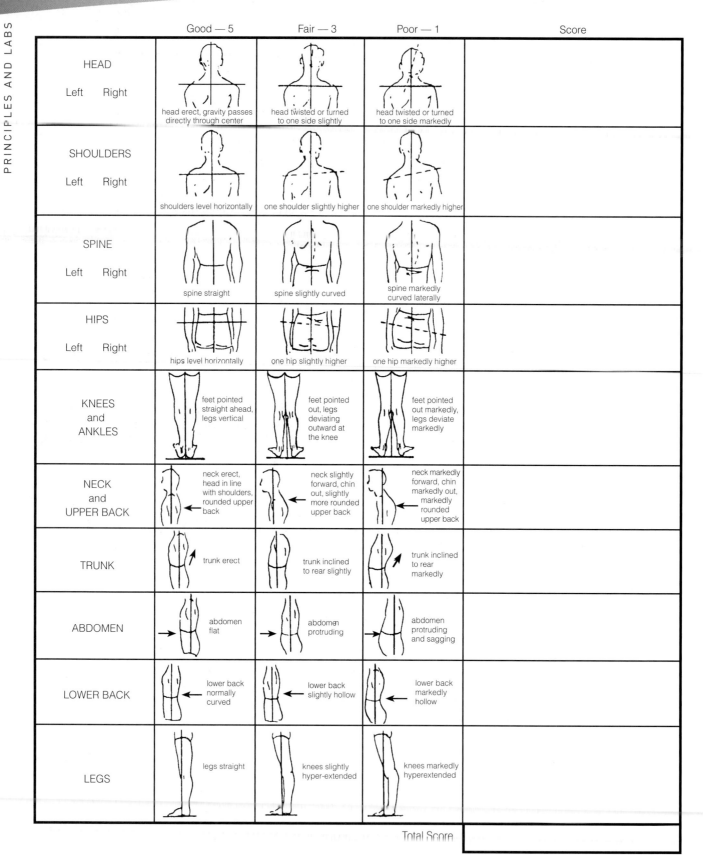

| | Good — 5 | Fair — 3 | Poor — 1 | Score |
|---|---|---|---|---|
| **HEAD** Left Right | head erect, gravity passes directly through center | head twisted or turned to one side slightly | head twisted or turned to one side markedly | |
| **SHOULDERS** Left Right | shoulders level horizontally | one shoulder slightly higher | one shoulder markedly higher | |
| **SPINE** Left Right | spine straight | spine slightly curved | spine markedly curved laterally | |
| **HIPS** Left Right | hips level horizontally | one hip slightly higher | one hip markedly higher | |
| **KNEES and ANKLES** | feet pointed straight ahead, legs vertical | feet pointed out, legs deviating outward at the knee | feet pointed out markedly, legs deviate markedly | |
| **NECK and UPPER BACK** | neck erect, head in line with shoulders, rounded upper back | neck slightly forward, chin out, slightly more rounded upper back | neck markedly forward, chin markedly out, markedly rounded upper back | |
| **TRUNK** | trunk erect | trunk inclined to rear slightly | trunk inclined to rear markedly | |
| **ABDOMEN** | abdomen flat | abdomen protruding | abdomen protruding and sagging | |
| **LOWER BACK** | lower back normally curved | lower back slightly hollow | lower back markedly hollow | |
| **LEGS** | legs straight | knees slightly hyper-extended | knees markedly hyperextended | |
| | | | Total Score | |

Adapted from *The New York Physical Fitness Test: A Manual for Teachers of Physical Education,* New York State Education Department (Division of HPER), 1958.

# LAB 8C: Flexibility Development and Low-Back Conditioning

Name _____   Date _____   Grade _____

Instructor _____   Course _____   Section _____

### Necessary Lab Equipment
Minor implements such as a chair, a table, an elastic band (surgical tubing or a wood or aluminum stick), and a stool or steps.

### Objective
To develop a flexibility exercise program and a conditioning program for the prevention and rehabilitation of low-back pain.

### Lab Preparation
Wear exercise clothing and prepare to participate in a sample stretching exercise session. All of the flexibility and low-back conditioning exercises are illustrated on pages 307–314.

### I. Stage of Change for Flexibility Training
Using Figure 2.5 (page 57) and Table 2.3 (page 57), identify your current stage of change for participation in a muscular stretching program:

### II. Instruction
Perform all of the recommended flexibility exercises given on pages 307–314. Use a combination of slow-sustained and proprioceptive neuromuscular facilitation stretching techniques. Indicate the technique(s) used for each exercise and, where applicable, the number of repetitions performed and the length of time that the final degree of stretch was held.

**Stretching Exercises**

| Exercise | Stretching Technique | Repetitions | Length of Final Stretch |
|---|---|---|---|
| Lateral head tilt | | | NA* |
| Arm circles | | | NA |
| Side stretch | | | |
| Body rotation | | | |
| Chest stretch | | | |
| Shoulder hyperextension stretch | | | |
| Shoulder rotation stretch | | | NA |
| Quad stretch | | | |
| Heel cord stretch | | | |
| Adductor stretch | | | |
| Sitting adductor stretch | | | |
| Sit-and-reach stretch | | | |
| Triceps stretch | | | |

*Not Applicable

Stretching Schedule (Indicate days, time, and place where you will stretch):

Flexibility-training days: M ☐ T ☐ W ☐ Th ☐ F ☐ Sa ☐ Su ☐ Time of day: ☐ Place: ☐

## Low-Back Conditioning Program

Perform all of the recommended exercises for the prevention and rehabilitation of low-back pain given on pages 311–314. Indicate the number of repetitions performed for each exercise.

| Flexibility Exercises | Repetitions | Strength/Endurance Exercises | Repetitions | Seconds Held |
|---|---|---|---|---|
| Hip flexor stretch | ☐ | Pelvic tilt | ☐ | ☐ |
| Single-knee-to-chest stretch | ☐ | The cat | ☐ | ☐ |
| Double-knee-to-chest stretch | ☐ | Abdominal crunch or abdominal curl-up | ☐ | |
| Upper- and lower-back stretch | ☐ | Reverse crunch | ☐ | |
| Sit-and-reach stretch | ☐ | Supine bridge | ☐ | ☐ |
| Gluteal stretch | ☐ | Pelvic clock | ☐ | ☐ |
| Back extension stretch | ☐ | Lateral bridge | ☐ | ☐ |
| Trunk rotation and lower back stretch | ☐ | Prone bridge | ☐ | ☐ |
| | | Leg press | ☐ | |
| | | Seated back | ☐ | |
| | | Lat pull-down | ☐ | |
| | | Back extension | ☐ | ☐ |

## Proper Body Mechanics

Perform the following tasks using the proper body mechanics given in Figure 8.7 (pages 301–302). Check off each item as you perform the task:

☐ Standing (carriage) position

☐ Sitting position

☐ Bed posture

☐ Resting position for tired and painful back

☐ Lifting an object

## "Rules to Live By — From Now On"

Read the 18 "Rules to Live By—From Now On" given in Figure 8.7 (page 302) and indicate below those rules that you need to work on to improve posture and body mechanics and prevent low-back pain.

_____

_____

_____

_____

_____

_____

_____

# Skill Fitness and Fitness Programming

**9**

## Objectives

- Learn the benefits of good skill-related fitness
- Identify and define the six components of skill-related fitness
- Become familiar with performance tests to assess skill-related fitness
- Dispel common misconceptions related to physical fitness and wellness
- Become aware of safety considerations for exercising
- Learn concepts for preventing and treating injuries
- Describe the relationship between fitness and aging
- Be able to write a comprehensive fitness program
- Obtain your personal prescription for improving cardiorespiratory fitness. Get on the road to a wellness way of life by chronicling your daily activities.

**CENGAGENOW™**

Check your understanding of the chapter contents by logging on to CengageNOW and accessing the pre-test, personalized learning plan, and post-test for this chapter.

# FAQ

### What is the best fitness activity?

No single physical activity, sport, or exercise contributes to the development of overall fitness (see Chapter 6, Table 6.10, page 217). Most people who exercise pick and adhere to a single mode, such as walking, swimming, or jogging. Many activities will contribute to cardiorespiratory development. The extent of contribution to other fitness components, though, varies among the activities. For total fitness, aerobic activities should be supplemented with strength and flexibility programs. Cross-training—that is, selecting different activities for fitness development and maintenance (jogging, swimming, spinning)—adds enjoyment to the program, decreases the risk of incurring injuries from overuse, and keeps exercise from becoming monotonous.

### Is it best not to eat before exercise?

Despite popular belief, research indicates that eating some food, liquid or solid, prior to physical activity provides energy and nutrients that improve endurance and exercise performance. Of course, how long before exercise, how much food, and what type of food you eat depends on the intensity of exercise and your stomach's tolerance to pre-exercise food. The primary fuel for exercise is provided by carbohydrates, which the body converts to glucose and stores as glycogen. Some protein along with carbohydrates is also recommended (see next question).

Aim to consume 1 gram of carbohydrate per kilogram of body weight (.5 gram of carbohydrate per pound of body weight) within the hour prior to exercise. For high-intensity aerobic activities, sports drinks that are consumed 30 to 60 minutes prior to exercise are best because they are rapidly absorbed by the body. Solid foods (granola bars, energy bars, bagels, sugar wafers, crackers) or semi-liquid solid foods (yogurt, gelatin, pudding) are acceptable for lower-intensity aerobic exercise or strength training. Even a snack consumed a few minutes before exercise will help you, as long as you exercise longer than 30 minutes. Through trial and error you will learn which sport snacks best suit your stomach without interfering with exercise performance.

### Are there specific nutrient requirements for optimal development and recovery following exercise?

Carbohydrates with some protein appear to be best. Protein is recommended prior to and immediately following high-intensity aerobic or strength-training exercise. Intense exercise causes microtears in muscle tissue, and the presence of amino acids (the building blocks of proteins) in the blood contributes to the healing process and subsequent development and strengthening of the muscle fibers. Protein consumption along with carbohydrates also accelerates glycogen replenishment in the body after intense or prolonged exercise. Thus, carbohydrates provide energy for exercise and replenishment of glycogen stores after exercise, while protein optimizes muscle repair, growth, glycogen replenishment, and recovery following exercise. Aim for a ratio of 4 to 1 grams of carbohydrates to protein. For example, you may consume a snack that contains 40 grams of carbohydrates (160 calories) and 10 grams of protein (40 calories). Examples of good recovery foods include milk and cereal, a tuna fish sandwich, a peanut butter and jelly sandwich, and pasta with turkey meat sauce.

**Skill-related fitness** is needed for success in athletics and in lifetime sports and activities such as basketball, racquetball, golf, hiking, soccer, and water skiing. While most exercise programs are designed to enhance the health-related components of fitness, skill-related sports participation also contributes to health-related fitness, enhances quality of life, and helps people cope more effectively in emergency situations.

Outstanding gymnasts, for example, must achieve good skill-related fitness in all components. A significant amount

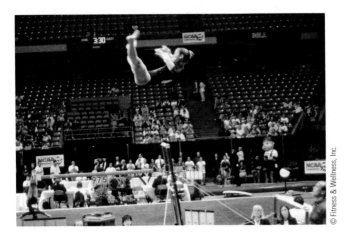

Successful gymnasts demonstrate high levels of skill fitness

of agility is necessary to perform a double back somersault with a full twist—a skill during which the athlete must simultaneously rotate around one axis and twist around a different one. Static balance is essential for maintaining a handstand or a scale. Dynamic balance is needed to perform many of the gymnastics routines (such as those on the balance beam, parallel bars, and pommel horse).

Coordination is important to successfully integrate multiple skills, each with its own degree of difficulty, into one routine. Power and speed are needed to propel the body into the air, such as when tumbling or vaulting. Quick reaction time is necessary to determine when to end rotation upon a visual cue, such as spotting the floor on a dismount.

The principle of specificity of training applies to skill-related components just as it does to health-related fitness components. The development of agility, balance, coordination, and reaction time is highly task specific. That is, to develop a certain task or skill, the individual must practice that same task many times. There seems to be very little crossover learning effect.

For instance, properly practicing a handstand (balance) will lead eventually to successfully performing the skill, but complete mastery of this skill does not ensure that the person will have immediate success when attempting to perform other static-balance positions in gymnastics. In contrast, power and speed may improve with a specific strength-training program or frequent repetition of the specific task to be improved, or both.

The rate of learning in skill-related fitness varies from person to person, mainly because these components seem to be determined to a large extent by genetics. Individuals with good skill-related fitness tend to do better and learn faster when performing a wide variety of skills. Nevertheless, few individuals enjoy complete success in all skill-related components. Furthermore, though skill-related fitness can be enhanced with practice, improvements in reaction time and speed are limited and seem to be related to genetic endowment.

Although we do not know how much skill-related fitness is desirable, everyone should attempt to develop and maintain a better-than-average level. As pointed out earlier, this type of fitness is crucial for athletes, and it also enables fitness participants to lead a better and happier life. Improving skill-related fitness not only affords an individual more enjoyment and success in lifetime sports (for example, tennis, golf, racquetball, basketball), but it also can help a person cope more effectively in emergency situations. Some of the benefits are as follows:

1. Good reaction time, balance, coordination, and/or agility can help you avoid a fall or break a fall and thereby minimize injury.

2. The ability to generate maximum force in a short time (power) may be crucial to ameliorate injury or even preserve life if you ever have to lift a heavy object that has fallen on another person or even on yourself.

3. In our society, where the average lifespan continues to expand, maintaining speed can be especially important for elderly people. Many of these individuals and, for that matter, many unfit/overweight young people no longer have the speed they need to cross an intersection safely before the light changes or run for help if someone else needs assistance.

Regular participation in a health-related fitness program can heighten performance of skill-related components. For example, significantly overweight people do not have good agility or speed. Because participating in aerobic and strength-training programs helps take off body fat, an overweight individual who loses weight through such an exercise program can improve agility and speed. A sound flexibility program decreases resistance to motion about body joints, which may increase agility, balance, and overall coordination. Improvements in strength definitely help develop power. People who have good skill-related fitness usually participate in lifetime sports and games, which in turn helps develop and/or maintain health-related fitness.

## Critical Thinking

If you are interested in health fitness, should you participate in skill-fitness activities? Explain the pros and cons of participating in skill-fitness activities. Should you participate in skill-fitness activities to get fit, or should you get fit to participate in skill-fitness activities?

**Skill-related fitness** Fitness components important for success in skillful activities and athletic events; encompasses agility, balance, coordination, power, reaction time, and speed.

# Performance Tests for Skill-Related Fitness

Several performance tests will assess the various components of skill-related fitness. Results of the performance tests, expressed in percentile ranks, are given in Table 9.1 (men) and Table 9.2 (women) on pages 327–328. Fitness categories for skill-fitness components are established according to percentile rankings only. These rankings fall into categories that are similar to those given for muscular strength and endurance and for flexibility (see Table 9.3 on page 328). You can record the results of your skill-related fitness tests in Lab 9A.

## Agility
**Agility** is the ability to quickly and efficiently change body position and direction. Agility is important in sports such as basketball, soccer, and racquetball, in which the participant must change direction rapidly and also maintain proper body control.

**Agility Test**
SEMO (Southeast Missouri) Agility Test[1]
**Objective**
To measure general body agility
**Procedure** The free-throw area of a basketball court or any other smooth area 12 by 19 feet with adequate running space around it can be used for this test. Four plastic cones or similar objects are placed on each corner of the free-throw lane, as shown in Figure 9.1.

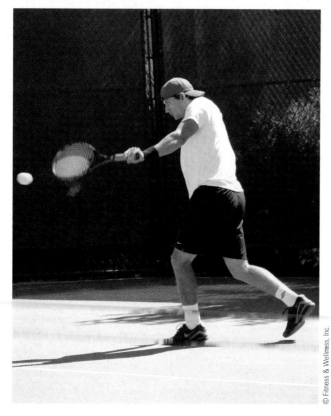

Good tennis players have excellent agility and reaction time.

Start on the outside of the free-throw lane at point A, with your back to the free-throw line. When given the "go" command, sidestep from A to B (do not make crossover steps), backpedal from B to D, sprint forward from D to A, again backpedal from A to C, sprint forward from C to B, and sidestep from B to the finish line at A.

During the test, always go outside each corner cone. A stopwatch is started at the "go" command and stopped when you cross the finish line. Take a practice trial and then use the best of two trials as the final test score. Record the time to the nearest tenth of a second.

## Balance
**Balance** is the ability to maintain the body in proper equilibrium and is vital in activities such as gymnastics, diving, ice skating, skiing, and even football and wrestling, in which the athlete attempts to upset the opponent's equilibrium.

**Balance Test**
One-Foot Stand Test (preferred foot, without shoes)
**Objective**
To measure the static balance of the participant
**Procedure** A flat, smooth floor, not carpeted, is used for this test. Remove your shoes and socks and stand on your preferred foot, placing the other foot on the inside of the supporting knee, and the hands on the sides of the hips. When the "go" command is given, raise your heel off the floor and balance yourself as long as possible without moving the ball of the foot from its initial position.

The test is terminated when any of the following conditions occur:

1. The supporting foot moves (shuffles).
2. The raised heel touches the floor.
3. The hands are moved from the hips.
4. A minute has elapsed.

**FIGURE 9.1  Graphic description of the SEMO test for agility.**

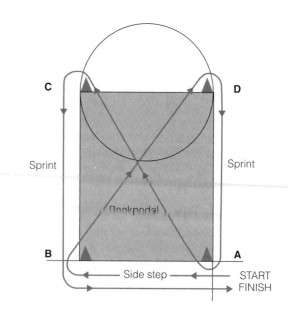

One-Foot Stand test for balance.

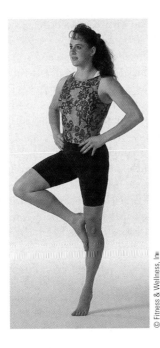

**FIGURE 9.2  Graphic illustration of the "Soda Pop" test**

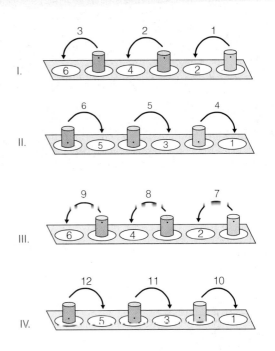

The test is scored by recording the number of seconds that the testee maintains balance on the selected foot, starting with the "go" command. After a practice trial, use the best of two trials as the final performance score. Record the time to the nearest tenth of a second.

## Coordination

**Coordination** is the integration of the nervous and muscular systems to produce correct, graceful, and harmonious body movements. This component is important in a wide variety of motor activities, such as golf, baseball, karate, soccer, and racquetball, in which hand–eye and/or foot–eye movements, or both, must be integrated.

**Coordination Test**

Soda Pop Test

**Objective**

To assess overall motor/muscular control and movement time

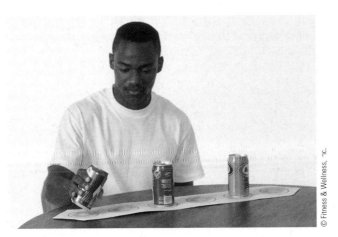

"Soda Pop" test for coordination.

### Procedure

**Administrator:** Homemade equipment is necessary to perform this test. Draw a straight line lengthwise through the center of a piece of cardboard approximately 32 inches long by 5 inches wide. Draw six marks exactly 5 inches away from each other on this line (draw the first mark about 2½ inches from the edge of the cardboard). Using a compass, draw six circles, each 3¼ inches in diameter (a radius of 1 centimeter larger than a can of soda pop), which must be centered on the six marks along the line. See Figure 9.2.

For the purpose of this test, each circle is assigned a number, starting with 1 for the first circle on the right of the test taker and ending with 6 for the last circle on the left. The cardboard, three unopened (full) cans of soda pop, a table, a chair, and a stopwatch are needed to perform the test.

Place the cardboard on a table and have the person sit in front of it with the center of the cardboard bisecting the body. Use the preferred hand for this test. If this is the right hand, place the three cans of soda pop on the cardboard in the following manner: can 1 centered in circle 1 (farthest to the right); can 2 in circle 3; and can 3 in circle 5.

---

**Agility**  The ability to quickly and efficiently change body position and direction.

**Balance**  The ability to maintain the body in proper equilibrium.

**Coordination**  The integration of the nervous and muscular systems to produce correct, graceful, and harmonious body movements.

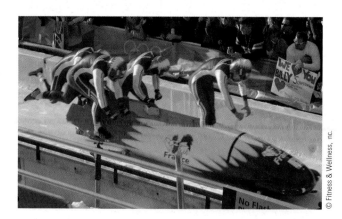

Fast starts in bob sleigh require exceptional leg power.

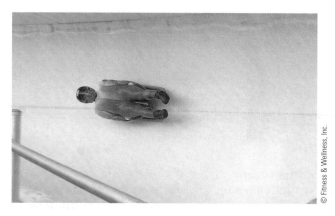

Luge athletes exhibit excellent reaction time and coordination.

**Participant:** To start the test, place the right hand, with the thumb up, on can 1 with the elbow joint bent at about 100°–120°. When the tester gives the signal and the stopwatch is started, turn the cans of soda pop upside down, placing can 1 inside circle 2, followed by can 2 inside circle 4, and then can 3 inside circle 6. Immediately return all three cans, starting with can 1, then can 2, and can 3, turning them right side up to their original placement. On this "return trip," grasp the cans with the hand in a thumb-down position.

**FIGURE 9.3 Correct placement of the feet for start of standing long jump.**

The entire procedure is done twice, without stopping, and is counted as one trial. Two "trips" down and up are required to complete one trial. The watch is stopped when the last can of soda pop is returned to its original position, following the second trip back. The preferred hand (in this case, the right hand) is used throughout the entire task, and the objective of the test is to perform the task as fast as possible, making sure the cans are always placed within each circle.

If the person misses a circle at any time during the test (that is, if a can is placed on a line or outside a circle), the trial must be repeated from the start. A graphic illustration of this test is provided in Figure 9.2.

If using the left hand, the participant follows the same procedure, except the cans are placed starting from the left, with can 1 in circle 6, can 2 in circle 4, and can 3 in circle 2. The procedure is initiated by turning can 1 upside down onto circle 5, can 2 onto circle 3, and so on.

Prior to initiating the test, two practice trials are allowed. Two test trials then are administered, and the best time, recorded to the nearest tenth of a second, is used as the test score. If the person has a mistrial (misses a circle), the test is repeated until two consecutive successful trials are accomplished.

## Power

**Power** is defined as the ability to produce maximum force in the shortest time. The two components of power are speed and force (strength). An effective combination of these two components allows a person to produce explosive movements such as in jumping, putting the shot, and spiking/throwing/hitting a ball.

Power is necessary to perform many activities of daily living that require strength and speed, such as climbing stairs, lifting objects, preventing falls, or hurrying to catch a bus. Power is also beneficial in sports such as soccer, tennis, softball, golf, and volleyball.

**Power Test**
Standing Long Jump Test[2]
**Objective**
To measure leg power
**Procedure**
**Administrator:** Draw a takeoff line on the floor and place a 10-foot-long tape measure perpendicular to this line. Have the participant stand with feet several inches apart, centered on the tape measure, and toes just behind the takeoff line (see Figure 9.3).

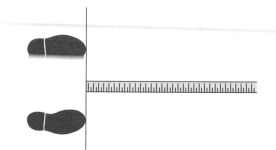

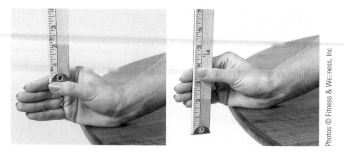

"Yardstick" Reaction Time Test.

**Participant:** Prior to the jump, swing your arms backward and bend your knees. Perform the jump by extending your knees and swinging your arms forward at the same time.

The distance is recorded from the takeoff line to the heel or other body part that touches the floor nearest the takeoff line. Three trials are allowed, and the best trial, measured to the nearest inch, becomes the final test score.

## Reaction Time
**Reaction time** is defined as the time required to initiate a response to a given stimulus. Good reaction time is important for starts in track and swimming, when playing tennis at the net, and in sports such as ping pong, boxing, and karate.

**Reaction Time Test** Yardstick Test (preferred hand)

**Objective** To measure hand reaction time in response to a visual stimulus

**Procedure**

**Administrator:** For this test you will need a regular yardstick with a shaded "concentration zone" marked on the first 2 inches of the stick (see the photo on the previous page). Administer the test with the participant sitting in a chair adjacent to a table and the preferred forearm and hand resting on the table.

**Participant:** Hold the tips of the thumb and fingers in a "ready-to-pinch" position, about 1 inch apart and 3 inches beyond the edge of the table, with the upper edges of the thumb and index finger parallel to the floor. With the person administering the test holding the yardstick near the upper end and the zero point of the stick even with the upper edge of your thumb and index finger (the administrator may steady the middle of the stick with the other hand), look at the "concentration zone" and react by catching the stick when it is dropped. Do not look at the administrator's hand or move your hand up or down while trying to catch the stick.

Twelve trials make up the test, each preceded by the preparatory command "ready." The administrator makes a random 1- to 3-second count between the "ready" command and each drop of the stick. Each trial is scored to the nearest half inch, read just above the upper edge of the thumb.

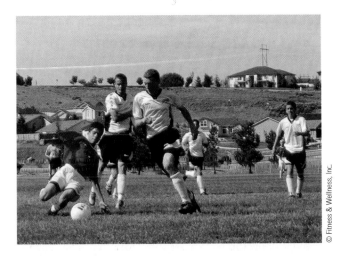

Speed is essential in the sport of soccer.

© Fitness & Wellness, Inc.

**TABLE 9.1** Percentile Rank and Fitness Category for the Skill-Related Fitness Components—Men

|  | Agility* | Balance* | Coordination* | Power* | Reaction Time* | Speed** |
|---|---|---|---|---|---|---|
| 99 | 9.5 | 59.8 | 5.8 | 9'10" | 3.5 | 5.4 |
| 95 | 10.3 | 46.9 | 7.5 | 8'5" | 4.2 | 5.9 |
| 90 | 10.6 | 41.1 | 7.7 | 8'2" | 4.5 | 6.0 |
| 80 | 11.1 | 24.9 | 8.5 | 7'10" | 4.9 | 6.3 |
| 70 | 11.5 | 15.4 | 8.9 | 7'7" | 5.3 | 6.4 |
| 60 | 11.7 | 12.0 | 9.3 | 7'5" | 5.5 | 6.5 |
| 50 | 11.9 | 9.2 | 9.6 | 7'2" | 5.8 | 6.6 |
| 40 | 12.1 | 7.3 | 9.9 | 7'0" | 6.1 | 6.8 |
| 30 | 12.4 | 5.8 | 10.2 | 6'8" | 6.5 | 7.0 |
| 20 | 12.9 | 4.3 | 10.7 | 6'4" | 6.7 | 7.1 |
| 10 | 13.7 | 3.1 | 11.3 | 5'10" | 7.2 | 7.5 |
| 5 | 14.0 | 2.6 | 11.8 | 5'3" | 7.4 | 7.9 |

*Norms developed at Boise State University, Department of Kinesiology.
**From *AAHPERD Youth Fitness: Test Manual.* 1976.

Three practice trials are given before the actual test, to be sure the subject understands the procedure. The three lowest and the three highest scores are discarded, and the average of the middle six is used as the final test score. The testing area should be as free from distractions as possible.

## Speed
**Speed** is the ability to rapidly propel the body or a part of the body from one point to another. Examples of activities that require good speed for success are soccer, basketball, sprints in track, and stealing a base in baseball. In everyday life, speed can be important in a wide variety of emergency situations.

**Speed Test** 50-Yard Dash[3]

**Objective** To measure speed

**Procedure** Two participants take their positions behind the starting line. The starter raises one arm and asks, "Are you ready?" and the gives the command "go" while swinging the raised arm downward as a signal for the timer(s) at the finish line to start the stopwatch(es).

The score is the time that elapses between the starting signal and the moment the participant crosses the finish line, recorded to the nearest tenth of a second.

## Interpreting Test Results
Look up your score for each test in Table 9.1 or 9.2, then use Table 9.3 to see your level of fitness in that particular skill.

**Power** The ability to produce maximum force in the shortest time.

**Reaction time** The time required to initiate a response to a given stimulus.

**Speed** The ability to rapidly propel the body or a part of the body from one point to another.

**TABLE 9.2** Percentile Rank and Fitness Category for the Skill-Related Fitness Components—Women

| | Agility* | Balance* | Coordination* | Power* | Reaction Time* | Speed** |
|---|---|---|---|---|---|---|
| 99 | 11.1 | 59.9 | 7.5 | 7'6" | 3.3 | 6.4 |
| 95 | 12.0 | 39.1 | 8.0 | 6'9" | 4.5 | 6.8 |
| 90 | 12.2 | 25.8 | 8.2 | 6'6" | 4.7 | 7.0 |
| 80 | 12.5 | 16.7 | 8.6 | 6'2" | 5.1 | 7.3 |
| 70 | 12.9 | 11.9 | 9.0 | 5'11" | 5.3 | 7.5 |
| 60 | 13.2 | 9.8 | 9.2 | 5'9" | 5.9 | 7.6 |
| 50 | 13.4 | 7.6 | 9.5 | 5'5" | 6.1 | 7.9 |
| 40 | 13.9 | 6.2 | 9.6 | 5'3" | 6.4 | 8.0 |
| 30 | 14.2 | 5.0 | 9.9 | 5'0" | 6.7 | 8.2 |
| 20 | 14.8 | 4.2 | 10.3 | 4'9" | 7.2 | 8.5 |
| 10 | 15.5 | 2.9 | 10.7 | 4'4" | 7.8 | 9.0 |
| 5 | 16.2 | 1.8 | 11.2 | 4'1" | 8.4 | 9.5 |

*Norms developed at Boise State University, Department of Kinesiology.
**From *AAHPERD Youth Fitness: Test Manual*. 1976.

**TABLE 9.3** Skill-Fitness Categories

| Percentile Rank | Fitness Category |
|---|---|
| ≥81 | Excellent |
| 61–80 | Good |
| 41–60 | Average |
| 21–40 | Fair |
| ≤20 | Poor |

**TABLE 9.4** Contribution of Selected Activities to Skill-Related Components

| Activity | Agility | Balance | Coordination | Power | Reaction Time | Speed |
|---|---|---|---|---|---|---|
| Alpine skiing | 4 | 5 | 4 | 2 | 3 | 2 |
| Archery | 1 | 2 | 4 | 2 | 3 | 1 |
| Badminton | 4 | 3 | 4 | 2 | 4 | 3 |
| Baseball | 3 | 2 | 4 | 4 | 5 | 4 |
| Basketball | 4 | 3 | 4 | 3 | 4 | 3 |
| Bowling | 2 | 2 | 4 | 1 | 1 | 1 |
| Cross-country skiing | 3 | 4 | 3 | 2 | 2 | 1 |
| Football | 4 | 4 | 4 | 4 | 4 | 3 |
| Golf | 1 | 2 | 5 | 3 | 1 | 3 |
| Gymnastics | 5 | 5 | 5 | 4 | 3 | 3 |
| Ice skating | 5 | 5 | 5 | 3 | 3 | 3 |
| In-line skating | 4 | 4 | 4 | 3 | 2 | 4 |
| Judo/Karate | 5 | 5 | 5 | 4 | 5 | 4 |
| Racquetball | 5 | 4 | 4 | 4 | 5 | 4 |
| Soccer | 5 | 3 | 5 | 5 | 3 | 4 |
| Table tennis | 5 | 3 | 5 | 3 | 5 | 3 |
| Tennis | 4 | 3 | 5 | 3 | 5 | 3 |
| Volleyball | 4 | 3 | 5 | 4 | 5 | 3 |
| Water skiing | 3 | 4 | 3 | 2 | 2 | 1 |
| Wrestling | 5 | 5 | 5 | 4 | 5 | 4 |

1 = Low, 2 = Fair, 3 = Average, 4 = Good, 5 = Excellent.

# Team Sports

Choosing activities that you enjoy will greatly enhance your adherence to exercise. People tend to repeat things they enjoy doing. Enjoyment by itself is a reward. In this regard, combining individual activities (such as jogging, swimming, cycling) can deepen your commitment to fitness.

People with good skill-related fitness usually participate in lifetime sports and games, which in turn helps develop health-related fitness. Individuals who enjoyed basketball or soccer in their youth tend to stick to those activities later in life. The availability of teams and community leagues may be all that is needed to stop contemplating and start participating. The social element of team sports provides added incentive to participate. Team sports offer an opportunity to interact with people who share a common interest. Being a member of a team creates responsibility—another incentive to exercise because you are expected to be there. Furthermore, team sports foster lifetime friendships, strengthening the social and emotional dimensions of wellness.

For those who were not able to participate in youth sports, it's never too late to start (see the discussion of behavior modification and motivation in Chapter 2). Don't be afraid to select a new activity, even if that means learning new skills. The fitness and social rewards will be ample.

Similar to the fitness benefits of the aerobic activities discussed in Chapter 6 (see Table 6.10), the contributions of skill-related activities also vary among activities and individuals. The extent to which an activity helps develop each skill-related component varies by the effort the individual makes and, most important, by proper execution (technique) of the skill (correct coaching is highly recommended) and the individual's potential based on genetic endowment. As with aerobic activities, a summary of potential contributions to skill-related fitness for selected activities is provided in Table 9.4.

## Critical Thinking

Sports participation is a good predictor of adherence to exercise later in life. What previous experiences have you had with participation in sports? Were these experiences positive? What effect do they have on your current physical activity patterns?

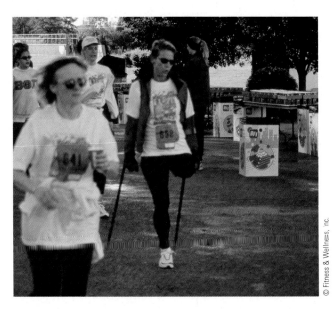

Physically challenged people can participate in and derive health and fitness benefits from a high-intensity exercise program.

# Specific Exercise Considerations

In addition to the exercise-related issues already discussed in this book, many other concerns require clarification or are somewhat controversial. Let's examine some of these issues.

1. **Do people get a "physical high" during aerobic exercise?**

   During vigorous exercise, **endorphins** are released from the pituitary gland in the brain. Endorphins can create feelings of euphoria and natural well-being. Higher levels of endorphins often result from aerobic endurance activities and may remain elevated for as long as 30 to 60 minutes after exercise. Many experts believe these higher levels explain the physical high that some people get during and after prolonged exercise.

   Endorphin levels also have been shown to increase during pregnancy and childbirth. Endorphins act as painkillers. The higher levels could explain a woman's greater tolerance for the pain and discomfort of natural childbirth and her pleasant feelings shortly after the baby's birth. Several reports have indicated that well-conditioned women have shorter and easier labor. These women may attain higher endorphin levels during delivery, making childbirth less traumatic than it is for untrained women.

2. **Can people with asthma exercise?**

   Asthma, a condition that causes difficult breathing, is characterized by coughing, wheezing, and shortness of breath induced by narrowing of the airway passages because of contraction (bronchospasm) of the airway muscles, swelling of the mucous membrane, and excessive secretion of mucus. In a few people, asthma can be triggered by exercise itself, particularly in cool and dry environments. This condition is referred to as exercise-induced asthma (EIA).

   People with asthma need to obtain proper medication from a physician prior to initiating an exercise program. A regular program is best, because random exercise bouts are more likely to trigger asthma attacks. In the initial stages of exercise, an intermittent program (with frequent rest periods during the exercise session) is recommended. Gradual warm-up and cool-down are essential to reduce the risk of an acute attack. Furthermore, exercising in warm and humid conditions (such as swimming) is better because it helps to moisten the airways and thereby minimizes the asthmatic response. For land-based activities (such as walking and aerobics), drinking water before, during, and after exercise helps to keep the airways moist, decreasing the risk of an attack. During the winter months, wearing an exercise mask is recommended to increase the warmth and humidity of inhaled air. People with asthma should not exercise alone and should always carry their medication with them during workouts.

3. **What types of activities are recommended for people with arthritis?**

   Individuals who have arthritis should participate in a combined stretching, aerobic, and strength-training program. The participant should do mild stretching prior to aerobic exercise to relax tight muscles. A regular flexibility program following aerobic exercise is encouraged to help maintain good joint mobility. During the aerobic portion of the exercise program,

---

**Endorphins** Morphine-like substances released from the pituitary gland (in the brain) during prolonged aerobic exercise; thought to induce feelings of euphoria and natural well-being.

individuals with arthritis should avoid high-impact activities because these may cause greater trauma to arthritic joints. Low-impact activities such as swimming, water aerobics, and cycling are recommended. A complete strength-training program also is recommended, with special emphasis on exercises that will support the affected joint(s). As with any other program, individuals with arthritis should start with low-intensity or resistance exercises and build up gradually to a higher fitness level.

**4. What precautions should people with diabetes take with respect to exercise?**

According to the Centers for Disease Control and Prevention, there are more than 20 million diabetics in the United States, and more than 1 million new cases are diagnosed each year. At the current rate, one in three children born in the United States will develop the disease.

There are two types of diabetes: type 1, or insulin-dependent diabetes mellitus (IDDM); and type 2, or non-insulin-dependent diabetes mellitus (NIDDM). In type 1, an autoimmune-related disease found primarily in young people, the pancreas produces little or no insulin. Like everyone else, people with type 1 diabetes benefit from physical activity, but such does not prevent or cure the disease.

Physical activity does help in the prevention and treatment of type 2 diabetes. With type 2, the pancreas may not produce enough insulin or the cells may become insulin resistant, thereby keeping glucose from entering the cell. Type 2 accounts for more than 90 percent of all cases of diabetes, and it occurs mainly in overweight people. (A more thorough discussion of the types of diabetes is given in Chapter 11.)

If you have diabetes, consult your physician before you start exercising. You may not be able to begin until the diabetes is under control. Never exercise alone, and always wear a bracelet that identifies your condition. If you take insulin, the amount and timing of each dose may have to be regulated with your physician. If you inject insulin, do so over a muscle that won't be exercised, then wait an hour before exercising.

Both types of diabetes improve with exercise, although the results are more notable in patients with type 2 diabetes. Exercise usually lowers blood sugar and helps the body use food more effectively. The extent to which the blood glucose level can be controlled in overweight people with NIDDM seems to be related directly to how long and how hard a person exercises. Normal or near-normal blood glucose levels can be achieved through a proper exercise program.

As with any fitness program, the exercise must be done regularly to be effective against diabetes. The benefits of a single exercise bout on blood glucose are highest between 12 and 24 hours following exercise. These benefits are completely lost within 72 hours

after exercise. Thus, regular participation is crucial to derive ongoing benefits. In terms of fitness, all diabetic patients can achieve higher fitness levels, including reductions in weight, blood pressure, and total cholesterol and triglycerides.

The biggest concern for people with diabetes is exercise-induced hypoglycemia during, immediately following, or even a day after the exercise session. Common symptoms of hypoglycemia include weakness, confusion, shakiness, anxiousness, tiredness, hunger, increased perspiration, headaches, and even loss of consciousness. Physical activity increases insulin sensitivity and muscle glucose uptake, thus lowering blood glucose, an effect that may last several hours after exercise. With enhanced insulin sensitivity, a unit of insulin lowers blood glucose to a much greater extent during and following exercise than under nonexercise conditions. Typically, the longer and more intense the exercise bout, the greater the effect on insulin sensitivity.

According to the American College of Sports Medicine (ACSM),[4] along with other health organizations, patients with type 2 diabetes should adhere to the following guidelines to make their exercise program safe and derive the most benefit:

- Expend a minimum of 1,000 calories per week through your exercise program.
- Exercise at a level of 40–70 percent of heart-rate reserve intensity. Start your program with 10 to 15 minutes per session, on at least three nonconsecutive days, but preferably exercise five days per week. Gradually increase the time you exercise to 30 minutes until you achieve your goal of at least 1,000 calories weekly. Diabetic individuals with a weight problem should build up daily physical activity to 60 minutes per session.
- Choose an activity that you enjoy doing, and stay with it. As you select your activity, be aware of your condition. For example, if you have lost sensation in your feet, swimming or stationary cycling is better than walking or jogging to minimize the risk for injury.
- Check your blood glucose levels before and after exercise. Do not exercise if your blood glucose is above 300 mg/dL or fasting blood glucose is above 250 mg/dL and you have ketones in your urine. If your blood glucose is below 100 mg/dL, eat a small carbohydrate snack before exercise.
- If you are on insulin or diabetes medication, monitor your blood glucose regularly and check it at least twice within 30 minutes of starting exercise.
- Schedule your exercise 1 to 3 hours after a meal, and avoid exercise when your insulin is peaking. If you are going to exercise 1 to 2 hours following a meal, you may have to reduce your insulin or blood glucose–reducing medication.
- To prevent hypoglycemia, consume between .15 and .20 gram of carbohydrates per pound of body

weight for each hour of moderate-intensity activity. This amount, however, should be adjusted based on your blood glucose monitoring. Up to .25 gram of carbohydrates per pound of body weight may be required for vigorous exercise. Your goal should be to regulate carbohydrate intake and medication dosage so as to maintain blood glucose level between 100 and 200 mg/dL. With physical activity and exercise, you will probably need to reduce your insulin or oral medication, increase carbohydrate consumption, or do both.

- Be ready to treat low blood sugar with a fast-acting source of sugar, such as juice, raisins, or other source recommended by your doctor.
- If you feel that a reaction is about to occur, discontinue exercise immediately. Check your blood glucose level and treat the condition as needed.
- When you exercise outdoors, always do so with someone who knows what to do in a diabetes-related emergency.
- Stay well-hydrated. Dehydration can have a negative effect on blood glucose, heart function, and performance. Consume adequate amounts of fluids before and after exercise. Drink about 8 ounces of water before you start each exercise session. If you are going to exercise for longer than an hour, drink 8 ounces (one cup) of a 6 to 8 percent carbohydrate sports drink every 15 to 20 minutes.

People with type 1 diabetes should ingest 15 to 30 grams of carbohydrates during each 30 minutes of intense exercise and follow it with a carbohydrate snack after exercise. In addition, strength training twice per week using 8 to 10 exercises with a minimum of one set of 10 to 15 repetitions to near fatigue is recommended for individuals with diabetes. A complete description of strength-training programs is provided in Chapter 7.

### 5. Is exercise safe during pregnancy?

Exercise is beneficial during pregnancy. According to the American College of Obstetricians and Gynecologists (ACOG), in the absence of contraindications, healthy pregnant women are encouraged to participate in regular, moderate-intensity physical activities to continue to derive health benefits during pregnancy.[5] Pregnant women, however, should consult their physicians to ensure that they have no contraindications to exercise during pregnancy.

As a general rule, healthy pregnant women can also accumulate 30 minutes of moderate-intensity physical activity on most, if not all, days of the week. Physical activity strengthens the body and helps prepare for the challenges of labor and childbirth.

The average labor and delivery lasts 10–12 hours. In most cases, labor and delivery are highly intense, with repeated muscular contractions interspersed with short rest periods. Proper conditioning will better prepare the body for childbirth. Moderate exercise

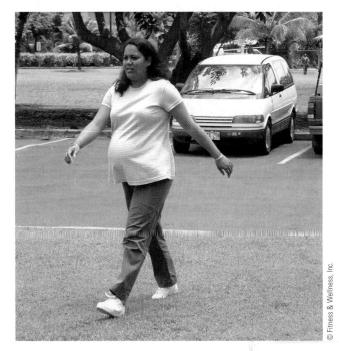

Low- to moderate-intensity exercise is recommended throughout pregnancy.

during pregnancy also helps to prevent back pain and excessive weight gain, and it speeds recovery following childbirth.

The most common recommendations for exercise during pregnancy for healthy pregnant women with no additional risk factors are as follows:

- Don't start a new or more rigorous exercise program without proper medical clearance.
- Accumulate 30 minutes of moderate-intensity physical activities on most days of the week.
- Instead of using heart rate to monitor intensity, exercise at an intensity level between "low" and "somewhat hard," using the Physical Activity Perceived Exertion (H-PAPE) scale in Chapter 6, Figure 6.7 (see page 212).
- Gradually switch from weight-bearing and high-impact activities, such as jogging and aerobics, to non-weight-bearing/lower-impact activities, such as walking, stationary cycling, swimming, and water aerobics. The latter activities minimize the risk for injury and may allow exercise to continue throughout pregnancy.
- Avoid exercising at an altitude above 6,000 feet (1,800 meters), as well as scuba diving, because either may compromise the availability of oxygen to the fetus.
- Women who are accustomed to strenuous exercise may continue in the early stages of pregnancy but should gradually decrease the amount, intensity, and exercise mode as pregnancy advances (most healthy pregnant women, however, slow down during the first few weeks of pregnancy until morning sickness and fatigue subside).

- Pay attention to the body's signals of discomfort and distress, and never exercise to exhaustion. When fatigued, slow down or take a day off. Do not stop exercising altogether unless you experience any of the contraindications for exercise listed in the adjacent box.
- To prevent fetal injury, avoid activities that involve potential contact or loss of balance or that cause even mild trauma to the abdomen. Examples of these activities are basketball, soccer, volleyball, Nordic or water skiing, ice skating, road cycling, horseback riding, and motorcycle riding.
- During pregnancy, don't exercise for weight loss purposes.
- Get proper nourishment (pregnancy requires between 150 and 300 extra calories per day), and eat a small snack or drink some juice 20 to 30 minutes prior to exercise. Prevent dehydration by drinking a cup of fluids 20 to 30 minutes before exercise, and drink 1 cup of liquid every 15 to 20 minutes during exercise.
- During the first 3 months in particular, don't exercise in the heat. Wear clothing that allows for proper dissipation of heat. A body temperature above 102.6°F (39.2°C) can harm the fetus.
- After the first trimester, avoid exercises that require lying on the back. This position can block blood flow to the uterus and the baby.
- Perform stretching exercises gently because hormonal changes during pregnancy increase the laxity of muscles and connective tissue. Although these changes facilitate delivery, they also make women more susceptible to injuries during exercise.

**6. Does exercise help relieve dysmenorrhea?**

Although exercise has not been shown to either cure or aggravate **dysmenorrhea**, it has been shown to relieve menstrual cramps because it improves circulation to the uterus. Less severe menstrual cramps also could be caused by higher levels of endorphins produced during prolonged physical activity, which may counteract pain. Particularly, stretching exercises of the muscles in the pelvic region seem to reduce and prevent painful menstruation that is not the result of disease.[6]

**7. Does participation in exercise hinder menstruation?**

In some instances, highly trained athletes develop **amenorrhea** during training and competition. This condition is seen most often in extremely lean women who also engage in sports that require strenuous physical effort over a sustained time. It is by no means irreversible. At present, we do not know whether the condition is caused by physical or emotional stress related to high-intensity training, excessively low body fat, or other factors.

Although, on the average, women have a lower physical capacity during menstruation, medical sur-

## Contraindications to Exercise During Pregnancy

Stop exercise and seek medical advice if you experience any of the following symptoms:

- Unusual pain or discomfort, especially in the chest or abdominal area
- Cramping, primarily in the pelvic or lower back areas
- Muscle weakness, excessive fatigue, or shortness of breath
- Abnormally high heart rate or a pounding (palpitations) heart rate
- Decreased fetal movement
- Insufficient weight gain
- Amniotic fluid leakage
- Nausea, dizziness, or headaches
- Persistent uterine contractions
- Vaginal bleeding or rupture of the membranes
- Swelling of ankles, calves, hands, or face

veys at the Olympic Games have shown that women have broken Olympic and world records at all stages of the menstrual cycle. Menstruation should not keep a woman from exercising, and it will not necessarily have a negative impact on performance.

**8. Does exercise offset the detrimental effects of cigarette smoking?**

Physical exercise often motivates a person to stop smoking, but it does not offset any ill effects of smoking. Smoking greatly decreases the ability of the blood to transport oxygen to working muscles.

Oxygen is carried in the circulatory system by hemoglobin, the iron-containing pigment of the red blood cells. Carbon monoxide, a by-product of cigarette smoke, has 210 to 250 times greater affinity for hemoglobin over oxygen. Consequently, carbon monoxide combines much faster with hemoglobin, decreasing the oxygen-carrying capacity of the blood.

Chronic smoking also increases airway resistance, requiring the respiratory muscles to work much harder and consume more oxygen just to ventilate a given amount of air. If a person quits smoking, exercise does help increase the functional capacity of the pulmonary system.

A regular exercise program seems to be a powerful incentive to quit smoking. A random survey of 1,250 runners conducted at the 6.2-mile Peachtree Road Race in Atlanta provided impressive results. The sur-

FIGURE 9.4  What to look for in a good pair of shoes.

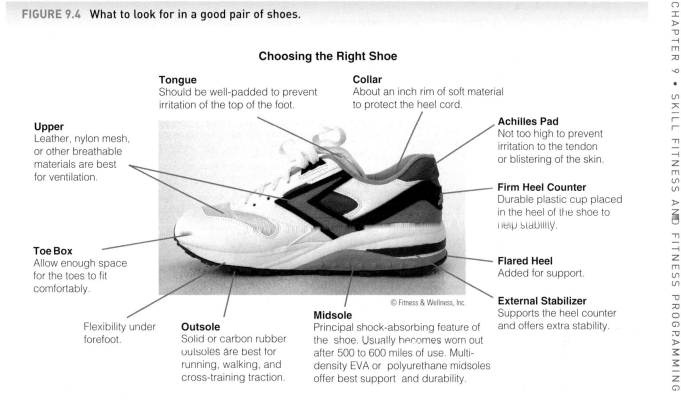

**Choosing the Right Shoe**

**Tongue**
Should be well-padded to prevent irritation of the top of the foot.

**Collar**
About an inch rim of soft material to protect the heel cord.

**Upper**
Leather, nylon mesh, or other breathable materials are best for ventilation.

**Achilles Pad**
Not too high to prevent irritation to the tendon or blistering of the skin.

**Firm Heel Counter**
Durable plastic cup placed in the heel of the shoe to help stability.

**Toe Box**
Allow enough space for the toes to fit comfortably.

**Flared Heel**
Added for support.

© Fitness & Wellness, Inc.

**External Stabilizer**
Supports the heel counter and offers extra stability.

Flexibility under forefoot.

**Outsole**
Solid or carbon rubber outsoles are best for running, walking, and cross-training traction.

**Midsole**
Principal shock-absorbing feature of the shoe. Usually becomes worn out after 500 to 600 miles of use. Multi-density EVA or polyurethane midsoles offer best support and durability.

vey indicated that of the men and women who smoked cigarettes when they started running, 81 percent and 75 percent, respectively, had quit before the date of the race.

**9. How long should a person wait after a meal before exercising strenuously?**

The length of time to wait before exercising after a meal depends on the amount of food eaten. On the average, after a regular meal, you should wait about 2 hours before participating in vigorous physical activity. But a walk or some other low to moderate physical activity is fine following a meal. If anything, it helps burn extra calories and may help the body metabolize fats more efficiently.

**10. What type of clothing should I wear when I exercise?**

The type of clothing you wear during exercise is important. In general, clothing should fit comfortably and allow free movement of the various body parts. Select clothing according to air temperature, humidity, and exercise intensity. Avoid nylon and rubberized materials and tight clothes that interfere with the cooling mechanism of the human body or obstruct normal blood flow. Choose fabrics made of polypropylene, Capilene, Thermax, or any synthetic that draws (wicks) moisture away from the skin, enhancing evaporation and cooling of the body. It's also important to consider your exercise intensity, because the harder you exercise, the more heat your body produces.

When exercising in the heat, avoid the hottest time of the day, between 11:00 a.m. and 5:00 p.m. Surfaces such as asphalt, concrete, and artificial turf absorb heat, which then radiates to the body. Therefore, these surfaces are not recommended. (Also see the discussion about heat and humidity in Question 12.)

Only a minimal amount of clothing is necessary during exercise in the heat, to allow for maximal evaporation. Clothing should be lightweight, light-colored, loose-fitting, airy, and absorbent. Examples of commercially available products that can be used during exercise in the heat are Asics's Perma Plus, COOLMAX, and Nike's Dri-FIT.

Double-layer acrylic socks are more absorbent than cotton and help to prevent blistering and chafing of the feet. A straw-type hat can be worn to protect the eyes and head from the sun. (Clothing for exercise in the cold is discussed in Question 14, page 335.)

A good pair of shoes is vital to prevent injuries to lower limbs. Shoes manufactured specifically for your choice of activity are a must (see Figure 9.4). When selecting proper footwear, you should consider body type, tendency toward pronation (rotating the foot outward) or supination (rotating the foot inward), and exercise surfaces. Shoes should have good stability, motion control, and comfortable fit. Purchase shoes in the middle of the day when your feet have expanded and might be one half size larger. For increased breathability, choose shoes with nylon or mesh uppers.

**Dysmenorrhea** Painful menstruation.

**Amenorrhea** Cessation of regular menstrual flow.

Generally, salespeople at reputable athletic shoe stores are knowledgeable and can help you select a good shoe that fits your needs. After 300 to 500 miles or 6 months, examine your shoes and obtain a new pair if they are worn out. Old shoes are frequently responsible for injuries to the lower limbs.

**11. What time of the day is best for exercise?**

You can do intense exercise almost any time of the day, with the exception of about 2 hours following a heavy meal or the midday and early afternoon hours on hot, humid days. Moderate exercise seems to be beneficial shortly after a meal, because exercise enhances the **thermogenic response**. A walk shortly after a meal burns more calories than a walk several hours after a meal.

Many people enjoy exercising early in the morning because it gives them a boost to start the day. People who exercise in the morning also seem to stick with it more than others, because the chances of putting off the exercise session for other reasons are minimized. Some prefer the lunch hour for weight-control reasons. By exercising at noon, they do not eat as big a lunch, which helps keep down the daily caloric intake. Highly stressed people seem to like the evening hours because of the relaxing effects of exercise.

**12. Why is exercising in hot and humid conditions unsafe?**

When a person exercises, only 30 to 40 percent of the energy the body produces is used for mechanical work or movement. The rest of the energy (60 to 70 percent) is converted into heat. If this heat cannot be dissipated properly because the weather is too hot or the relative humidity is too high, body temperature increases, and in extreme cases, it can result in death.

The specific heat of body tissue (the heat required to raise the temperature of the body by 1°C) is .38 calorie per pound of body weight (.38 cal/lb). This indicates that if no body heat is dissipated, a 150-pound person has to burn only 57 calories (150 × .38) to increase total body temperature by 1°C. If this person were to conduct an exercise session requiring 300 calories (e.g., running about 3 miles) without any dissipation of heat, the inner body temperature would increase by 5.3°C (300 ÷ 57), which is the equivalent of going from 98.6°F to 108.1°F.

This example illustrates clearly the need for caution when exercising in hot or humid weather. If the relative humidity is too high, body heat cannot be lost through evaporation because the atmosphere already is saturated with water vapor. In one instance, a football casualty occurred when the temperature was only 64°F, but the relative humidity was 100 percent. People must be cautious when air temperature is above 90°F and the relative humidity is above 60 percent.

The ACSM recommends avoiding strenuous physical activity when the readings of a wet-bulb globe thermometer exceed 82.4°F. With this type of thermometer, the wet bulb is cooled by evaporation, and on dry days it shows a lower temperature than the regular (dry) thermometer. On humid days, the cooling effect is less because of less evaporation; hence, the difference between the wet and dry readings is not as great.

Following are descriptions of, and first-aid measures for, the three major signs of heat illness:

- **Heat cramps**. Symptoms include cramps, spasms, and muscle twitching in the legs, arms, and abdomen. To relieve heat cramps, stop exercising, get out of the heat, massage the painful area, stretch slowly, and drink plenty of fluids (water, fruit drinks, or electrolyte beverages).

- **Heat exhaustion**. Symptoms include fainting, dizziness, profuse sweating, cold and clammy skin, weakness, headache, and a rapid, weak pulse. If you incur any of these symptoms, stop and find a cool place to rest. If conscious, drink cool water. Do not give water to an unconscious person. Loosen or remove clothing and rub your body with a cool, wet towel or apply ice packs. Place yourself in a supine position with the legs elevated 8 to 12 inches. If you are not fully recovered in 30 minutes, seek immediate medical attention.

- **Heat stroke**. Symptoms include serious disorientation; warm, dry skin; no sweating; rapid, full pulse; vomiting; diarrhea; unconsciousness; and high body temperature. As the body temperature climbs, unexplained anxiety sets in. When the body temperature reaches 104–105°F, the individual may feel a cold sensation in the trunk of the body, goosebumps, nausea, throbbing in the temples, and numbness in the extremities. Most people become incoherent after this stage.

## Symptoms of Heat Illness

If any of these symptoms occur, stop physical activity, get out of the sun, and start drinking fluids.

- Decreased perspiration
- Cramping
- Weakness
- Flushed skin
- Throbbing head
- Nausea/vomiting
- Diarrhea
- Numbness in the extremities
- Blurred vision
- Unsteadiness
- Disorientation
- Incoherency

- When body temperature reaches 105–107°F, disorientation, loss of fine-motor control, and muscular weakness set in. If the temperature exceeds 106°F, serious neurological injury and death may be imminent.

- Heat stroke requires immediate emergency medical attention. Request help and get out of the sun and into a cool, humidity-controlled environment. While you are waiting to be taken to the hospital emergency room, you should be placed in a semiseated position, and your body should be sprayed with cool water and rubbed with cool towels. If possible, cold packs should be placed in areas that receive an abundant blood supply, such as the head, neck, armpits, and groin. Fluids should not be given if you are unconscious. In any case of heat-related illness, if the person refuses water, vomits, or starts to lose consciousness, an ambulance should be summoned immediately. Proper initial treatment of heat stroke is vital.

**13. What should a person do to replace fluids lost during prolonged aerobic exercise?**

The main objective of fluid replacement during prolonged aerobic exercise is to maintain the blood volume so circulation and sweating can continue at normal levels. Adequate water replacement is the most important factor in preventing heat disorders. Drinking about 6 to 8 ounces of cool water every 15 to 20 minutes during exercise is recommended to prevent dehydration. Cold fluids seem to be absorbed more rapidly from the stomach. Other relevant points are the following:

- Drinking commercially prepared sports drinks is recommended when exercise will be strenuous and carried out for more than an hour. For exercise lasting less than an hour, water is just as effective in replacing lost fluid. The sports drinks you select may be based on your personal preference. Try different drinks at 6 to 8 percent glucose concentration to see which drink you tolerate best and suits your taste as well.

- Commercial fluid-replacement solutions (such as Powerade® and Gatorade®) contain about 6 to 8 percent glucose, which seems to be optimal for fluid absorption and performance. Sugar does not become available to the muscles until about 30 minutes after consumption of a glucose solution.

- Drinks high in fructose or with a glucose concentration above 8 percent are not recommended because they slow water absorption during exercise in the heat.

- Most sodas (both cola and non-cola) contain between 10 and 12 percent glucose, which is too high for proper rehydration during exercise in the heat.

- Do not overhydrate with just water during a very or ultra long distance event, as such can lead to

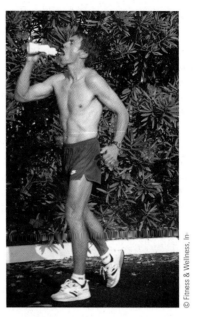

Fluid and carbohydrate replacement are essential when exercising in the heat or for a prolonged period.

hyponatremia (see also "Hyponatremia" in Chapter 3, page 103) or low sodium concentration in the blood. When water loss through sweat during prolonged exercise is replaced by water alone, blood sodium is diluted to the point where it creates serious health problems, including seizures and coma in severe cases.

**14. What precautions must a person take when exercising in the cold?**

When exercising in the cold, the two factors to consider are frostbite and **hypothermia**. In contrast to hot and humid conditions, cold weather usually does not threaten health because clothing can be selected for heat conservation, and exercise itself increases the production of body heat.

Most people actually overdress for exercise in the cold. Because exercise increases body temperature, a moderate workout on a cold day makes a person feel that the temperature is 20 to 30 degrees warmer than it actually is. Overdressing for exercise can make the clothes damp from excessive perspiration. The risk for hypothermia increases when a person is wet or after exercise stops, when the person is not moving around sufficiently to increase (or maintain) body heat.

**Thermogenic response** Amount of energy required to digest food.

**Heat cramps** Muscle spasms caused by heat-induced changes in electrolyte balance in muscle cells.

**Heat exhaustion** Heat-related fatigue.

**Heat stroke** Emergency situation resulting from the body being subjected to high atmospheric temperatures.

**Hypothermia** A breakdown in the body's ability to generate heat; a drop in body temperature below 95°F.

Initial warning signs of hypothermia include shivering, losing coordination, and having difficulty speaking. With a continued drop in body temperature, shivering stops, the muscles weaken and stiffen, and the person feels elated or intoxicated and eventually loses consciousness. To prevent hypothermia, use common sense, dress properly, and be aware of environmental conditions.

The popular belief that exercising in cold temperatures (32°F and lower) freezes the lungs is false, because the air is warmed properly in the air passages before it reaches the lungs. Cold is not what poses a threat; wind velocity is what increases the chill factor most.

For example, a temperature of 25°F is not too cold to exercise with adequate clothing, but if the wind is blowing at 25 miles per hour, the chill factor lowers the actual temperature to 15°F. This effect is even worse if a person is wet and exhausted. When the weather is windy, the individual should exercise (jog or cycle) against the wind on the way out and with the wind upon returning.

Even though the lungs are under no risk when you exercise in the cold, your face, head, hands, and feet should be protected because they are subject to frostbite. Watch for numbness and discoloration—the signs of frostbite. In cold temperatures, as much as half of the body's heat can be lost through an unprotected head and neck. A wool or synthetic cap, hood, or hat will help to hold in body heat. Mittens are better than gloves, because they keep the fingers together so the surface area from which to lose heat is less. Inner linings of synthetic material to wick moisture away from the skin are recommended. Avoid cotton next to the skin, because once cotton gets wet, whether from perspiration, rain, or snow, it loses its insulating properties.

Wearing several layers of lightweight clothing is preferable to wearing one single, thick layer because warm air is trapped between layers of clothes, enabling greater heat conservation. As body temperature increases, you can remove layers as necessary.

The first layer of clothes should wick moisture away from the skin. Polypropylene, Capilene, and Thermax are recommended materials. Next, a layer of wool, Dacron, or polyester fleece insulates well even when wet. Lycra tights or sweatpants help protect the legs. The outer layer should be waterproof, wind resistant, and breathable. A synthetic material such as Gore-Tex is best, so moisture can still escape from the body. A ski mask or face mask helps protect the face. In extremely cold conditions, exposed skin, such as the nose, cheeks, and around the eyes, can be insulated with petroleum jelly.

For lengthy or long-distance workouts (cross-country skiing or long runs), take a small backpack to carry the clothing you removed. You also can carry extra warm and dry clothes in case you stop exercising away from shelter. If you remain outdoors following exercise, added clothing and continuous body movement are essential to maintain body temperature and avoid hypothermia.

**15. Can I exercise when I have a cold or the flu?**
The most important consideration is to use common sense and pay attention to your symptoms. Usually, you may continue to exercise if your symptoms include a runny nose, sneezing, or a scratchy throat. But, if your symptoms include fever, muscle ache, vomiting, diarrhea, or a hacking cough, you should avoid exercise. After an illness, be sure to ease back gradually into your program. Do not attempt to return at the same intensity and duration that you were used to prior to your illness.

# Exercise-Related Injuries

To enjoy and maintain physical fitness, preventing injury during a conditioning program is essential. Exercise-related injuries, nonetheless, are common in individuals who participate in exercise programs. Surveys indicate that more than half of all new participants incur injuries during the first 6 months of the conditioning program. The four most common causes of injuries are:

1. High-impact activities
2. Rapid conditioning programs (doing too much too quickly)
3. Improper shoes or training surfaces
4. Anatomical predisposition (that is, body propensity)

High-impact activities and a significant increase in quantity, intensity, or duration of activities are by far the most common causes of injuries. The body requires time to adapt to more intense activities. Most of these injuries can be prevented through a more gradual and correct conditioning (low-impact) program.

Proper shoes for specific activities are essential. Shoes should be replaced when they show a lot of wear and tear. Softer training surfaces, such as grass and dirt, produce less trauma than asphalt and concrete.

Because few people have perfect body alignment, injuries associated with overtraining may occur eventually. In case of injury, proper treatment can avert a lengthy recovery process. A summary of common exercise-related injuries and how to manage them follows.

**Acute Sports Injuries** The best treatment always has been prevention. If an activity causes unusual discomfort or chronic irritation, you need to treat the cause by decreasing the intensity, switching activities, substituting equipment, or upgrading clothing (such as buying proper-fitting shoes).

In cases of acute injury, the standard treatment is rest, cold application, compression or splinting (or both), and

**TABLE 9.5** Reference Guide for Exercise-Related Problems

| Injury | Signs/Symptoms | Treatment* |
|---|---|---|
| Bruise (contusion) | Pain, swelling, discoloration | Cold application, compression, rest |
| Dislocations/Fracture | Pain, swelling, deformity | Splinting, cold application, seek medical attention |
| Heat cramp | Cramps, spasms, and muscle twitching in the legs, arms, and abdomen | Stop activity, get out of the heat, stretch, massage the painful area, drink plenty of fluids |
| Heat exhaustion | Fainting, profuse sweating, cold/clammy skin, weak/rapid pulse, weakness, headache | Stop activity, rest in a cool place, loosen clothing, rub body with cool/wet towel, drink plenty of fluids, stay out of heat for 2–3 days |
| Heat stroke | Hot/dry skin, no sweating, serious disorientation, rapid/full pulse, vomiting, diarrhea, unconsciousness, high body temperature | **Seek immediate medical attention,** request help and get out of the sun, bathe in cold water/spray with cold water/rub body with cold towels, drink plenty of cold fluids |
| Joint sprains | Pain, tenderness, swelling, loss of use, discoloration | Cold application, compression, elevation, rest; heat after 36–48 hours (if no further swelling) |
| Muscle cramps | Pain, spasm | Stretch muscle(s), use mild exercises for involved area |
| Muscle soreness and stiffness | Tenderness, pain | Mild stretching, low-intensity exercise, warm bath |
| Muscle strains | Pain, tenderness, swelling, loss of use | Cold application, compression, elevation, rest; heat after 36–48 hours (if no further swelling) |
| Shin splints | Pain, tenderness | Cold application prior to and following any physical activity, rest; heat (if no activity is carried out) |
| Side stitch | Pain on the side of the abdomen below the rib cage | Decrease level of physical activity or stop altogether, gradually increase level of fitness |
| Tendinitis | Pain, tenderness, loss of use | Rest, cold application, heat after 48 hours |

*Cold should be applied three to five times a day for 15 minutes. Heat can be applied three times a day for 15 to 20 minutes.

elevation of the affected body part. This is commonly referred to as **RICE:**

R = rest
I = ice (cold) application
C = compression
E = elevation

Cold should be applied three to five times a day for 15 minutes at a time during the first 36 to 48 hours, by submerging the injured area in cold water, using an ice bag, or applying ice massage to the affected part. An elastic bandage or wrap can be used for compression. Elevating the body part decreases blood flow (and therefore swelling) in that body part.

The purpose of these treatment modalities is to minimize swelling in the area and thus hasten recovery time. After the first 36 to 48 hours, heat can be used if the injury shows no further swelling or inflammation. If you have doubts as to the nature or seriousness of the injury (such as suspected fracture), you should seek a medical evaluation.

Obvious deformities (exhibited by fractures, dislocations, or partial dislocations, for example) call for splinting, cold application with an ice bag, and medical attention. Do not try to reset any of these conditions by yourself, because you could further damage muscles, ligaments, and nerves. Treatment of these injuries should always be left to specialized medical personnel. A quick reference guide for the signs or symptoms and treatment of exercise-related problems is provided in Table 9.5.

## Muscle Soreness and Stiffness
Individuals who begin an exercise program or participate after a long layoff from exercise often develop muscle soreness and stiffness. The acute soreness that sets in during the first few hours after exercise is thought to be related to general fatigue of the exercised muscles.

**RICE** An acronym used to describe the standard treatment procedure for acute sports injuries: *r*est, *i*ce (cold) application, *c*ompression, and *e*levation.

Delayed muscle soreness that appears several hours after exercise (usually about 12 hours later) and lasts 2 to 4 days may be related to actual micro-tears in muscle tissue, muscle spasms that increase fluid retention (stimulating the pain nerve endings), and overstretching or tearing of connective tissue in and around muscles and joints.

Mild stretching before and adequate stretching after exercise help to prevent soreness and stiffness. Gradually progressing into an exercise program is important, too. A person should not attempt to do too much too quickly. To relieve pain, mild stretching, low-intensity exercise to stimulate blood flow, and a warm bath are recommended.

### Exercise Intolerance

When starting an exercise program, participants should stay within the safe limits. The best method to determine whether you are exercising too strenuously is to check your heart rate and make sure it does not exceed the limits of your target zone. Exercising above this target zone may not be safe for unconditioned or high-risk individuals. You do not have to exercise beyond your target zone to gain the desired cardiorespiratory benefits.

Several physical signs will tell you when you are exceeding your functional limitations—that is, experiencing **exercise intolerance**. Signs of intolerance include rapid or irregular heart rate, difficult breathing, nausea, vomiting, lightheadedness, headache, dizziness, unusually flushed or pale skin, extreme weakness, lack of energy, shakiness, sore muscles, cramps, and tightness in the chest. Learn to listen to your body. If you notice any of these symptoms, seek medical attention before continuing your exercise program.

Recovery heart rate is another indicator of overexertion. To a certain extent, recovery heart rate is related to fitness level. The higher your cardiorespiratory fitness level, the faster your heart rate will decrease following exercise. As a rule, heart rate should be below 120 bpm 5 minutes into recovery. If your heart rate is above 120, you most likely have overexerted yourself or possibly could have some other cardiac abnormality. If you lower the intensity or the duration of exercise, or both, and you still have a fast heart rate 5 minutes into recovery, you should consult your physician.

### Side Stitch

**Side stitch** is a cramp-like pain in the lower area of the ribcage that can develop in the early stages of participation in exercise. It occurs primarily in unconditioned beginners and in trained individuals when they exercise at higher intensities than usual. As one's physical condition improves, this condition tends to disappear unless training is intensified. A few people have a life-long susceptibility to side stitches regardless of fitness level or training intensity. In such cases, the condition is most likely genetically related.

The exact cause is unknown. Some experts suggest that it could relate to a lack of blood flow to the respiratory muscles during strenuous physical exertion. Some people encounter side stitch during downhill running. If you experience side stitch during exercise, slow down. If it persists, stop altogether. Lying down on your back and gently bringing both knees to the chest and holding that position for 30 to 60 seconds also helps.

Some people get side stitch if they drink juice or eat anything shortly before exercise. Drinking only water 1–2 hours prior to exercise sometimes prevents side stitch. Other individuals have problems with commercially available sports drinks during high-intensity exercise. Unless carbohydrate replacement is crucial to complete a long-distance event (over 90 minutes, such as road cycling, a marathon, or a triathlon), drink cool water for fluid replacement or try a different carbohydrate solution.

### Shin Splints

**Shin splints**, one of the most common injuries to the lower limbs, usually results from one or more of the following: (a) lack of proper and gradual conditioning, (b) doing physical activities on hard surfaces (wooden floors, hard tracks, cement, or asphalt), (c) fallen arches, (d) chronic overuse, (e) muscle fatigue, (f) faulty posture, (g) improper shoes, (h) participating in weight-bearing activities when excessively overweight.

The following are options to manage shin splints:

1. Remove or reduce the cause (exercise on softer surfaces, wear better shoes or arch supports, or completely stop exercise until the shin splints heal).
2. Do stretching exercises before and after physical activity.
3. Use ice massage for 10 to 20 minutes before and after exercise.
4. Apply active heat (whirlpool and hot baths) for 15 minutes, two to three times a day.
5. Use supportive taping during physical activity (a qualified athletic trainer can teach you the proper taping technique).

### Muscle Cramps

Muscle cramps are caused by the body's depletion of essential electrolytes or a breakdown in the coordination between opposing muscle groups. If you have a muscle cramp, you should first attempt to stretch the muscles involved. In the case of the calf muscle, for example, pull your toes up toward the knees. After stretching the muscle, rub it down gently, and, finally, do some mild exercises requiring the use of that muscle.

In pregnant and lactating women, muscle cramps often are related to a lack of calcium. If women get cramps during these times, calcium supplements usually relieve the problem. Tight clothing also can cause cramps by decreasing blood flow to active muscle tissue.

# Exercise and Aging

The elderly constitute the fastest-growing segment of the population. The number of Americans ages 65 and older increased from 3.1 million in 1900 (4.1 percent of the population) to about 36 million (12 percent) in 2003. By the year 2030, more than 72 million people, or 20 percent of the U.S. population, are expected to be older than 65.

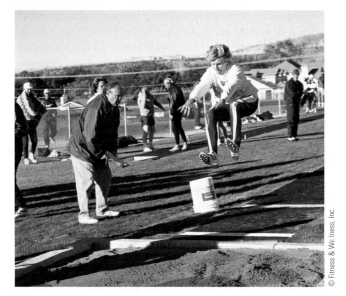

Older adults who exercise enjoy better health, increase their quality of life, and live longer than physically inactive adults.

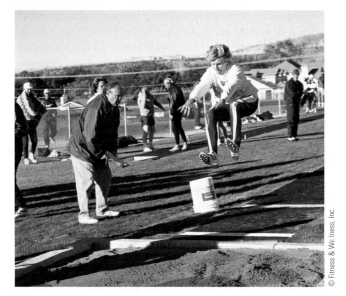 © Fitness & Wellness, Inc.

**TABLE 9.6** Effects of Physical Activity and Inactivity on Older Men

| | Exercisers | Non-exercisers |
|---|---|---|
| Age (yrs) | 68.0 | 69.8 |
| Weight (lbs) | 160.3 | 186.3 |
| Resting heart rate (bpm) | 55.8 | 66.0 |
| Maximal heart rate (bpm) | 157.0 | 146.0 |
| Heart rate reserve* (bpm) | 101.2 | 80.0 |
| Blood pressure (mm Hg) | 120/78 | 150/90 |
| Maximal oxygen uptake (mL/kg/min) | 38.6 | 20.3 |

*Heart rate reserve = maximal heart rate − resting heart rate.
Data from F. W. Kash, J. L. Boyer, S. P. Van Camp, L. S. Verity, and J. P. Wallace, "The Effect of Physical Activity on Aerobic Power in Older Men (A Longitudinal Study)," *The Physician and Sports Medicine* 18, no. 4 (1990): 73–83.

The main objectives of fitness programs for older adults should be to help them improve their functional status and contribute to healthy aging. This implies the ability to maintain independent living status and to avoid disability. Older adults are encouraged to participate in programs that will help develop cardiorespiratory endurance, muscular strength and endurance, muscular flexibility, agility, balance, and motor coordination.

**Physical Training in the Older Adult** Regular participation in physical activity provides both physical and psychological benefits to older adults.[7] Cardiorespiratory endurance training helps to increase functional capacity, decrease the risk for disease, improve health status, and increase life expectancy. Strength training decreases the rate at which strength and muscle mass are lost. Among the psychological benefits are preserved cognitive function, reduced symptoms and behaviors related to depression, and improved self-confidence and self-esteem.

The trainability of older men and women alike and the effectiveness of physical activity in enhancing health have been demonstrated in research. Older adults who increase their physical activity experience significant changes in cardiorespiratory endurance, strength, and flexibility. The extent of the changes depends on their initial fitness level and the types of activities they select for their training (walking, cycling, strength training, and so on).

Improvements in maximal oxygen uptake in older adults are similar to those of younger people, although older people seem to require a longer training period to achieve these changes. Declines in maximal oxygen uptake average about 1 percent per year between ages 25 and 75.[8] A slower rate of decline is seen in people who maintain a lifetime aerobic exercise program.

Results of research on the effects of aging on the cardiorespiratory systems of male exercisers versus male nonexercisers has showed that the maximal oxygen uptake of regular exercisers was almost twice that of the nonexercisers (see Table 9.6).[9] The study revealed a decline in maximal oxygen uptake between ages 50 and 68 of only 13 percent in the active group, compared with 41 percent in the inactive group. These changes indicate that about one-third of the loss in maximal oxygen uptake results from aging, and two-thirds of the loss comes from inactivity. Blood pressure, heart rate, and body weight also were remarkably better in the exercising group. Furthermore, aerobic training seems to decrease high blood pressure in older patients at the same rate as in young hypertensive people.[10]

In terms of aging, muscle strength declines by 10 to 20 percent between ages 20 and 50; but between ages 50 and 70, it drops by another 25 to 30 percent. Through strength training, frail adults in their 80s or 90s can double or triple their strength in just a few months. The amount of muscle hypertrophy achieved, however, decreases with age. Strength gains close to 200 percent have been found in previously inactive adults over age 90.[11] In fact, research has shown that regular strength training improves balance, gait, speed, **functional independence**, morale, depression symptoms, and energy intake.[12]

Although muscle flexibility drops by about 5 percent per decade of life, 10 minutes of stretching every other day can prevent most of this loss as a person ages.[13] Improved

**Exercise intolerance** Inability to function during exercise because of excessive fatigue or extreme feelings of discomfort.

**Side stitch** A sharp pain in the side of the abdomen.

**Shin splints** Injury to the lower leg characterized by pain and irritation in the shin region of the leg.

**Functional independence** Ability to carry out activities of daily living without assistance from other individuals.

flexibility also enhances mobility skills.[14] The latter promotes independence because it helps older adults successfully perform activities of daily living.

In terms of body composition, inactive adults continue to gain body fat after age 60 despite their tendency toward lower body weight. The increase in body fat is likely related to a decrease in physical activity, lean body mass, and basal metabolic rate, along with increased caloric intake above that required to maintain daily energy requirements.[15]

Older adults who wish to initiate or continue an exercise program are strongly encouraged to have a complete medical exam, including a stress electrocardiogram test. Recommended activities for older adults include calisthenics, walking, jogging, swimming, cycling, and water aerobics.

Older people should avoid isometric and very high intensity weight-training exercises. Activities that require all-out effort or participants to hold their breaths tend to lessen blood flow to the heart, cause a significant increase in blood pressure, and increase the load placed on the heart. Older adults should participate in activities that require continuous and rhythmic muscular activity (about 40 to 60 percent of heart rate reserve). These activities do not cause large increases in blood pressure or overload the heart.

# Preparing for Sports Participation

To enhance your participation in sports, keep in mind that in most cases it is better to get fit before playing sports rather than playing sports to get fit.[16] A good preseason training program will help make the season more enjoyable and prevent exercise-related injuries.

Properly conditioned individuals can participate safely in sports and enjoy the activities to their fullest with few or no limitations. Unfortunately, sports injuries are often the result of poor fitness and a lack of sport-specific conditioning. Many injuries occur when fatigue sets in following overexertion by unconditioned individuals.

**Base Fitness Conditioning** Pre-activity screening that includes a health history (see "Health History Questionnaire," page 35) and/or a medical evaluation appropriate to your sport selection is recommended. Once cleared for exercise, start by building a base of general athletic fitness that includes the four health-related fitness components: cardiorespiratory fitness, muscular strength and endurance, flexibility, and recommended body composition. The base fitness conditioning program should last a minimum of 6 weeks.

As explained in Chapter 6, for cardiorespiratory fitness select an activity that you enjoy (such as walking, jogging, cycling, **step aerobics**, cross-country skiing, stair climbing) and train three to five times per week at a minimum of 20 minutes of continuous activity per session. Exercise between 60 percent and 80 percent intensity for adequate conditioning. You should feel as though you are training "somewhat hard" to "hard" at these intensity levels.

Strength (resistance) training helps maintain and increase muscular strength and endurance. Following the guidelines provided in Chapter 7, select 10 to 12 exercises that involve the major muscle groups and train two or three times per week on nonconsecutive days. Select a resistance (weight) that allows you to do 3 to 20 repetitions to near fatigue (3 to 20 RM based on your fitness goals—see Chapter 7). That is, the resistance will be heavy enough so that when you perform one set of an exercise, you will not be able to do more than the predetermined number of repetitions at that weight. Begin your program slowly and perform between one and three sets of each exercise. Recommended exercises include the bench press, lat pull-down, leg press, leg curl, triceps extension, arm curl, rowing torso, heel raise, abdominal crunch, and back extension.

Flexibility is important in sports participation to enhance the range of motion in the joints. Using the guidelines from Chapter 8, schedule flexibility training two or three days per week. Perform each stretching exercise four times, and hold each stretch for 15 to 30 seconds. Examples of stretching exercises include the side body stretch, body rotation, chest stretch, shoulder stretch, sit-and-reach stretch, adductor stretch, quad stretch, heel cord stretch, and knee-to-chest stretch.

In terms of body composition, excess body fat hinders sports performance and increases the risk for injuries. Depending on the nature of the activity, fitness goals for body composition range from 12 percent to 20 percent body fat for men and 17 percent to 25 percent for most women.

**Sport-Specific Conditioning** Once you have achieved the general fitness base, continue with the program but make adjustments to add sport-specific training. This training should match the sport's requirements for aerobic/anaerobic capabilities, muscular strength and endurance, and range of motion.

During the sport-specific training, about half of your aerobic/anaerobic training should involve the same muscles used during your sport. Ideally, allocate 4 weeks of sport-specific training before you start participating in the sport. Then continue the sport-specific training on a more limited basis throughout the season. Depending on the nature of the sport (aerobic versus anaerobic), once the season starts, sports participation itself can take the place of some or all of your aerobic workouts.

The next step is to look at the demands of the sport. For example, soccer, bicycle racing, cross-country skiing, and snowshoeing are aerobic activities, whereas basketball, racquetball, alpine skiing, snowboarding, and ice hockey are stop-and-go sports that require a combination of aerobic and anaerobic activity. Consequently, aerobic training may be appropriate for cross-country skiing, but it will do little to prepare your muscles for the high-intensity requirements of combined aerobic and anaerobic sports.

Adapted with permission of the American College of Sports Medicine, from W. W. K. Hoeger and J. R. Moore, "Preparing for Outdoor Winter Sports," ACSM Fit Society® Page, Fall 2008, p. 3. (www.acsm.org).

**Interval training**, performed twice per week, is added to the program at this time. The intervals consist of a 1:3 work-to-rest ratio. This means you'll work at a fairly high intensity for, say, 15 seconds and then spend 45 seconds on low-intensity recovery. Be sure to keep moving during the recovery phase. Perform four or five intervals at first, then gradually progress to 10 intervals. As your fitness improves, lengthen the high-intensity proportion of the intervals progressively to 1 minute and use a 1:2 work-to-rest ratio, in which you work at high intensity for 1 minute and then at low intensity for 2 minutes.

For aerobic sports, interval training once a week also improves performance. These intervals, however, can be done on a 3-minute to 3-minute work-to-rest ratio. You also can do a 5- to 10-minute work interval followed by 1 to 2 minutes of recovery, but the intensity of these longer intervals should not be as high, and only three to five intervals are recommended. The interval-training workouts are not performed in addition to the regular aerobic workouts but, instead, take the place of one of these workouts.

Consider sport-specific strength requirements as well. Look at the primary muscles used in your sport, and make sure your choice of exercises works those muscles. Try to perform your strength training through a range of motions similar to those used in your sport.

Aerobic/anaerobic sports require greater strength; during the season, the recommendation is three sets of 8 to 12 repetitions to near fatigue, two or three times per week. For aerobic endurance sports, the recommendation is a minimum of one set of 8 to 12 repetitions to near fatigue, once or twice per week during the season.

Stop-and-go sports (basketball, racquetball, soccer) require greater strength than pure endurance sports (triathlon, long-distance running, cross-country skiing). For example, recreational participants during the sport-specific training phase for stop-and-go sports perform three sets of 8 to 12 repetitions to near fatigue, two to three times per week. Competitive athletes and those desiring greater strength gains typically conduct three to five sets of 4 to 12 repetitions to near fatigue three times per week.

For some winter sports, such as alpine skiing and snowboarding, gravity supplies most of the propulsion, and the body acts more as a shock absorber. Muscles in the hips, knees, and trunk are used to control the forces on the body and equipment. Multi-joint exercises, such as the leg press, squats, and lunges, are suggested for these activities.

Before the season starts, make sure your equipment is in proper working condition. For example, alpine skiers' bindings should be cleaned and adjusted properly so they will release as needed. This is one of the most important things you can do to help prevent knee injuries. A good pair of bindings is cheaper than knee surgery.

The first few times you participate in the sport of your choice, go easy, practice technique, and do not continue once you are fatigued. Gradually increase the length and intensity of your workouts. Consider taking some lessons, to have someone watch your technique and help correct flaws early in the season. Even Olympic athletes have

## Behavior Modification Planning

### COMMON SIGNS AND SYMPTOMS OF OVERTRAINING

- ☐ Decreased fitness
- ☐ Decreased sports performance
- ☐ Increased fatigue
- ☐ Loss of concentration
- ☐ Staleness and burnout
- ☐ Loss of competitive drive
- ☐ Increased resting and exercise heart rate
- ☐ Decreased appetite
- ☐ Loss of body weight
- ☐ Altered sleep patterns
- ☐ Decreased sex drive
- ☐ Generalized body aches and pains
- ☐ Increased susceptibility to illness and injury
- ☐ Mood disturbances
- ☐ Depression

### Try It

If following several weeks or months of hard training you experience some of the above symptoms, you need to substantially decrease training volume and intensity for a week or two. This recovery phase will allow the body to recover, strengthen, and prepare for the next training phase. In your Behavior Change Tracker or your Online Journals, modify your training program to allow a light week of training following each 5 to 8 weeks of hard exercise training.

coaches watching them. Proper conditioning allows for a more enjoyable and healthier season.

**Overtraining** Rest is important in any fitness conditioning program. Although the term **overtraining** is associated most frequently with athletic performance, it

---

**Step aerobics** A form of exercise that combines stepping up and down from a bench accompanied by arm movements.

**Interval training** A system of exercise in which a short period of intense effort is followed by a specified recovery period according to a prescribed ratio; for instance, a 1:3 work-to-recovery ratio.

**Overtraining** An emotional, behavioral, and physical condition marked by increased fatigue, decreased performance, persistent muscle soreness, mood disturbances, and feelings of "staleness" or "burnout" as a result of excessive physical training.

applies just as well to fitness participants. We all know that hard work improves fitness and performance. Hard training without adequate recovery, however, breaks down the body and leads to loss of fitness.

Physiological improvements in fitness and conditioning programs occur during the rest periods following training. As a rule, a hard day of training must be followed by a day of light training. Equally, a few weeks of increased training **volume** are to be followed by a few days of light recovery work. During these recovery periods, body systems strengthen and compensate for the training load, leading to a higher level of fitness. If proper recovery is not built into the training routine, overtraining occurs. Decreased performance, staleness, and injury are frequently seen with overtraining. Thus, to obtain optimal results, training regimens are altered during different phases of the year.

## Periodization

**Periodization** is a training approach that uses a systematic variation in intensity and volume to enhance fitness and performance. This model was designed around the premise that the body becomes stronger as a result of training, but if similar workouts are constantly repeated, the body tires and enters a state of staleness and fatigue.

Periodization is used most frequently for athletic conditioning. Because athletes cannot maintain peak fitness during an entire season, most athletes seeking peak performance use a periodized training approach. Studies have documented that greater improvements in fitness are achieved by using a variety of training loads. Using the same program and attempting to increase volume and intensity over a prolonged time will be manifested in overtraining.

The periodization training system involves three cycles:

1. Macrocycles
2. Mesocycles
3. Microcycles

These cycles vary in length depending on the requirements of the sport. Typically, the overall training period (season or year) is referred to as a macrocycle. For athletes who need to peak twice a year, such as cross-country and track runners, two macrocycles can be developed within the year.

Macrocycles are divided into smaller weekly or monthly training phases known as mesocycles. A typical season, for example, is divided into the following mesocycles: base fitness conditioning (off-season), preseason or sport-specific conditioning, competition, peak performance, and transition (active recovery from sport-specific training and competition). In turn, mesocycles are divided into smaller weekly or daily microcycles. During microcycles, training follows the general objective of the mesocycle, but the workouts are altered to avoid boredom and fatigue.

The concept behind periodizing can be used in both aerobic and anaerobic sports. In the case of a long-distance runner, for instance, training can start with a general strength-conditioning program and cardiorespiratory endurance **cross-training** (jogging, cycling, swimming) during the off-season. In preseason, the volume of strength training is decreased, and the total weekly running mileage, at moderate intensities, is progressively increased. During the competitive season, the athlete maintains a limited strength-training program but now increases the intensity of the runs while decreasing the total weekly mileage. During the peaking phase, volume (miles) of training is reduced even further, while the intensity is maintained at a high level. At the end of the season, a short transition period of 2 to 4 weeks, involving low- to moderate-intensity activities other than running and lifting weights, is recommended.

Periodization is frequently used for development of muscular strength, progressively cycling through the various components (hypertrophy, strength, and power) of strength training. Research indicates that varying the volume and intensity over time is more effective for long-term progression than are either single- or multiple-set programs with no variations. Training volume and intensity are typically increased only for large muscle/multijoint lifts (for example, bench press, squats, and lat pulldowns). Single-joint lifts (triceps extension, biceps curls, hamstring curls) usually remain in the range of three sets of 8 to 12 repetitions.

A sample sequence—one macrocycle—of periodized training is provided in Table 9.7. The program starts with high volume and low intensity. During subsequent mesocycles (divided among the objectives of hypertrophy, strength, and power), the volume is decreased, and the intensity (resistance) increases. Following each mesocycle, the recommendation is up to seven days of very light training. This brief resting period allows the body to fully recuperate, preventing overtraining and risk for injury. Other models of periodization are available, but the example provided is the most commonly used.

For aerobic endurance sports, one to three sets of 8 to 12 repetitions to near fatigue performed once or twice a week is recommended. Although strength training does not enhance maximal oxygen uptake, and strength requirements are not as high with endurance sports, data indicate that strength training does help the individual sustain submaximal exercise for longer periods of time.

In recent years, the practice of altering or cycling workouts has become popular among fitness participants. Research indicates that periodization is not limited to athletes but has been used successfully by fitness enthusiasts who are preparing for special events such as a 10K run, a triathlon, or a bike race and by those who are simply aiming for higher fitness. Altering training is also recommended for people who progressed nicely in the initial weeks of a fitness program but now feel "stale" and "stagnant." Studies indicate that even among general fitness participants, systematically altering volume and intensity of training is most effective for progress in long-term fitness. Because training phases change continually during

**TABLE 9.7** Periodization Program for Strength

| | One Macrocycle | | | |
| --- | --- | --- | --- | --- |
| | Mesocycle 1* | Mesocycle 2* | Mesocycle 3* | Mesocycle 4* |
| | Hypertrophy | Strength & Hypertrophy | Strength & Power | Peak Performance |
| Sets per exercise | 3–5 | 3–5 | 3–5 | 1–3 |
| Repetitions | 8–12 | 6–9 | 1–5 | 1–3 |
| Intensity (resistance) | Low | Moderate | High | Very High |
| Volume | High | Moderate | Low | Very Low |
| Weeks (microcycles) | 6–8 | 4–6 | 3–5 | 1–2 |

*Each mesocycle is followed by several days of light training.

a macrocycle, periodization breaks the staleness and the monotony of repeated workouts.

For the nonathlete, a periodization program does not have to account for every detail of the sport. You can periodize workouts by altering mesocycles every 2 to 8 weeks. You can use different exercises, change the number of sets and repetitions, vary the speed of the repetitions, alter recovery time between sets, and even cross-train.

Periodization is not for everyone. People who are starting an exercise program, who enjoy a set routine, or who are satisfied with their fitness routine and fitness level do not need to periodize. For new participants, the goal is to start and adhere to exercise long enough to adopt the exercise behavior.

# Personal Fitness Programming: An Example

Now that you understand the principles of fitness assessment and exercise prescription given in Chapters 6 through 8 and this chapter, you can review this program to cross-check and improve the design of your own fitness program. Let's look at an example.

Mary is 20 years old and 5 feet 6 inches tall. She participated in organized sports on and off throughout high school. During the last 2 years, however, she has participated only minimally in physical activity. She was not taught the principles for exercise prescription and has not participated in regular exercise to improve and maintain the various health-related components of fitness.

Mary became interested in fitness and contemplated signing up for a fitness and wellness course. As she was preparing her class schedule for the semester, she noted a "Lifetime Fitness and Wellness" course. In registering for the course, Mary anticipated some type of structured aerobic exercise. She knew that good fitness was important to health and weight management, but she didn't quite know how to plan and implement a program.

Once the new course started, she and her classmates received the "Stages of Change Questionnaire." Mary learned that she was in the Preparation stage for cardiorespiratory endurance, the Precontemplation stage for muscular strength and endurance, the Maintenance stage for flexibility, and the Preparation stage for body composition (see the discussion of the transtheoretical model in Chapter 2, pages 49–52). Various fitness assessments determined that her cardiorespiratory endurance level was fair, her muscular strength and endurance were poor, her flexibility was good, and her percent body fat was 25 (the Moderate category).

## Critical Thinking

In your own experience with personal fitness programs throughout the years, what factors have motivated you and helped you the most to stay with a program? What factors have kept you from being physically active, and what can you do to change these factors?

**Cardiorespiratory Endurance** At the beginning of the semester, the instructor informed the students that the course would require self-monitored participation

**Volume (of training)** The total amount of training performed in a given work period (day, week, month, or season).

**Periodization** A training approach that divides the season into three cycles (macrocycles, mesocycles, and microcycles) using a systematic variation in intensity and volume of training to enhance fitness and performance.

**Cross-training** A combination of aerobic activities that contribute to overall fitness.

in activities outside the regularly scheduled class hours. Thus, Mary was in the Preparation stage for cardiorespiratory endurance. She knew she would be starting exercise in the next couple of weeks.

While in this Preparation stage, Mary chose three processes of change to help her implement her program (see Chapter 2, Table 2.1, page 50). She thought she could adopt an aerobic exercise program (Positive Outlook process of change) and set a realistic goal to reach the "Good" category for cardiorespiratory endurance by the end of the semester (Goal Setting). By staying in this course, she committed to go through with exercise (Commitment). She prepared a 12-week Personalized Cardiorespiratory Exercise Prescription (see Figure 9.5), wrote down her goal, signed the prescription (now a contract), and shared the program with her instructor and roommates.

As her exercise modalities, Mary selected walking/jogging and aerobics. Initially she walked/jogged twice a week and did aerobics once a week. By the 10th week of the program, she was jogging three times per week and participating in aerobics twice a week. She also selected Self-monitoring, Self-reevaluation, and Countering as techniques of change (see Chapter 2, Table 2.2, page 56). Using the exercise log in Figure 6.10 in Chapter 6 (page 220) and the online exercise log (see Figure 9.6), she monitored her exercise program. At the end of 6 weeks, she scheduled a follow-up cardiorespiratory assessment test (Self-reevaluation process of change), and she replaced her evening television hour with aerobic training (Countering).

Mary also decided to increase her daily physical activity. She chose to walk 10 minutes to and from school, take the stairs instead of elevators whenever possible, and add 5-minute walks every hour during study time. On Saturdays, she cleaned her apartment and went to a school-sponsored dance at night. On Sundays, she opted to walk to and from church and took a 30-minute leisurely walk after the dinner meal. Mary now was fully in the Action stage of change for cardiorespiratory endurance.

## Muscular Strength and Endurance

After Mary had started her fitness and wellness course, she wasn't yet convinced that she wanted to strength train. Still, she contemplated strength training because a small part of her grade depended on it. When she read the information on the effect of lean body mass on basal metabolic rate and weight maintenance (Consciousness-raising), she thought that perhaps it would be good to add strength training to her program. She also was contemplating the long-term consequences of loss of lean body mass, its effect on her personal appearance, and the potential for decreased independence and quality of life (Emotional Arousal).

Mary visited her course instructor for additional guidance. Following this meeting, Mary committed herself to strength train. While yet in the Preparation stage, she outlined a 10-week periodized training program (see Figure 9.7) and opted to aim for the "Good" strength category by the end of it.

Because this was the first time Mary had lifted weights, the course instructor introduced her to two other students who were already lifting (Helping Relationships). She also monitored her program with the form provided in Chapter 7, Figure 7.8. Mary promised herself a movie and dinner out if she completed the first 5 weeks of strength training, and a new blouse if she made it through 10 weeks (Rewards process and technique for change).

## Muscular Flexibility

Good flexibility is not a problem for Mary because she regularly stretched 15 to 30 minutes while watching the evening news on television. She had developed this habit the last 2 years of high school to maintain flexibility as a member of the dance-drill team (Environment Control—as a team member, she'd needed good flexibility).

Because Mary had been stretching regularly for more than 3 years, she was in the Maintenance stage for flexibility. The flexibility fitness tests revealed that she had good flexibility. These results allowed her to pursue her stretching program because she thought she would be excellent for this fitness component (Self-evaluation).

To gain greater improvements in flexibility, Mary chose slow-sustained stretching and proprioceptive neuromuscular facilitation (PNF). She would need help to carry out the PNF technique. She spoke to one of her lifting classmates; together they decided to allocate 20 minutes at the end of strength training to stretching (Helping Relationships), and they chose the sequence of exercises presented in Chapter 8, Lab 8C (Consciousness-raising and Goal Setting).

## Body Composition

One of the motivational factors to enroll in a fitness course was Mary's desire to learn how to better manage her weight. She had gained a few pounds since entering college. To prevent further weight gain, she thought it was time to learn sound principles for weight management (Behavior Analysis). She was in the Preparation stage of change because she was planning to start a diet and exercise program but wasn't sure how to get it done. All Mary needed was a little consciousness-raising to get her into the Action stage.

With the knowledge she had now gained, Mary planned her program. At 25 percent body fat and 140 pounds, she decided to aim for 23 percent body fat so she would be in the "Good" category for body composition (Goal Setting). This meant that she would have to lose about 4 pounds (see Chapter 4, Lab 4B). Mary's daily estimated energy requirement was about 2,027 calories (see Chapter 5, Table 5.3). Mary also figured out that she was expending an additional 400 calories per day through her newly adopted exercise program and increased level of daily physical activity. Thus, her total daily energy intake would be around 2,427 calories (2,027 + 400).

To lose weight, Mary could decrease her caloric intake by 700 calories per day (body weight × 5) (see Chapter 5, Lab 5A), yielding a target daily intake of 1,727 calories. By decreasing the intake by 700 calories daily, Mary should achieve her target weight in about 20 days

**FIGURE 9.5** Sample online cardiorespiratory exercise prescription.

# Personalized Cardiorespiratory Exercise Prescription
Fitness & Wellness Series
Wadsworth Cengage Learning

**Mary Johnson**  September 1, 2009
Maximal heart rate: 200 bpm  Resting heart rate: 76 bpm
Present cardiorespiratory fitness level: Fair  Age: 20

*The following is your personal program for cardiorespiratory fitness development and maintenance. If you have been exercising regularly and you are in the average or good category, you may start at week 5. If you are in the excellent category, you can start at week 10.*

| Week | Time (min.) | Frequency (per week) | Training Intensity (beats per minute) | Pulse (10 sec. count) |
|---|---|---|---|---|
| 1 | 15 | 3 | 126–138 | 21–23 beats |
| 2 | 15 | 4 | 126–138 | 21–23 beats |
| 3 | 20 | 4 | 126–138 | 21–23 beats |
| 4 | 20 | 5 | 126–138 | 21–23 beats |
| 5 | 20 | 4 | 138–150 | 23–25 beats |
| 6 | 20 | 5 | 138–150 | 23–25 beats |
| 7 | 30 | 4 | 138–150 | 23–25 beats |
| 8 | 30 | 5 | 138–150 | 23–25 beats |
| 9 | 30 | 4 | 150–181 | 25–30 beats |
| 10 | 30 | 5 | 150–181 | 25–30 beats |
| 11 | 30–40 | 5 | 150–181 | 25–30 beats |
| 12 | 30–40 | 5–6 | 150–181 | 25–30 beats |

*You may participate in any combination of activities that are aerobic and continuous in nature such as walking, jogging, swimming, cross-country skiing, aerobic exercise, rope skipping, cycling, aerobic dancing, racquetball, stair climbing, stationary running or cycling, etc. As long as the heart rate reaches the desired rate, and it stays at that level for the period of time indicated, the cardiorespiratory system will improve.*

*Following the 12-week program, in order to maintain your fitness level, you should exercise to reach between 150 and 181 bpm for about 30 minutes, a minimum of three times per week on nonconsecutive days. When you exercise, allow about 5 minutes for a gradual warm-up period and another 5 for gradual cool-down. Also, when you check your exercise heart rate, only count your pulse for 10 seconds (start counting with 0) and then refer to the above 10-second pulse count. You may also multipy by 6 to obtain your rate in beats per minute.*

*Good cardiorespiratory fitness will greatly contribute to the enhancement and maintenance of good health. It is especially important in the prevention of cardiovascular disease. We encourage you to be persistent in your exercise program and to participate regularly.*

Training days: ✓M ✓T __W __Th ✓F ✓S __S   Training time: *7:00 am*

Signature: *Mary Johnson*   Goal: *Good*   Date: *9/01/09*

FIGURE 9.6 Sample exercise record using the online exercise option at CengageNOW.

# Exercise Log
Fitness & Wellness Series
Wadsworth Cengage Learning

## Mary Johnson

| Date | Exercise | Body Weight (lbs) | Heart Rate (bpm) | Duration (min) | Distance (miles) | Calories Burned |
|------|----------|-------------------|------------------|----------------|------------------|-----------------|
| 09/01/2009 | Walking (4.5 mph) | 140.0 | 138 | 15 | 1.00 | 95 |
| 09/03/2009 | Aerobics/Moderate | 140.0 | 144 | 20 | | 182 |
| 09/05/2009 | Walking (4.5 mph) | 141.0 | 138 | 15 | 1.00 | 95 |
| 09/06/2009 | Dance/Moderate | 141.0 | 100 | 60 | | 254 |
| 09/07/2009 | Walking (4.5 mph) | 140.0 | 132 | 30 | 2.00 | 189 |
| 09/08/2009 | Jogging (11 min/mile) | 140.0 | 138 | 15 | 1.25 | 147 |
| 09/10/2009 | Aerobics/Moderate | 140.0 | 138 | 20 | | 182 |
| 09/11/2009 | Jogging (11 min/mile) | 139.0 | 138 | 15 | 1.25 | 146 |
| 09/12/2009 | Jogging (11 min/mile) | 139.0 | 134 | 15 | 1.25 | 146 |
| 09/13/2009 | Dance/Moderate | 140.0 | 96 | 75 | | 315 |
| 09/14/2009 | Walking (4.5 mph) | 139.0 | 126 | 30 | 2.50 | 188 |
| 09/15/2009 | Jogging (11 min/mile) | 139.0 | 134 | 20 | 2.00 | 195 |
| 09/16/2009 | Strength Training | 138.0 | 96 | 30 | | 207 |
| 09/17/2009 | Step-Aerobics | 139.0 | 138 | 30 | | 292 |
| 09/18/2009 | Jogging (11 min/mile) | 138.0 | 138 | 20 | 2.00 | 193 |
| 09/19/2009 | Jogging (11 min/mile) | 138.0 | 138 | 20 | 2.00 | 193 |
| | Strength Training | 138.0 | 96 | 30 | | 207 |
| 09/20/2009 | Dance/Moderate | 138.0 | 90 | 30 | | 124 |
| 09/21/2009 | Walking (4.5 mph) | 138.0 | 126 | 30 | 2.50 | 186 |
| 09/22/2009 | Jogging (11 min/mile) | 137.0 | 136 | 20 | 2.00 | 192 |
| 09/23/2009 | Step-Aerobics | 138.0 | 138 | 30 | | 290 |
| | Strength Training | 138.0 | 96 | 40 | | 276 |
| 09/24/2009 | Jogging (8.5 min/mile) | 138.0 | 144 | 20 | 2.50 | 248 |
| 09/25/2009 | Step-Aerobics | 137.0 | 136 | 20 | | 192 |
| 09/26/2009 | Strength Training | 137.0 | 92 | 40 | | 274 |
| | Jogging (8.5 min/mile) | 137.0 | 140 | 20 | 2.50 | 247 |
| 09/27/2009 | Dance/Moderate | 136.0 | 94 | 90 | | 367 |
| 09/28/2009 | Walking (4.5 mph) | 136.0 | 120 | 30 | 2.50 | 184 |

## Totals

| | | | | 13 hr 50 min | 28.25 | 5806 |
|--|--|--|--|--------------|-------|------|

## Average per exercise session

| | | 138.5 | 124 | 30 | 1.88 | 207 |
|--|--|-------|-----|----|------|-----|

Number of exercise sessions: 28

## Average per day exercised

| | | | | 33 | | 232 |
|--|--|--|--|----|--|-----|

Number of days exercised: 25

## Distance summary

| | |
|--|--|
| Total miles run: | 16.8 |
| Total miles walked: | 11.5 |

**FIGURE 9.7** Sample starting muscular strength and endurance periodization program.

|  | Learning Lifting Technique | Muscular Strength | Muscular Endurance | Muscular Strength |
|---|---|---|---|---|
| Sets per exercise | 1–2 | 2 | 2 | 3 |
| Repetitions | 10 | 12 | 18–20 | 8–12 (RM) |
| Intensity (resistance) | Very low | Moderate | Low | High |
| Volume | Low | Moderate | Moderate | High |
| Sessions per week | 2 | 2 | 2 | 3 |
| Weeks | 2 | 3 | 2 | 1 |

Selected exercises: Bench press, leg press, leg curl, lat pull-down, rowing torso, rotary torso, seated back, and abdominal crunch.

Training days: ☐ M ☐ T ☐ W ☐ Th ☐ F ☐ S ☐ S    Training time: *3:00 pm*

Signature: *Mary Johnson*    Goal: *Average*    Date: *9-10-09*

(4 pounds of fat × 3,500 calories per pound of fat ÷ 700 fewer calories per day = 20 days). Mary picked the 1,800-calorie diet and eliminated one daily serving of grains (80 calories) to avoid exceeding her target 1,727 daily calorie intake.

The processes of change that will help Mary in the Action stage for weight management are Goal Setting, Countering (exercising instead of watching television), Monitoring, Environment Control, and Rewards. To monitor her daily caloric intake, Mary uses the 1,800-calorie diet plan in Chapter 5, Lab 5C. To further exert control over her environment, she gave away all of her junk food. She determined that she would not eat out while on the diet, and she bought only low- to moderate-fat/complex carbohydrate foods during the 3 weeks. As her reward, she achieved her target body weight of 136 pounds.

# You Can Get It Done

Once they understand the proper exercise, nutrition, and behavior modification guidelines, people find that implementing a fitness lifestyle program is not as difficult as they thought. With adequate preparation and a personal behavioral analysis, you are now ready to design, implement, evaluate, and adhere to a lifetime fitness program that can enhance your functional capacity and zest for life.

Using the concepts provided thus far in this book and the exercise prescription principles that you have learned, you should now update your personal fitness program in Lab 9B. You also have an opportunity to revise your current stage of change, fitness category for each health-related component of physical fitness, and number of daily steps taken. You have the tools—the rest is up to you!

# ASSESS YOUR BEHAVIOR

Log on to http://www.cengage.com/sso/ to create or update your personal log to include all your fitness activities.

1. Do you participate in recreational sports as a means to further improve your fitness and add enjoyment to training?

2. Have you been able to meet your cardiorespiratory endurance, muscular strength, muscular flexibility, and recommended body composition goals?

3. Are you able to incorporate a variety of activities into your fitness program, and do you vary exercise intensity and duration from time to time in your training?

# ASSESS YOUR KNOWLEDGE

Log on to http://www.cengage.com/sso/ to assess your understanding of this chapter's topics by taking the Student Practice Test and exploring the modules recommended in your Personalized Study Plan.

1. Which of the following is *not* a skill-related fitness component?
   a. Agility
   b. Speed
   c. Power
   d. Strength
   e. Balance

2. The ability to quickly and efficiently change body position and direction is known as
   a. agility.
   b. coordination.
   c. speed.
   d. reaction time.
   e. mobility.

3. The two components of power are
   a. strength and endurance.
   b. speed and force.
   c. speed and endurance.
   d. strength and force.
   e. endurance and force.

4. People with diabetes should
   a. not exercise alone.
   b. wear a bracelet that identifies their condition.
   c. exercise at a low-to-moderate intensity.
   d. check blood glucose levels before and after exercise.
   e. follow all four guidelines above.

5. During pregnancy a woman should
   a. accumulate 30 minutes of moderate-intensity activity on most days of the week.
   b. exercise between "low" and "somewhat hard."
   c. avoid exercising at an altitude above 6,000 feet.
   d. All of the above choices are correct.
   e. None of the choices is correct.

6. During exercise in the heat, drinking about a cup of cool water every _____ minutes seems to be ideal to prevent dehydration.
   a. 5
   b. 15 to 20
   c. 30
   d. 30 to 45
   e. 60

7. One of the most common causes of activity-related injuries is
   a. high impact.
   b. low level of fitness.
   c. exercising without stretching.
   d. improper warm-up.
   e. All the choices cause about an equal number of injuries.

8. Improvements in maximal oxygen uptake in older adults (as compared with younger adults) as a result of cardiorespiratory endurance training are
   a. lower.
   b. higher.
   c. difficult to determine.
   d. nonexistent.
   e. similar.

9. To participate in sports, it is recommended that you have
   a. base fitness and sport-specific conditioning.
   b. at least a good rating on skill fitness.
   c. good-to-excellent agility.
   d. basic speed.
   e. all of the above.

10. Periodization is a training approach that
    a. uses a systematic variation in intensity and volume.
    b. helps enhance fitness and performance.
    c. is commonly used by athletes.
    d. helps prevent staleness and overtraining.
    e. All are correct choices.

Correct answers can be found at the back of the book.

# MEDIA MENU

You can find the links below at the book companion site: www.cengage.com/health/hoeger/plfw10e

- American Council of Exercise. This site features "Fit Facts," covering sports and outdoor activities, youth fitness, and exercise information for people with health challenges. *http://www.acefitness.com*

- Fitness Jumpsite. This site features information on nutrition, weight management, fitness equipment, and healthy lifestyles. A comprehensive search engine is also available. *http://www.primusweb.com/fitnesspartner*

- President's Council on Physical Fitness and Sports. This site features fitness basics, workout plans, and exercise principles. *http://www.hoptechno.com/book11.htm*

- Fitness Online. This site features information on fitness goals and programs, fitness adventures, injury prevention, nutrition, and mental fitness. *http://www.fitnessonline.com*

# NOTES

1. Kirby, R. F. "A Simple Test of Agility," *Coach and Athlete*, June 1971: 30–31.

2. American Alliance for Health, Physical Education, Recreation and Dance (AAHPERD). *Youth Fitness: Test Manual*. Reston, VA: AAHPERD, 1976.

3. See note 2.

4. American College of Sports Medicine, "Position Stand: Exercise and Type 2 Diabetes," *Medicine and Science in Sports and Exercise* 32 (2000): 1345–1360.

5. American College of Obstetricians and Gynecologists, "Exercise During Pregnancy and the Postpartum Period. ACOG Committee Opinion No. 267," *International Journal of Gynecology and Obstetrics* 77 (2002): 79–81.

6. University of California at Berkeley, *The Wellness Guide to Lifelong Fitness* (New York: Random House, 1993): 198.

7. American College of Sports Medicine, "Position Stand: Exercise and Physical Activity for Older Adults," *Medicine and Science in Sports and Exercise* 30 (1998): 992–1008.

8. R. J. Shephard, "Exercise and Aging: Extending Independence in Older Adult," *Geriatrics* 48 (1993): 61–64.

9. F. W. Kash, J. L. Boyer, S. P. Van Camp, L. S. Verity, and J. P. Wallace, "The Effect of Physical Activity on Aerobic Power in Older Men (A Longitudinal Study)," *Physician and Sports Medicine* 18, no. 4 (1990): 73–83.

10. J. Hagberg, S. Blair, A. Ehsani, N. Gordon, N. Kaplan, C. Tipton, and E. Zambraski, "Position Stand: Physical Activity, Physical Fitness, and Hypertension," *Medicine and Science in Sports and Exercise* 25 (1993): i–x.

11. W. S. Evans, "Exercise, Nutrition and Aging," *Journal of Nutrition* 122 (1992): 796–801.

12. See note 7.

13. The Editors, "Exercise for the Ages," *Consumer Reports on Health* (Yonkers, NY: July 1996).

14. J. M. Walker, D. Sue, N. Miles-Elkousy, G. Ford, and H. Trevelyan, "Active Mobility of the Extremities in Older Subjects," *Physical Therapy* 64 (1994): 919–923.

15. S. B. Roberts, et al., "What Are the Dietary Needs of Adults?" *International Journal of Obesity* 16 (1992): 969–976.

16. J. M. Moore and W. W. K. Hoeger, "Game On! Preparing Your Clients for Recreational Sports," *ACSM's Health & Fitness Journal* 9 no. 3 (2005): 14–19.

# SUGGESTED READINGS

American College of Obstetricians and Gynecologists. "Exercise During Pregnancy and the Postpartum Period." ACOG Committee Opinion No. 267. *International Journal of Gynecology and Obstetrics* 77 (2002): 79–81.

Coleman, E. *Eating for Endurance*. Palo Alto, CA: Bull Publishing, 2003.

Pfeiffer, R. P., and B. C. Mangus. *Concepts of Athletic Training*. Boston: Jones and Bartlett, 2005.

Unruh, N., S. Unruh, and E. Scantling. "Heat Can Kill: Guidelines to Prevent Heat Illness in Athletics and Physical Education." *Journal of Physical Education, Recreation & Dance* 73 no. 6 (2002): 36–38.

# LAB 9A: Assessment of Skill Fitness

Name _____  Date _____  Grade _____

Instructor _____  Course _____  Section _____

### Necessary Lab Equipment

**Agility:** Free-throw area of a basketball court (or any smooth area 12 by 19 feet with sufficient running space around it), four plastic cones, and a stopwatch.

**Balance:** Any flat, smooth floor (not carpeted) and a stopwatch.

**Coordination:** A 32-inch–long by 5 inch wide piece of cardboard with six circles drawn on it as explained in Figure 9.2, page 325, three full cans of soda pop (12 oz), and a stopwatch.

**Power:** A flat, smooth surface, and a 10-foot tape measure (or two standard cloth measuring tapes, each 60 inches long).

**Reaction Time:** A standard yardstick with a shaded "concentration zone" drawn on the first 2 inches of the stick.

**Speed:** A school track or premeasured 50-yard straightaway.

### Objective

To assess the fitness level for each skill-related fitness component.

### Lab Preparation

Wear exercise clothing, including running shoes. Do not exercise strenuously several hours prior to this lab.

### Instructions

Perform all six tests for the fitness-related components as outlined in Chapter 9. Report the results below and answer the questions given at the end of this lab.

### Skill-Related Fitness: Test Results

|  | |  | | |
|---|---|---|---|---|
| Agility | Trials: | 1. ☐☐.☐ | | 2. ☐☐.☐ |
| Balance | Trials: | 1. ☐☐.☐ | | 2. ☐☐.☐ |
| Coordination | Trials: | 1. ☐☐.☐ | | 2. ☐☐.☐ |
| Power | Trials: | 1. ☐ | | 2. ☐  3. ☐ |
| Reaction Time | Trials: | 1. ☐☐.☐ | | 2. ☐☐.☐  3. ☐☐.☐ |

4. ☐☐.☐  5. ☐☐.☐  6. ☐☐.☐  7. ☐☐.☐

8. ☐☐.☐  9. ☐☐.☐  10. ☐☐.☐  11. ☐☐.☐

12. ☐☐.☐  Average of 6 middle scores = ☐☐.☐

Speed  Trial:  1. ☐☐.☐

| Fitness Component/Test | Percentile Rank* | Category* |
|---|---|---|
| Agility: SEMO test | | |
| Balance: One-foot stand | | |
| Coordination: Soda pop test | | |
| Power: Standing long jump | | |
| Reaction Time: Yardstick test | | |
| Speed: 50-yard dash | | |

See Tables 9.1, 9.2, and 9.3, pages 327–328 Skill-Related Fitness Categories

## Interpretation of Test Results

**1.** What conclusions can you draw from your test results?

_____

_____

_____

_____

_____

**2.** Briefly state how you could improve your test results and what activities you could engage in to obtain the desired results.

_____

_____

_____

_____

_____

**3.** Did you ever participate in organized sports, or have you found success in a particular game or sport?  ☐ Yes  ☐ No

    **3a.** If your answer is yes, list the sports, games, or events in which you enjoy(ed) success.

_____

_____

    **3b.** Is there a relationship between your answers to question 3a and your test results in this lab?

_____

_____

_____

# LAB 9B: Personal Fitness Plan

Name _____  Date _____  Grade _____

Instructor _____  Course _____  Section _____

### Assignment
This laboratory experience should be carried out as a homework assignment to be completed over the next 7 days.

### Lab Resources
Be sure to understand the assessment techniques for the various health related components of physical fitness; the ACSM exercise prescription guidelines provided in Chapters 6, 7, and 8; the stages of change model and goal setting guidelines explained in Chapter 2; and contributions of different activities to the health-related components of fitness.

### Objective
To update your personal fitness program according to personal goals, interests, and current exercise prescription guidelines.

### I. Exercise Clearance
Is it safe for you to participate in an exercise program?   ☐ Yes   ☐ No

### II. Fitness Evaluation

| | Current | | Fitness Category Goal | | |
| --- | --- | --- | --- | --- | --- |
| Component | Test Results | Fitness Category | Training Frequency per Week | Stage of Change | Fitness Goal |
| Cardiorespiratory endurance | | | | | |
| Muscular strength and endurance | | | | | |
| Muscular flexibility | | | | | |
| Body composition | | | NA | | |

## III. Cardiorespiratory Endurance

Outline your cardiorespiratory endurance program according to ACSM guidelines. Include intensity, frequency, duration, aerobic activities, time of day for training, facility where you will perform the training, and reward for accomplishing your goal.

_____

_____

_____

_____

_____

_____

_____

_____

_____

_____

_____

_____

## IV. Muscular Strength and Endurance

Using ACSM guidelines, outline your muscular strength/endurance training program. List the exercises used, sets and repetitions, amount of resistance to be used, frequency per week, training facility, and reward for accomplishing your goal.

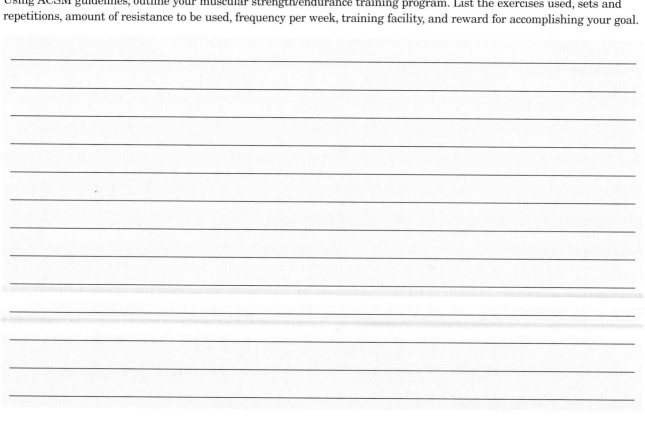

## V. Muscular Flexibility

Design your flexibility training program to include the selected exercises, technique used, number of repetitions for each exercise, length of final hold, site for training, and reward for accomplishing your goal.

_____

_____

_____

_____

_____

_____

_____

_____

_____

## VI. Recreational Activities

List any other sports or recreational activities in which you participate and include how often and how long you participate. Indicate also the primary reason for participation in these activities (physical activity, fitness, competition, skill development, recreation, stress management) and your future goals for these activities.

_____

_____

_____

_____

## VII. Daily Physical Activity

Indicate the efforts that you are making to increase daily physical activity, your feelings about your choice of activities, and what future goals you have regarding daily physical activities.

_____

_____

_____

_____

Total number of daily steps: [_____]

## VIII. Body Composition and Fitness Benefits

List all of the activities in which you participate regularly and rate the respective contribution to body composition and other fitness components. Use the following rating scale: 1 = low, 2 = fair, 3 = average, 4 = good, and 5 = excellent.

| Activity | Body Composition | Cardiorespiratory | Musc. Strength | Musc. Flexibility | Agility | Balance | Coordination | Power | Reaction Time | Speed |
|---|---|---|---|---|---|---|---|---|---|---|
| *Example: Jogging* | 5 | 5 | 2 | 1 | 2 | 2 | 1 | 2 | 1 | 2 |
| | | | | | | | | | | |
| | | | | | | | | | | |
| | | | | | | | | | | |
| | | | | | | | | | | |
| | | | | | | | | | | |
| | | | | | | | | | | |
| | | | | | | | | | | |
| | | | | | | | | | | |
| | | | | | | | | | | |
| | | | | | | | | | | |
| | | | | | | | | | | |
| | | | | | | | | | | |
| | | | | | | | | | | |

## IX. Contract

I hereby commit to carry out the above described fitness plan and complete my goals by _____ .

Upon completion of all my fitness goals I will present my results to _____ and will

reward myself with _____ .

_____  _____

My signature  Date

_____  _____

Witness signature  Date

# Stress Assessment and Management Techniques

# 10

## Objectives

- Define stress, eustress, and distress
- Explain the role of stress in maintaining health and optimal performance
- Identify the major sources of stress in life
- Define the two major types of behavior patterns
- Learn to lower your vulnerability to stress
- Develop time management skills
- Define the role of physical exercise in reducing stress
- Describe and learn to use various stress management techniques
- Learn how you're affected by stress. Find out how vulnerable you are to stress.

Ryan McVay/PhotoDisc/Getty Images

Check your understanding of the chapter contents by logging on to CengageNOW and accessing the pre-test, personalized learning plan, and post-test for this chapter.

# FAQ

### Is all stress detrimental to health and performance?

Living in today's world is nearly impossible without encountering stress. The good news is that stress can be self-controlled. Unfortunately, most people have accepted stress as a normal part of daily life, and even though everyone has to face it, few seem to understand it or know how to cope with it effectively. It is difficult to succeed and have fun in life without "runs, hits, and errors." In fact, stress should not be avoided entirely, because a certain amount is necessary for motivation, performance, and optimum health and well-being. When stress levels push you to the limit, however, stress becomes distress and you will no longer function effectively.

### How can I most effectively deal with negative stress?

Feelings of stress are the result of the body's instinct to defend itself. If you start to experience mental, social, and physical symptoms such as exhaustion, headaches, sleeplessness, frustration, apathy, loneliness, and changes in appetite, you are most likely under excessive stress and need to take action to overcome the stress-causing event(s). Do not deal with these symptoms through alcohol, drugs, or other compulsive behaviors, as such will not get rid of the stressor that is causing the problem. Stress management is best accomplished by maintaining a sense of control when excessive demands are placed upon you.

First, recognize when you are feeling stressed. Early warning signs include tension in your shoulders and neck and clenching of your fists or teeth. Now, determine if there is something that you can do to control, change, or remove yourself from the situation. Most importantly, change how you react to stress. Be positive, avoid extreme reactions (anger, hostility, hatred, depression), try to change the way you see things, work off stress through physical activity, and master one or more stress management techniques to help you in situations where it is necessary to cope effectively. Finally, take steps to reduce the demands placed on you by prioritizing your activities—"don't sweat the small stuff." Realize that it is not stress that makes you ill, but the manner in which you react to stress that leads to illness and disease.

According to a growing body of evidence, virtually every illness known to modern humanity—from arthritis to migraine headaches, from the common cold to cancer—appears to be influenced for good or bad by our emotions. To a profound extent, emotions affect our susceptibility to disease and our **immunity.** The way we react to what comes along in life can determine in great measure how we will react to the disease-causing organisms that we face. The feelings we have and the way we express them can either boost our immune system or weaken it.

Emotional health is a key part of total wellness. Most emotionally healthy people take care of themselves physically—they eat well, exercise, and get enough rest. They work to develop supportive personal relationships. In contrast, many people who are emotionally unhealthy are self-destructive. For example, they may abuse alcohol and other drugs or may overwork and not have balance in their lives. Emotional health is so important that it affects what we do, who we meet, who we marry, how we look, how we feel, the course of our lives, and even how long we live.

# The Mind/Body Connection

Emotions cause physiologic responses that can influence health. Certain parts of the brain are associated with specific emotions and specific hormone patterns. The release of certain hormones is associated with various emotional responses, and those hormones affect health. These responses may contribute to development of disease. Emotions have to be expressed somewhere, somehow. If they are suppressed repeatedly, and/or if a person feels conflict about controlling them, they often reveal themselves through physical symptoms. These physiologic responses may weaken the immune system over time.

**The Brain** The brain is the most important part of the nervous system. For the body to survive, the brain must be maintained. All other organs sacrifice to keep the brain alive and functioning when the entire body is under severe stress.

The brain directs nerve impulses that are carried throughout the body. It controls voluntary processes, such as the direction, strength, and coordination of muscle movements; the processes involved in smelling, touching, and seeing; and involuntary functions over which you have no conscious control. Among the latter are many automatic, vital functions in the body, such as breathing, heart rate, digestion, control of the bowels and bladder, blood pressure, and release of hormones.

The brain is the cognitive center of the body, the place where ideas are generated, memory is stored, and emotions are experienced. The brain has a powerful influence over the body via the link between the emotions and the immune system. That link is extremely complex.

The emotions that the brain produces are a mixture of feelings and physical responses. Every time the brain manufactures an emotion, physical reactions accompany it. The brain's natural chemicals form literal communication links among the brain, its thought processes, and the cells of the body, including those of the immune system.

### The Immune System
The immune system patrols and guards the body against attackers. This system consists of about a trillion cells called **lymphocytes** (the cells responsible for waging war against disease or infection) and about a hundred million trillion molecules called **antibodies.** The brain and the immune system are closely linked in a connection that allows the mind to influence both susceptibility and resistance to disease. A number of immune system cells—including those in the thymus gland, spleen, bone marrow, and lymph nodes—are laced with nerve cells.

Cells of the immune system are equipped to respond to chemical signals from the central nervous system. For example, the surface of the lymphocytes contains receptors for a variety of central nervous system chemical messengers, such as catecholamines, prostaglandins, serotonin, endorphins, sex hormones, the thyroid hormone, and the growth hormone. Certain white blood cells possess the ability to receive messages from the brain.

Because of these receptors on the lymphocytes, physical and psychological stress alters the immune system. Stress causes the body to release several powerful neurohormones that bind with the receptors on the lymphocytes and suppress immune function.

# Stress

Living in today's world is nearly impossible without encountering **stress.** In an unpredictable world that changes with every new day, most people find that working under pressure has become the rule rather than the exception. As a result, stress has become one of the most common problems we face and undermines our ability to stay well. Current estimates indicate that the annual cost of stress and stress-related diseases in the United States exceeds $100 billion, a direct result of health care costs, lost productivity, and absenteeism. Many medical and stress researchers believe that "stress should carry a health warning" as well.

The good news is that stress can be self-controlled. Unfortunately, most people have accepted stress as a normal part of daily life, and even though everyone has to deal with it, few seem to understand it or know how to cope effectively. It is difficult to succeed and have fun in life without "runs, hits, and errors." In fact, stress should not be avoided entirely, because a certain amount is necessary for optimum health, performance, and well-being.

Just what is stress? Dr. Hans Selye, one of the foremost authorities on stress, defined it as "the nonspecific response of the human organism to any demand that is placed upon it."[1] "Nonspecific" indicates that the body reacts in a similar fashion, regardless of the nature of the event that leads to the stress response. In simpler terms, stress is the body's mental, emotional, and physiologic response to any situation that is new, threatening, frightening, or exciting.

The body's response to stress has been the same ever since humans were first put on the earth. Stress prepares the organism to react to the stress-causing event, also called the **stressor.** The problem arises in the way in which we react to stress. Many people thrive under stress; others under similar circumstances are unable to handle it. An individual's reaction to a stress-causing agent determines whether that stress is positive or negative.

Dr. Selye defined the ways in which we react to stress as either eustress or distress. In both cases, the nonspecific response is almost the same. In the case of **eustress**, health and performance continue to improve even as stress increases. On the other hand, **distress** refers to the unpleasant or harmful stress under which health and performance begin to deteriorate. The relationship between stress and performance is illustrated in Figure 10.1.

Stress is a fact of modern life, and every person does need an optimal level of stress that is most conducive to

---

**Immunity** The function that guards the body from invaders, both internal and external.

**Lymphocytes** Immune system cells responsible for waging war against disease or infection.

**Antibodies** Substances produced by the white blood cells in response to an invading agent.

**Stress** The mental, emotional, and physiologic response of the body to any situation that is new, threatening, frightening, or exciting.

**Stressor** Stress-causing event.

**Eustress** Positive stress: Health and performance continue to improve, even as stress increases.

**Distress** Negative stress: Unpleasant or harmful stress under which health and performance begin to deteriorate.

**FIGURE 10.1** Relationship between stress and health and performance.

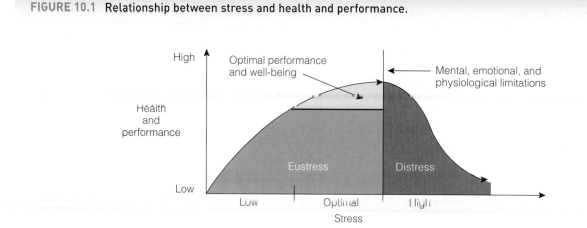

adequate health and performance. When stress levels reach mental, emotional, and physiologic limits, however, stress becomes distress and the person no longer functions effectively.

Chronic distress raises the risk for many health disorders—among them, coronary heart disease, hypertension, eating disorders, ulcers, diabetes, asthma, depression, migraine headaches, sleep disorders, and chronic fatigue—and may even play a role in the development of certain types of cancers.[2] Recognizing this and overcoming the problem quickly and efficiently are crucial in maintaining emotional and physiologic stability.

## Critical Thinking

Can you identify sources of eustress and distress in your personal life during this past year? Explain your emotional and physical response to each stressor and how the two differ.

# Stress Adaptation

The body continually strives to maintain a constant internal environment. This state of physiologic balance, known as **homeostasis**, allows the body to function as effectively as possible. When a stressor triggers a nonspecific response, homeostasis is disrupted. This reaction to stressors, best explained by Dr. Selye through the **general adaptation syndrome (GAS)**, is composed of three stages: alarm reaction, resistance, and exhaustion/recovery.

**Alarm Reaction**  The alarm reaction is the immediate response to a stressor (whether positive or negative). During the alarm reaction, the body evokes an instant physiologic reaction that mobilizes internal systems and processes to minimize the threat to homeostasis (see also "Coping with Stress" on page 368). If the stressor subsides, the body recovers and returns to homeostasis.

**Resistance**  If the stressor persists, the body calls upon its limited reserves to build up its resistance as it strives to maintain homeostasis. For a short while, the body copes effectively and meets the challenge of the stressor until it can be overcome (see Figure 10.2).

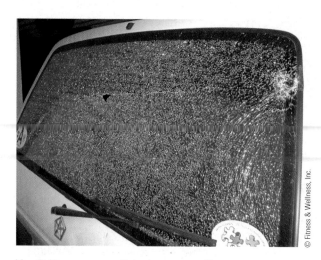

Vandalism causes distress or negative stress.

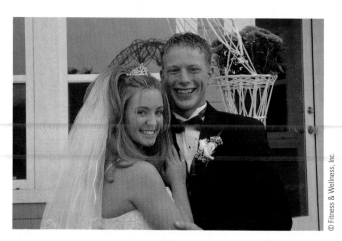

Marriage is an example of positive stress, also known as eustress.

**FIGURE 10.2** General adaptation syndrome: The body's response to stress can end in exhaustion, illness, or recovery.

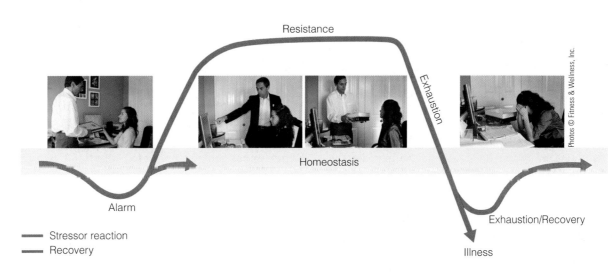

— Stressor reaction
— Recovery

### Exhaustion/Recovery

If stress becomes chronic and intolerable, the body spends its limited reserves and loses its ability to cope, entering the exhaustion/recovery stage. During this stage, the body functions at a diminished capacity while it recovers from stress. In due time, following an "adequate" recovery period (which varies greatly), the body recuperates and is able to return to homeostasis. If chronic stress persists during the exhaustion stage, however, immune function is compromised, which can damage body systems and lead to disease.

An example of the stress response through the general adaptation syndrome can be illustrated in college test performance. As you prepare to take an exam, you experience an initial alarm reaction. If you understand the material, study for the exam, and do well (eustress), the body recovers and stress is dissipated. If, however, you are not adequately prepared and fail the exam, you trigger the resistance stage. You are now concerned about your grade, and you remain in the resistance stage until the next

exam. If you prepare and do well, the body recovers. But, if you fail once again and can no longer bring up the grade, exhaustion sets in and physical and emotional breakdowns may occur. Exhaustion may be further aggravated if you are struggling in other courses as well.

The exhaustion stage is often manifested by athletes and the most ardent fitness participants. Staleness is usually a manifestation of overtraining. Peak performance can be sustained for only about 2 to 3 weeks at a time. Any attempts to continue intense training after peaking leads to exhaustion, diminished fitness, and mental and physical problems associated with overtraining (see Chapter 9). Thus, athletes and some fitness participants also need an active recovery phase following the attainment of peak fitness.

## Perceptions and Health

The habitual manner in which people explain the things that happen to them is their **explanatory style.** It is a way of thinking when all other factors are equal and when there are no clear-cut right and wrong answers. The contrasting explanatory styles are pessimism and optimism. People with a pessimistic explanatory style interpret events negatively; people with an optimistic explanatory style interpret events in a positive light (every cloud has a silver lining).

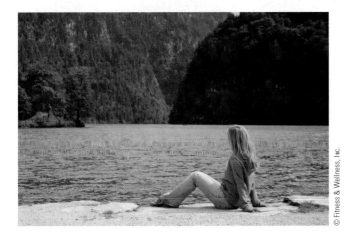

Taking time out during stressful life events is critical for good health and wellness.

**Homeostasis** A natural state of equilibrium; the body attempts to maintain this equilibrium by constantly reacting to external forces that attempt to disrupt this fine balance.

**General adaptation syndrome (GAS)** A theoretical model that explains the body's adaptation to sustained stress which includes three stages: alarm reaction, resistance, and exhaustion/recovery.

**Explanatory style** The way people perceive the events in their lives, from an optimistic or a pessimistic perspective.

A pessimistic explanatory style can delay healing time and worsen the course of illness in several major diseases. For example, it can affect the circulatory system and general outlook for people with coronary heart disease. Blood flow actually changes as thoughts, feelings, and attitudes change. People with a pessimistic explanatory style have a higher risk of developing heart disease.

Studies of explanatory style verify that a negative explanatory style also compromises immunity. Blood samples taken from people with a negative explanatory style revealed suppressed immune function, a low ratio of helper/suppressor T-cells, and fewer lymphocytes.

In contrast, an optimistic style tends to increase the strength of the immune system. An optimistic explanatory style and the positive attitude it fosters can also enhance the ability to resist infections, allergies, autoimmunities, and even cancer. A change in explanatory style can lead to a remarkable change in the course of disease. An optimistic explanatory style and the positive emotions it embraces—such as love, acceptance, and forgiveness—stimulate the body's healing systems.

### Self-esteem

**Self-esteem** is a way of viewing and assessing yourself. Positive self-esteem is a sense of feeling good about one's capabilities, goals, accomplishments, place in the world, and relationship to others. People with high self-esteem respect themselves. Self-esteem is a powerful determinant of health behavior and, therefore, of health status. Healthy self-esteem is one of the best things a person can develop for overall health, both mental and physical. A good, strong sense of self can boost the immune system, protect against disease, and aid in healing.

Whether people get sick—and how long they stay that way—may depend in part on the strength of their self-esteem. For example, low self-esteem worsens chronic pain. The higher the self-esteem, the more rapid the recovery. If we have strong self-esteem, the outlook is good. If our self-esteem is poor, however, our health can decline in direct proportion as our attitude and negative perceptions worsen.

Belief in oneself is one of the most powerful weapons people have to protect health and live longer, more satisfying lives. It has a dramatic and positive impact on wellness, and we can work to harness it to our advantage.

### A Fighting Spirit

A **fighting spirit** involves the healthy expression of emotions, whether they are negative or positive. At the other extreme is hopelessness, a surrender to despair. Fighting spirit can play a major role in recovery from disease. People with a fighting spirit accept their disease diagnosis, adopt an optimistic attitude filled with faith, seek information about how to help themselves, and are determined to fight the disease. A fighting spirit makes a person take charge.

A fighting spirit may be the underlying factor in what is called **spontaneous remission** from incurable illness. More and more physicians believe that the phenomenon is real and that the patient is the key in spontaneous remission. They believe the patient's attitude, especially the presence of a fighting spirit, is responsible for victory over disease. Fighters are not stronger or more capable than others—they simply do not give up as easily. They enjoy better health and live longer even when physicians and laboratory tests say they should not. Fighters are intrinsically different from people who give up, and their health status reflects those differences.

# Sources of Stress

Several instruments have been developed to assess sources of stress in life. The most practical instrument is the **Life Experiences Survey**, presented in Lab 10A, which identifies the life changes within the last 12 months that may have an impact on your physical and psychological well-being.

The Life Experiences Survey is divided into two sections. Section 1, to be completed by all respondents, contains a list of 47 life events plus three blank spaces for other events experienced but not listed in the survey. Section 2 contains an additional 10 questions designed for students only (students should fill out both sections). Common stressors in the lives of college students are depicted in Figure 10.3.

The survey requires testees to rate the extent to which their life events had a positive or negative impact on their lives at the time these events occurred. The ratings are on a 7-point scale. A rating of −3 indicates an extremely undesirable impact. A rating of zero (0) suggests neither a positive nor a negative impact (**neustress**). A rating of +3 indicates an extremely desirable impact.

**FIGURE 10.3  Stressors in the lives of college students.**

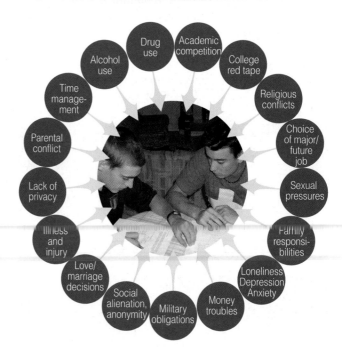

Adapted from W. W. K. Hoeger, L. W. Turner, and B. Q. Hafen. *Wellness Guidelines for a Healthy Lifestyle.* Wadsworth/Thomson Learning, 2007.

After the person evaluates his or her life events, the negative and the positive points are totaled separately. Both scores are expressed as positive numbers (for example, positive ratings of 2, 1, 3, and 3 = 9 points positive score; negative ratings of −3, −2, −2, −1, and −2 = 10 points negative score). A final "total life change" score can be obtained by adding the positive score and the negative score together as positive numbers (total life change score: 9 + 10 = 19 points).

Because negative and positive changes alike can produce nonspecific responses, the total life change score is a good indicator of total life stress. Most research in this area, however, suggests that the negative change score is a better predictor of potential physical and psychological illness than the total change score. More research is necessary to establish the role of total change and the role of the ratio of positive to negative stress.

# Behavior Patterns

Common life events are not the only source of stress in life. All too often, individuals bring on stress as a result of their behavior patterns. The two main types of behavior patterns, Type A and Type B, are based on several observable characteristics.

Several attempts have been made to develop an objective scale to identify Type A individuals properly, but these questionnaires are not as valid and reliable as researchers would like them to be. Consequently, the main assessment tool to determine behavioral type is still the **structured interview**, during which a person is asked to reply to several questions that describe Type A and Type B behavior patterns. The interviewer notes not only the responses to the questions but also the individual's mental, emotional, and physical behaviors as he or she replies to each question.

Based on the answers and the associated behaviors, the interviewer rates the person along a continuum from Type A to Type B. Along this continuum behavioral patterns are classified into five categories: A-1, A-2, X (a mix of Type A and Type B), B-3, and B-4. Type A-1 people exhibit all of the Type A characteristics, and B-4 people show a relative absence of Type A behaviors. Type A-2 people do not exhibit a complete Type A pattern, and Type B-3 people exhibit only a few Type A characteristics.

**Type A** behavior characterizes a primarily hard-driving, overambitious, aggressive, and at times hostile and overly competitive person. Type A individuals often set their own goals, are self-motivated, try to accomplish many tasks at the same time, are excessively achievement oriented, and have a high degree of time urgency.

In contrast, **Type B** behavior is characteristic of calm, casual, relaxed, easygoing individuals. Type B people take one thing at a time, do not feel pressured or hurried, and seldom set their own deadlines.

Over the years, experts have indicated that individuals classified as Type A are under too much stress and have a significantly higher incidence of coronary heart disease. Based on these findings, Type A individuals have been counseled to lower their stress level by modifying many of their Type A behaviors.

Many of the Type A characteristics are learned behaviors. Consequently, if people can learn to identify the sources of stress and make changes in their behavioral responses, they can move along the continuum and respond with more Type B behavior. The debate, however, has centered on which Type A behaviors should be changed, because not all of them are undesirable.

Even though personality questionnaires are not as valid and reliable as structured interviews in identifying Type A individuals, Drs. Meyer Friedman and Ray Rosenman, two San Francisco scientists, constructed a Type A personality assessment form, adapted from the structured interview method, to give people a general idea of Type A behavioral patterns. This assessment form is found in Lab 10B. You can use it to understand your own behavioral patterns better. If you obtain a high rating, you probably are a Type A person.

We also know that many individuals perform well under pressure. They typically are classified as Type A but do not demonstrate any of the detrimental effects of stress. Drs. Robert and Marilyn Kriegel came up with the term "Type C" to characterize people with these behaviors.[3]

**Self-esteem** A sense of positive self-regard and self-respect.

**Fighting spirit** Determination; the open expression of emotions, whether negative or positive.

**Spontaneous remission** Inexplicable recovery from incurable disease.

**Life Experiences Survey** A questionnaire used to assess sources of stress in life.

**Neustress** Neutral stress; stress that is neither harmful nor helpful.

**Structured interview** Assessment tool used to determine behavioral patterns that define Type A and B personalities.

**Type A** Behavior pattern characteristic of a hard-driving, overambitious, aggressive, at times hostile, and overly competitive person.

**Type B** Behavior pattern characteristic of a calm, casual, relaxed, and easygoing individual.

# Behavior Modification Planning

## CHANGING A TYPE A PERSONALITY

☐ I PLAN TO    ☐ I DID IT

☐ ☐ Make a contract with yourself to slow down and take it easy. Put it in writing. Post it in a conspicuous spot, then stick to the terms you set up. Be specific. Abstracts ("I'm going to be less uptight") don't work.

☐ ☐ Work on only one or two things at a time. Wait until you change one habit before you tackle the next one.

☐ ☐ Eat more slowly and eat only when you are relaxed and sitting down.

☐ ☐ If you smoke, quit.

☐ ☐ Cut down on your caffeine intake, because it increases the tendency to become irritated and agitated.

☐ ☐ Take regular breaks throughout the day, even as brief as 5 or 10 minutes, when you totally change what you're doing. Get up, stretch, get a drink of cool water, walk around for a few minutes.

☐ ☐ Work on fighting your impatience. If you're standing in line at the grocery store, study the interesting things people have in their carts instead of getting upset.

☐ ☐ Work on controlling hostility. Keep a written log. When do you flare up? What causes it? How do you feel at the time? What preceded it? Look for patterns and figure out what sets you off. Then do something about it. Either avoid the situations that cause you hostility or practice reacting to them in different ways.

☐ ☐ Plan some activities just for the fun of it. Load a picnic basket in the car and drive to the country with a friend. After a stressful physics class, stop at a theater and see a good comedy.

☐ ☐ Choose a role model, someone you know and admire who does not have a Type A personality. Observe the person carefully, then try out some techniques the person demonstrates.

☐ ☐ Simplify your life so you can learn to relax a little bit. Figure out which activities or com-

mitments you can eliminate right now, then get rid of them.

☐ ☐ If morning is a problem time for you and you get too hurried, set your alarm clock half an hour earlier.

☐ ☐ Take time out during even the most hectic day to do something truly relaxing. Because you won't be used to it, you may have to work at it at first. Begin by listing things you'd really enjoy that would calm you. Include some things that take only a few minutes: Watch a sunset, lie out on the lawn at night and look at the stars, call an old friend and catch up on news, take a nap, sauté a pan of mushrooms and savor them slowly.

☐ ☐ If you're under a deadline, take short breaks. Stop and talk to someone for 5 minutes, take a short walk, or lie down with a cool cloth over your eyes for 10 minutes.

☐ ☐ Pay attention to what your own body clock is saying. You've probably noticed that every 90 minutes or so, you lose the ability to concentrate, get a little sleepy, and have a tendency to daydream. Instead of fighting the urge, put down your work and let your mind wander for a few minutes. Use the time to imagine and let your creativity run wild.

☐ ☐ Learn to treasure unplanned surprises: a friend dropping by unannounced, a hummingbird outside your window, a child's tightly clutched bouquet of wildflowers.

☐ ☐ Savor your relationships. Think about the people in your life. Relax with them and give yourself to them. Give up trying to control others and resist the urge to end relationships that don't always go as you'd like them to.

From W. W. K. Hoeger, L. W. Turner, and B. Q. Hafen, *Wellness: Guidelines for a Healthy Lifestyle* (4th ed.) (Belmont, CA: Thomson Wadsworth, 2007).

## Try It

If Type A describes your personality, pick three of the above strategies and apply them in your life this week. At the end of each day determine how well you have done that day and evaluate how you can improve the next day.

## Behavior Modification Planning

### TIPS TO MANAGE ANGER

**I PLAN TO**
**I DID IT**

☐ ☐ Commit to change and gain control over the behavior.

☐ ☐ Remind yourself that chronic anger leads to illness and disease and may eventually kill you.

☐ ☐ Recognize when feelings of anger are developing and ask yourself the following questions:

- Is the matter really that important?
- Is the anger justified?
- Can I change the situation without getting angry?
- Is it worth risking my health over it?
- How will I feel about the situation in a few hours?

☐ ☐ Tell yourself, "Stop, my health is worth it" every time you start to feel anger.

☐ ☐ Prepare for a positive response: Ask for an explanation or clarification of the situation, walk away and evaluate the situation, exercise, or use appropriate stress management techniques (breathing, meditation, imagery) before you become angry and hostile.

☐ ☐ Manage anger at once; do not let it build up.

☐ ☐ Never attack anyone verbally or physically.

☐ ☐ Keep a journal and ponder the situations that cause you to be angry.

☐ ☐ Seek professional help if you are unable to overcome anger by yourself: You are worth it.

### Try It

If you and others feel that anger is disrupting your health and relationships, the above management strategies are critical to help restore a sense of well-being in your life. In your Online Journal or class notebook, list all of the strategies on a separate sheet of paper, study them each morning, and then evaluate yourself every night for the next week. If you gain control over the behavior, continue with the exercise until it becomes a healthy behavior. If you still struggle, professional help is recommended. "You are worth it."

**Type C** individuals are just as highly stressed as those classified as Type A but do not seem to be at higher risk for disease than those classified as Type B. The keys to successful Type C performance seem to be commitment, confidence, and control. Type C people are highly committed to what they are doing, have a great deal of confidence in their ability to do their work, and are in constant control of their actions. In addition, they enjoy their work and

maintain themselves in top physical condition to be able to meet the mental and physical demands of their work.

Type A behavior by itself is no longer viewed as a major risk factor for coronary heart disease, but Type A individuals who commonly express anger and hostility are at higher risk. Therefore, many behavioral modification counselors now work on changing the latter behaviors to prevent disease. The questionnaire provided in Lab 10B will help you determine whether you have a hostile personality as well as your anger score.

Next time you feel like "killing" someone for what he or she has done to you, you may want to consider that your anger may be more likely to kill *you*. Anger increases heart rate and blood pressure and leads to constriction of blood vessels. Over time, these changes can cause damage to the arteries and eventually lead to a heart attack. Studies indicate that hostile people who get angry often, more

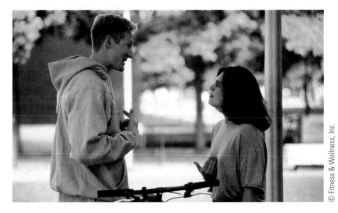

© Fitness & Wellness, Inc.

Anger and hostility can increase the risk for disease.

**Type C** Behavior pattern of individuals who are just as highly stressed as the Type A but do not seem to be at higher risk for disease than the Type B.

intensely, and for longer periods of time have up to a threefold increased risk for CHD and are seven times more likely to suffer a fatal heart attack by age 50.

Many experts also believe that emotional stress is far more likely than physical stress to trigger a heart attack. People who are impatient and readily annoyed when they have to wait for someone or something—an employee, a traffic light, a table in a restaurant—are especially vulnerable.

Research is also focusing on individuals who have anxiety, depression, and feelings of helplessness when they encounter setbacks and failures in life. People who lose control of their lives or who give up on their dreams in life, knowing that they could and should be doing better, probably are more likely to have heart attacks than hard-driving people who enjoy their work.

# Vulnerability to Stress

Researchers have identified a number of factors that can affect the way in which people handle stress. How people deal with these factors can actually increase or decrease vulnerability to stress. The questionnaire provided in Lab 10C lists these factors so you can determine your vulnerability rating. Many of the items on this questionnaire are related to health, social support, self-worth, and nurturance (sense of being needed). All of these factors are crucial to a person's physical, social, mental, and emotional well-being and are essential to their coping effectively with stressful life events. The more integrated people are in society, the less vulnerable they are to stress and illness.

Positive correlations have been found between social support and health outcomes. People can draw upon social support to weather crises. Knowing that someone else cares, that people are there to lean on, that support is out there, is valuable for survival (or growth) in times of need.

The health benefits of physical fitness have already been discussed extensively. The questionnaire in Lab 10C will help you identify specific areas in which you can make improvements to help you cope more efficiently.

As you complete Lab 10C, you will notice that many of the items describe situations and behaviors that are within your own control. To make yourself less vulnerable to stress, you will want to improve the behaviors that are the basis of this vulnerability. You should start by modifying the behaviors that are easiest to change before undertaking some of the most difficult ones.

# Time Management

According to Benjamin Franklin, "Time is the stuff life is made of." The present hurry-up style of American life is not conducive to wellness. The hassles involved in getting through a routine day often lead to stress-related illnesses. People who do not manage their time properly will quickly experience chronic stress, fatigue, despair, discouragement, and illness.

Surveys indicate that most Americans think time moves too fast for them, and more than half of those surveyed think they have to get *everything* done. The younger the respondents, the more they struggle with lack of time. Almost half wish they had more time for exercise and recreation, hobbies, and family. Healthy and successful people are good time managers, able to maintain a pace of life within their comfort zone, and attribute their success to *smart* work, not necessarily hard work.

**Five Steps to Time Management** Trying to achieve one or more goals in a limited time can create a tremendous amount of stress. Many people just don't seem to have enough hours in the day to accomplish their tasks. The greatest demands on our time, nonetheless, frequently are self-imposed: trying to do too much, too fast, too soon.

Some time killers, such as eating, sleeping, and recreation, are necessary for health and wellness, but, in excess, they'll lead to stress in life. You can follow five basic steps to make better use of your time (also see Lab 10D):

1. Find the time killers. Many people do not know how they spend each part of the day. Keep a 4- to 7-day log and record your activities at half-hour intervals as you go through your typical day, so that you will remember them all. At the end of each day, decide when you wasted time. You may be shocked by the amount of time you spent on the phone, on the Internet, sleeping (more than 8 hours per night), or watching television.

2. Set long-range and short-range goals. Setting goals requires some in-depth thinking and helps put your life and daily tasks in perspective. What do I want out of life? Where do I want to be 10 years from now? Next year? Next week? Tomorrow? You can use Lab 10D to list these goals.

3. Identify your immediate goals and prioritize them for today and this week (use Lab 10D—make as many copies as necessary). Each day sit down and determine what you need to accomplish that day and that week. Rank your "today" and "this week" tasks in four categories: (a) top-priority, (b) medium-priority, (c) low-priority, and (d) trash.

   Top-priority tasks are the most important ones. If you were to reap most of your productivity from 30 percent of your activities, which would they be? Medium-priority activities are those that must be done but can wait a day or two. Low-priority activities are those to be done only upon completing all top- and middle-priority activities. Trash activities are not worth your time (for example, cruising the hallways, channel-surfing).

4. Use a daily planner to help you organize and simplify your day. In this way you can access your priority list, appointments, notes, references, names, places, phone numbers, and addresses conveniently from your coat pocket or purse. Many individuals think that planning daily and weekly activities is a waste of time. A few

## Behavior Modification Planning

### COMMON TIME KILLERS

Have you minimized the role of these time killers in your life?

| I PLAN TO | I DID IT | |
|---|---|---|
| ☐ | ☐ | Watching television |
| ☐ | ☐ | Listening to radio/music |
| ☐ | ☐ | Sleeping |
| ☐ | ☐ | Eating |
| ☐ | ☐ | Daydreaming |
| ☐ | ☐ | Shopping |
| ☐ | ☐ | Socializing/parties |
| ☐ | ☐ | Recreation |
| ☐ | ☐ | Talking on the telephone |
| ☐ | ☐ | Worrying |
| ☐ | ☐ | Procrastinating |
| ☐ | ☐ | Drop-in visitors |
| ☐ | ☐ | Confusion (unclear goals) |
| ☐ | ☐ | Indecision (what to do next) |
| ☐ | ☐ | Interruptions |
| ☐ | ☐ | Perfectionism (every detail must be done) |

### Try It

Using Lab 10D, find the time killers in your life and make the necessary changes as required.

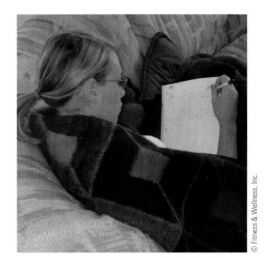

Planning and prioritizing activities will simplify your days.

minutes to schedule your time each day, however, may pay off in hours saved.

As you plan your day, be realistic and find your comfort zone. Determine what is the best way to organize your day. Which is the most productive time for work, study, errands? Are you a morning person, or are you getting most of your work done when people are quitting for the day? Pick your best hours for top-priority activities. Be sure to schedule enough time for exercise and relaxation. Recreation is not necessarily wasted time. You need to take care of your physical and emotional well-being. Otherwise your life will be seriously imbalanced.

5. Conduct nightly audits. Take 10 minutes each night to figure out how well you accomplished your goals that day. Successful time managers evaluate themselves daily. This simple task will help you see the entire picture. Cross off the goals you accomplished, and carry over to the next day those you did not get done. You also may realize that some goals can be moved down to low-priority or be trashed.

**Time management Skills** In addition to the five major steps, the following can help you make better use of your time:

- Delegate. If possible, delegate activities that someone else can do for you. Having another person type your paper while you prepare for an exam might be well worth the expense and your time.

- Say no. Learn to say no to activities that keep you from getting your top priorities done. You can do only so much in a single day. Nobody has enough time to do everything he or she would like to get done. Don't overload either. Many people are afraid to say no because they feel guilty if they do. Think ahead, and think of the consequences. Are you doing it to please others? What will it do to your well-being? Can you handle one more task? At some point you have to balance your activities and look at life and time realistically.

- Protect against boredom. Doing nothing can be a source of stress. People need to feel that they are contributing and that they are productive members of society. It is also good for self-esteem and self-worth. Set realistic goals and work toward them each day.

- Plan ahead for disruptions. Even a careful plan of action can be disrupted. An unexpected phone call or visitor can ruin your schedule. Planning your response ahead will help you deal with these saboteurs.

- Get it done. Select only one task at a time, concentrate on it, and see it through. Many people do a little here, a little there, then do something else. In the end, nothing gets done. But an exception to working on just one task at a time is when you are doing a difficult task. Rather than "killing yourself," interchange with another activity that is not as hard.

- Eliminate distractions. If you have trouble adhering to a set plan, remove distractions and trash activities from your eyesight. Television, radio, magazines, open doors, or studying in a park might distract you and become time killers.
- Set aside "overtimes." Regularly schedule time you did not think you would need as overtime to complete unfinished projects. Most people underschedule rather than overschedule time. The result is usually late-night burnout! If you schedule overtimes and get your tasks done, enjoy some leisure time, get ahead on another project, or work on some of your trash activities.
- Plan time for you. Set aside special time for yourself daily. Life is not meant to be all work. Use your time to walk, read, or listen to your favorite music.
- Reward yourself. As with any other healthy behavior, positive change or a job well done deserves a reward. We often overlook the value of rewards, even if they are self-given. People practice behaviors that are rewarded and discontinue those that are not.

One more activity that you should perform weekly is to go through the list of strategies in Lab 10D to determine if you are becoming a good time manager. Provide a yes or no answer to each statement. If you are able to answer yes to most questions, congratulations. You are becoming a good time manager.

# Coping with Stress

The ways in which people perceive and cope with stress seem to be more important in the development of disease than the amount and type of stress itself. If individuals perceive stress as a definite problem in their lives or if it interferes with their optimal level of health and performance, they can call upon several excellent stress management techniques that can help them cope more effectively.

First, of course, the person must recognize the presence of a problem. Many people either do not want to believe they are under too much stress or they fail to recognize some of the typical symptoms of distress. Noting some of the stress-related symptoms (see "Common Symptoms of Stress") will help a person respond more objectively and initiate an adequate coping response.

When people have stress-related symptoms, they should first try to identify and remove the stressor or stress-causing agent. This is not as simple as it may seem, because in some situations, eliminating the stressor is not possible, or a person may not even know the exact causing agent. If the cause is unknown, keeping a log of the time and days when the symptoms occur, as well as the events preceding and following the onset of symptoms, may be helpful.

For instance, a couple noted that every afternoon around 6 o'clock, the wife became nauseated and had abdominal pain. After seeking professional help, both spouses were instructed to keep a log of daily events. It soon became clear that the symptoms did not occur on weekends but always started just before the husband came home from work during the week. Following some personal interviews with the couple, it was determined that the wife felt a lack of attention from her husband and responded subconsciously by becoming ill to the point at which she

## Behavior Modification Planning

### COMMON SYMPTOMS OF STRESS
Check those symptoms you experience regularly.
- Headaches
- Muscular aches (mainly in neck, shoulders, and back)
- Grinding teeth
- Nervous tic, finger tapping, toe tapping
- Increased sweating
- Increase in or loss of appetite
- Insomnia
- Nightmares
- Fatigue
- Dry mouth
- Stuttering
- High blood pressure
- Tightness or pain in the chest
- Impotence
- Hives
- Dizziness
- Depression
- Irritation
- Anger
- Hostility
- Fear, panic, anxiety
- Stomach pain, flutters
- Nausea
- Cold, clammy hands
- Poor concentration
- Pacing
- Restlessness
- Rapid heart rate
- Low-grade infection
- Loss of sex drive
- Rash or acne

### Try It
If you regularly experience some of the above symptoms, use your Online Journal or class notebook to keep a log of when these symptoms occur and under what circumstances. You may find out that a pattern emerges when experiencing distress in life.

required personal care and affection from her husband. Once the stressor was identified, appropriate behavior changes were initiated to correct the situation.

In many instances, the stressor cannot be removed. Examples of such situations are the death of a close family member, the first year on the job, an intolerable boss, or a change in work responsibility. Nevertheless, stress can be managed through relaxation techniques.

The body responds to stress by activating the **fight-or-flight** mechanism, which prepares a person to take action by stimulating the vital defense systems. This stimulation originates in the hypothalamus and the pituitary gland in the brain. The hypothalamus activates the sympathetic nervous system, and the pituitary activates the release of catecholamines (hormones) from the adrenal glands.

These hormonal changes increase heart rate, blood pressure, blood flow to active muscles and the brain, glucose levels, oxygen consumption, and strength—all necessary for the body to fight or flee. For the body to relax, one of these actions must take place. However, if the person is unable to take action, the muscles tense up and tighten (see Figure 10.4). This increased tension and tightening can be dissipated effectively through some coping techniques.

**Physical Activity** The benefits of physical activity in reducing the physiologic and psychological responses to stress are well established.[4] Exercise is one of the simplest tools to control stress. The value of exercise in reducing stress is related to several factors, the main one being a decrease in muscular tension. For example, a person can be distressed because he or she has had a miserable 8 hours of work with an intolerable boss. To make matters worse, it is late and, on the way home, the car in front is going much slower than the speed limit. The fight-or-flight mechanism—already activated during the stressful day—begins again: catecholamines rise, heart rate and blood pressure shoot up, breathing quickens and deepens, muscles tense up, and all systems say "go." No action can be initiated or stress dissipated, though, because the person cannot just hit the boss or the car in front.

A real remedy would be to take action by "hitting" the swimming pool, the tennis ball, the weights, or the jogging trail. Engaging in physical activity reduces the muscular tension and metabolizes the increased catecholamines (which were triggered by the fight-or-flight mechanism and brought about the physiologic changes). Although exercise does not solve problems at work or take care of slow drivers, it certainly can help a person cope with stress and can prevent stress from becoming a chronic problem.

The early evening hours are a popular time to exercise for a lot of highly stressed executives. On the way home from work, they stop at the health club or the fitness center. Exercising at this time helps them to dissipate the stress accumulated during the day. Not only does evening exercise help to get rid of the stress, but it also provides an opportunity to enjoy the evening more. At home, the family will appreciate Dad or Mom coming home more relaxed, leaving work problems behind, and being able to dedicate all energy to family activities.

Many people can relate to exercise as a means of managing stress by remembering how good they felt the last time they concluded a strenuous exercise session after a long, difficult day at the office. A fatigued muscle is a relaxed muscle. For this reason, many people have said that the best part of exercise is the shower afterward.

Research also has shown that physical exercise requiring continuous and rhythmic muscular activity, such as aerobic exercise, stimulates alpha-wave activity in the brain. These are the same wave patterns seen commonly during meditation and relaxation.

Further, during vigorous aerobic exercise lasting 30 minutes or longer, morphine-like substances referred to as **endorphins** are thought to be released from the

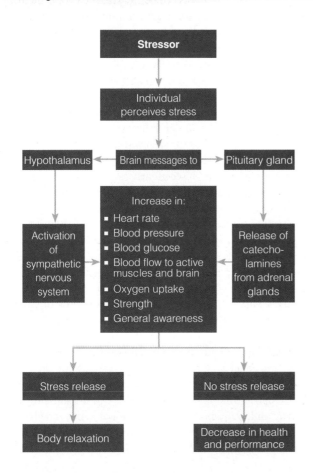

**FIGURE 10.4** Physiologic response to stress: fight-or-flight mechanism.

```
                    Stressor
                       │
                       ▼
                  Individual
                perceives stress
                       │
                       ▼
Hypothalamus ◄──► Brain messages to ──► Pituitary gland
     │                                        │
     ▼                                        ▼
Activation     Increase in:              Release of
of             ■ Heart rate              catecho-
sympathetic    ■ Blood pressure          lamines
nervous        ■ Blood glucose           from adrenal
system         ■ Blood flow to active    glands
               muscles and brain
               ■ Oxygen uptake
               ■ Strength
               ■ General awareness
                       │
          ┌────────────┴────────────┐
          ▼                         ▼
    Stress release            No stress release
          │                         │
          ▼                         ▼
    Body relaxation          Decrease in health
                             and performance
```

**Fight or flight** Physiologic response of the body to stress that prepares the individual to take action by stimulating the body's vital defense systems.

**Endorphins** Morphine-like substances released from the pituitary gland in the brain during prolonged aerobic exercise, thought to induce feelings of euphoria and natural well-being.

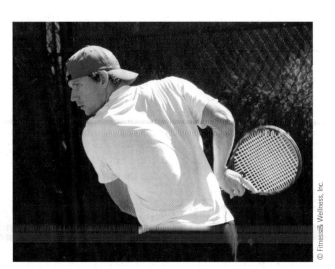

Physical activity: An excellent tool to control stress.

pituitary gland in the brain. These substances not only act as painkillers but also seem to induce the soothing, calming effect often associated with aerobic exercise.

Another way by which exercise helps lower stress is to deliberately divert stress to various body systems. Dr. Hans Selye explains in his book *Stress Without Distress* that when one specific task becomes difficult, a change in activity can be as good or better than rest itself.[5] For example, if a person is having trouble with a task and does not seem to be getting anywhere, jogging or swimming for a while is better than sitting around and getting frustrated. In this way the mental strain is diverted to the working muscles, and one system helps the other to relax.

Other psychologists indicate that when muscular tension is removed from the emotional strain, the emotional strain disappears. In many cases, the change of activity suddenly clears the mind and helps put the pieces together.

Researchers have found that physical exercise gives people a psychological boost because exercise does all of the following:

- Lessens feelings of anxiety, depression, frustration, aggression, anger, and hostility
- Alleviates insomnia
- Provides an opportunity to meet social needs and develop new friendships
- Allows the person to share common interests and problems
- Develops discipline

- Provides the opportunity to do something enjoyable and constructive that will lead to better health and total well-being

Beyond the short-term benefits of exercise in lessening stress, a regular aerobic exercise program actually strengthens the cardiovascular system itself. Because the cardiovascular system seems to be affected seriously by stress, a stronger system should be able to cope more effectively. For instance, good cardiorespiratory endurance has been shown to lower resting heart rate and blood pressure. Because both heart rate and blood pressure rise in stressful situations, initiating the stress response at a lower baseline will counteract some of the negative effects of stress. Cardiorespiratory-fit individuals can cope more effectively and are less affected by the stresses of daily living.

# Relaxation Techniques

Although benefits are reaped immediately after engaging in any of the several relaxation techniques, several months of regular practice may be necessary for total mastery. The relaxation exercises that follow should not be considered cure-alls. If these exercises do not prove to be effective, more specialized textbooks and professional help are called for. (Some symptoms may not be caused by stress but may be related to a medical disorder.)

**Biofeedback** Clinical application of **biofeedback** has been used for many years to treat various medical disorders. Besides its successful application in managing stress, it is commonly used to treat medical disorders such as essential hypertension, asthma, heart rhythm and rate disturbances, cardiac neurosis, eczematous dermatitis, fecal incontinence, insomnia, and stuttering. Biofeedback as a treatment modality has been defined as a technique in which a person learns to influence physiologic responses that are not typically under voluntary control or that normally are regulated but whose regulation has broken down as a result of injury, trauma, or illness.

In simpler terms, biofeedback is the interaction with the interior self. This interaction enables a person to learn the relationship between the mind and the biological response. The person actually can "feel" how thought processes influence biological responses (such as heart rate, blood pressure, body temperature, and muscle tension) and how biological responses influence the thought process.

As an illustration of this interaction, consider the association between a strange noise in the middle of a dark, quiet night and the heart rate response. At first the heart rate shoots up because of the stress the unknown noise induces. The individual may even feel the heart palpitating in the chest and, while still uncertain about the noise, may attempt not to panic to prevent an even faster heart rate. Upon realizing that all is well, the person can take control and influence the heart rate to come down. The mind, now calm, is able to exert almost complete control over the biological response.

**Biofeedback** A stress management technique in which a person learns to influence physiologic responses that are not typically under voluntary control or responses that typically are regulated but for which regulation has broken down as a result of injury, trauma, or illness.

**Progressive muscle relaxation** A stress management technique that involves sequential contraction and relaxation of muscle groups throughout the body.

**FIGURE 10.5** Biofeedback mechanism.

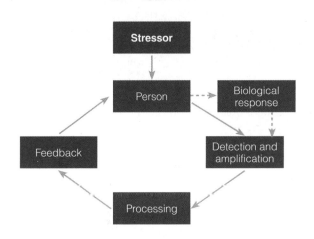

Complex electronic instruments are required to conduct biofeedback. The process itself entails a three-stage, closed-loop feedback system:

1. A biological response to a stressor is detected and amplified.
2. The response is processed.
3. Results of the response are fed back to the individual immediately.

The person uses this new input and attempts to change the physiologic response voluntarily—this attempt, in turn, is detected, amplified, and processed. The results then are fed back to the person. The process continues with the intent of teaching the person to reliably influence the physiologic response for the better (see Figure 10.5). The most common methods used to measure physiologic responses are monitoring of the heart rate, finger temperature, and blood pressure; electromyograms; and electroencephalograms. The goal of biofeedback training is to transfer the experiences learned in the laboratory to everyday living.

Although biofeedback has significant applications in treating various medical disorders, including stress, it requires adequately trained personnel and, in many cases, costly equipment. Therefore, several alternative methods that yield similar results are frequently substituted for biofeedback. For example, research has shown that exercise and progressive muscle relaxation, used successfully in stress management, seem to be just as effective as biofeedback in treating essential hypertension.

## Progressive Muscle Relaxation
**Progressive muscle relaxation,** developed by Dr. Edmund Jacobson in the 1930s, enables individuals to relearn the sensation of deep relaxation. The technique involves progressively contracting and relaxing muscle groups throughout the body. Because chronic stress leads to high levels of muscular tension, acute awareness of how progressively tightening and relaxing the muscles feels can release the tension in the muscles and teach the body to relax at will.

## Behavior Modification Planning
### CHARACTERISTICS OF GOOD STRESS MANAGERS
Do you have the habits and characteristics of someone who manages stress well?

I PLAN TO / I DID IT

Good stress managers
- are physically active, eat a healthy diet, and get adequate rest every day.
- believe they have control over events in their life (have an internal locus of control, see page 47).
- understand their own feelings and accept their limitations.
- recognize, anticipate, monitor, and regulate stressors within their capabilities.
- control emotional and physical responses when distressed.
- use appropriate stress management techniques when confronted with stressors.
- recognize warning signs and symptoms of excessive stress.
- schedule daily time to unwind, relax, and evaluate the day's activities.
- control stress when called upon to perform.
- enjoy life despite occasional disappointments and frustrations.
- look success and failure squarely in the face and keep moving along a predetermined course.
- move ahead with optimism and energy and do not spend time and talent worrying about failure.
- learn from previous mistakes and use them as building blocks to prevent similar setbacks in the future.
- give of themselves freely to others.
- have a deep meaning in life.

### Try It
Change for many people is threatening, but often required. Pick three of the above strategies and apply them in your life. After several days, determine the usefulness of these strategies to your physical, mental, social, and emotional well-being.

Feeling the tension during the exercises also helps the person to be more alert to signs of distress, because this tension is similar to that experienced in stressful situations. In everyday life, these feelings then can cue the person to do relaxation exercises.

Relaxation exercises should be done in a quiet, warm, well-ventilated room. The recommended exercises and the duration of the routine vary from one person to the next. Most important is that the individual pay attention to the sensation he or she feels each time the muscles are tensed and relaxed.

The exercises should encompass all muscle groups of the body. Following is an example of a sequence of progressive muscle relaxation exercises. The instructions for these exercises can be read to the person, memorized, or tape-recorded. At least 20 minutes should be set aside to complete the entire sequence. Doing the exercises any faster will defeat their purpose. Ideally, the sequence should be done twice a day.

The individual performing the exercises stretches out comfortably on the floor, face up, with a pillow under the knees, and assumes a passive attitude, allowing the body to relax as much as possible. Each muscle group is to be contracted in sequence, taking care to avoid any strain. Muscles should be tightened to only about 70 percent of the total possible tension to avoid cramping or some type of injury to the muscle itself.

To produce the relaxation effects, the person must pay attention to the sensation of tensing up and relaxing. The person holds each contraction about 5 seconds and then allows the muscles to go totally limp. The person should take enough time to contract and relax each muscle group before going on to the next. An example of a complete progressive muscle relaxation sequence is as follows:

1. Point your feet, curling the toes downward. Study the tension in the arches and the top of the feet. Hold, continue to note the tension, then relax. Repeat once.

2. Flex the feet upward toward the face and note the tension in your feet and calves. Hold and relax. Repeat once.

3. Push your heels down against the floor as if burying them in the sand. Hold and note the tension at the back of the thigh. Relax. Repeat once.

4. Contract the right thigh by straightening the leg, gently raising the leg off the floor. Hold and study the tension. Relax. Repeat with the left leg. Hold and relax. Repeat each leg.

5. Tense the buttocks by raising your hips ever so slightly off the floor. Hold and note the tension. Relax. Repeat once.

6. Contract the abdominal muscles. Hold them tight and note the tension. Relax. Repeat once.

7. Suck in your stomach. Try to make it reach your spine. Flatten your lower back to the floor. Hold and feel the tension in the stomach and lower back. Relax. Repeat once.

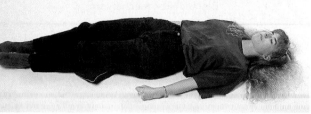

Practicing progressive muscle relaxation on a regular basis helps reduce stress.

8. Take a deep breath and hold it, then exhale. Repeat. Note your breathing becoming slower and more relaxed.

9. Place your arms at the sides of your body and clench both fists. Hold, study the tension, and relax. Repeat.

10. Flex the elbow by bringing both hands to the shoulders. Hold tight and study the tension in the biceps. Relax. Repeat.

11. Place your arms flat on the floor, palms up, and push the forearms hard against the floor. Note the tension on the triceps. Hold, and relax. Repeat.

12. Shrug your shoulders, raising them as high as possible. Hold and note the tension. Relax. Repeat.

13. Gently push your head backward. Note the tension in the back of the neck. Hold, relax. Repeat.

14. Gently bring the head against the chest, push forward, hold, and note the tension in the neck. Relax. Repeat.

15. Press your tongue toward the roof of your mouth. Hold, study the tension, and relax. Repeat.

16. Press your teeth together. Hold, and study the tension. Relax. Repeat.

17. Close your eyes tightly. Hold them closed and note the tension. Relax, leaving your eyes closed. Do this one more time.

18. Wrinkle your forehead and note the tension. Hold and relax. Repeat.

When time is a factor during the daily routine and an individual is not able to go through the entire sequence, he or she may do only the exercises specific to the area that feels most tense. Performing a partial sequence is better than not doing the exercises at all. Completing the entire sequence, of course, yields the best results.

## Breathing Techniques for Relaxation

**Breathing exercises** also can be an antidote to stress. These exercises have been used for centuries in the Orient and India to improve mental, physical, and emotional stamina. In breathing exercises, the person concentrates on "breathing away" the tension and inhaling a large amount of air with each breath. Breathing exercises can be learned in only a few minutes and require considerably less time than the progressive muscle relaxation exercises.

As with any other relaxation technique, these exercises should be done in a quiet, pleasant, well-ventilated room. Any of the three examples of breathing exercises presented here will help relieve tension induced by stress.

1. *Deep breathing.* Lie with your back flat against the floor and place a pillow under your knees. Feet are slightly separated, with toes pointing outward. (The exercise also may be done while sitting up in a chair or standing straight up.) Place one hand on your abdomen and the other hand on your chest.

   Slowly breathe in and out so the hand on your abdomen rises when you inhale and falls as you exhale. The hand on the chest should not move much at all. Repeat the exercise about ten times. Next, scan your body for tension and compare your present tension with the tension you felt at the beginning of the exercise. Repeat the entire process once or twice.

2. *Sighing.* Using the abdominal breathing technique, breathe in through your nose to a specific count (e.g., 4, 5, 6). Now exhale through pursed lips to double the intake count (e.g., 8, 10, 12). Repeat the exercise eight to ten times whenever you feel tense.

3. *Complete natural breathing.* Sit in an upright position or stand straight up. Breathing through your nose, gradually fill your lungs from the bottom up. Hold your breath for several seconds. Now exhale slowly by allowing your chest and abdomen to relax completely. Repeat the exercise eight to ten times.

## Critical Thinking

List the three most common stressors that you face as a college student. What techniques have you used to manage these situations, and in what way have they helped you cope?

## Visual Imagery

Visual or mental **imagery** has been used as a healing technique for centuries in various cultures around the world. In Western medicine, the practice of imagery is relatively new and not widely accepted among health care professionals.

Research is now being done to study the effects of imagery on the treatment of conditions such as cancer, hypertension, asthma, chronic pain, and obesity. Imagery induces a state of relaxation that rids the body of the stress that leads to illness. It improves circulation and increases the delivery of healing antibodies and white blood cells to the site of illness.[6] Imagery also helps with self-confidence, to regain control and power over the body, and to lower feelings of hopelessness, fear, and depression.

Visual imagery involves the creation of relaxing visual images and scenes in times of stress to elicit body and

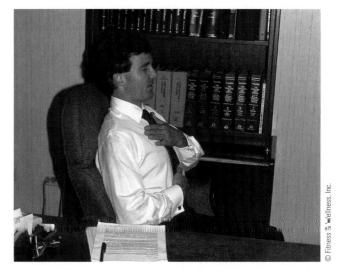

Breathing exercises help dissipate stress.

mind relaxation. Imagery works by offsetting the stressor with the visualization of relaxing scenes such as a sunny beach, a beautiful meadow, a quiet mountaintop, or some other peaceful setting. If you are ill, you can also visualize your white blood cells attacking an infection or a tumor. Imagery can also be used in conjunction with breathing exercises, meditation, and yoga.

As with other stress management techniques, imagery should be performed in a quiet and comfortable environment. You can either sit or lie down for the exercise. If you lie down, use a soft surface and place a pillow under your knees. Be sure that your clothes are loose and that you are as comfortable as you can be.

To start the exercise, close your eyes and take a few breaths using one of the breathing techniques previously described. You then can proceed to visualize one of your favorite scenes in nature. Place yourself into the scene and visualize yourself moving about and experiencing nature to its fullest. Enjoy the people, the animals, the colors, the sounds, the smells, and even the temperature in your scene. After 10 to 20 minutes of visualization, open your eyes and compare the tension in your body and mind at this point with how you felt prior to the exercise. You can repeat this exercise as often as you deem necessary when you are feeling tension or stress.

You may not always be able to find a quiet/comfortable setting in which to sit or lie down for 10 to 20 minutes. If you think imagery works for you, however, you can perform this technique while standing or sitting in an active

**Breathing exercises** A stress management technique wherein the individual concentrates on "breathing away" the tension and inhaling fresh air to the entire body.

**Imagery** Mental visualization of relaxing images and scenes to induce body relaxation in times of stress or as an aid in the treatment of certain medical conditions such as cancer, hypertension, asthma, chronic pain, and obesity.

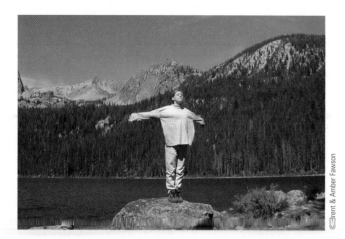

©Brent & Amber Fawson

Visual imagery of beautiful and relaxing scenes helps attenuate the stress response.

setting. If you are able, close your eyes and disregard your surroundings for a short moment and visualize one of your favorite scenes. Once you feel that you have regained some control over the stressor, open your eyes and continue with your assigned tasks.

## Autogenic Training

**Autogenic training** is a form of self-suggestion in which people place themselves in an autohypnotic state by repeating and concentrating on feelings of heaviness and warmth in the extremities. This technique was developed by Johannes Schultz, a German psychiatrist who noted that hypnotized individuals developed sensations of warmth and heaviness in the limbs and torso. The sensation of warmth is caused by dilation of blood vessels, which increases blood flow to the limbs. Muscular relaxation produces the feeling of heaviness.

In this technique the person lies down or sits in a comfortable position, eyes closed, concentrates progressively on six fundamental stages, and says (or thinks) the following:

1. Heaviness

   My right (left) arm is heavy.

   Both arms are heavy.

   My right (left) leg is heavy.

   Both legs are heavy.

   My arms and legs are heavy.

2. Warmth

   My right (left) arm is warm.

   Both arms are warm.

   My right (left) leg is warm.

   Both legs are warm.

   My arms and legs are warm.

3. Heart

   My heartbeat is calm and regular. (Repeat four or five times.)

4. Respiration

   My body breathes itself. (Repeat four or five times.)

5. Abdomen

   My abdomen is warm. (Repeat four or five times.)

6. Forehead

   My forehead is cool. (Repeat four or five times.)

The autogenic training technique is more difficult to master than any of those mentioned previously. The person should not move too fast through the entire exercise, because this actually may interfere with learning and relaxation. Each stage must be mastered before proceeding to the next.

## Meditation

**Meditation** is a mental exercise that can bring about psychological and physical benefits. Regular meditation has been shown to decrease blood pressure, stress, anger, anxiety, fear, negative feelings, and chronic pain and to increase activity in the brain's left frontal region—an area associated with positive emotions.[7] The objective of meditation is to gain control over one's attention by clearing the mind and blocking out the stressor(s) responsible for the higher tension.

This technique can be learned rather quickly, but first-time users often drop out before reaping benefits because they feel intimidated, confused, bored, or frustrated. In such cases, a group setting is best to get started. Many colleges, community programs, health clubs, and hospitals offer classes.

Initially the person who is learning to meditate should choose a room that is comfortable, quiet, and free of all disturbances (including telephones). After learning the technique, the person will be able to meditate just about anywhere. A time block of approximately 10 to 15 minutes is adequate to start, but as you become more comfortable with meditation you can lengthen the time to 30 minutes or longer. To use meditation effectively, meditate daily, as just once or twice per week may not provide noticeable benefits.

Of the several forms of meditation, the following routine is recommended to get started.

1. Sit in a chair in an upright position with the hands resting either in your lap or on the arms of the chair. Close your eyes and focus on your breathing. Allow your body to relax as much as possible. Do not try to consciously relax, because trying means work. Rather, assume a passive attitude and concentrate on your breathing.

2. Allow the body to breathe regularly, at its own rhythm, and repeat in your mind the word "one" every time you inhale, and the word "two" every time you exhale. Paying attention to these two words keeps distressing thoughts from entering into your mind.

3. Continue to breathe in this way about 15 minutes. Because the objective of meditation is to bring about a hypometabolic state leading to body relaxation, do not use an alarm clock to remind you that the 15 minutes have expired. The alarm will only trigger your stress response again, defeating the purpose of the exercise.

## Stress Coping Strategies

- Balance personal, work, and family needs and obligations.
- Have a sense of purpose in life.
- Get adequate sleep.
- Eat well-balanced meals.
- Be physically active every day.
- Do not worry about things that you cannot control (the weather, for example).
- Actively strive to resolve conflicts with other people.
- Prepare for stressful events the best possible way (public speaking, job interviews, exams).
- Limit or abstain from alcohol intake.
- Do not use tobacco in any form.
- View change as positive and not as a threat.
- Obtain social support from family members and friends.
- Use stress management programs and counselors available through work and school programs.
- Seek help from church leaders.
- Engage in nonstressful activities (reading, sports, hobbies, and social events).
- Practice stress management techniques.

Opening your eyes once in a while to keep track of the time is fine, but do not rush or anticipate the end of the session. This time has been set aside for meditation, and you need to relax, take your time, and enjoy the exercise.

Yoga **Yoga** is an excellent stress-coping technique. It is a school of thought in the Hindu religion that seeks to help the individual attain a higher level of spirituality and peace of mind. Although its philosophical roots can be considered spiritual, yoga is based on principles of self-care.

Practitioners of yoga adhere to a specific code of ethics and a system of mental and physical exercises that promote control of the mind and the body. In Western countries, many people are familiar mainly with the exercise portion of yoga. This system of exercises (postures, or *asanas*) can be used as a relaxation technique for stress management. The exercises include a combination of postures, diaphragmatic breathing, muscle relaxation, and meditation that help buffer the biological effects of stress.

Western interest in yoga exercises developed gradually over the last century, particularly since the 1970s. The practice of yoga exercises helps align the musculoskeletal system and increases muscular flexibility, muscular strength and endurance, and balance.[8] People pursue yoga exercises to help dispel stress by raising self-esteem, clearing the mind, slowing respiration, promoting neuro-muscular relaxation, and increasing body awareness. In addition, the exercises help relieve back pain and control involuntary body functions like heart rate, blood pressure, oxygen consumption, and metabolic rate. Yoga also is used in many hospital-based programs for cardiac patients to help manage stress and decrease blood pressure.

In addition, yoga exercises have been used to help treat chemical dependency and insomnia and to prevent injury. Research on patients with coronary heart disease who practiced yoga (among other lifestyle changes) has shown that it slows down or even reverses atherosclerosis. These patients were compared with others who did not use yoga as one of the lifestyle changes.[9]

Of the many different styles of yoga, more than 60 are presently taught in the United States. Classes vary according to their emphasis. Some styles of yoga are athletic, others are passive in nature.

The most popular variety of yoga in the Western world is **hatha yoga**, which incorporates a series of static-stretching postures performed in specific sequences (*asanas*) that help induce the relaxation response. The postures are held for several seconds while participants concentrate on breathing patterns, meditation, and body awareness.

Most yoga classes now are variations of hatha yoga, from which many of the typical stretches used in flexibility exercises today have been adapted. Examples include:

1. *Integral yoga* and *viny yoga,* which focus on gentle/static stretches
2. *Iyengar yoga,* which promotes muscular strength and endurance
3. *Yogalates,* incorporating Pilates exercises to increase muscular strength
4. *Power yoga* or *yogarobics,* a high-energy form that links many postures together in a dance-like routine to promote cardiorespiratory fitness.

---

**Autogenic training** A stress management technique using a form of self-suggestion, wherein an individual is able to place himself or herself in an autohypnotic state by repeating and concentrating on feelings of heaviness and warmth in the extremities.

**Meditation** A stress management technique used to gain control over one's attention by clearing the mind and blocking out the stressor(s) responsible for the increased tension.

**Yoga** A school of thought in the Hindu religion that seeks to help the individual attain a higher level of spirituality and peace of mind.

**Hatha yoga** A form of yoga that incorporates specific sequences of static-stretching postures to help induce the relaxation response.

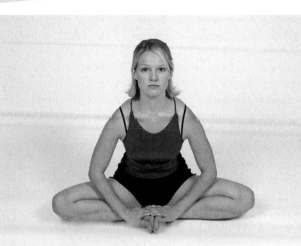

Yoga exercises help induce the relaxation response.

© Fitness & Wellness, Inc.

As with flexibility exercises, the stretches in hatha yoga should not be performed to the point of discomfort. Instructors should not push participants beyond their physical limitations. Similar to other stress management techniques, yoga exercises are best performed in a quiet place for 15 to 60 minutes per session. Many yoga participants like to perform the exercises daily.

To appreciate yoga exercises, a person has to experience them. The discussion here serves only as an introduction. Although yoga exercises can be practiced with the instruction of a book or video, most participants take classes. Many of the postures are difficult and complex, and few individuals can master the entire sequence in the first few weeks.

Individuals who are interested in yoga exercises should initially pursue them under qualified instruction. Many universities offer yoga courses, and you also can check the phone book for a listing of yoga instructors or classes. Yoga courses are offered at many health clubs and recreation centers. Because instructors and yoga styles vary, you may want to sit in on a class before enrolling. The most important thing is to look for an instructor whose views on wellness parallel your own. Instructors are not subject to any national certification standards. If you are new to yoga, you are encouraged to compare a couple of instructors before you select a class.

## Which Technique Is Best?

Each person reacts to stress differently. Therefore, the best coping strategy depends mostly on the individual. Which technique is used does not really matter, as long as it works. An individual may want to experiment with several or all of them to find out which works best. A combination of two or more is best for many people.

All of the coping strategies discussed here help to block out stressors and promote mental and physical relaxation by diverting the attention to a different, nonthreatening action. Some of the techniques are easier to learn and may take less time per session. As a part of your class experience, you may participate in a stress management session (see Lab 10E). Regardless of which technique you select, the time spent doing stress management exercises (several times a day, as needed) is well worth the effort when stress becomes a significant problem in life.

Keep in mind that most individuals need to learn to relax and take time for themselves. Stress is not what makes people ill; it's the way they react to the stress-causing agent. Individuals who learn to be diligent and start taking control of themselves find that they can enjoy a better, happier, and healthier life.

## ASSESS YOUR BEHAVIOR

Log on to http://www.cengage.com/sso/ and take the stress inventory to identify the main stressors in your life and to create a plan for dealing more effectively with those stressors.

1. Are you able to channel your emotions and feelings to exert a positive effect on your mind, health, and wellness?

2. Do you use time management strategies on a regular basis?

3. Do you use stress management techniques and do they allow you to be in control over the daily stresses of life?

# ASSESS YOUR KNOWLEDGE

Log on to http://www.cengage.com/sso/ to assess your understanding of this chapter's topics by taking the Student Practice Test and exploring the modules recommended in your Personalized Study Plan.

1. Positive stress is also referred to as
   a. eustress.
   b. posstress.
   c. functional stress.
   d. distress.
   e. physiostress.

2. Which of the following is *not* a stage of the general adaptation syndrome?
   a. Alarm reaction
   b. Resistance
   c. Compliance
   d. Exhaustion/recovery
   e. All are stages of the general adaptation syndrome.

3. The behavior pattern of highly stressed individuals who do not seem to be at higher risk for disease is known as Type
   a. A.
   b. B.
   c. C.
   d. X.
   e. Z.

4. Effective time managers
   a. delegate.
   b. learn to say "no."
   c. protect themselves from boredom.
   d. set aside "overtimes."
   e. do all of the above.

5. Hormonal changes that occur during a stress response
   a. decrease heart rate.
   b. sap the body's strength.
   c. diminish blood flow to the muscles.
   d. induce relaxation.
   e. increase blood pressure.

6. Exercise decreases stress levels by
   a. deliberately diverting stress to various body systems.
   b. metabolizing excess catecholamines.
   c. diminishing muscular tension.
   d. stimulating alpha-wave activity in the brain.
   e. doing all of the above.

7. Biofeedback is
   a. the interaction with the interior self.
   b. the biological response to stress.
   c. the nonspecific response to a stress-causing agent.
   d. used to identify biological factors that cause stress.
   e. most readily achieved while in a state of self-hypnosis.

8. The technique in which a person breathes in through the nose to a specific count and then exhales through pursed lips to double the intake count is known as
   a. sighing.
   b. deep breathing.
   c. meditation.
   d. autonomic ventilation.
   e. release management.

9. During autogenic training, a person
   a. contracts each muscle to about 70 percent of capacity.
   b. concentrates on feelings of warmth and heaviness.
   c. visualizes relaxing scenes to induce body relaxation.
   d. learns to reliably influence physiologic responses.
   e. notes the positive and negative impact of frequent stressors on various body systems.

10. Yoga exercises have been successfully used to
    a. stimulate ventilation.
    b. increase metabolism during stress.
    c. slow down atherosclerosis.
    d. decrease body awareness.
    e. accomplish all of the above.

Correct answers can be found at the end of the book.

# MEDIA MENU

You can find the links below at the book companion site: www.cengage.com/health/hoeger/plfw10e

- Identify the stressors in your life and develop a change plan to deal more effectively with them.

- Check how well you understand the chapter's concepts.

## Internet Connections

- Stress: Who Has Time for It? This is a visually appealing site that describes the symptoms of stress and how to daily manage it. *http://www.familydoctor.org/handouts/278.html*

- Workplace Stress. This site, sponsored by the American Institute of Stress, provides research-based, practical information on occupational stress and its effect on health. *http://www.stress.org/job.htm*

- Mind Tools. This site covers a variety of topics on stress management, including recognizing stress, exercise, time management, self-hypnosis, meditation, breathing exercises, coping mechanisms, and more. The site also features a free comprehensive personal self-assessment with questions pertaining to work and home stressors, physical and behavioral signs and symptoms, and personal coping skills and resources. *http://www.mindtools.com/smpage.html*

# NOTES

1. H. Selye, *Stress Without Distress* (New York: Signet, 1974).

2. E. Gullete, et al., "Effects of Mental Stress on Myocardial Ischemia during Daily Life," *Journal of the American Medical Association* 277 (1997): 1521–1525; C. A. Lengacher, et al., "Psycho-neuroimmunology and Immune System Link for Stress, Depression, Health Behaviors, and Breast Cancer," *Alternative Health Practitioner* 4 (1998): 95–108.

3. R. J. Kriegel and M. H. Kriegel, *The C Zone: Peak Performance Under Stress* (Garden City, NY: Anchor Press/Doubleday, 1985).

4. See note 2, Lengacher; J. Moses, et al., "The Effects of Exercise Training on Mental Well-Being in the Normal Population: A Controlled Trial," *Journal of Psychosomatic Research* 33 (1989): 47–61; C. Shang, "Emerging Paradigms in Mind-Body Medicine," *Journal of Complementary and Alternative Medicine* 7 (2001): 83–91.

5. See note 1.

6. M. Samuels, "Use Your Mind to Heal Your Body," *Bottom Line/Health* 19 (February 2005): 13–14.

7. S. Bodian, "Meditate Your Way to Much Better Health," *Bottom Line/Health* 18 (June 2004): 11–13.

8. D. Mueller, "Yoga Therapy," *ACSM's Health & Fitness Journal* 6 (2002): 18–24.

9. S. C. Manchanda, et al., "Retardation of Coronary Atherosclerosis with Yoga Lifestyle Intervention," *Journal of the Association of Physicians of India* 48 (2000): 687–694.

# SUGGESTED READINGS

Girdano, D. A., D. E. Dusek, and G. S. Everly. *Controlling Stress and Tension.* San Francisco: Benjamin Cummings, 2005.

Greenberg, J. S. *Comprehensive Stress Management.* New York: McGraw-Hill/Primis Custom Publishing, 2002.

Olpin, M., and M. Hesson. *Stress Management for Life.* Belmont, CA: Wadsworth/Thomson Learning, 2007.

Schwartz, M. S., and F. Andrasik. *Biofeedback: A Practitioner's Guide.* New York: Guilford Press, 2004.

Selye, H. *The Stress of Life.* New York: McGraw-Hill, 1978.

# LAB 10A: Life Experiences Survey

Name _____    Date _____    Grade _____

Instructor _____    Course _____    Section _____

**Necessary Lab Equipment**

None required.

**Objective**

To determine stressful life experiences within the last 12 months that may affect your physical and psychological well-being and your Type A personality rating.

## I. Life Experiences Survey

**Introduction**

The Life Experiences Survey contains a list of events that sometimes bring about change in the lives of those who experience them and that necessitate social readjustment. Please check events that you have experienced in the past 12 months. Be sure all checkmarks are directly across from the items to which they correspond (check only those that apply). For each item checked, please indicate the type and extent of impact the event had on your life at the time the event occurred. Rate yourself on a 7-point scale (−3, −2, −1, 0, +1, +2, +3). A rating of −3 would indicate an extremely negative impact. A rating of 0 suggests no impact either positive or negative. A rating of +3 would indicate an extremely positive impact.

**Section 1**

1. Marriage ☐
2. Detention in jail or comparable institution ☐
3. Death of spouse ☐
4. Major change in sleeping habits (much more or much less sleep) ☐
5. Death of close family member:
   a. mother ☐
   b. father ☐
   c. brother ☐
   d. sister ☐
   e. grandmother ☐
   f. grandfather ☐
   g. other (specify) ☐
6. Major change in eating habits (much more or much less food intake) ☐
7. Foreclosure on mortgage or loan ☐
8. Death of close friend ☐
9. Outstanding personal achievement ☐
10. Minor law violations (traffic tickets, disturbing the peace, etc.) ☐
11. Male: Wife/girlfriend's pregnancy ☐
12. Female: Pregnancy ☐
13. Changed work situation (different work responsibility, major change in working conditions or working hours, etc.) ☐
14. New job ☐
15. Serious illness or injury of close family member:
    a. father ☐
    b. mother ☐
    c. sister ☐

d. brother ☐
e. grandfather ☐
f. grandmother ☐
g. spouse ☐
h. other (specify) ☐
16. Sexual difficulties ☐
17. Trouble with employer (in danger of losing job or of being suspended or demoted, etc.) ☐
18. Trouble with in-laws ☐
19. Major change in financial status (a lot better off or a lot worse off) ☐
20. Major change in closeness of family members (increased or decreased closeness) ☐
21. Gaining a new family member (through birth, adoption, family member moving in, etc.) ☐
22. Change of residence ☐
23. Marital separation from mate (due to conflict) ☐
24. Major change in church activities (increased or decreased attendance) ☐
25. Marital reconciliation with mate ☐
26. Major change in number of arguments with spouse (a lot more or a lot less arguments) ☐
27. Married male: Change in wife's work outside the home (beginning work, ceasing work, changing to a new job, etc.) ☐
28. Married female: Change in husband's work (loss of job, beginning new job, retirement, etc.) ☐
29. Major change in usual type and/or amount of recreation ☐
30. Borrowing more than $10,000 (buying home, business, etc.) ☐

*Continued*

From Sarason, I. G., et al., "Assessing the Impact of Life Changes: Development of the Life Experiences Survey," *Journal of Consulting and Clinical Psychology* 46 (1978): 932–946. Copyright 1978 by the American Psychological Association. Adapted with permission.

31. Borrowing less than $10,000 (buying car or TV, getting school loan, etc.)

32. Being fired from job

33. Male: Wife/girlfriend having abortion

34. Female: Having abortion

35. Major personal illness or injury

36. Major change in social activities (participation in parties, movies, visiting, etc.)

37. Major change in living conditions of family (building new home or remodeling, deterioration of home or neighborhood, etc.)

38. Divorce

39. Serious injury or illness of close friend

40. Retirement from work

41. Son or daughter leaving home (because of marriage, college, etc.)

42. End of formal schooling

43. Separation from spouse (because of work, travel, etc.)

44. Engagement

45. Breaking up with boyfriend/girlfriend

46. Leaving home for the first time

47. Reconciliation with boyfriend/girlfriend

48. Others _____

49. _____

50. _____

**Section 2**

51. Beginning a new school experience at a higher academic level (college, graduate school, professional school, etc.)

52. Changing to a new school at the same academic level (undergraduate, graduate, etc.)

53. Academic probation

54. Being dismissed from dormitory or other residence

55. Failing an important exam

56. Changing a major

57. Failing a course

58. Dropping a course

59. Joining a fraternity/sorority

60. Financial problems concerning school (in danger of not having sufficient money to continue)

## How to Score

After determining the life events that have taken place, sum the negative and the positive points separately (e.g., positive ratings: 3, 2, 1, 2 = 8 points positive score; negative ratings: −1, −3, −1, −3, −2, −3 = 13 negative points score). A final "total life change" score is obtained by adding the positive and negative scores together as positive numbers (e.g., total life change score: 8 + 13 = 21 points). The various stress ratings for the Life Experiences Survey are given below. Your negative score is the best indicator of stress (distress or negative stress) in your life.

## Score Interpretation*

| Stress Category | Negative Score | | Total Score | |
|---|---|---|---|---|
| | **Men** | **Women** | **Men** | **Women** |
| Poor | ≥13 | ≥15 | ≥27 | ≥27 |
| Fair | 7–12 | 8–14 | 17–26 | 18–26 |
| Average | 6 | 7 | 16 | 17 |
| Good | 1–5 | 1–6 | 5–15 | 6–16 |
| Excellent | 0 | 0 | 1–4 | 1–5 |

## Life Experiences Survey Results

| | **Points** | **Stress Category** |
|---|---|---|
| Negative score: | _____ | _____ |
| Positive score: | _____ | _____ |
| Total life change score: | _____ | _____ |

# LAB 10B: Type A Personality and Hostility Assessment

Name _____  Date _____  Grade _____

Instructor _____  Course _____  Section _____

**Necessary Lab Equipment**
None required.

**Objective**
To determine your Type A personality and hostility ratings.

## I. Type A Behavior

**Instructions**
Please answer "yes" or "no" for each of the items listed below. For questions 7, 15, and 16, give yourself one point for each "yes" answer. For the rest of the questions, give yourself one point for each "no" answer.

**Yes   No**

1. Do you feel your job carries heavy responsibility?
2. Would you describe yourself as a hard-driving, ambitious type of person?
3. Do you usually try to get things done as quickly as possible?
4. Would family members and close friends describe you as hard-driving and ambitious?
5. Have people close to you ever asked you to slow down in your work?
6. Do you think you drive harder to accomplish things than most of your associates do?
7. When you play games with people your own age, do you play just for the fun of it?
8. If there's competition in your job, do you enjoy this?
9. When you are driving and there is a car in your lane going much too slowly for you, do you mutter and complain? Would anyone riding with you know you are annoyed?
10. If you make an appointment with someone, are you there on time in almost all cases?
11. If you are kept waiting, do you resent it?
12. If you see someone doing a job rather slowly and you know you could do it faster and better yourself, does it make you restless to watch him or her?
13. Would you be tempted to step in and do it yourself?
14. Do you eat rapidly? Walk rapidly?
15. After you've finished eating, do you like to sit around the table and chat?
16. When you go out to a restaurant and find eight or ten people waiting ahead of you for a table, will you wait?
17. Do you really resent having to wait in line at the bank or post office?
18. Do you always feel anxious to get going and finish whatever you have to do?
19. Do you have the feeling that time is passing too rapidly for you to accomplish all the things you'd like to get done in one day?
20. Do you often feel a sense of time urgency or time pressure?
21. Do you hurry in doing most things?

Form revised from The Structured Interview from the Forum on Type A Behavior, National Heart/Lung/Blood Institute, Ray M. Rosenman, MD, 1981. This form is reprinted from R. W. Patton, et al., *Implementing Health/Fitness Programs* (Champaign, IL: Human Kinetics Publisher, 1986).

## How to Score

**Results**                     **Points**

Questions 7, 15, 16: [_____] (1 point for each "yes" answer)

All other questions: [_____] (1 point for each "no" answer)

Total score: [_____]

Your level of Type A: [_____]

**Score Interpretation**

| Rating | Points |
|--------|--------|
| High | 0–7 |
| Medium | 8–13 |
| Low | 14–21 |

## II. Hostile Personality Assessment

Hostility could harm your heart. Experts now conclude that feelings of hostility increase your risk of heart disease. Dr. Redford Williams, of Duke University Medical Center, designed a questionnaire to help you determine whether you have a hostile personality. Circle the answer that most closely fits how you would respond to the given situation:

1. **A teenager drives by my yard blasting the car stereo:**
   A. I begin to understand why teenagers can't hear.
   B. I can feel my blood pressure starting to rise.

2. **A boyfriend/girlfriend calls at the last minute "too tired to go out tonight." I'm stuck with two $15 tickets:**
   A. I find someone else to go with.
   B. I tell my friend how inconsiderate he/she is.

3. **Waiting in the express checkout line at the supermarket where a sign says "No More Than 10 Items Please":**
   A. I pick up a magazine and pass the time.
   B. I glance to see if anyone has more than 10 items.

4. **Most homeless people in large cities:**
   A. Are down and out because they lack ambition.
   B. Are victims of illness or some other misfortune.

5. **At times when I've been very angry with someone:**
   A. I was able to stop short of hitting him/her.
   B. I have, on occasion, hit or shoved him/her.

6. **When I am stuck in a traffic jam:**
   A. I am usually not particularly upset.
   B. I quickly start to feel irritated and annoyed.

7. **When there's a really important job to be done:**
   A. I prefer to do it myself.
   B. I am apt to call on my friends to help.

8. **The cars ahead of me start to slow and stop as they approach a curve:**
   A. I assume there is a construction site ahead.
   B. I assume someone ahead had a fender-bender.

9. **An elevator stops too long above where I'm waiting:**
   A. I soon start to feel irritated and annoyed.
   B. I start planning the rest of my day.

10. **When a friend or co-worker disagrees with me:**
    A. I try to explain my position more clearly.
    B. I am apt to get into an argument with him or her.

11. **At times when I was really angry in the past:**
    A. I have never thrown things or slammed a door.
    B. I've sometimes thrown things or slammed a door.

12. **Someone bumps into me in a store:**
    A. I pass it off as an accident.
    B. I feel irritated at their clumsiness.

13. **When my spouse (significant other) is fixing a meal:**
    A. I keep an eye out to make sure nothing burns.
    B. I talk about my day or read the paper.

14. **Someone is hogging the conversation at a party:**
    A. I look for an opportunity to put him/her down.
    B. I soon move to another group.

15. **In most arguments:**
    A. I am the angrier one.
    B. The other person is angrier than I am.

### How to Score

Score one point for each of these answers: 1. B, 2. B, 3. B, 4. A, 5. B, 6. B, 7. A, 8. B, 9. A, 10. B, 11. B, 12. B, 13. A, 14. A, 15. A. If you scored 4 or more points you may be hostile. Questions 1, 6, 9, 12, and 15 reflect anger. Questions 2, 5, 10, 11, and 14 reflect aggression. Questions 3, 4, 7, 8, and 13 reflect cynicism. If you scored 2 points in any category, you should work on that area of your personality.

Hostility score [ ]    Anger score [ ]    Aggression score [ ]    Cynicism score [ ]

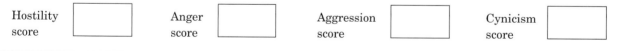

# LAB 10C: Stress Vulnerability Questionnaire

Name _____   Date _____   Grade _____

Instructor _____   Course _____   Section _____

**Necessary Lab Equipment**
None required.

**Objective**
To determine your stress vulnerability rating and identify areas where you can reduce your vulnerability to stress.

**Instructions**
Carefully read each statement and circle the number that best describes your feelings or behavior. Please be completely honest with your answers.

## I. Stress Vulnerability Questionnaire

| Item | Strongly Agree | Mildly Agree | Mildly Disagree | Strongly Disagree |
|------|------|------|------|------|
| 1. I try to incorporate as much physical activity as possible in my daily schedule. | 1 | 2 | 3 | 4 |
| 2. I accumulate a minimum of 30 minutes of moderate-intensity physical activity at least five times per week, and I exercise aerobically for 20 minutes or more at least three times per week. | 1 | 2 | 3 | 4 |
| 3. I regularly sleep 7 to 8 hours per night. | 1 | 2 | 3 | 4 |
| 4. I take my time eating at least one hot, balanced meal a day. | 1 | 2 | 3 | 4 |
| 5. I drink fewer than two cups of coffee (or equivalent) per day. | 1 | 2 | 3 | 4 |
| 6. I am at recommended body weight. | 1 | 2 | 3 | 4 |
| 7. I enjoy good health. | 1 | 2 | 3 | 4 |
| 8. I do not use tobacco in any form. | 1 | 2 | 3 | 4 |
| 9. I limit my alcohol intake to no more than one drink per day. | 1 | 2 | 3 | 4 |
| 10. I do not use hard drugs (chemical dependency). | 1 | 2 | 3 | 4 |
| 11. There is someone I love, trust, and can rely on for help if I have a problem or need to make an essential decision. | 1 | 2 | 3 | 4 |
| 12. There is love in my family. | 1 | 2 | 3 | 4 |
| 13. I routinely give and receive affection. | 1 | 2 | 3 | 4 |
| 14. I have close personal relationships with other people that provide me with a sense of emotional security. | 1 | 2 | 3 | 4 |
| 15. There are people close by whom I can turn to for guidance in time of stress. | 1 | 2 | 3 | 4 |
| 16. I can speak openly about feelings, emotions, and problems with people I trust. | 1 | 2 | 3 | 4 |
| 17. Other people rely on me for help. | 1 | 2 | 3 | 4 |
| 18. I am able to keep my feelings of anger and hostility under control. | 1 | 2 | 3 | 4 |
| 19. I have a network of friends who enjoy the same social activities that I do. | 1 | 2 | 3 | 4 |
| 20. I take time to do something fun at least once a week. | 1 | 2 | 3 | 4 |
| 21. My religious beliefs provide guidance and strength in my life. | 1 | 2 | 3 | 4 |
| 22. I often provide service to others. | 1 | 2 | 3 | 4 |
| 23. I enjoy my job (or major or school). | 1 | 2 | 3 | 4 |
| 24. I am a competent worker. | 1 | 2 | 3 | 4 |
| 25. I get along well with co-workers (or students). | 1 | 2 | 3 | 4 |

*Continued*

| Item | Strongly Agree | Mildly Agree | Mildly Disagree | Strongly Disagree |
|---|---|---|---|---|
| 26. My income is sufficient for my needs. | 1 | 2 | 3 | 4 |
| 27. I manage time adequately. | 1 | 2 | 3 | 4 |
| 28. I have learned to say "no" to additional commitments when I already am pressed for time. | 1 | 2 | 3 | 4 |
| 29. I take daily quiet time for myself. | 1 | 2 | 3 | 4 |
| 30. I practice stress management as needed. | 1 | 2 | 3 | 4 |

Total Points: _____

## Test Interpretation

| Rating | Points |
|---|---|
| Excellent (great stress resistance) | 0–30 points |
| Good (little vulnerability to stress) | 31–40 points |
| Average (somewhat vulnerable to stress) | 41–50 points |
| Fair (vulnerable to stress) | 51–60 points |
| Poor (very vulnerable to stress) | ≥61 points |

This questionnaire helps you identify areas where improvements can be made to help you cope with stress more effectively. As you take this test, you will notice that most of the items describe situations and behaviors that are within your control. To make yourself less vulnerable to stress, improve the behaviors that make you more vulnerable to stress. Start by modifying behaviors that are easiest to change before undertaking the most difficult ones.

II. In the space provided below, list, in order of priority, behaviors that you would like to change to help you decrease your vulnerability to stress. Also, briefly outline how you intend to accomplish these changes.

# LAB 10D: Goals and Time Management Skills

Name _____    Date _____    Grade _____

Instructor _____    Course _____    Section _____

### Necessary Lab Equipment
None required.

### Objective
To help you develop time management skills.

### Instructions
If you think you don't have enough hours during the day to get everything done, this lab is for you. Be sure to read the Time Management section and fill out all the forms provided with this lab.

### I. Long- and Short-Term Goals
In the spaces provided below, list your goals as indicated. You may want to keep this form and review it in years to come.

1. List three goals you wish to accomplish in this life:

_____

_____

_____

2. List three goals you wish to see accomplished 10 years from now:

_____

_____

_____

3. List three goals you wish to accomplish this year:

_____

_____

_____

4. List three goals you wish to accomplish this month:

_____

_____

_____

5. List three goals you wish to accomplish this week:

_____

_____

_____

Signature: _____    Date: _____

## II. Finding Time Killers

Keep a 4- to 7-day log and record at half-hour intervals the activities you do (make additional copies of this form as needed). Record the activities as you go through your typical day, so you will remember them all. At the end of each day, decide when you wasted time. Using a highlighter, identify the time killers on this form and plan necessary changes for the next day.

| | |
|---|---|
| 6:00 | |
| 6:30 | |
| 7:00 | |
| 7:30 | |
| 8:00 | |
| 8:30 | |
| 9:00 | |
| 9:30 | |
| 10:00 | |
| 10:30 | |
| 11:00 | |
| 11:30 | |
| 12:00 | |
| 12:30 | |
| 1:00 | |
| 1:30 | |
| 2:00 | |
| 2:30 | |
| 3:00 | |
| 3:30 | |
| 4:00 | |
| 4:30 | |
| 5:00 | |
| 5:30 | |
| 6:00 | |
| 6:30 | |
| 7:00 | |
| 7:30 | |
| 8:00 | |
| 8:30 | |
| 9:00 | |
| 9:30 | |
| 10:00 | |
| 10:30 | |

## III. Daily and Weekly Goals and Priorities

**Daily Goals:** Take 10 minutes each morning to write down the goals or tasks you wish to accomplish that day. Rank them as top, medium, low, or "trash" priorities. (Make as many copies of this form as needed.) At the end of the day, evaluate how well you accomplished your tasks for the day. Cross off the goals you accomplished and carry over to the next day those you did not get done.

Date: [   /   /   ]   Day of the Week: [      ]

### Top-Priority Goals

1. _____
2. _____
3. _____
4. _____

### Medium-Priority Goals

1. _____
2. _____
3. _____
4. _____

### Low-Priority Goals

1. _____
2. _____
3. _____
4. _____

### Trash (do only after all other goals have been accomplished)

1. _____
2. _____
3. _____
4. _____

**Weekly Goals:** Take a few minutes each Sunday night to write down the goals or tasks you wish to accomplish that week. As with your daily goals, rank them as top, medium, low, or "trash" priorities. (Make as many copies of this form as needed.) At the end of the week, evaluate how well you accomplished your goals. Cross off the goals you accomplished and carry over to the next week those you did not get done.

Week: [   /   /   ] to [   /   /   ]

### Top-Priority Goals

1. _____
2. _____
3. _____
4. _____

### Medium-Priority Goals

1. _____
2. _____
3. _____
4. _____

### Low-Priority Goals

1. _____
2. _____
3. _____
4. _____

### Trash (do only after all other goals have been accomplished)

1. _____
2. _____
3. _____
4. _____

## IV. Time Management Evaluation

On a weekly basis, go through the list of strategies below and provide a "yes" or "no" answer to each statement. If you are able to answer "yes" to most questions, congratulations, you are becoming a good time manager.

| Strategy      Date: | | | | | | | | | | | | | | | | |
|---|---|---|---|---|---|---|---|---|---|---|---|---|---|---|---|---|
| 1. I evaluate my time killers periodically. | | | | | | | | | | | | | | | | |
| 2. I have written down my long-range goals. | | | | | | | | | | | | | | | | |
| 3. I have written down my short-term goals. | | | | | | | | | | | | | | | | |
| 4. I use a daily planner. | | | | | | | | | | | | | | | | |
| 5. I conduct nightly audits. | | | | | | | | | | | | | | | | |
| 6. I conduct weekly audits. | | | | | | | | | | | | | | | | |
| 7. I delegate activities that others can do. | | | | | | | | | | | | | | | | |
| 8. I have learned to say "no" to additional tasks when I'm already in overload. | | | | | | | | | | | | | | | | |
| 9. I plan activities to avoid boredom. | | | | | | | | | | | | | | | | |
| 10. I plan ahead for distractions. | | | | | | | | | | | | | | | | |
| 11. I work on one task at a time until it's done. | | | | | | | | | | | | | | | | |
| 12. I have removed distractions from my work. | | | | | | | | | | | | | | | | |
| 13. I set aside overtimes. | | | | | | | | | | | | | | | | |
| 14. I set aside special time for myself daily. | | | | | | | | | | | | | | | | |
| 15. I reward myself for a job well done. | | | | | | | | | | | | | | | | |

# LAB 10E: Stress Management

Name _____  Date _____  Grade _____

Instructor _____  Course _____  Section _____

## Necessary Lab Equipment
None required.

## Objective
To participate in a stress management session.

## I. Stage of Change for Stress Management
Using Figure 2.5 (page 57) and Table 2.3 (page 57), identify your current stage of change for a stress management program:

|  |
|--|
|  |

## II. Stress Management
**Instructions:** The class should be divided into groups of about five students per group. Each group should select and go through a minimum of two of the following stress management techniques outlined in Chapter 10:

1. Progressive Muscle Relaxation
2. Breathing Techniques for Relaxation
3. Visual Imagery
4. Autogenic Training
5. Meditation
6. Yoga

A group leader is chosen who will lead the exercise according to the instructions provided for each relaxation technique in Chapter 10. Be sure this experience is conducted in a comfortable room that is as free of noise as possible. If trained personnel or a tape-recording for progressive muscle relaxation exercises is available, the entire class may participate in this experience at once. Institutions that have biofeedback equipment may use it in this laboratory as well. After completing this lab, answer the four questions given below.

1. Indicate the two relaxation techniques used in your lab:

   A. _____   B. _____

2. In your own words, relate your feelings as you were going through exercises A and B above:

   Exercise A: _____

   _____

   Exercise B: _____

   _____

3. Indicate how you felt mentally, emotionally, and physically after participating in this experience:

   _____

   _____

4. Are there situations in your daily life in which you think you would benefit from practicing the selected stress management exercises?

   _____

   _____

## III. Self-Assessment Stress Evaluation

1. Do you currently perceive stress to be a problem in your life? ☐ Yes ☐ No

2. Do you experience any of the typical stress symptoms listed in the box on page 368? If so, which ones?

|  |  |  |
|---|---|---|
|  |  |  |

3. Indicate any specific events in your life that trigger a stress response.

_____

_____

_____

_____

4. Write specific objectives to either avoid or help you manage the various stress-inducing events listed above, including one or more stress management techniques.

_____

_____

_____

_____

5. Do you have any behavior patterns you would like to modify? List those you would like to change.

_____

_____

_____

_____

6. List specific techniques of change you will use to change undesirable behaviors (see Table 2.2, page 56).

_____

_____

_____

_____

# Preventing Cardiovascular Disease

**11**

© Fitness & Wellness, Inc.

## Objectives

- Define cardiovascular disease and coronary heart disease
- Explain the importance of a healthy lifestyle in preventing cardiovascular disease
- Become familiar with the major risk factors that lead to the development of coronary heart disease, including physical inactivity, an abnormal cholesterol profile, hypertension, homocysteine, C-reactive protein, diabetes, and smoking
- Assess your own risk for developing coronary heart disease
- Outline a comprehensive program for reducing the risk for coronary heart disease and managing the overall risk for cardiovascular disease
- Determine your risk for heart disease
- Check how well you understand the chapter's concepts

Check your understanding of the chapter contents by logging on to CengageNOW and accessing the pre-test, personalized learning plan, and post-test for this chapter.

# FAQ

**As a young college student, why should I have to worry about heart disease?**

Young people should not think that heart disease will not affect them. The process begins early in life, as shown in American soldiers who died during the Korean and Vietnam conflicts. Autopsies conducted on soldiers killed at 22 years of age and younger revealed that approximately 70 percent had early stages of atherosclerosis. Other studies found elevated blood cholesterol levels in children as young as 10 years old. Overall risk factor management and positive lifestyle habits are the best ways to prevent disease. The choices you make today will affect your health and well-being in middle age and older life.

**How much aerobic exercise is required to decrease the risk for cardiovascular disease?**

This is a difficult question to answer, and the amount most likely varies due to genetics, age, gender, body composition, health status, and personal lifestyle, among other factors. What may be sufficient for a low-risk individual may not be enough for someone else with disease risk factors. For example, an apparently healthy individual at recommended body weight may not need more than 30 daily minutes of accumulated moderate-intensity physical activity. Another person with a weight problem and other risk factors such as high blood pressure, cholesterol abnormalities, and borderline high blood sugar may need a much greater amount of activity to counteract these risk factors.

Although research may never indicate the exact amount of aerobic exercise required to lower the risk for cardiovascular disease, pioneer research in this area conducted in the 1980s showed that expending 2,000 calories per week as a result of physical activity yielded the lowest risk for cardiovascular disease among a group of almost 17,000 Harvard alumni. Expending 2,000 calories per week represents about 300 calories per daily exercise session or the equivalent of jogging 3 miles in 30 minutes or walking 3 miles in about 45 minutes.

**Trans fats have been debated extensively lately. What foods are most likely to contain trans fats?**

With extensive media coverage of their potential harmfulness, the amount of trans fats in foods is decreasing significantly. Trans fats are found primarily in fried foods such as french fries, doughnuts, and apple fritters, but they are also found in baked foods, including pastries, biscuits, crackers, pie crusts, and pizza crust. Stick margarine and shortenings also contain trans fats.

Trans fats increase the risk for heart disease and stroke by increasing the LDL ("bad") cholesterol and decreasing the cardioprotective HDL ("good") cholesterol. To decrease consumption of trans fats, always read the food label for trans fat content and look for "hydrogenated fat/oil" or "partially hydrogenated fat/oil" (the latter are trans fats) on the list of ingredients. The FDA does not require food companies to list trans fat content on the label if it is less than .5 gram per serving. The American Heart Association recommends that on average we keep trans fat intake below 2 grams per day. Four servings of a product that contains .49 gram of partially hydrogenated oil, not listed on the food label, provide almost the entire daily allowance of trans fats.

# Prevalence of Cardiovascular Disease

More than 35 percent of all deaths in the United States are attributable to **cardiovascular diseases**, the most prevalent degenerative condition in the United States.[1]

More than a third of the adult population has some form of these diseases of the heart and blood vessels. According to the Centers for Disease Control and Prevention (CDC), about 60 percent of deaths from heart disease are sudden and unexpected, with no previous symptoms of the disease. Almost half of these deaths occur outside of the hospital, most likely because the individuals failed to recognize early warning symptoms of a heart attack.

**TABLE 11.1** Stroke Risk Factors

| Unchangeable factors |
| --- |
| Age: Increased risk after age 55 |
| Gender: Higher risk in men |
| Race: African Americans are at greater risk |
| Family history |

| Manageable Factors |
| --- |
| Tobacco use: Stop! |
| Blood pressure: Maintain in normal range |
| Diet: Decrease fat and sodium consumption and increase potassium, fruit, and vegetable intake |
| Activity level: Increase frequency and intensity |
| Weight: Maintain within recommended range |
| Cholesterol: Maintain normal levels |
| Diabetes: Prevent or manage condition |

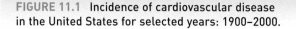

**FIGURE 11.1** Incidence of cardiovascular disease in the United States for selected years: 1900–2000.

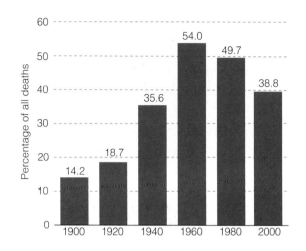

***Source:*** Centers for Disease Control, Atlanta.

Some examples of cardiovascular diseases are coronary heart disease, stroke, **peripheral vascular disease**, congenital heart disease, rheumatic heart disease, atherosclerosis, high blood pressure, and congestive heart failure. According to CDC estimates, if all deaths from the major cardiovascular diseases were eliminated, life expectancy in the United States would increase by about 7 years.

The American Heart Association (AHA) estimated the cost of heart and blood vessel disease in the United States at $448.5 billion in 2008. About one million people have new or recurrent heart attacks each year, and over 45 percent of them will die as a result. More than half of these deaths occur within 1 hour of the onset of symptoms, before the person reaches the hospital.

## Stroke
When cardiovascular diseases are separated by categories, **stroke** becomes the third leading cause of death in the United States, accounting for approximately 150,000 deaths each year. About 700,000 new stroke victims are reported each year, and of these, 266,000 survivors are left with permanent disabilities. About 20 percent of those who survive require institutional care.[2]

Stroke is the most significant contributor to mental and physical disability in the United States, yet it does not draw the same attention as coronary heart disease, high blood pressure, diabetes, or cancer. Similar to those for coronary heart disease, most risk factors for stroke are preventable. Table 11.1 lists the major risk factors; the first four factors are beyond a person's control, whereas the latter seven are fully manageable.

## Coronary Heart Disease
Although heart and blood vessel disease is still the number one health problem in the United States, the incidence declined by 28 percent between 1960 and 2000 (see Figure 11.1), in large part because of health education. More people now are aware of the risk factors for cardiovascular disease and are changing their lifestyles to lower their potential risk for these diseases.

The heart and the coronary arteries are illustrated in Figure 11.2. The major form of cardiovascular disease is **coronary heart disease (CHD)**, in which the arteries that supply the heart muscle with oxygen and nutrients are narrowed by fatty deposits, such as cholesterol and triglycerides. Narrowing of the coronary arteries diminishes the blood supply to the heart muscle, which can precipitate a heart attack.

CHD is the single leading cause of death in the United States, accounting for about 20 percent of all deaths and approximately half of all deaths from cardiovascular disease. Approximately 80 percent of deaths from CHD in people under age 65 occur during the first heart attack. CHD is the leading cause of sudden cardiac deaths. More than one half of people who die suddenly of CHD have no previous symptoms of the disease. The risk of death is also greater in the least educated segment of the population. Each year, more than 500,000 coronary bypass operations and more than 1 million coronary **angioplasty** procedures are performed in the United States.

**Cardiovascular diseases** The array of conditions that affect the heart and the blood vessels.

**Peripheral vascular disease** Narrowing of the peripheral blood vessels.

**Stroke** Condition in which a blood vessel that feeds the brain ruptures or is clogged, leading to blood flow disruption to the brain.

**Coronary heart disease (CHD)** Condition in which the arteries that supply the heart muscle with oxygen and nutrients are narrowed by fatty deposits, such as cholesterol and triglycerides.

**Angioplasty** A procedure in which a balloon-tipped catheter is inserted, then inflated, to widen the inner lumen of the artery.

FIGURE 11.2 The heart and its blood vessels.

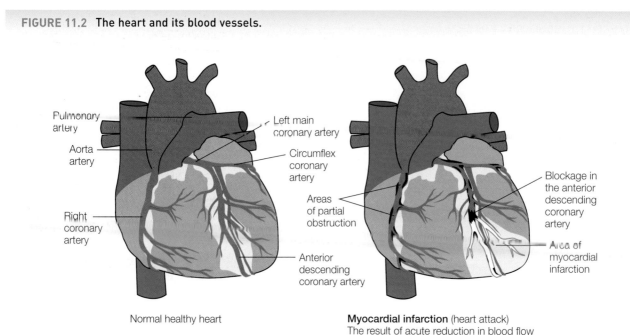

Normal healthy heart

Myocardial infarction (heart attack)
The result of acute reduction in blood flow
through the anterior descending coronary artery.

## Signs of Heart Attack and Stroke

Any or all of the following signs may occur during a heart attack or a stroke. If you experience any of these and they last longer than a few minutes, call 911 and seek medical attention immediately. Failure to do so may cause irreparable damage and even result in death.

### Warning Signs of a Heart Attack

- Chest pain, discomfort, pressure, or squeezing that lasts for several minutes. These feelings may go away and return later.
- Pain or discomfort in the shoulders, neck, or arms or between the shoulder blades
- Chest discomfort with shortness of breath, lightheadedness, cold sweats, nausea and/or vomiting, a feeling of indigestion, sudden fatigue or weakness, fainting, or sense of impending doom

### Warning Signs of Stroke

- Sudden weakness or numbness of the face, arm, or leg—particularly on one side of the body
- Sudden severe headache
- Sudden confusion, dizziness, or difficulty with speech and understanding
- Sudden difficulty walking; loss of balance or coordination
- Sudden visual difficulty

# Coronary Heart Disease Risk Profile

Although genetic inheritance plays a role in CHD, the most important determinant is personal lifestyle. Several of the major **risk factors** for CHD are preventable and reversible. CHD risk factor analyses are administered to evaluate the impact of a person's lifestyle and genetic endowment as potential contributors to the development of coronary disease. The specific objectives of a CHD risk factor analysis are:

- To screen individuals who may be at high risk for the disease
- To educate people regarding the leading risk factors for developing CHD
- To implement programs aimed at reducing the risks
- To use the analysis as a starting point from which to compare changes induced by the intervention program.

Leading Risk Factors for CHD  The leading risk factors contributing to CHD are listed in Table 11.2. A self-assessment of risk factors for CHD is given in Lab 11A. This analysis can be done by people who have little or no medical information about their cardiovascular health, as well as those who have had a thorough medical examination. The guidelines for zero risk are outlined for each factor, making this self-analysis a valuable tool for managing the risk factors for CHD.

For example, a person who fills out the form learns that recommended blood pressure is less than 120/80, that risk is reduced by smoking less or quitting altogether, that **high-density lipoprotein (HDL) cholesterol** should be

**TABLE 11.2** Weighing System for Coronary Heart Disease Risk Factors

| Risk Factors | Maximal Risk Points |
|---|---|
| Abnormal cholesterol profile | 12 |
| Low HDL cholesterol | 6 |
| High LDL cholesterol | 6 |
| High-sensitivity C-reactive protein | 8 |
| Physical inactivity | 8 |
| Smoking | 8 |
| Body mass index | 8 |
| Hypertension | 8 |
| Systolic blood pressure | 4 |
| Diastolic blood pressure | 4 |
| Personal history of heart disease | 8 |
| Abnormal stress electrocardiogram | 8 |
| Diabetes | 6 |
| High blood glucose | 3 |
| Known diabetes | 3 |
| Family history of heart disease | 8 |
| Elevated homocysteine | 4 |
| Age | 4 |
| Tension and stress | 3 |
| Abnormal resting electrocardiogram | 3 |
| Elevated triglycerides | 2 |

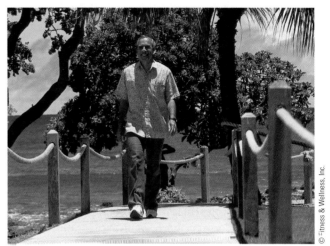

Regular physical activity helps to control most of the major risk factors that lead to heart disease.

40 mg/dL (milligrams per deciliter) or higher, and that **low-density lipoprotein (LDL) cholesterol** should be less than 100 mg/dL (if unknown, basic nutritional guidelines are also given). (The respective roles of HDL and LDL cholesterol in protecting against and causing heart disease are discussed later in this chapter.)

To provide a meaningful score for CHD risk, a weighting system was developed to show the impact of each risk factor on developing the disease (see Table 11.2 and Lab 11A). This system is based on current research and on the work done at leading preventive medical facilities in the United States. The most significant risk factors are given the heaviest numerical weight.

For example, a poor cholesterol profile is one of the best predictors for developing CHD. Up to 12 risk points are assigned to individuals with very high LDL cholesterol and low HDL cholesterol levels. The least heavily weighted risk factor is triglycerides, with a maximum of only 2 risk points assigned to this factor. Each risk factor is also assigned a zero risk level—the level at which it apparently does not increase the risk for disease at all.

Based on actual test results, a person receives a score anywhere from zero to the maximum number of points for each factor. When the risk points from all of the risk factors are totaled, the final number is used to place an individual in one of five overall risk categories for potential development of CHD (see Lab 11A).

The "Very Low" CHD risk category designates the group at lowest risk for developing heart disease based on age and gender. "Low" CHD suggests that even though people in this category are taking good care of their cardiovascular health, they can improve it (unless all of the risk points come from age and family history). "Moderate" CHD risk means that the person can definitely improve his or her lifestyle to lower the risk for disease, or medical treatment may be required. A score in the "High" or "Very High" CHD risk category points to a strong probability of developing heart disease within the next few years and calls for immediate implementation of a personal risk-reduction program, including professional medical, nutritional, and physical activity intervention.

The leading risk factors for CHD are discussed next, along with the general recommendations for risk reduction.

## Critical Thinking

What do you think of your own risk for diseases of the cardiovascular system? Is this something you need to concern yourself with at this point in your life? Why or why not?

**Risk factors** Lifestyle and genetic variables that may lead to disease.

**High-density lipoproteins (HDLs)** Cholesterol-transporting molecules in the blood ("good" cholesterol) that help clear cholesterol from the blood.

**Low-density lipoproteins (LDLs)** Cholesterol-transporting molecules in the blood ("bad" cholesterol) that tend to increase blood cholesterol.

**Physical Inactivity** Physical inactivity is responsible for low levels of cardiorespiratory endurance (the ability of the heart, lungs, and blood vessels to deliver enough oxygen to the cells to meet the demands of prolonged physical activity). The level of cardiorespiratory endurance (or fitness) is given most commonly by the maximal amount of oxygen (in milliliters) that every kilogram (2.2 pounds) of body weight is able to utilize per minute of physical activity (mL/kg/min). As maximal oxygen uptake ($VO_{2max}$) increases, so does efficiency of the cardiorespiratory system.

Even though physical inactivity has not been assigned the most risk points (8 points for a poor level of fitness versus 12 for a poor cholesterol profile—see Table 11.2), improving cardiorespiratory endurance through daily physical activity and aerobic exercise greatly reduces the overall risk for heart disease.

Although specific recommendations can be followed to improve each risk factor, daily physical activity and a regular aerobic exercise program help to control most of the major risk factors that lead to heart disease. Physical activity and aerobic exercise will:

- Increase cardiorespiratory endurance
- Decrease and control blood pressure
- Reduce body fat
- Lower blood lipids (cholesterol and triglycerides)
- Improve HDL cholesterol
- Prevent and help control diabetes
- Decrease low-grade (hidden) inflammation in the body
- Increase and maintain good heart function, sometimes improving certain electrocardiogram abnormalities
- Motivate toward smoking cessation
- Alleviate tension and stress
- Counteract a personal history of heart disease

Data from the research summarized in Figure 1.10 in Chapter 1 clearly show the tie between physical activity

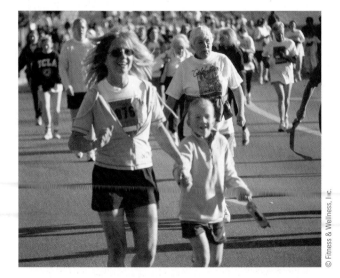

Lifetime participation in physical activity is one of the most important factors in the prevention of cardiovascular disease.

and mortality, regardless of age and other risk factors.[3] A higher level of physical fitness benefits even those who exhibit other risk factors, such as high blood pressure and serum cholesterol, cigarette smoking, and a family history of heart disease. In most cases, less fit people in the study without these risk factors had higher death rates than highly fit people with these same risk factors.

The findings show that the higher the level of cardiorespiratory fitness, the longer the life, but the largest drop in premature death is seen between the "Unfit" and the "Moderately Fit" groups. Even small improvements in cardiorespiratory endurance greatly decrease the risk for cardiovascular mortality. Most adults who engage in a moderate exercise program can attain these fitness levels easily. A 2-mile walk in 30 to 40 minutes, five to seven days a week, is adequate to decrease risk.

Subsequent research published in the *New England Journal of Medicine* substantiated the importance of exercise in preventing CHD.[4] The benefits to previously inactive adults of starting a moderate to vigorous physical activity program were as important as quitting smoking, managing blood pressure, or controlling cholesterol. In relative risk for death from CHD, the increase in physical activity led to the same decrease as giving up cigarette smoking.

The scientific data are quite clear that moderate-intensity physical activity provides substantial benefits in terms of overall cardiovascular risk reduction. Scientific studies indicate, however, that when feasible, vigorous-intensity activity is preferable because of greater improvements in aerobic fitness, blood pressure, and glucose control and a larger reduction in CHD risk.[5] A note of caution: Do not engage in vigorous exercise without proper clearance and a minimum of six weeks of proper conditioning through moderate-intensity activity.

While aerobically fit individuals have a lower incidence of cardiovascular disease, regular physical activity and aerobic exercise by themselves do not guarantee a lifetime free of cardiovascular problems. Poor lifestyle habits—such as smoking, eating too many fatty/salty/sweet foods, being overweight, and having high stress levels—increase cardiovascular risk, and their effects will not be eliminated completely through an active lifestyle.

Overall management of risk factors is the best guideline to lower the risk for cardiovascular disease. Still, aerobic exercise is one of the most important factors in preventing and reducing cardiovascular problems. Based on the overwhelming amount of scientific data in this area, evidence of the benefits of aerobic exercise in reducing heart disease is far too impressive to be ignored. The basic principles for cardiorespiratory exercise are given in Chapter 6.

As more research studies are conducted, the addition of strength training is increasingly recommended for good heart function. The AHA recommends strength training even for individuals who have had a heart attack or have high blood pressure, as long as they strength train under a physician's advice. Strength training helps control body weight and blood sugar and lowers cholesterol and blood pressure.

FIGURE 11.3 Normal electrocardiogram.

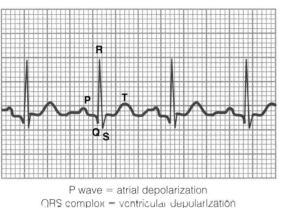

P wave = atrial depolarization
QRS complex = ventricular depolarization
T wave = ventricular repolarization

FIGURE 11.4 Abnormal electrocardiogram showing a depressed S-T segment.

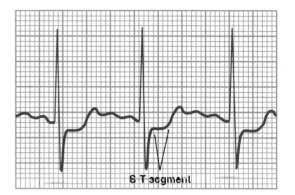

S-T segment

## Abnormal Electrocardiograms

The **electrocardiogram (ECG or EKG)** is a valuable measure of the heart's function. The ECG provides a record of the electrical impulses that stimulate the heart to contract (see Figure 11.3). In reading an ECG, doctors interpret five general areas: heart rate, heart rhythm, axis of the heart, enlargement or hypertrophy of the heart, and myocardial infarction.

During a standard 12-lead ECG, 10 electrodes are placed on the person's chest. From these 10 electrodes, 12 tracings, or "leads," of the electrical impulses as they travel through the heart muscle, or **myocardium**, are studied from 12 different positions. By looking at ECG tracings, medical professionals can identify abnormalities in heart functioning (see Figure 11.4). Based on the findings, the ECG may be interpreted as normal, equivocal, or abnormal. An ECG will not always identify problems, so a normal tracing is not an absolute guarantee. Conversely, an abnormal tracing does not necessarily signal a serious condition.

ECGs are taken at rest, during the stress of exercise, and during recovery. A **stress electrocardiogram** is also known as a "graded exercise stress test" or a "maximal exercise tolerance test." Similar to a high-speed test on a car, a stress ECG reveals the tolerance of the heart to increased physical activity. It is a much better test than a resting ECG to discover CHD.

Stress ECGs also are used to assess cardiorespiratory fitness levels, to screen individuals for preventive and cardiac rehabilitation programs, to detect abnormal blood pressure response during exercise, and to establish actual or functional maximal heart rate for exercise prescription. The recovery ECG is another important diagnostic tool to monitor the return of the heart's activity to normal conditions.

Not every adult who wishes to start or continue an exercise program needs a stress ECG. This type of test is recommended for symptomatic and diseased individuals, asymptomatic individuals with CHD risk factors, those who are going to start a vigorous exercise program, and those in occupations in which cardiovascular problems affect public safety.[6] In terms of risk factors, a stress ECG is recommended for:

1. Men over age 45 and women over age 55

2. Anyone with total cholesterol level above 240 mg/dL, LDL cholesterol above 160, or HDL cholesterol below 40 mg/dL

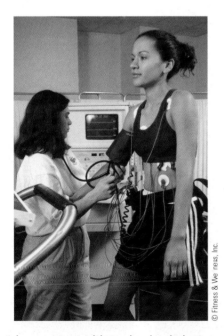

Exercise tolerance test with twelve-lead electrocardiographic monitoring (an exercise-stress ECG).

**Electrocardiogram (ECG or EKG)** A recording of the electrical activity of the heart.

**Myocardium** Heart muscle.

**Stress electrocardiogram** An exercise test during which the workload is increased gradually until the individual reaches maximal fatigue, with blood pressure and 12-lead electrocardiographic monitoring throughout the test.

3. Hypertensive and diabetic patients

4. Cigarette smokers

5. Individuals with a family history of CHD, syncope, or sudden death before age 60

6. People with an abnormal resting ECG

7. All individuals with symptoms of chest discomfort, dysrhythmias (abnormal heartbeat), syncope (brief loss of consciousness), or chronotropic incompetence (heart rate that increases slowly during exercise and never reaches maximum)

At times, the stress ECG has been questioned as a reliable predictor of CHD. Nevertheless, it remains the most practical and inexpensive noninvasive procedure available to diagnose latent (undiagnosed/unknown) CHD. The test is accurate in diagnosing CHD about 65 percent of the time. The sensitivity of the test increases along with the severity of the disease, and more accurate results are seen in people who are at high risk for cardiovascular disease—in particular, men over age 45 and women over age 55.

### Abnormal Cholesterol Profile

**Cholesterol** receives much attention because of its direct relationship to heart disease. **Blood lipids** (cholesterol and triglycerides) are carried in the bloodstream by protein molecules of HDLs, LDLs, **very-low-density lipoproteins (VLDLs)**, and **chylomicrons**. An increased risk for CHD has been established in individuals with high total cholesterol, high LDL cholesterol, and low HDL cholesterol.

An abnormal cholesterol profile contributes to **atherosclerosis**, the buildup of fatty tissue in the walls of the arteries (see Figures 11.5 and 11.6). As the plaque builds up, it blocks the blood vessels that supply the myocardium with oxygen and nutrients (the coronary arteries), and these obstructions can trigger a **myocardial infarction**, or heart attack.

Unfortunately, the heart disguises its problems quite well, and typical symptoms of heart disease, such as **angina pectoris**, do not start until the arteries are about 75 percent blocked. In many cases, the first symptom is sudden death.

The recommendation of the National Cholesterol Education Program (NCEP) is to keep total cholesterol levels below 200 mg/dL. Cholesterol levels between 200 and 239 mg/dL are borderline high, and levels of 240 mg/dL and above indicate high risk for disease (see Table 11.3). The risk for heart attack increases 2 percent for every 1 percent increase in total cholesterol.[7] About 105.2 million U.S. adults (49 percent) have total cholesterol values of 200 mg/dL or higher. Of these, more than 36.6 million have values at or above 240 mg/dL.[8]

Preventive medicine practitioners often recommend a range between 160 and 180 mg/dL as best for total cholesterol. Furthermore, in the Framingham Heart Study (a 60-year ongoing project in the community of Framingham, Massachusetts), not a single individual with a total cholesterol level of 150 mg/dL or lower has had a heart attack.

As important as it is, total cholesterol is not the best predictor for cardiovascular risk. Many heart attacks oc-

**FIGURE 11.5 The atherosclerotic process.**

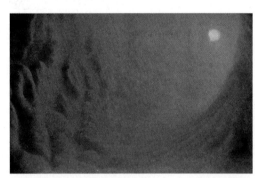

Early stage of atherosclerosis

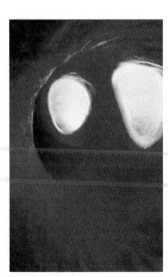

Normal artery

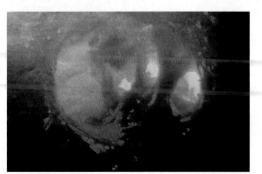

Progression of the atherosclerotic plaque

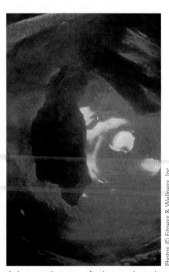

Advanced stage of atherosclerosis

**FIGURE 11.6** Comparison of a normal healthy artery (A) and diseased arteries (B and C).

**The Atherosclerotic Process**

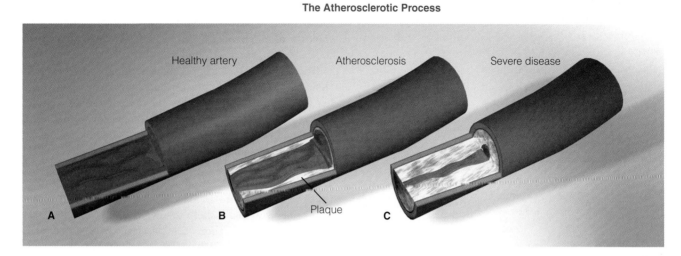

cur in people with only slightly elevated total cholesterol. More significant is the way in which cholesterol is carried in the bloodstream. Cholesterol is transported primarily in the form of LDL and HDL.

LDL ("bad") cholesterol tends to release cholesterol, which then may penetrate the lining of the arteries and speed the process of atherosclerosis. The NCEP guidelines given in Table 11.3 state that an LDL cholesterol value below 100 mg/dL is optimal.

Even when more LDL cholesterol is present than the cells can use, cholesterol seems not to cause a problem until it is oxidized by free radicals (see discussion under "Antioxidants" in Chapter 3, pages 95–97). After cholesterol is oxidized, white blood cells invade the arterial wall, take up the cholesterol, and clog the arteries.

LDL cholesterol particles are of two types: large, or pattern A; and small, or pattern B. Small particles are

thought to pass through the inner lining of the coronary arteries more readily, thereby increasing the risk for a heart attack. A predominance of small particles can lead to a sixfold increase in the risk for CHD.[9]

A genetic variation of LDL cholesterol, known as lipoprotein-a, or Lp(a), is also noteworthy because a high level of these particles promotes blood clots and earlier development of atherosclerosis. It is thought that certain substances in the arterial wall interact with Lp(a) and lead to premature formation of plaque. About 10 percent of the population has elevated levels of Lp(a). Only medications help decrease Lp(a), and drug options should be discussed with a physician.

Intermediate-density lipoprotein (IDL) is also of concern because these mid-sized particles are more likely to cause atherosclerosis than a similar amount of LDL cholesterol. For individuals at risk for heart disease, a comprehensive blood lipid profile that includes total cholesterol, HDL cholesterol, LDL cholesterol, Lp(a), IDL, and size pattern (A and B) is recommended.

**TABLE 11.3** Cholesterol Guidelines

| | Amount | Rating |
|---|---|---|
| Total cholesterol | <200 mg/dL | Desirable |
| | 200–239 mg/dL | Borderline high |
| | ≥240 mg/dL | High risk |
| LDL cholesterol | <100 mg/dL | Optimal |
| | 100–129 mg/dL | Near or above optimal |
| | 130–159 mg/dL | Borderline high |
| | 160–189 mg/dL | High |
| | ≥190 mg/dL | Very high |
| HDL cholesterol | <40 mg/dL | Low (high risk) |
| | ≥60 mg/dL | High (low risk) |

From National Cholesterol Education Program.

**Cholesterol** A waxy substance, technically a steroid alcohol, found only in animal fats and oil; used in making cell membranes, as a building block for some hormones, in the fatty sheath around nerve fibers, and other necessary substances.

**Blood lipids (fat)** Cholesterol and triglycerides.

**Very-low-density lipoproteins (VLDLs)** Triglyceride-, cholesterol-, and phospholipid-transporting molecules in the blood that tend to increase blood cholesterol.

**Chylomicrons** Triglyceride-transporting molecules.

**Atherosclerosis** Fatty/cholesterol deposits in the walls of the arteries leading to formation of plaque.

**Myocardial infarction** Heart attack; damage to or death of an area of the heart muscle as a result of an obstructed artery to that area.

**Angina pectoris** Chest pain associated with coronary heart disease.

**TABLE 11.4** Cholesterol and Saturated Fat Content of Selected Foods

| Food | Serving Size | Cholesterol (mg) | Sat. Fat (gr) |
|---|---|---|---|
| Avocado | ⅛ med. | — | 3.2 |
| Bacon | 2 slices | 30 | 2.7 |
| Beans (all types) | any | — | — |
| Beef—lean, fat trimmed off | 3 oz | 75 | 6.0 |
| Beef heart (cooked) | 3 oz | 150 | 1.6 |
| Beef liver (cooked) | 3 oz | 255 | 1.3 |
| Butter | 1 tsp | 12 | 0.4 |
| Caviar | 1 oz | 85 | — |
| Cheese | | | |
| American | 2 oz | 54 | 11.2 |
| Cheddar | 2 oz | 60 | 12.0 |
| Cottage (1% fat) | 1 cup | 10 | 0.4 |
| Cottage (4% fat) | 1 cup | 31 | 6.0 |
| Cream | 2 oz | 62 | 6.0 |
| Muenster | 2 oz | 54 | 10.8 |
| Parmesan | 2 oz | 38 | 9.3 |
| Swiss | 2 oz | 52 | 10.0 |
| Chicken (no skin) | 3 oz | 45 | 0.4 |
| Chicken liver | 3 oz | 472 | 1.1 |
| Chicken thigh, wing | 3 oz | 69 | 3.3 |
| Egg (yolk) | 1 lrg | 218 | 1.6 |
| Frankfurter | 2 | 90 | 11.2 |
| Fruits | any | — | — |
| Grains (all types) | any | — | — |
| Halibut, flounder | 3 oz | 43 | 0.7 |
| Ice cream | ½ cup | 27 | 4.4 |
| Lamb | 3 oz | 60 | 7.2 |
| Lard | 1 tsp | 5 | 1.9 |
| Lobster | 3 oz | 170 | 0.5 |
| Margarine (all vegetable) | 1 tsp | — | 0.7 |
| Mayonnaise | 1 tbsp | 10 | 2.1 |
| Milk | | | |
| Skim | 1 cup | 5 | 0.3 |
| Low fat (2%) | 1 cup | 18 | 2.9 |
| Whole | 1 cup | 34 | 5.1 |
| Nuts | 1 oz | — | 1.0 |
| Oysters | 3 oz | 42 | — |
| Salmon | 3 oz | 30 | 0.8 |
| Scallops | 3 oz | 29 | — |
| Sherbet | ½ cup | 7 | 1.2 |
| Shrimp | 3 oz | 128 | 0.1 |
| Trout | 3 oz | 45 | 2.1 |
| Tuna (canned—drained) | 3 oz | 55 | — |
| Turkey dark meat | 3 oz | 60 | 0.6 |
| Turkey light meat | 3 oz | 50 | 0.4 |
| Vegetables (except avocado) | any | — | — |

In a process known as **reverse cholesterol transport**, HDLs act as "scavengers," removing cholesterol from the body and preventing plaque from forming in the arteries. The strength of HDL is in the protein molecules found in its coating. When HDL comes in contact with cholesterol-filled cells, these protein molecules attach to the cells and take their cholesterol.

The more HDL ("good") cholesterol, the better. HDL cholesterol offers some protection against heart disease. A low level of HDL cholesterol is one of the strongest predictors of CHD at all levels of total cholesterol, including levels below 200 mg/dL. Data suggest that for every 1 mg/dL increase in HDL cholesterol, the risk for CHD drops up to 3 percent in men and 5 percent in women.[10] The recommended HDL cholesterol values to minimize the risk for CHD are at least 40 mg/dL. HDL cholesterol levels above 60 mg/dL help to lower the risk for CHD.

Similar to LDL, there are two known types of HDL particles, $HDL_2$ and $HDL_3$. $HDL_2$ are larger particles that carry cholesterol from the arterial wall to the liver for disposal. These particles also have antioxidant and anti-inflammatory effects. $HDL_3$ also transports cholesterol out of the arterial wall but may not be as effective as $HDL_2$. $HDL_3$, however, seems to protect against cholesterol oxidation that results in atherosclerosis.[11]

For the most part, HDL cholesterol is determined genetically. Generally, women have higher levels than men. Because the female sex hormone estrogen tends to raise HDL, premenopausal women have a much lower incidence of heart disease. African American children and adult men have higher HDL values than Caucasians. HDL cholesterol also decreases with age.

Increasing HDL cholesterol improves the cholesterol profile and lessens the risk for CHD. Habitual aerobic exercise, weight loss, and nonsmoking help raise HDL cholesterol. Drug therapy may also promote higher HDL cholesterol levels. Niacin helps convert $HDL_3$ to $HDL_2$.

Improved HDL cholesterol is clearly related to a regular aerobic exercise program (preferably high intensity, or above 6 metabolic equivalents [METs], for at least 20 minutes three times per week—see Chapter 6). Individual responses to aerobic exercise differ, but generally, the more you exercise, the higher your HDL cholesterol level.

**Counteracting Cholesterol** The average adult in the United States consumes between 400 and 600 mg of cholesterol daily. The body, however, manufactures more than that. Saturated and trans fats (trans fatty acids) raise cholesterol levels more than anything else in the diet. These fats produce approximately 1,000 mg of cholesterol per day. Because of individual differences, some people can have a higher than normal intake of saturated and trans fats and still maintain normal levels. Others, who have a lower intake, can have abnormally high levels.

Saturated fats are found mostly in meats and dairy products and seldom in foods of plant origin (see Table 11.4). Poultry and fish contain less saturated fat than does beef but should be eaten in moderation (about 3 to

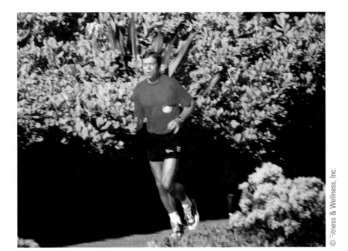

Habitual aerobic exercise helps increase HDL cholesterol ("good" cholesterol).

6 ounces per day—see Chapter 3). Unsaturated fats are mainly of plant origin and cannot be converted to cholesterol. Two or three omega-3–rich fish meals per week also help lower LDL cholesterol and **triglycerides**.

The antioxidant effect of vitamins C and E, obtained from food sources, may provide benefits. Data suggest that a single unstable free radical (an oxygen compound produced during metabolism—see Chapter 3) can damage LDL particles, accelerating the atherosclerotic process. Vitamin C may inactivate free radicals and slow the oxidation of LDL cholesterol. Vitamin E may protect LDL from oxidation, preventing heart disease, but studies suggest that it does not seem to be helpful in reversing damage once it has taken place.

**Trans Fats** Foods that contain trans fatty acids, hydrogenated fat, or partially hydrogenated vegetable oil should be avoided. Studies indicate that these foods elevate LDL cholesterol as much as saturated fats do. Trans fats also increase triglycerides and lower HDL cholesterol. These changes contribute not only to heart disease, but also to gallstone formation. Trans fats are found primarily in processed foods.

Food companies use trans fats because they are inexpensive to produce and easy to use, last a long time, and add taste and texture to food. Restaurants and fast-food chains choose oils with trans fats because they can be used repeatedly in commercial fryers.

Hydrogen frequently is added to monounsaturated and polyunsaturated fats to increase shelf life and to solidify them so they are more spreadable. Hydrogenation can change the position of hydrogen atoms along the carbon chain, transforming the fat into a trans fatty acid. Margarine and spreads, chips, commercially produced crackers and cookies, and fast foods often contain trans fatty acids. Small amounts of trans fats are also found naturally in some meats, dairy products, and other animal-based foods.

In 2006, the AHA became the first major health organization to issue dietary guidelines for trans fat intake. In the 2006 revision of its Diet and Lifestyle Recommendations, the AHA limits trans fat intake to less than 1 percent of total daily calories.[12] This amount represents about 1.5 grams of trans fats a day for a 1,500-calorie diet, 2 grams for 2,000 calories, and 3 grams for 3,000 calories. Because the U.S. Food and Drug Administration (FDA) now requires that all food labels list the trans fat content, you can keep better track of your daily trans fat intake by paying attention to food labels. Additional information on trans fats is found under the "Trans Fatty Acids" section in Chapter 3 (see page 75).

The FDA allows food manufacturers to label any product that has less than half a gram of trans fat per serving as zero. Be aware that if you eat three or four servings of a particular food near a half a gram of trans fat, you may be getting your maximum daily allowance (1 gram per 1,000 calories of daily caloric intake). Thus, you are encouraged to look at the list of ingredients and search for the words "partially hydrogenated" as an indicator of hidden trans fats.

The labels "partially hydrogenated" and "trans fatty acids" indicate that the product carries a health risk just as high as that of saturated fat. Now that trans fats are listed on food labels, companies are looking to reformulate their products to reduce or eliminate these fats. Some products that once had high trans fat content now have none. As a consumer, you are encouraged to check food labels often to obtain current information. Table 11.5 lists the average trans fat content of some foods. These values may vary among brands according to food formulation and ingredients and may change in the near future as manufacturers alter food formulations to decrease or eliminate trans fat content.

**Lowering LDL Cholesterol** LDL cholesterol levels higher than ideal can be lowered through dietary changes, by losing body fat, by taking medication, and by participating in a regular aerobic exercise program. Research conducted at the Aerobics Research Institute in Dallas, Texas, showed a higher relative risk of mortality in unfit individuals with low cholesterol than fit people with high cholesterol.[13] The lowest mortality rate, of course, is seen in fit people with low total cholesterol levels.

In terms of dietary modifications, a diet lower in saturated fat, trans fats, and cholesterol and high in fiber is recommended. Saturated fat should be replaced with monounsaturated and polyunsaturated fats (preferably omega-3 fatty acids) because the latter tend to decrease LDL cholesterol and increase HDL cholesterol (see the discussion of "Simple Fats" in Chapter 3, pages 73–74). Total saturated fat intake should be less than 7 percent of

**Reverse cholesterol transport** A process in which HDL molecules attract cholesterol and carry it to the liver, where it is changed to bile and eventually excreted in the stool.

**Triglycerides** Fats formed by glycerol and three fatty acids; also called free fatty acids.

**TABLE 11.5** Average Trans Fat Content of Selected Foods*

| Food Item | Amount | Grams |
|---|---|---|
| **Fats/Oils** | | |
| Margarine, stick | 1 tbsp | 2.0 |
| Margarine, tub | 1 tbsp | 0.5 |
| Butter | 1 tbsp | 0.3 |
| Shortening | 1 tbsp | 4.0 |
| Mayonnaise | 1 tbsp | 0.0 |
| **Snacks** | | |
| Oreo cookies | 3 | 2.5 |
| Chips Ahoy Chocolate Chip Cookies | 3 | 1.5 |
| Ritz crackers | 5 | 1.5 |
| Flavorite Honey Maid Grahams | 8 sections | 1.5 |
| Fig Newtons | 2 | 1.0 |
| Potato chips | 2 oz | 3.0 |
| Cake, pound | 1 slice (3 oz) | 4.5 |
| Candy bar | 1 | 3.0 |
| **Fast Foods** | | |
| Dunkin' Donuts Apple Fritter | 1 | 2.5 |
| Krispy Kreme Apple Fritter | 1 | 7.0 |
| Krispy Kreme Doughnut, glazed | 1 | 4.0 |
| McDonald's Biscuit | 1 | 5.0 |
| McDonald's Cinnamon Roll | 1 | 4.5 |
| McDonald's Baked Apple Pie | 1 | 4.0 |
| McDonald's Chicken McNuggets | 10 pieces | 2.5 |
| Burger King French Toast Sticks | 5 pieces | 4.5 |
| Burger King Chicken Tenders | 5 pieces | 2.5 |
| Burger King Big Fish Sandwich | 1 | 1.5 |
| KFC Extra Crispy Breast | 6 oz | 4.5 |
| KFC Breast, original recipe | 6 oz | 2.5 |
| French fries | 1 med (4 oz) | 5.0 |
| Taco Bell, Taco | 1 | 0.5 |
| Taco Bell, Taco Supreme | 1 | 1.0 |
| Taco Bell, Burrito | 1 | 2.0 |
| Taco Bell, Burrito Supreme, beef | 1 | 2.0 |

*Note:* Trans fat intake should be limited to no more than 1 percent of total daily caloric intake or the equivalent of 1 gram per 1,000 calories of energy intake.

*Trans fat content in food items may decrease significantly in the near future as food manufacturers are looking to lower the amount in their products because of FDA regulations that require trans fats to be listed on food labels. Trans fat content also varies between different brands based on food formulation and ingredients. Check food labels regularly to obtain current information.

## Behavior Modification Planning

### 2006 AMERICAN HEART ASSOCIATION DIET AND LIFESTYLE RECOMMENDATIONS FOR CARDIOVASCULAR DISEASE RISK REDUCTION

I PLAN TO | I DID IT

☐ ☐ Balance caloric intake and physical activity to achieve or maintain a healthy body weight.

☐ ☐ Consume a diet rich in vegetables and fruits.

☐ ☐ Consume whole-grain, high-fiber foods.

☐ ☐ Consume fish, especially oily fish, at least twice a week.

☐ ☐ Limit your intake of saturated fat to less than 7 percent and trans fat to less than 1 percent of total daily caloric intake.

☐ ☐ Limit cholesterol intake to less than 300 mg per day.

☐ ☐ Minimize your intake of beverages and foods with added sugars.

☐ ☐ Choose and prepare foods with little or no salt.

☐ ☐ If you consume alcohol, do so in moderation.

☐ ☐ When you eat food that is prepared outside of the home, follow the above recommendations.

☐ ☐ Avoid use of and exposure to tobacco products.

### Try It

In your Online Journal or class notebook, record which of the above recommendations you fall short on and propose at least one thing you could do to improve.

the total daily caloric intake, preferably much lower while on a cholesterol-lowering diet. Trans fat intake should be less than 1 percent of the daily caloric intake. Exercise is important because dietary manipulation by itself is not as effective in lowering LDL cholesterol as a combination of diet plus aerobic exercise.

To lower LDL cholesterol significantly, total daily fiber intake must be in the range of 25 to 38 grams per day (see "Fiber" in Chapter 3), and total fat consumption can be in the range of 30 percent of total daily caloric intake—as long as most is unsaturated fat and the average cholesterol consumption is lower than 300 mg per day (preferably less than 200 mg). Increasing consumption of vegetables, fruits, whole grains, and beans further accelerates the rate of LDL cholesterol reduction.[14]

Among people in the United States, the average fiber intake is less than 15 grams per day. Fiber, in particular the soluble type, has been shown to lower cholesterol. Soluble fiber dissolves in water and forms a gel-like substance that encloses food particles. This property helps bind and excrete fats from the body. Soluble fibers also bind intestinal bile acids that could be recycled into additional cholesterol. Soluble fibers are found primarily in oats, fruits, barley, legumes, and psyllium.

Psyllium, a grain that is added to some multigrain breakfast cereals, also helps lower LDL cholesterol. As little as 3 daily grams of psyllium can lower LDL cholesterol by 20 percent. Commercially available fiber supplements that contain psyllium (such as Metamucil) can be used to increase soluble fiber intake. Three tablespoons daily will add about 10 grams of soluble fiber to the diet.

The incidence of heart disease is very low in populations in which daily fiber intake exceeds 30 grams per day. Further, a Harvard University Medical School study of 43,000 middle-aged men who were followed for more than 6 years showed that increasing daily fiber intake to 30 grams resulted in a 41 percent reduction in heart attacks.[15]

Research on the effects of a "typical" 30 percent fat diet (including saturated fat) has shown that it has little or no effect in lowering cholesterol and that CHD actually continues to progress in people who have the disease. Thus, some practitioners recommend a 10 percent or less fat-calorie diet combined with a regular aerobic exercise program if you are trying to lower cholesterol.

A daily 10 percent total fat diet requires the person to limit fat intake to an absolute minimum. Some health care professionals contend that a diet like this is difficult to follow indefinitely. People with high cholesterol levels may not have to follow that diet indefinitely but should adopt the 10 percent fat diet while attempting to lower cholesterol. Thereafter, a 20 to 30 percent fat diet may be adequate to maintain recommended cholesterol levels, as long as most of the intake is from unsaturated fats (national data indicate that current fat consumption in the United States averages 34 percent of total calories—see Chapter 3, Table 3.5).

A drawback of very low fat diets (less than 25 percent fat) is that they tend to lower HDL cholesterol and increase triglycerides. If HDL cholesterol is already low, monounsaturated and polyunsaturated fats should be added to the diet. Examples of food items that are high in monounsaturated fats and polyunsaturated fats are olive and canola oils and nuts. The table of nutritive values in Appendix A can be used to determine food items that are high in monounsaturated and polyunsaturated fats (see also Chapter 3, Figure 3.9).

## Behavior Modification Planning

### BLOOD CHEMISTRY TEST GUIDELINES

People who have never had a blood chemistry test should do so to establish a baseline for future reference. The blood test should include total cholesterol, LDL cholesterol, HDL cholesterol, triglycerides, and blood glucose.

Following an initial normal baseline test no later than age 20, for a person who adheres to the recommended dietary and exercise guidelines, a blood analysis at least every 5 years prior to age 40 should suffice. Thereafter, a blood lipid test is recommended every year, in conjunction with a regular preventive medicine physical examination.

A single baseline test is not necessarily a valid measure. Cholesterol levels vary from month to month and sometimes even from day to day. If the initial test reveals cholesterol abnormalities, the test should be repeated within a few weeks to confirm the results.

### Try It

Blood chemistry tests are available at many wellness centers on college campuses for under $25 for a comprehensive test that includes total cholesterol, LDL cholesterol, HDL cholesterol, triglycerides, and blood glucose levels. Have you had your blood test done, and are you aware of your blood lipid profile?

❑ I PLAN TO  ❑ I DID IT

**NCEP Guidelines** The NCEP guidelines for people who are trying to decrease LDL cholesterol allow for a diet with up to 35 percent of calories from fat, including 10 percent from polyunsaturated fats and 20 percent from monounsaturated fats.[16] If you are attempting to lower LDL cholesterol, saturated fats should be kept to an absolute minimum. Carbohydrate intake can be in the range of 45 to 65 percent of total calories.

Margarines and salad dressings that contain stanol ester, a plant-derived compound that interferes with cholesterol absorption in the intestine, are now also on the market. Over the course of several weeks, daily intake of about 3 grams of margarine or 6 tablespoons of salad dressing containing stanol ester lowers LDL cholesterol by 14 percent. Dietary guidelines to lower LDL cholesterol levels are provided in the accompanying box.

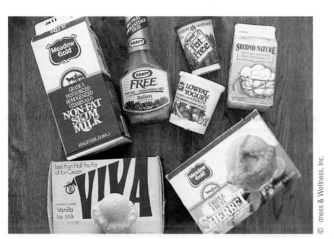

As long as the number of servings are not increased, substituting low-fat/cholesterol-free/trans-fat-free products for high-fat products in the diet significantly decreases the risk for disease.

The best prescription for controlling blood lipids is the combination of a healthy diet, a sound aerobic exercise program, and weight control. If this does not work, a physician can recommend appropriate drug therapies based upon a blood test to analyze the various subcategories of lipoproteins.

The NCEP guidelines recommend that people consider drug therapy if, after 6 months on a diet low in cholesterol and trans fat and saturated fat, cholesterol remains unacceptably high. An unacceptable level is an LDL cholesterol above 190 mg/dL for individuals with fewer than two risk factors and no signs of heart disease. For individuals with more than two risk factors and with a history of heart disease, LDL cholesterol above 160 mg/dL is unacceptable.

**Elevated Triglycerides** Triglycerides, also known as free fatty acids, make up most of the fat in our diet and most of the fat that circulates in the blood. In combination with cholesterol, triglycerides speed up formation of

## Behavior Modification Planning

### DIETARY GUIDELINES TO LOWER LDL CHOLESTEROL

I PLAN TO / I DID IT

- ❏ ❏ Consume between 25 and 38 grams of fiber daily, including a minimum of 10 grams of soluble fiber (good sources are oats, fruits, barley, legumes, and psyllium).
- ❏ ❏ Increase consumption of vegetables, fruits, whole grains, and beans.
- ❏ ❏ Do not consume more than 200 mg of dietary cholesterol a day.
- ❏ ❏ Consume red meats (3 ounces per serving) fewer than 3 times per week and no organ meats (such as liver and kidneys).
- ❏ ❏ Do not eat commercially baked foods.
- ❏ ❏ Avoid foods that contain trans fatty acids, hydrogenated fat, or partially hydrogenated vegetable oil.
- ❏ ❏ Increase intake of omega-3 fatty acids (see Chapter 3) by eating two to three omega-3-rich fish meals per week.
- ❏ ❏ Consume 25 grams of soy protein a day.
- ❏ ❏ Drink low-fat milk (1 percent or less fat, preferably) and use low-fat dairy products.
- ❏ ❏ Do not use coconut oil, palm oil, or cocoa butter.
- ❏ ❏ Limit egg consumption to fewer than three eggs per week (this is for people with high cholesterol only; others may consume eggs in moderation).
- ❏ ❏ Use margarines and salad dressings that contain stanol ester instead of butter and regular margarine.
- ❏ ❏ Bake, broil, grill, poach, or steam food instead of frying.
- ❏ ❏ Refrigerate cooked meat before adding to other dishes. Remove fat hardened in the refrigerator before mixing the meat with other foods.
- ❏ ❏ Avoid fatty sauces made with butter, cream, or cheese.
- ❏ ❏ Maintain recommended body weight.

### Try It

Dietary guidelines for health and wellness were thoroughly discussed in Chapter 3, "Nutrition for Wellness." How have your dietary habits changed since studying these guidelines, and how well do they support the above recommendations to lower LDL cholesterol?

plaque in the arteries. Triglycerides are carried in the bloodstream primarily by VLDLs and chylomicrons.

Although they are found in poultry skin, lunch meats, and shellfish, these fatty acids are manufactured mainly in the liver from refined sugars, starches, and alcohol. High intake of alcohol and sugars (honey and fruit juices included) significantly raises triglyceride levels.

To lower triglycerides, avoid pastries, candies, soft drinks, fruit juices, white bread, pasta, and alcohol. In addition, cutting down on overall fat consumption, quitting smoking, reducing weight (if overweight), and doing aerobic exercise are helpful measures. Omega-3 fatty acids also help, but doses higher than those found in fish are required. The AHA recommends 2 to 4 grams of fish oil daily under a physician's supervision.

The desirable blood triglyceride level is less than 150 mg/dL (see Table 11.6). For people with cardiovascular problems, this level should be below 100 mg/dL. Levels above 1,000 mg/dL pose an immediate risk for potentially fatal sudden inflammation of the pancreas.

**LDL Phenotype B** Some people consistently have slightly elevated triglyceride levels (above 140 mg/dL) and HDL cholesterol levels below 35 mg/dL. About 80 percent of these people have a genetic condition called LDL phenotype B. Although the blood lipids may not be notably high, these people are at higher risk for atherosclerosis and CHD.

## Critical Thinking

Are you aware of your blood lipid profile? If not, what is keeping you from getting a blood chemistry test? What are the benefits of having it done now rather than later in life?

**Cholesterol-Lowering Medications** Effective medications are available to treat elevated cholesterol and triglycerides. Most notable among them are the statins (Lipitor®, Mevacor®, Pravachol®, Lescol®, and Zocor®), which can lower cholesterol by up to 60 percent in 2 to 3 months. Statins slow down cholesterol production and

increase the liver's ability to remove blood cholesterol. They also decrease triglycerides and produce a small increase in HDL levels. The drug Tricor® is commonly used to lower triglycerides.

In general, it is better to lower LDL cholesterol without medication, because drugs often cause undesirable side effects. Many people with heart disease must take cholesterol-lowering medication, but medication is best combined with lifestyle changes to augment the cholesterol-lowering effect. For example, when Zocor was taken alone over 3 months, LDL cholesterol decreased by 30 percent; but when a Mediterranean diet was adopted in combination with Zocor therapy, LDL cholesterol decreased by 41 percent.[17]

Other drugs effective in reducing LDL cholesterol are bile acid sequestrants, which bind the cholesterol found in bile acids. Cholesterol subsequently is excreted in the stools. These drugs often are used in combination with statin drugs.

High dosages (1.5 to 3 grams per day) of nicotinic acid or niacin (a B vitamin) also help lower LDL cholesterol, Lp(a), and triglycerides and increase HDL cholesterol (change $HDL_3$ to $HDL_2$). Niacin in combination with some of the aforementioned drugs also exerts positive effects on IDL and pattern size. A fourth group of drugs, known as fibrates, is used primarily to lower triglycerides.

**Elevated Homocysteine** Clinical data indicating that many heart attack and stroke victims have normal cholesterol levels have led researchers to look for other risk factors that may contribute to atherosclerosis. Although it is not a blood lipid, one of these factors is a high concentration of the amino acid **homocysteine** in the blood. It is thought to enhance the formation of plaque and the subsequent blockage of arteries.

The body uses homocysteine to help build proteins and carry out cellular metabolism. It is an intermediate amino acid in the interconversion of two other amino acids—methionine and cysteine. This interconversion requires the B vitamin folate (folic acid) and vitamins $B_6$ and $B_{12}$. Typically, homocysteine is metabolized rapidly, so it does not accumulate in the blood or damage the arteries. Still, many people have high blood levels of homocysteine. This might result from either a genetic inability to metabolize homocysteine or a deficiency in the vitamins required for its conversion.

Homocysteine typically is measured in micromoles per liter (µmol/L). Guidelines to interpret homocysteine levels are provided in Table 11.7. A 10-year follow-up study of people with high homocysteine levels showed that those individuals with a level above 14.25 µmol/L had almost twice the risk for stroke compared with individuals whose level was below 9.25 µmol/L.[18]

### TABLE 11.6 Triglycerides Guidelines

| Amount | Rating |
| --- | --- |
| <150 mg/dL | Desirable |
| 150–199 mg/dL | Borderline high |
| 200–499 mg/dL | High |
| ≥500 mg/dL | Very high |

*Source:* National Heart, Lung and Blood Institute.

**Homocysteine** An amino acid that, when allowed to accumulate in the blood, may lead to plaque formation and blockage of arteries.

**TABLE 11.7** Homocysteine Guidelines

| Level | Rating |
|---|---|
| <9.0 μmol/L | Desirable |
| 9–12 μmol/L | Mild elevation |
| 13–15 μmol/L | Elevated |
| >15 μmol/L | Extreme elevation |

Adapted from K. S. McCully, "What You Must Know Now About Homocysteine," *Bottom Line/Health* 18 (January 2004): 7–9.

Homocysteine accumulation is theorized to be toxic because it may:

1. Cause damage to the inner lining of the arteries (the initial step in the process of atherosclerosis)

2. Stimulate the proliferation of cells that contribute to plaque formation

3. Encourage clotting, which could completely obstruct an artery and lead to a heart attack or stroke

Keeping homocysteine from accumulating in the blood seems to be as simple as eating the recommended daily servings of vegetables, fruits, grains, and some meat and legumes. Five servings of fruits and vegetables daily can provide sufficient levels of folate and vitamin $B_6$ to remove

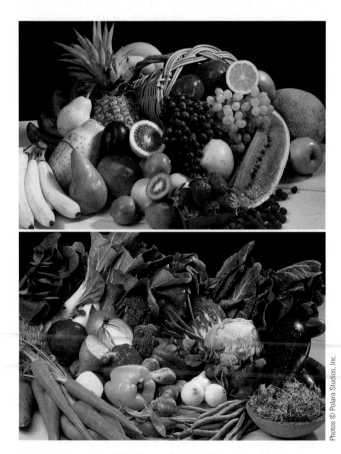

Ample amounts of fruits and vegetables provide the necessary nutrients to keep homocysteine from causing heart disease or stroke.

and clear homocysteine from the blood. Vitamin $B_{12}$ is found primarily in animal flesh and animal products. Vitamin $B_{12}$ deficiency is rarely a problem because 1 cup of milk or an egg provides the daily requirement. The body also recycles most of this vitamin; therefore, a deficiency takes years to develop. People who consume five servings of fruits and vegetables daily are unlikely to derive extra benefits from a vitamin-B-complex supplement.

Increasing evidence that folate can prevent heart attacks has led to the recommendation that people consume 400 mcg per day—obtainable from five daily servings of fruits and vegetables. Unfortunately, estimates indicate that more than 80 percent of Americans do not get 400 daily mcg of folate (adequate folate intake also is critical for women of childbearing age to prevent birth defects).

**Inflammation** In addition to homocysteine, scientists are looking at inflammation as a major risk factor for heart attacks. Low-grade inflammation can occur in a variety of places throughout the body. For years it has been known that inflammation plays a role in CHD and that inflammation hidden deep in the body is a common trigger of heart attacks, even when cholesterol levels are normal or low and arterial plaque is minimal.

To evaluate ongoing inflammation in the body, physicians have turned to **C-reactive protein (CRP)**, whose levels in the blood increase with inflammation. Individuals with elevated CRP are more prone to cardiovascular events, even in the absence of elevated LDL cholesterol. The evidence shows that CRP blood levels elevate years before a first heart attack or stroke and that individuals with elevated CRP have twice the risk for a heart attack. This risk is even higher in people with both elevated CRP and cholesterol, resulting in an almost ninefold increase in risk (see Figure 11.7).

Because high CRP levels might be a better predictor of future heart attacks than high cholesterol alone, a test

**FIGURE 11.7** Relationships between C-reactive protein, cholesterol, and risk for cardiovascular disease.

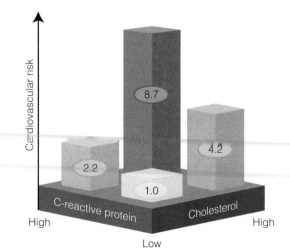

*Source:* Adapted from P. Libby, P. M. Ridker, and A. Maseri, "Inflammation and Atherosclerosis," *Circulation* 105 (2002): 1135–1143.

**TABLE 11.8** High-Sensitivity CRP Guidelines

| Amount | Rating |
| --- | --- |
| <1 mg/L | Low risk |
| 1–3 mg/L | Average risk |
| >3 mg/L | High risk |

*Source:* T.A. Pearson et al., "Markers of Inflammation and Cardiovascular Disease," *Circulation* 107 (2003): 499–511.

**TABLE 11.9** Blood Glucose Guidelines

| Amount | Rating |
| --- | --- |
| ≤100 mg/dL | Normal |
| 101–125 mg/dL | Pre-diabetes |
| ≥126 mg/dL | Diabetes* |

*Confirmed by two tests on different days.

known as high-sensitivity CRP (hs-CRP), which measures inflammation in the blood vessels, is commonly used. The term "high-sensitivity" was derived from the test's capability to detect small amounts of CRP in the blood. Hs-CRP test results provide a good measure of the probability of plaque rupturing within the arterial wall.

The two main types of plaque are soft and hard. Soft plaque is the most likely to rupture. Ruptured plaque releases clots into the bloodstream that can lead to a heart attack or a stroke. Other evidence has linked high CRP levels to high blood pressure and colon cancer.

Excessive intake of alcohol and high-protein diets also increase CRP. Evidence further indicates that high-fat fast food increases CRP levels for several hours following the meal.[19] And cooking meat and poultry at high temperatures creates damaged proteins called *advanced glycosylation end products* (AGEs), which trigger inflammation. Obesity increases inflammation. With weight loss, CRP levels decrease proportional to the amount of fat lost.

An hs-CRP test is relatively inexpensive and is highly recommended for individuals at risk for heart attack. A level above 2 mg/L appears to be a better predictor of a heart attack than an LDL cholesterol level above 130 mg/dL.[20] General guidelines for hs-CRP levels are given in Table 11.8.

A weakness of the hs-CRP test is that it does not detect differences between acute and chronic inflammation, and results may not be stable from day to day. An acute inflammation, for example, could be the result of a pulled muscle or a passing cold. It is chronic inflammation that increases heart disease risk. Thus, a new test that specifically detects chronic inflammation, lipoprotein phospholipase A2 (Lp-PLA2), may soon replace the hs-CRP test.

CRP levels decrease with statin drugs, which also lower cholesterol and reduce inflammation. Exercise, weight loss, proper nutrition, and not smoking are helpful in reducing hs-CRP.[21] Omega-3 fatty acids (found in salmon, tuna, and mackerel fish) inhibit proteins that cause inflammation. Aspirin therapy also helps by controlling inflammation.

## Diabetes

**Diabetes mellitus** is a condition in which blood glucose is unable to enter the cells because the pancreas totally stops producing **insulin**, or it does not produce enough to meet the body's needs, or the cells develop **insulin resistance**. The role of insulin is to "unlock" the cells and escort glucose into them.

As of 2006, diabetes affected about 20 million people in the United States, and about 1 million new cases are diagnosed each year. Between 1980 and 2003, the prevalence of diabetes more than doubled. The National Institutes of Health estimate the cost of diabetes to be in excess of $100 billion annually.

The incidence of cardiovascular disease and death in the diabetic population is quite high. Two of three people with diabetes will die from cardiovascular disease. People with chronically elevated blood glucose levels may have problems metabolizing fats, which can make them more susceptible to atherosclerosis, CHD, heart attacks, high blood pressure, and stroke. Diabetes is also marked by lower HDL cholesterol and higher triglyceride levels.

Further, chronic high blood sugar can lead to stroke, nerve damage, vision loss, kidney damage, sexual dysfunction, and decreased immune function (making the individual more susceptible to infections). Compared with nondiabetic people, those with diabetes are 4 times more likely to become blind and 20 times more likely to develop kidney failure. Nerve damage in the lower extremities decreases the person's awareness of injury and infection, and a small, untreated sore can result in severe infection and gangrene, which can even lead to an amputation.

An 8-hour fasting blood glucose level above 125 mg/dL on two separate tests confirms a diagnosis of diabetes (see Table 11.9). A level of 126 or higher should be brought to the attention of a physician.

**Types of Diabetes** Diabetes is of two types: **type 1**, or insulin-dependent diabetes mellitus (IDDM), and **type 2**,

**C-reactive protein (CRP)** A protein whose blood levels increase with inflammation, at times hidden deep in the body; elevation of this protein is an indicator of potential cardiovascular events.

**Diabetes mellitus** A disease in which the body doesn't produce or utilize insulin properly.

**Insulin** A hormone secreted by the pancreas; essential for proper metabolism of blood glucose (sugar) and maintenance of blood glucose level.

**Insulin resistance** Inability of the cells to respond appropriately to insulin.

**Type 1 diabetes** Insulin-dependent diabetes mellitus (IDDM), a condition in which the pancreas produces little or no insulin; also known as juvenile diabetes.

**Type 2 diabetes** Non-insulin-dependent diabetes mellitus (NIDDM), a condition in which insulin is not processed properly; also known as adult-onset diabetes.

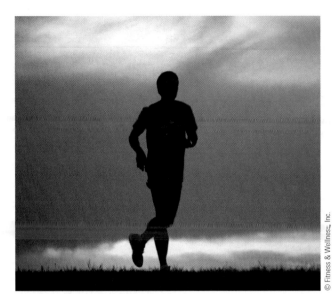

Habitual aerobic exercise increases insulin sensitivity and decreases risk for diabetes.

or non-insulin-dependent diabetes mellitus (NIDDM). Type 1 has also been called "juvenile diabetes," because it is found mainly in young people. With type 1, the pancreas produces little or no insulin. With type 2, either the pancreas does not produce sufficient insulin or it produces adequate amounts but the cells become insulin resistant, thereby keeping glucose from entering them. Type 2 accounts for 90 to 95 percent of all cases of diabetes.

Although diabetes has a genetic predisposition, 60 to 80 percent of type 2 diabetes is related closely to overeating, obesity, and lack of physical activity. Type 2 diabetes, once limited primarily to overweight adults, now accounts for almost half of the new cases diagnosed in children. According to the CDC, 1 in 3 children born in the United States today will develop diabetes.

More than 80 percent of all people with type 2 diabetes are overweight or have a history of excessive weight. In most cases, this condition can be corrected through regular exercise, a special diet, and weight loss.

Aerobic exercise helps prevent type 2 diabetes. The protective effect is even greater in those with risk factors such as obesity, high blood pressure, and family propensity. The preventive effect is attributed to less body fat and to better sugar and fat metabolism resulting from the regular exercise program. At 3,500 calories of energy expenditure per week through exercise, the risk is cut in half versus that of a sedentary lifestyle.

Both moderate- and vigorous-intensity physical activity are associated with increased insulin sensitivity and decreased risk for diabetes. The key to increase and maintain proper insulin sensitivity is regularity of the exercise program. Failing to maintain habitual physical activity voids these benefits. Thus, a simple aerobic exercise program (walking, cycling, or swimming four or five times per week) often is prescribed because it increases the body's sensitivity to insulin. Exercise guidelines for diabetic patients are discussed in detail in Chapter 9, page 330.

## Behavior Modification Planning

### GUIDELINES TO PREVENT AND MANAGE TYPE 2 DIABETES

Experts agree that the following healthy lifestyle strategies are effective in type 2 diabetes management:

| I PLAN TO | I DID IT | |
|---|---|---|
| ☐ | ☐ | Follow an overall healthful dietary pattern that includes |
| ☐ | ☐ | A minimum of five daily servings of fruits and vegetables |

- At least three daily servings of whole grains
- Consumption of at least two 3-oz servings of fatty fish per week
- A few small portions of nuts each week
- Skim milk and low-fat dairy products in your daily diet

| | | |
|---|---|---|
| ☐ | ☐ | Maintain recommended body weight |
| ☐ | ☐ | Increase daily physical activity (to at least 30 minutes of daily moderate-intensity activity) |

### Try It

Review your Behavior Change Plan and your Online Journal or class notebook. Are you following these guidelines? Are there changes you need to make to your Behavior Change Plan to bring yourself into closer compliance?

A diet high in complex carbohydrates (unrefined whole grains) and water-soluble fibers (found in fruits, vegetables, oats, beans, and psyllium) low in saturated fat and low in sugar is helpful in treating diabetes. Aggressive weight loss, especially if combined with exercise, often allows diabetic patients to normalize their blood sugar level without the use of medication.

Recent evidence also suggests that consumption of low-fat dairy products lowers the risk for type 2 diabetes. Research on more than 41,000 men showed that those who consumed the most dairy products had a 23 percent lower incidence of the disease. Furthermore, each additional daily serving of dairy products was associated with a 9 percent decrease in type 2 diabetes risk.[22]

**Glycemic Index** Although complex carbohydrates are recommended in the diet, people with diabetes need to pay careful attention to the glycemic index (explained in

Chapter 5 and detailed there in Table 5.1). Refined and starchy foods (small-particle carbohydrates, which are quickly digested) rank high in the glycemic index, whereas grains, fruits, and vegetables are low-glycemic foods.

Foods high in the glycemic index cause a rapid increase in blood sugar. A diet that includes many high-glycemic foods increases the risk for cardiovascular disease in people with high insulin resistance and **glucose intolerance**.[23] Combining a moderate amount of high-glycemic foods with low-glycemic foods or with some fat and protein, however, can bring down the average index.

**A1C Test** Individuals who have high blood glucose levels should consult a physician to decide on the best treatment. They also might obtain information about the test for hemoglobin A1c (also called HbA1c), which measures the amount of glucose that has been in a person's blood over the last 3 months. Blood glucose can become attached to hemoglobin in the red blood cells. Once attached, it remains there for the life of the red blood cell, which is about 3 months. The higher the blood glucose, the higher the concentration of glucose in the red blood cells. Results of this test are given in percentages.

The HbA1c goal for diabetic patients is to keep it under 7 percent. At this level and below, diabetic patients have a lower risk for developing diabetes-related problems of the eyes, kidneys, and nerves. Because the test tells a person how well blood glucose has been controlled over the last 3 months, a change in treatment is almost always recommended if the HbA1c results are above 8 percent. All people with type 2 diabetes should have an HbA1c test twice per year.

**Metabolic Syndrome** As the cells resist the actions of insulin, the pancreas releases even more insulin in an attempt to keep blood glucose from rising. A chronic rise in insulin seems to trigger a series of abnormalities referred to as the **metabolic syndrome.** These abnormal conditions include abdominal obesity, elevated blood pressure, high blood glucose, low HDL cholesterol, high triglycerides, and an increased blood-clotting mechanism. All of these conditions increase the risk for CHD and other diabetes-related conditions (blindness, infection, nerve damage, kidney failure). Approximately 50 million Americans are afflicted with this condition.

People with metabolic syndrome have an abnormal insulin response to carbohydrates, in particular high-glycemic foods. Research on metabolic syndrome indicates that a low-fat, high-carbohydrate diet may not be the best for preventing CHD and actually could increase the risk for the disease in individuals with high insulin resistance and glucose intolerance. It might be best for these people to distribute daily caloric intake so that 45 percent of the calories are derived from carbohydrates (primarily low-glycemic), 40 percent from fat, and 15 percent from protein.[24] Of the 40 percent fat calories, most of the fat should come from mono- and polyunsaturated fats and less than 7 percent from saturated fat.

Individuals with metabolic syndrome also benefit from weight loss (if overweight), exercise, and smoking cessation.

## Diagnosis of Metabolic Syndrome

| Components | Men | Women |
|---|---|---|
| Waist circumference | >40 inches | >35 inches |
| Blood pressure | >130/85 mm Hg | >130/85 mm Hg |
| Fasting blood glucose | >110 mg/dL | >110 mg/dL |
| Fasting HDL cholesterol | <40 mg/dL | <50 mg/dL |
| Fasting triglycerides | >150 mg/dL | >150 mg/dL |

Note: Metabolic syndrome is identified by the presence of at least three of the above components.

Insulin resistance drops by about 40 percent in overweight people who lose 20 pounds. Forty-five minutes of daily aerobic exercise enhances insulin efficiency by 25 percent. Quitting smoking also decreases insulin resistance.

**Hypertension** Some 60,000 miles of blood vessels run through the human body. As the heart forces the blood through these vessels, the fluid is under pressure. **Blood pressure** is measured in milliliters of mercury (mm Hg), usually expressed in two numbers: **Systolic blood pressure** is the higher number, and **diastolic blood pressure** is the lower number. Ideal blood pressure is 120/80 or lower.

**Standards** Statistical evidence indicates that damage to the arteries starts at blood pressures above 120/80. The risk for cardiovascular disease doubles with each increment of 20/10, starting with a blood pressure of 115/75.[25] All blood pressures above 140/90 are considered to be **hypertension** (see Table 11.10). Blood pressures ranging from 120/80 to 139/89 are referred to as prehypertension.

---

**Glucose intolerance** A condition characterized by slightly elevated blood glucose levels.

**Metabolic syndrome** An array of metabolic abnormalities that contribute to the development of atherosclerosis triggered by insulin resistance. These conditions include low HDL-cholesterol, high triglycerides, high blood pressure, and an increased blood-clotting mechanism.

**Blood pressure** A measure of the force exerted against the walls of the vessels by the blood flowing through them.

**Systolic blood pressure** Pressure exerted by blood against walls of arteries during forceful contraction (systole) of the heart; higher of the two numbers in blood pressure readings.

**Diastolic blood pressure** Pressure exerted by blood against walls of arteries during relaxation phase (diastole) of the heart; lower of the two numbers in blood pressure readings.

**Hypertension** Chronically elevated blood pressure.

**TABLE 11.10 Blood Pressure Guidelines (mm Hg)**

| Rating | Systolic | Diastolic |
|---|---|---|
| Normal | <120 | <80 |
| Prehypertension | 121–139 | 81–89 |
| Stage 1 hypertension | 140–159 | 90–99 |
| Stage 2 hypertension | ≥160 | ≥100 |

*Source:* National High Blood Pressure Education Program.

Based on estimates released in 2004, approximately 1 in every 3 adults is hypertensive, up from 1 in 4 a decade earlier. The incidence is higher among African Americans—in fact, it is among the highest in the world. Approximately 30 percent and 20 percent of all deaths in African American men and women, respectively, may be caused by high blood pressure.

Although the threshold for hypertension has been set at 140/90, many experts believe that the lower the blood pressure, the better. Even if the pressure is around 90/50, as long as that person does not have any symptoms of **hypotension**, he or she need not be concerned. Typical symptoms of hypotension are dizziness, lightheadedness, and fainting.

Blood pressure also may fluctuate during a regular day. Many factors affect blood pressure, and one single reading may not be a true indicator of the real pressure. For example, physical activity and stress increase blood pressure, and rest and relaxation decrease blood pressure. Consequently, several measurements should be taken before diagnosing high blood pressure.

**Incidence and Pathology** Based on estimates by the AHA, 73 million Americans are hypertensive (Figure 11.8), and more than 54,000 Americans die each year as a result of high blood pressure. The dramatic increase in hypertension seems to be linked to the growing epidemic of obesity and the aging of the U.S. population. Unless appropriate and healthy lifestyle strategies are implemented, people who do not have high blood pressure at age 55 have a 90 percent chance of developing it at some point in their lives.[26]

Hypertension has been referred to as "the silent killer." It does not hurt; it does not make you feel sick; and unless you check it, years may go by before you even realize you have a problem. High blood pressure is a risk factor for CHD, congestive heart failure, stroke, kidney failure, and osteoporosis.

All inner walls of arteries are lined by a layer of smooth endothelial cells. Blood lipids cannot penetrate the healthy lining and start to build up on the walls unless the cells are damaged. High blood pressure is thought to be a leading contributor to destruction of this lining. As blood pressure rises, so does the risk for atherosclerosis. The higher the pressure, the greater is the damage to the arterial wall, making the vessels susceptible to fat deposits, espe-

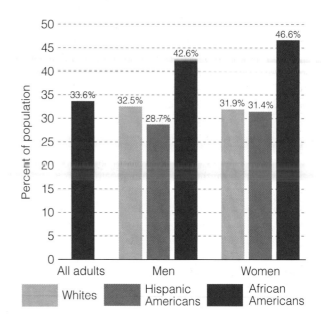

**FIGURE 11.8  Incidence of high blood pressure in the United States, 2007.**

*Source:* American Heart Association, *Heart Disease and Stroke Statistics: 2008 Update at-a-Glance* (Dallas: AHA, 2007).

cially if serum cholesterol is also high. Blockage of the coronary vessels decreases blood supply to the heart muscle and can lead to heart attacks. When brain arteries are involved, a stroke may follow.

A clear example of the connection between high blood pressure and atherosclerosis can be seen by comparing blood vessels in the human body. Even when atherosclerosis is present throughout major arteries, fatty plaques rarely are seen in the pulmonary artery, which goes from the right part of the heart to the lungs. The pressure in this artery normally is below 40 mm Hg, and at such a low pressure, significant deposits do not occur. This is one of the reasons that people with low blood pressure have a lower incidence of cardiovascular disease.

Constantly elevated blood pressure also causes the heart to work much harder. At first the heart does well, but in time this continual strain produces an enlarged heart, followed by congestive heart failure. Furthermore, high blood pressure damages blood vessels to the kidneys and eyes, which can result in kidney failure and loss of vision.

**Treatment** Of all hypertension, 90 percent has no definite cause. Called "essential hypertension," it is treatable. Aerobic exercise, weight reduction, a low-salt/low-fat and high-potassium/high-calcium diet, lower alcohol and caffeine intake, smoking cessation, stress management, and antihypertensive medication all have been used effectively to treat essential hypertension.

The remaining 10 percent of hypertensive cases are caused by pathological conditions, such as narrowing of the kidney arteries, glomerulonephritis (a kidney disease), tumors of the adrenal glands, and narrowing of the aortic

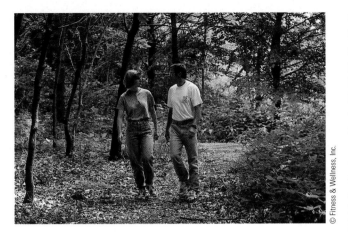

Regular physical activity is an important way to maintain healthy blood pressure.

artery. With this type of hypertension, the pathological cause has to be treated before the blood pressure problem can be corrected.

Antihypertensive medicines often are the first choice of treatment, but they produce many side effects. These include lethargy, sleepiness, sexual difficulties, higher blood cholesterol and glucose levels, lower potassium levels, and elevated uric acid levels. A physician may end up treating these side effects as much as the hypertension itself. Because of the many side effects, about half of the patients stop taking the medication within the first year of treatment.

Another factor contributing to elevated blood pressure is too much sodium in the diet (salt, or sodium chloride, contains approximately 40 percent sodium). With a high sodium intake, the body retains more water, which increases the blood volume and, in turn, drives up the pressure. High intake of potassium seems to regulate water retention and lower the pressure slightly. According to the Institute of Medicine of the National Academy of Sciences, we need to consume at least 4,700 mg of potassium per day. Most Americans get only half that amount.[27] Foods high in potassium include vegetables (especially leafy green), citrus fruit, dairy products, fish, beans, and nuts.

## Critical Thinking

Do you know what your most recent blood pressure reading was, and did you know at the time what the numbers meant? How would you react if your doctor were to instruct you to take blood pressure medication?

Although sodium is essential for normal body functions, the body can function with as little as 200 mg, or a tenth of a teaspoon, daily. Even under strenuous conditions in jobs and sports that incite heavy perspiration, the amount of sodium required is seldom more than 3,000 mg per day. Yet, sodium intake in the typical U.S. diet ranges between 3,100 and 4,700 mg per day in men and 2,300 to 3,100 mg in women (the average daily intake is lower in women because they tend to eat fewer calories than men, not because they limit their sodium intake).

A government report indicated that to either prevent or postpone the onset of hypertension and to help control existing hypertension, we should consume even less sodium than previously recommended.[28] These new guidelines are provided in Table 11.11. The upper limit has been set at 2,300 mg per day. Among North Americans, about 95 percent of men and 75 percent of women exceed this limit. Where does all the sodium come from? Part of the answer is given in Table 11.12. People do not realize the amount of sodium in various foods (the list in Table 11.12 does not include salt added at the table). Unfortunately, most of the sodium in our diets comes from prepared foods, over whose ingredients the consumer has no control.

When treating high blood pressure (unless it is extremely high), before recommending medication, many sports medicine physicians suggest a combination of aerobic exercise, weight loss, and less sodium in the diet. In most instances, this treatment brings blood pressure under control.

The relative risk for mortality based on blood pressure and fitness levels is similar to that of physical fitness and cholesterol. In men and women alike, the relative risk for early mortality is lower in fit people with high systolic blood pressure (140 mm Hg or higher) than in unfit people with a healthy systolic blood pressure (120 mm Hg or lower).[29]

The link between hypertension and obesity seems to be quite strong. Blood volume increases with excess body fat, and each additional pound of fat requires an estimated extra mile of blood vessels to feed this tissue. Furthermore, blood capillaries are constricted by the adipose tissues because these vessels run through them. As a result, the heart muscle must work harder to pump the blood through a longer, constricted network of blood vessels.

Regular physical activity plays a large role in managing blood pressure. On the average, fit individuals have a lower blood pressure than unfit people. Aerobic exercise of moderate intensity supplemented by strength training is recommended for individuals with high blood pressure.[30]

Comprehensive reviews of the effects of aerobic exercise on blood pressure have found that in general, an individual can expect exercise-induced reductions of approximately 4 to 5 mm Hg in resting systolic blood pressure and 3 to 4 mm Hg in resting diastolic blood pressure.[31]

**Hypotension** Low blood pressure.

**TABLE 11.11** Daily Sodium Recommendations for the Prevention and Treatment of High Blood Pressure

| Age | Sodium (mg/day) |
| --- | --- |
| 19–50 | 1,500 |
| 51–70 | 1,300 |
| >70 | 1,200 |

Although these reductions do not seem large, a decrease of about 5 mm Hg in resting diastolic blood pressure has been associated with a 40 percent decrease in the risk for stroke and a 15 percent reduction in the risk for CHD.[32] Even in the absence of any decrease in resting blood pressure, hypertensive individuals who exercise have a lower risk for all-cause mortality compared with normotensive/sedentary individuals. The research data also show that exercise, not weight loss, is the major contributor to the lower blood pressure of exercisers. If they discontinue aerobic exercise, they do not maintain these changes.

Another extensive review of research studies on the effects of at least 4 weeks of strength training on resting blood pressure yielded similar results.[33] Both systolic and diastolic blood pressures decreased by an average of 3 mm Hg. Participants in these studies, however, were primarily individuals with normal blood pressure. Of greater significance, the results showed that strength training did not cause an increase in resting blood pressure. More research remains to be done on hypertensive subjects.

The effects of long-term participation in exercise are apparently much more remarkable. An 18-year follow-up study on exercising and nonexercising subjects showed much lower blood pressures in the active group.[34] The exercise group had an average resting blood pressure of 120/78 compared with 150/90 for the nonexercise group (see Table 11.13).

Aerobic exercise programs for hypertensive patients should be of moderate intensity. Training at 40 to 60 percent intensity seems to have the same effect as training at 70 percent in lowering blood pressure. High-intensity training (above 70 percent) in hypertensive patients may not lower the blood pressure as much as moderate-intensity exercise. Even so, a person may be better off being highly fit and having high blood pressure than being unfit and having low blood pressure. The death rates for unfit individuals with low systolic blood pressure are much higher than for highly fit people with high systolic blood pressure. Strength training for hypertensive individuals calls for a minimum of one set of 10 to 15 repetitions that elicit a "somewhat hard" perceived exertion rating, using eight to ten multi-joint exercises two or three times per week.

Most important is a preventive approach. Keeping blood pressure under control is easier than trying to bring it down once it is high. Regardless of your blood pressure history, high or low, you should have it checked routinely. To keep your blood pressure as low as possible, exercise

**TABLE 11.12** Sodium and Potassium Levels of Selected Foods

| Food | Serving Size | Sodium (mg) | Potassium (mg) |
| --- | --- | --- | --- |
| Apple | 1 med | 1 | 102 |
| Asparagus | 1 cup | 2 | 330 |
| Avocado | ½ | 4 | 680 |
| Banana | 1 med | 1 | 440 |
| Beans | | | |
| Kidney (canned) | ½ cup | 436 | 330 |
| Lima (cooked) | ½ cup | 2 | 478 |
| Pinto (cooked) | ½ cup | 2 | 398 |
| Refried (canned) | ½ cup | 377 | 336 |
| Bologna | 3 oz | 1,107 | 133 |
| Bouillon cube | 1 | 960 | 4 |
| Cantaloupe | ¼ | 17 | 341 |
| Carrot (raw) | 1 | 34 | 225 |
| Cheese | | | |
| American | 2 oz | 614 | 93 |
| Cheddar | 2 oz | 342 | 56 |
| Muenster | 2 oz | 356 | 77 |
| Parmesan | 2 oz | 1,056 | 53 |
| Swiss | 2 oz | 148 | 64 |
| Chicken (light meat) | 6 oz | 108 | 700 |
| Corn (natural) | ½ up | 3 | 136 |
| Corn (canned) | ½ cup | 195 | 80 |
| Frankfurter | 1 | 627 | 136 |
| Haddock | 6 oz | 300 | 594 |
| Hamburger (reg) | 1 | 500 | 321 |
| Milk (whole) | 1 cup | 120 | 351 |
| Milk (skim) | 1 cup | 126 | 406 |
| Nuts | | | |
| Brazil | 1 nut | 1 | 120 |
| Walnuts | ½ cup | 1 | 327 |
| Orange | 1 med | 1 | 263 |
| Peach | 1 med | 2 | 308 |
| Peas (canned) | ½ cup | 200 | 82 |
| Pizza (cheese—14" diam.) | ⅛ | 456 | 85 |
| Potato | 1 med | 6 | 763 |
| Salami | 3 oz | 1,047 | 170 |
| Salmon (baked) | 4 oz | 75 | 424 |
| Salmon (canned) | 6 oz | 198 | 756 |
| Salt | 1 tsp | 2,132 | 0 |
| Soups | | | |
| Chicken Noodle | 1 cup | 979 | 55 |
| Cream of Mushroom | 1 cup | 955 | 98 |
| Vegetable Beef | 1 cup | 1,046 | 162 |
| Soy sauce | 1 tsp | 1,123 | 22 |
| Spaghetti (tomato sauce and cheese) | 6 oz | 648 | 276 |
| Spinach (cooked, fresh) | 1 cup | 126 | 838 |
| Strawberries | 1 cup | 1 | 244 |
| Tomato (raw) | 1 med | 3 | 444 |
| Tuna (drained) | 3 oz | 38 | 255 |

## Behavior Modification Planning

### GUIDELINES TO STOP HYPERTENSION

☐ I PLAN TO   ☐ I DID IT

☐ ☐ Participate in a moderate-intensity aerobic exercise program (50% intensity) for 30 to 45 minutes 5 to 7 times per week.

☐ ☐ Participate in a moderate-resistance strength-training program (use 12 to 15 repetitions to near-fatigue on each set) 2 times per week (seek your physician's approval and advice for this program).

☐ ☐ Lose weight if you are above recommended body weight.

☐ ☐ Eat less salt- and sodium-containing foods.

☐ ☐ Do not smoke cigarettes or use tobacco in any other form.

☐ ☐ Practice stress management.

☐ ☐ Do not consume more than two alcoholic beverages a day if you are a man or one if you are a woman.

☐ ☐ Consume more potassium-rich foods.

☐ ☐ Follow the Dietary Approach to Stop Hypertension (DASH) diet:

| Food Group | Servings |
|---|---|
| Whole grains | 7–8 per day |
| Fruits and vegetables | 8–10 per day |
| Low-fat or fat-free dairy foods | 2–13 per day |
| Meat, poultry, or fish* | 2 or less per day |
| Beans, peas, nuts, or seeds | 4–15 *per week* |
| Fats and oils | 2–3 servings per day |
| Snacks and sweets | 4–5 *per week* |

*Less than 3 ounces per serving

### Try It

In your Online Journal or class notebook, make a comparison of the goals of the DASH diet and Dietary Guidelines for Americans. How do they differ?

regularly, lose excess weight, eat less salt and sodium-containing foods, do not smoke, practice stress management, do not consume more than two alcoholic beverages a day if you are a man, or one if you are a woman, and

**TABLE 11.13** Effects of Long-Term (14–18 years) Aerobic Exercise on Resting Blood Pressure

| | Initial | Final |
|---|---|---|
| **Exercise Group** | | |
| Age | 44.6 | 68.0 |
| Blood Pressure | 120/79 | 120/78 |
| **Non-Exercise Group** | | |
| Age | 51.6 | 69.7 |
| Blood Pressure | 135/85 | 150/90 |

NOTE: The aerobic exercise program consisted of an average of four training sessions per week, each 66 minutes long, at about 76 percent of heart rate reserve.
Based on data from F. W. Kash, J. L. Boyer, S. P. Van Camp, L. S. Verity, and J. P. Wallace, "The Effect of Physical Activity on Aerobic Power in Older Men (A Longitudinal Study)," *The Physician and Sports Medicine* 18, no. 4 (1990): 73–83.

consume more potassium-rich foods such as potatoes, bananas, orange juice, cantaloupe, tomatoes, and beans (see the box "Guidelines to Stop Hypertension"). The Dietary Approach to Stop Hypertension (DASH)—which emphasizes fruits, vegetables, grains, and dairy products—lowers systolic blood pressure by 11 points and diastolic pressure by 5.5 points.[35]

Those who are taking medication for hypertension should not stop without the approval of the prescribing physician. If it is not treated properly, high blood pressure can kill. By combining medication with the other treatments, one might eventually reduce or eliminate the need for drug therapy.

**Excessive Body Fat** Although experts recognize obesity as an independent risk factor for CHD, the risks attributed to obesity actually may be augmented by other risk factors that usually accompany excessive body fat. Risk factors such as high blood lipids, hypertension, and diabetes typically are seen in conjunction with obesity. All of these risk factors usually improve with increased physical activity.

Attaining recommended body composition helps to improve some of the CHD risk factors and also helps one to reach a better state of health and wellness. People who have a weight problem and want to get down to recommended weight must:

1. Increase daily physical activity up to 90 minutes a day, including aerobic and strength-training programs

2. Follow a diet lower in fat and refined sugars and high in complex carbohydrates and fiber

3. Reduce total caloric intake moderately while getting the necessary nutrients to sustain normal body functions

A comprehensive weight reduction and weight control program is discussed in detail in Chapter 5.

**Cigarette Smoking** More than 46 million adults and 3.5 million adolescents in the United States smoke cigarettes. Smoking is the single largest preventable cause of illness and premature death in the United States. It has been linked to cardiovascular disease, cancer, bronchitis, emphysema, and peptic ulcers. In relation to coronary disease, smoking speeds the process of atherosclerosis and carries a threefold increase in the risk of sudden death after a myocardial infarction.

According to estimates, about 20 percent of all deaths from cardiovascular diseases are attributable to smoking. Smoking prompts the release of nicotine and another 1,200 toxic compounds into the bloodstream. Similar to hypertension, many of these substances are destructive to the inner membrane that protects the walls of the arteries. Once the lining is damaged, cholesterol and triglycerides can be deposited readily in the arterial wall. As the plaque builds up, it obstructs blood flow through the arteries.

Furthermore, smoking encourages the formation of blood clots, which can completely block an artery already narrowed by atherosclerosis. In addition, carbon monoxide, a by-product of cigarette smoke, decreases the blood's oxygen-carrying capacity. A combination of obstructed arteries, less oxygen, and nicotine in the heart muscle heightens the risk for a serious heart problem.

Smoking also increases heart rate, raises blood pressure, and irritates the heart, which can trigger fatal cardiac **arrhythmias**. Another harmful effect is a decrease in HDL cholesterol, the "good" type that helps control blood lipids. Smoking actually presents a much greater risk of death from heart disease than from lung disease.

Pipe and cigar smoking and tobacco chewing also increase the risk for heart disease. Even if the tobacco user inhales no smoke, he or she absorbs toxic substances through the membranes of the mouth, and these end up in the bloodstream. Individuals who use tobacco in any of these three forms also have a much greater risk for cancer of the oral cavity.

The risks for both cardiovascular disease and cancer start to decrease the moment a person quits smoking. One year after quitting, the risk for CHD decreases by half, and within 15 years, the relative risk of dying from cardiovascular disease and cancer approaches that of a lifetime nonsmoker. A more thorough discussion of the harmful effects of cigarette smoking, the benefits of quitting, and a complete program for quitting are detailed in Chapter 13.

**Tension and Stress** Tension and stress have become part of contemporary life. Everyone has to deal daily with goals, deadlines, responsibilities, and pressures. Almost everything in life (whether positive or negative) can be a source of stress. What creates the health hazard is not the stressor itself but, rather, the individual's response to it.

The human body responds to stress by producing more **catecholamines**, which prepare the body for quick physical action—often called "fight or flight." These hormones increase heart rate, blood pressure, and blood glucose levels, enabling the person to take action. If the person actu-

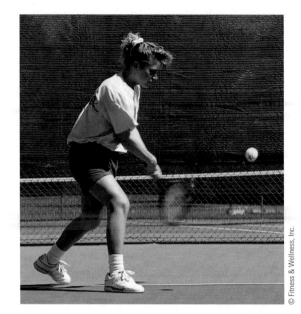

Physical activity, one of the best ways to relieve stress.

ally fights or flees, the higher levels of catecholamines are metabolized and the body can return to a normal state. If, however, a person is under constant stress and is unable to take action (as in the death of a close relative or friend, loss of a job, trouble at work, or financial insecurity), the catecholamines remain elevated in the bloodstream.

People who are not able to relax place a constant low-level strain on the cardiovascular system that could manifest itself as heart disease. Higher levels of the hormones epinephrine and cortisol in highly stressed people may raise blood pressure and cholesterol by 20 to 50 percent.[36] In addition, when a person is in a stressful situation, the coronary arteries that feed the heart muscle constrict, reducing the oxygen supply to the heart. If the blood vessels are largely blocked by atherosclerosis, arrhythmias or even a heart attack may follow.

Anger and hostility also contribute to heart disease by increasing heart rate, blood pressure, blood glucose, cholesterol, and interleukin-6 (a marker for arterial inflammation). Angina risk increases following an outburst of anger and doubles the risk for a heart attack in the first two hours thereafter.[37] Depression and isolation have also been linked to higher death rates from heart disease.

Individuals who are under a lot of stress and do not cope well with it need to take measures to counteract the effects of stress in their lives. One way is to identify the sources of stress and learn how to cope with them. People need to take control of themselves, examine and act upon the things that are most important in their lives, and ignore less meaningful details.

Physical activity is one of the best ways to relieve stress. When a person takes part in physical activity, the body metabolizes excess catecholamines and is able to return to a normal state. Exercise also steps up muscular activity, which contributes to muscular relaxation after completing the physical activity.

Many executives in large cities are choosing the evening hours for their physical activity programs, stopping after work at the health or fitness club. In doing this, they are able to "burn up" the excess tension accumulated during the day and enjoy the evening hours. This has proved to be one of the best stress management techniques. More information on stress management techniques is presented in Chapter 10.

**Personal and Family History** Individuals who have had cardiovascular problems are at higher risk than those who have never had a problem. People with this history should control other risk factors as much as they can. Many of the risk factors are reversible, so this will greatly decrease the risk for future problems. The more time that passes after the occurrence of the cardiovascular problem, the lower the risk for recurrence.

A genetic predisposition to heart disease has been demonstrated clearly. All other factors being equal, a person with blood relatives who now have or did have heart disease runs a greater risk than someone with no such history. Premature CHD is defined as a heart attack before age 55 in a close male relative or before age 65 in a close female relative. The younger the age at which the relative incurred the cardiovascular incident, the greater is the risk for the disease.

In some cases, there is no way of knowing whether the heart problem resulted from a person's genetic predisposition or simply poor lifestyle habits. A person may have been physically inactive and overweight and may have smoked and had bad dietary habits—all of which contributed to a heart attack. Regardless, blood relatives fall in the "family history" category. Because we have no reliable way to differentiate all the factors contributing to cardiovascular disease, a person with a family history should watch all other factors closely and maintain the lowest risk level possible. In addition, the person should have a blood chemistry analysis annually to make sure the body is handling blood lipids properly.

**Age** Age is a risk factor because of the higher incidence of heart disease as people get older. This tendency may be induced partly by other factors stemming from changes in lifestyle as we get older—less physical activity, poorer nutrition, obesity, and so on. Young people should not think that they are exempt from heart disease, though. The process begins early in life. Autopsies conducted on American soldiers killed at age 22 and younger revealed that approximately 70 percent had early stages of atherosclerosis. Other studies found elevated blood cholesterol levels in children as young as 10 years old.

Although the aging process cannot be stopped, it certainly can be slowed. Physiologic age versus chronological age is important in preventing disease. Some individuals in their 60s and older have the bodies of 30 year olds. And 30 year olds often are in such poor condition and health that they almost seem to have the bodies of 60 year olds. The best way to slow the natural aging process is to engage in risk factor management and positive lifestyle habits.

## Behavior Modification Planning

### AMERICAN HEART ASSOCIATION DIET AND LIFESTYLE GOALS FOR CARDIOVASCULAR DISEASE RISK REDUCTION

☐ I PLAN TO  ☐ I DID IT

- ☐ ☐ Consume an overall healthy diet.
- ☐ ☐ Aim for a healthy body weight.
- ☐ ☐ Aim for recommended levels of LDL cholesterol, HDL cholesterol, and triglycerides.
- ☐ ☐ Aim for a normal blood pressure.
- ☐ ☐ Aim for normal blood glucose levels.
- ☐ ☐ Be physically active.
- ☐ ☐ Avoid use of and exposure to tobacco products.

### Try It

To significantly offset the risk of cardiovascular disease, you need to aim for all of the above goals. You are now aware of the necessary lifestyle and dietary guidelines to do so. In your Online Journal or class notebook, outline the lifestyle changes that are required for you to meet the above goals.

**Other Risk Factors for Coronary Heart Disease** Additional evidence points to a few other factors that may be linked to CHD. One of these factors is gum disease. The oral bacteria that build up with dental plaque can enter the bloodstream and contribute to inflammation, formation of blood vessel plaque, and blood clotting and thus increase the risk for heart attack. Data on women who have periodontal disease indicate that they also have higher blood levels of CRP and lower HDL cholesterol. Daily flossing, using a power brush, scraping the tongue, and irrigating the gums with water are all preventive measures that will help protect you from gum disease.

Another factor that has been linked to cardiovascular disease is loud snoring. People who snore heavily may suf-

**Arrhythmias** Irregular heart rhythms.

**Catecholamines** "Fight-or-flight" hormones, including epinephrine and norepinephrine.

fer from sleep apnea, a sleep disorder in which the throat closes for a brief moment, causing breathing to stop. Individuals who snore heavily may triple their risk for a heart attack and quadruple the risk for a stroke.

Low birth weight, considered to be under 5.5 pounds, also has been linked to heart disease, hypertension, and diabetes. Individuals with low birth weight should bring this information to the attention of their personal physician and regularly monitor the risk factors for CHD.

Aspirin therapy is recommended to prevent heart disease. For individuals at moderate risk or higher, an aspirin dosage of about 81 mg per day (the equivalent of a baby aspirin) can prevent or dissolve clots that cause heart attack or stroke. With such daily use, the incidence of nonfatal heart attack decreases by about a third.

# Cardiovascular Risk Reduction

Most of the risk factors are reversible and preventable. Having a family history of heart disease and some of the other risk factors because of neglect in lifestyle does not mean you are doomed. A healthier lifestyle—free of cardiovascular problems—is something over which you have extensive control. Be persistent! Willpower and commitment are required to develop patterns that eventually will turn into healthy habits and contribute to your total well-being and longevity.

## ASSESS YOUR BEHAVIOR

Log on to http://www.cengage.com/sso/ to determine your risk for heart disease and to modify your Behavior Change Plan to incorporate at least on new activity that is heart-healthy.

1. Do you make a conscious effort to increase daily physical activity, and are you able to accumulate at least 30 minutes of moderate-intensity activity a minimum of five days per week?

2. Is your diet fundamentally low in saturated fat, and do you meet the daily suggested amounts of fruits, vegetables, and fiber?

3. Have you recently had your blood pressure measured, and established your blood lipid profile? Do you know what the results mean, and are you aware of strategies to manage them effectively?

## ASSESS YOUR KNOWLEDGE

Log on to http://www.cengage.com/sso/ to assess your understanding of this chapter's topics by taking the Student Practice Test and exploring the modules recommended in your Personalized Study Plan.

1. Coronary heart disease
   a. is the single leading cause of death in the United States.
   b. is the leading cause of sudden cardiac deaths.
   c. is a condition in which the arteries that supply the heart muscle with oxygen and nutrients are narrowed by fatty deposits.
   d. accounts for approximately 20 percent of all deaths in the United States.
   e. All of the above are correct.

2. The incidence of cardiovascular disease during the past 40 years in the United States has
   a. increased.
   b. decreased.
   c. remained constant.
   d. increased in some years and decreased in others.
   e. fluctuated according to medical technology.

3. Regular aerobic activity helps
   a. lower LDL cholesterol.
   b. lower HDL cholesterol.
   c. increase triglycerides.

   d. decrease insulin sensitivity.
   e. all of the above.

4. The risk for heart disease increases with
   a. high LDL cholesterol.
   b. low HDL cholesterol.
   c. high concentration of homocysteine.
   d. high levels of hs-CRP.
   e. all of the above factors.

5. An optimal level of LDL cholesterol is
   a. between 200 and 239 mg/dL.
   b. about 200 mg/dL.
   c. between 150 and 200 mg/dL.
   d. between 100 and 150 mg/dL.
   e. below 100 mg/dL.

6. As part of a CHD prevention program, saturated fat intake should be kept below
   a. 35 percent.
   b. 30 percent.
   c. 22 percent.
   d. 15 percent.
   e. 7 percent.

7. Statin drugs
   a. increase the liver's ability to remove blood cholesterol.
   b. decrease LDL cholesterol.
   c. slow cholesterol production.
   d. help reduce inflammation.
   e. accomplish all of the above.

8. Type 2 diabetes is related closely to
   a. overeating.
   b. obesity.
   c. lack of physical activity.
   d. insulin resistance.
   e. all of the above factors.

9. Metabolic syndrome is related to
   a. low HDL cholesterol.
   b. high triglycerides.

   c. increased blood-clotting mechanism.
   d. an abnormal insulin response to carbohydrates.
   e. all of the above.

10. Comprehensive reviews on the effects of aerobic exercise on blood pressure found that in general, an individual can expect exercise-induced reductions of
    a. approximately 3 to 5 mm Hg.
    b. approximately 5 to 10 mm Hg.
    c. approximately 10 to 15 mm Hg.
    d. over 15 mm Hg.
    e. There is no significant change in blood pressure with exercise.

Correct answers can be found at the back of the book.

# MEDIA MENU

You can find the links below at the book companion site: www.cengage.com/health/hoeger/plfw10e

- Determine your risk for heart disease.
- Check how well you understand the chapter's concepts.

## Internet Connections

- **American Heart Association.** This comprehensive site provides research, cardiac information for health professionals and the general public, and advocacy. The site features information on a variety of cardiovascular illnesses, healthy lifestyles, and cardiopulmonary resuscitation (CPR). It also offers a heart- and stroke-searchable encyclopedia and a 10-question "Healthy Heart Workout" quiz. *http://www.americanheart.org*

- **National Cholesterol Education Program.** This comprehensive site features interactive sessions on planning a low-cholesterol diet and lots more. It provides you with information to prevent heart disease as well as information for people who already have heart disease. You can hear radio messages from the Heart Beat Radio Network—a site highly recommended. *http://rover.nhlbi.nih.gov/chd*

- **The Heart: An Online Exploration.** This informative and interesting site, developed by the Franklin Institute of Science, provides an interactive multimedia tour of the heart, statistical information, resources, and links. You can learn how to monitor your heart's health by becoming aware of your vital signs, read more about diagnostic tests, and listen to heart sounds via the site's audio and video clips. *http://www.fi.edu/biosci/heart.html*

- **Check Your Healthy Heart I.Q.** Hosted by Infoplease. Test your knowledge about heart disease and its risk factors (high blood pressure, high blood cholesterol, smoking, lack of exercise, and overweight) and learn ways to reduce your risk. *http://www.infoplease.com/ipa/A0762279.html*

- **Lower Your Blood Pressure with DASH.** This part of the National Heart, Lung, and Blood Institute site introduces DASH—Dietary Approaches to Stop Hypertension—a plan that has been clinically proven to reduce blood pressure. *http://www.nhlbi.nih.gov/health/public/heart/hbp/dash/how_plan.html*

# NOTES

1. U.S. Department of Health and Human Services, Centers for Disease Control and Prevention, National Center for Health Statistics, *National Vital Statistics Reports, Deaths: Leading Causes for 2003* 55, no. 10 (March 15, 2007).

2. "Reducing Your Risk of a Stroke: The Latest Tips," *Environmental Nutrition* 29, no. 7 (July 2006): 3.

3. S. N. Blair, H. W. Kohl III, R. S. Paffenbarger, Jr., D. G. Clark, K. H. Cooper, and L. W. Gibbons, "Physical Fitness and All-Cause Mortality: A Prospective Study of Healthy Men and Women," *Journal of the American Medical Association* 262 (1989): 2395–2401.

4. R. S. Paffenbarger, Jr., R. T. Hyde, A. L. Wing, I. Lee, D. L. Jung, and J. B. Kampert, "The Association of Changes in Physical-Activity Level and Other Lifestyle Characteristics with Mortality Among Men," *New England Journal of Medicine* 328 (1993): 538–545.

5. D. P. Swain and B. A. Franklin, "Comparative Cardioprotective Benefits of Vigorous vs. Moderate Intensity Aerobic Exercise," *American Journal of Cardiology* 97, no. 1 (2006): 141–147.

6. American College of Sports Medicine, *ACSM's Guidelines for Exercise Testing and Prescription* (Philadelphia: Lippincott Williams & Wilkins, 2006).

7. "Lipid Research Clinics Program: The Lipid Research Clinic Coronary Primary Prevention Trial Results," *Journal of the American Medical Association* 251 (1984): 351–364.

8. See note 1.

9. M. D. Ozner, "The Ultimate Cholesterol Profile," *Bottom Line/Health* 21 (July 2007): 1–2.

10. "HDL on the Rise," *HealthNews* (September 10, 1999).

11. See note 9.

12. A. H. Lichtenstein, et al., "Diet and Lifestyle Recommendations Revision 2006: A Scientific Statement from the American Heart Association Nutrition Committee," *Circulation* 114 (2006): 82–96.

13. See note 3.

14. C. D. Gardner, et al., "The Effect of a Plant-Based Diet on Plasma Lipids in Hypercholesterolemic Adults," *Annals of Internal Medicine* 142 (2005): 725–733.

15. E. B. Rimm, A. Ascherio, E. Giovannucci, D. Spiegelman, M. J. Stampfer, and W. C. Willett, "Vegetable, Fruit, and Cereal Fiber Intake and Risk of Coronary Heart Disease Among Men," *Journal of the American Medical Association* 275 (1996): 447–451.

16. National Cholesterol Education Program Expert Panel, "Summary of the Third Report of the National Cholesterol Education Program (NCEP) Expert Panel on Detection, Evaluation, and Treatment of High Blood Cholesterol in Adults (Adult Treatment Panel III)," *Journal of the American Medical Association* 285 (2001): 2486–2497.

17. A. Jula, et al., "Effects of Diet and Simvastatin on Serum Lipids, Insulin, and Antioxidants in Hypercholesterolemic Men," *Journal of the American Medical Association* 287 (2002): 598–605.

18. "The Homocysteine-CVD Connection," *HealthNews* (October 25, 1999).

19. "Inflammation May Be Key Cause of Heart Disease and More: Diet's Role," *Environmental Nutrition* 27, no. 7 (July 2004): 1, 4.

20. H. R. Superko, "State-of-the Art Heart Tests," *Bottom Line/Health* 19 (February 2005): 3–5.

21. "Predict Heart Disease Better with CRP," *Environmental Nutrition* 28, no. 2 (February 2005): 3.

22. H. K. Choi, et al., "Dairy Consumption and Risk of Type 2 Diabetes Mellitus in Men," *Archives of Internal Medicine* 165 (2005): 997–1003.

23. S. Liu, et al., "A Prospective Study of Dietary Glycemic Load, Carbohydrate Intake, and Risk of Coronary Heart Disease in the U.S.," *American Journal of Clinical Nutrition* 71 (2000): 1455–1461.

24. G. M. Reaven, T. K. Strom, and B. Fox, *Syndrome X: Overcoming the Silent Killer That Can Give You a Heart Attack* (Englewood Cliffs, NJ: Simon & Schuster, 2000).

25. A. V. Chobanian, et al., "The Seventh Report of the Joint National Committee on Prevention, Detection, Evaluation, and Treatment of High Blood Pressure," *Journal of the American Medical Association* 289 (2003): 2560–2571.

26. L. E. Fields, et al., "The Burden of Adult Hypertension in the United States, 1999 to 2000: A Rising Tide," *Hypertension On Line First* (August 23, 2004).

27. "Water, Sodium, Potassium: The Verdict Is In," *University of California at Berkeley Wellness Letter* (Palm Coast, FL: The Editors, May 2004).

28. See note 27.

29. See note 3.

30. L. S. Pescatello, et al., "Exercise and Hypertension Position Stand," *Medicine and Science in Sports and Exercise* 36 (2004): 533–553.

31. G. Kelley, "Dynamic Resistance Exercise and Resting Blood Pressure in Adults: A Meta-analysis," *Journal of Applied Physiology* 82 (1997): 1559–1565; G. A. Kelley and Z. Tran, "Aerobic Exercise and Normotensive Adults: A Meta-analysis," *Medicine and Science in Sports and Exercise* 27 (1995): 1371–1377; G. Kelley and P. McClellan, "Antihypertensive Effects of Aerobic Exercise: A Brief Meta-analytic Review of Randomized Controlled Trials," *American Journal of Hypertension* 7 (1994): 115–119.

32. R. Collins, et al., "Blood Pressure, Stroke, and Coronary Heart Disease; Part 2, Short-term Reductions in Blood Pressure: Overview of Randomized Drug Trials in Their Epidemiological Context," *Lancet* 335 (1990): 827–838.

33. G. A. Kelley and K. S. Kelley, "Progressive Resistance Exercise and Resting Blood Pressure: A Meta-analysis of Randomized Controlled Trials," *Hypertension* 35 (2000): 838–843.

34. F. W. Kash, J. L. Boyer, S. P. Van Camp, L. S. Verity, and J. P. Wallace, "The Effect of Physical Activity on Aerobic Power in Older Men (A Longitudinal Study)," *Physician and Sports Medicine* 18, no. 4 (1990): 73–83.

35. S. G. Sheps, "High Blood Pressure Can Often Be Controlled Without Medication," *Bottom Line/Health* (November 1999).

36. M. Guarneri, "What Most People Don't Know About Heart Disease," *Bottom Line/Health* 21 (July 2007): 11–12.

37. See note 36.

# SUGGESTED READINGS

American Heart Association. *2009 Heart and Stroke Facts Statistical Update.* Dallas: AHA, 2009.

American Heart Association. *Heart and Stroke Facts.* Dallas: AHA, 2008.

National Cholesterol Education Program Expert Panel. "Summary of the Third Report of the National Cholesterol Education Program (NCEP) Expert Panel on Detection, Evaluation, and Treatment of High Blood Cholesterol in Adults (Adult Treatment Panel III)," *Journal of the American Medical Association* 285 (2001): 2486–2497.

# LAB 11A: Self-Assessment Coronary Heart Disease Risk Factor Analysis

Name _____     Date _____     Grade _____

Instructor _____     Course _____     Section _____

### Necessary Lab Equipment
Basic lab equipment to repeat the body composition and blood pressure tests. If possible, a blood chemistry analysis should be performed prior to this lab.

### Objective
To assess your current risk for coronary heart disease (CHD) and develop a behavior modification program.

### Instructions
The disease process for cardiovascular disease starts early in life, primarily as a result of poor lifestyle habits. Studies have shown beginning stages of atherosclerosis and elevated blood lipids in children as young as 10 years old. Consequently, the purpose of this activity is to establish a baseline CHD risk profile and to point out the "zero-risk" level for each coronary risk factor.

You may want to repeat the body composition and blood pressure tests to obtain current values for this activity. If you have had a blood chemistry analysis performed recently that included total cholesterol, HDL cholesterol, triglycerides, and glucose levels, you may use the results for this activity.

Score

| | | | |
|---|---|---|---|
| 1. Physical Activity | Do you get 30 or more minutes of moderate-intensity physical activity: | | |
| | Fewer than 3 times per week ...................................... | 8 | |
| | Between 3 and 4 times per week ................................ | 3 | [ ] |
| | 5 or more times per week ........................................ | 0 | |

| 2. Resting and Stress Electrocardiograms (ECGs) | Add scores for both ECGs | | | |
|---|---|---|---|---|
| | ECG | Resting | Stress | |
| | Normal | (0) | (0) ......................... | 0 |
| | Equivocal | (1) | (4) ......................... | 1–5 [ ] |
| | Abnormal | (3) | (8) ......................... | 3–11 |

| 3. HDL Cholesterol (If unknown, answer Question 6) | ≥40 ................................................. | 0 |
|---|---|---|
| | <40 ................................................. | 6 [ ] |

| 4. LDL Cholesterol (If unknown, answer Question 6) | <100 ................................................ | 0 |
|---|---|---|
| | 100–159 ............................................ | 3 [ ] |
| | ≥160 ............................................... | 6 |

| 5. Triglycerides (If unknown, answer Question 6) | ≤150 mg/dL ....................................... | 0 |
|---|---|---|
| | 150–199 mg/dL ................................... | .5 |
| | 200–499 mg/dL ................................... | 1 [ ] |
| | ≥500 mg/dL ...................................... | 2 |

| 6. Diet (Do not answer if Questions 3, 4, and 5 have been answered) | Does your regular diet include (high score if all apply): | |
|---|---|---|
| | 1 or more daily servings of red meat; 7 or more eggs/week; daily butter, cheese, whole milk, sweets, alcohol, and processed foods ............................................. | 10–14 |
| | 4 to 6 servings of red meat/week; 4–6 eggs per week; 1% or 2% milk, some cheese, sweets, alcohol, and processed foods........ | 4–10 |
| | Fish, poultry, red meat fewer than three times/week; fewer than 3 eggs/week; skim milk and skim milk products; moderate sweets and alcohol ...................... | 0–3 [ ] |

Subtotal Risk Score: [ ]

*(continued)*

420

Subtotal Risk Score (from previous page): [ ]

7. Homocysteine

Does your daily diet include:
2 and 3 servings of fruits and vegetables, respectively ............ 0
Fewer than 2 and 3 servings of fruits and vegetables respectively . 4 [ ]

8. Inflammation (as measured by High-Sensitivity C-Reactive Protein or hs-CRP)

<1 mg/L ............................................... 0
1–3 mg/L ............................................... 2
>3 mg/L ............................................... 8 [ ]

9. Diabetes/Glucose

≤120 .................................................... 0
121–128 .................................................. 1
129–136 .................................................. 1.5
107–144 .................................................. 2
145–149 .................................................. 2.5
≥150 .................................................... 3
Diabetics add another 3 points ............................... 3 [ ]

10. Blood Pressure

Add scores for both readings (e.g., 144/88 score = 5)

| Systolic | Diastolic | |
|---|---|---|
| <120 ........ (0) | <80 ......... (0) | 0 |
| 121–129 ....... (1) | 81–84 ........ (1) | 1–2 |
| 130–139 ....... (2) | 85–89 ........ (2) | 2–4 |
| 140–159 ....... (3) | 90–99 ........ (3) | 3–6 |
| ≥160 ........ (4) | ≥100 ........ (4) | 4–8 | [ ]

11. Body Mass Index (BMI)

≤25.0 ................................................... 0
25.0–29.99 .............................................. 2
30.0–39.99 .............................................. 4
≥40.0 ................................................... 8 [ ]

12. Smoking

Lifetime non-smoker ...................................... 0
Ex-smoker more than 1 year ............................... 0
Ex-smoker less than 1 year ............................... 1
Smoke 1 cigarette/day or none ............................. 1
Non-smoker, but live or work in smoking environment .......... 2
Pipe or cigar smoker, or chew tobacco ...................... 3
Smoke 1–9 cigarettes/day ................................. 3
Smoke 10–19 cigarettes/day ............................... 4
Smoke 20–29 cigarettes/day ............................... 5
Smoke 30–39 cigarettes/day ............................... 6
Smoke 40 or more cigarettes/day ........................... 8 [ ]

13. Tension and Stress

Are you:
Sometimes tense .......................................... 0
Often tense .............................................. 1
Nearly always tense ...................................... 2
Always tense ............................................ 3 [ ]

Subtotal Risk Score: [ ]

Subtotal Risk Score (from previous page): 

| | | |
|---|---|---|
| 14. Personal History | Have you had a heart attack, stroke, coronary disease, or any known heart problem: | |
| | During the last year .......................................... | 8 |
| | 1–2 years ago................................................ | 5 |
| | 2–5 years ago............................................... | 3 |
| | More than 5 years ago........................................ | 2 |
| | Never had heart disease....................................... | 0 |

| | | |
|---|---|---|
| 15. Family History | How many of your blood relatives (parents, uncles, brothers, sisters, grandparents) had cardiovascular disease (heart attack, strokes, bypass surgery): | |
| | One or more before age 51....................................... | 8 |
| | One or more between 51 and 60............................... | 4 |
| | One or more after age 60 ....................................... | 2 |
| | None had cardiovascular disease................................ | 0 |

| | | |
|---|---|---|
| 16. Age | 29 or younger................................................ | 0 |
| | 30–39 ....................................................... | 1 |
| | 40–49 ....................................................... | 2 |
| | 50–59 ....................................................... | 3 |
| | ≥60........................................................ | 4 |

Total Risk Score: 

How to Score

| Risk Category | Total Risk Score |
|---|---|
| Very Low ............................ 5 or fewer points |
| Low ........................ Between 6 and 15 points |
| Moderate................... Between 16 and 25 points |
| High ....................... Between 26 and 35 points |
| Very High .......................... 36 or more points |

## II. Stage of Change for Cardiovascular Disease Prevention

Using Figure 2.5 (page 57) and Table 2.3 (page 57), identify your current stage of change for participation in a cardiovascular disease risk-reduction program:

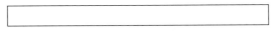

III. In a few sentences, discuss your family and personal risk for cardiovascular disease:

_____

_____

_____

_____

_____

_____

_____

_____

_____

_____

_____

IV. Discuss lifestyle changes that you have already implemented in this course, as well as additional changes that you can make to decrease your own risk of developing cardiovascular disease in the future.

_____

_____

_____

_____

_____

_____

_____

_____

_____

_____

_____

_____

V. Physical Activity Rating

Number of daily steps at the beginning of the term: [        ]    Current number of daily steps: [        ]

Current physical activity rating (use Table 1.2, page 10): [        ]

# Cancer Prevention

## 12

Mitch Hrdlicka/Photodisc/Getty Images

## Objectives

- Define cancer and understand how it starts and spreads
- Cite guidelines for preventing cancer
- Delineate the major risk factors that lead to specific types of cancer
- Assess the risk for developing certain types of cancer
- Learn everyday lifestyle strategies that you can use immediately to decrease overall cancer risk
- Assess your risk for cancer.

CENGAGENOW™

Check your understanding of the chapter contents by logging on to CengageNOW and accessing the pre-test, personalized learning plan, and post-test for this chapter.

# FAQ

### Can a healthy diet reduce cancer risk?

Much research is currently under way to examine the effects of foods in preventing and fighting off cancer. There is strong scientific evidence that a healthy diet and maintenance of recommended body weight reduce cancer risk. The current state of knowledge, however, cannot indicate that a certain dietary pattern will absolutely reduce your cancer risk. Years of research will be required to unravel most of this knowledge. Moreover, science may never be able to provide conclusive evidence that a certain diet will prevent cancer in most cases. Many of the foods that are currently recommended in a cancer-prevention diet, nonetheless, are similar to those encouraged to decrease disease risk and enhance health and overall well-being. If you are truly adhering to healthy dietary guidelines (see the Behavior Modification Planning box on page 429), you are most likely eating the right foods to decrease your cancer risk.

### Does regular physical activity affect cancer risk?

Regular physical activity has been shown to decrease the risk for developing certain types of cancer, in particular cancers of the colon, breast, endometrium, and prostate gland. Physical activity also prevents type 2 diabetes and obesity. The latter have been linked to colon, pancreatic, gallbladder, ovarian, thyroid, cervical, and possibly other types of cancers. The American Cancer Society recommends that you aim for at least 30 minutes of moderate to vigorous physical activity five or more days per week, although 45 to 60 minutes of intentional activity are preferable. For most non-tobacco users, a healthy dietary pattern and regular physical activity are the two most significant lifestyle behaviors that reduce cancer risk.

### Which is the biggest carcinogenic exposure in the environment?

Without question, tobacco use and exposure to secondhand smoke. Tobacco use in general is responsible for at least 30 percent of all cancer deaths and 87 percent of lung cancer deaths. Cigarette smoking causes more than 170,000 lung cancer deaths each year in the United States and contributes to at least 15 additional types of cancer, including oral, lip, nasal, pharyngeal, laryngeal, esophageal, uterine, stomach, and pancreatic. Worldwide, almost 5 million people die each year due to tobacco-related illnesses. If you smoke or use any other tobacco products, STOP NOW! If you do not smoke, DON'T EVER START. If you are ever around people who are smoking, claim your right to clean air, or distance yourself from them as much as you possibly can.

Under normal conditions, the 100 trillion cells in the human body reproduce themselves in an orderly way. Cell growth (cell reproduction) takes place to repair and replace old, worn-out tissue. Cell growth is controlled by **deoxyribonucleic acid (DNA)** and **ribonucleic acid (RNA),** found in the nucleus of each cell. When nuclei lose their ability to regulate and control cell growth, cell division is disrupted and mutant cells can develop (see Figure 12.1). Some of these cells might grow uncontrollably and abnormally, forming a mass of tissue called a tumor, which can be either **benign** or **malignant.** Benign tumors do not invade other tissues. Although they can interfere with normal bodily functions, they rarely cause death. A malignant tumor is a **cancer.** More than 100 types of cancer can develop in any tissue or organ of the human body.

The process of cancer actually begins with an alteration in DNA. Within DNA are **oncogenes** and tumor **suppressor genes,** which normally work together to repair and replace cells. Defects in these genes—caused by external factors such as radiation, chemicals, and viruses, as well as internal factors such as immune conditions, hormones, and genetic mutations—ultimately allow the cell to grow into a tumor.

A healthy cell can duplicate as many as 100 times in its lifetime. Normally, the DNA molecule is duplicated perfectly during cell division. In the few cases when the DNA molecule is not replicated exactly, specialized enzymes make repairs quickly. Occasionally, however, cells with defective DNA keep dividing and ultimately form a small tumor. As more mutations occur, the altered cells continue

FIGURE 12.1 Mutant (cancer) cells.

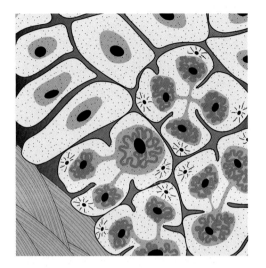

Adapted from American Cancer Society, *Youth Looks at Cancer* (New York: American Cancer Society, 1982) p. 4.

FIGURE 12.2 Erosion of chromosome telomeres in normal cells.

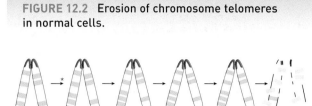

Telomeres    *Successive cell divisions

Death of cell

FIGURE 12.3 Action of the enzyme telomerase.

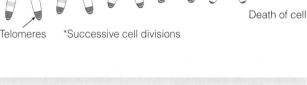

Telomeres    *Successive cell divisions

Telomerase

to divide and can become malignant. A decade or more might pass between exposure to carcinogens or mutations and the time cancer is diagnosed.

The process of abnormal cell division is related indirectly to chromosome segments called **telomeres** (Figure 12.2). Each time a cell divides, chromosomes lose some telomeres. After many cell divisions, chromosomes eventually run out of telomeres and the cell then invariably dies.

Human tumors make an enzyme known as **telomerase**. In cancer cells, telomerase keeps the chromosome from running out of telomeres entirely. The shortened strand of telomeres (Figure 12.3) now allows cells to reproduce indefinitely, creating a malignant tumor. Telomerase seems to have another function that is still under investigation: After many cell divisions, cancer cells grow old by nature, but telomerase is what apparently keeps them from dying. If scientists can confirm that telomerase plays such a crucial role in forming tumors, research will be directed to finding a way to block the action of telomerase, thereby making cancerous cells die.

Cancer starts with the abnormal growth of one cell, which then can multiply into billions of cancerous cells. A critical turning point in the development of cancer is when a tumor reaches about a million cells. At this stage, it is referred to as **carcinoma in situ**. The undetected tumor may go for months or years without any significant growth. While it remains encapsulated, it does not pose a serious threat to human health. To grow, however, the tumor requires more oxygen and nutrients.

In time, a few of the cancer cells start producing chemicals that enhance **angiogenesis**, or capillary (blood vessel) formation into the tumor. Angiogenesis is the precursor of **metastasis**. Through the new blood vessels formed by angiogenesis, cancerous cells now can break away from a malignant tumor and migrate to other parts of the body, where they can cause new cancer (Figure 12.4).

Most adults have precancerous or cancerous cells in their bodies. By middle age, our bodies contain millions of precancerous cells. The immune system and blood turbulence destroy most cancer cells, but only one abnormal cell lodging elsewhere is enough to start a new cancer. These cells grow and multiply uncontrollably, invading and destroying normal tissue. The rate at which cancer cells grow varies from one type to another. Some types grow fast, and others take years.

Once cancer cells metastasize, treatment becomes more difficult. Although therapy can kill most cancer cells, a few cells might become resistant to treatment. These cells then can grow into a new tumor that will not respond to the same treatment.

**Deoxyribonucleic acid (DNA)** Genetic substance of which genes are made; molecule that contains cell's genetic code.

**Ribonucleic acid (RNA)** Genetic material that guides the formation of cell proteins.

**Benign** Noncancerous.

**Malignant** Cancerous.

**Cancer** Group of diseases characterized by uncontrolled growth and spread of abnormal cells.

**Oncogenes** Genes that initiate cell division.

**Suppressor genes** Genes that deactivate the process of cell division.

**Telomeres** A strand of molecules at both ends of a chromosome.

**Telomerase** An enzyme that allows cells to reproduce indefinitely.

**Carcinoma in situ** Encapsulated malignant tumor that has not spread.

**Angiogenesis** Formation of blood vessels (capillaries).

**Metastasis** The movement of cells from one part of the body to another.

**FIGURE 12.4** How cancer starts and spreads.

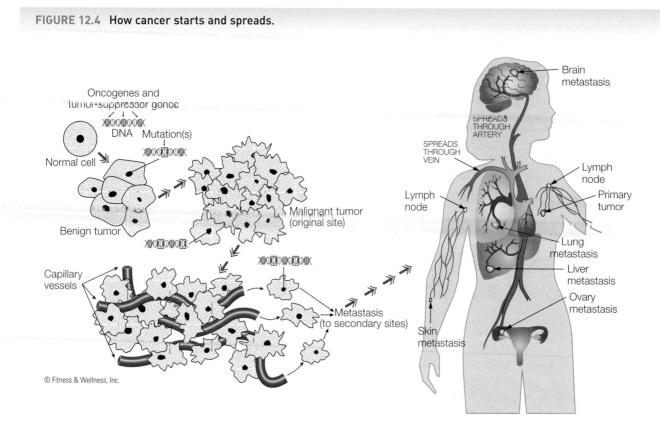

© Fitness & Wellness, Inc.

# Incidence of Cancer

According to mortality statistics for 2005 from the National Center for Health Statistics, cancer was the cause of almost 23 percent of all deaths in the United States. It is the second leading cause of death in the country and the leading cause in children between ages 1 and

14. The major contributor to the increase in incidence of cancer during the last five decades is lung cancer. Tobacco use alone is responsible for 30 percent of all deaths from cancer. Another third of all deaths from cancer are related to unhealthy nutrition, physical inactivity, and excessive body fat. Death rates for most major cancer sites are declining, except lung cancer in women (Figure 12.5).

**FIGURE 12.5** Death rates* for major cancer sites 1930–2004.

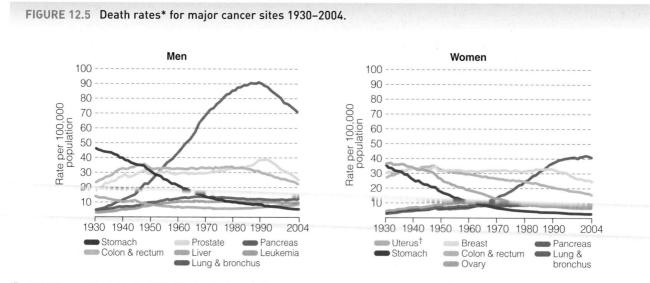

*Per 100,000, age-adjusted to the 1970 U.S. standard population.
†Uterus cancer deaths are for uterine cervix and uterine corpus combined.
*Note:* Due to changes in ICD coding, numerator information has changed over time. Rates for cancers of the liver, lung and bronchus, and colon and rectum are affected by these coding changes.
***Source:*** American Cancer Society, *Cancer Facts and Figures 2008.* Atlanta: American Cancer Society, Inc. Reprinted by permission.

FIGURE 12.6  2008 estimated cancer incidence and deaths by site and sex.*

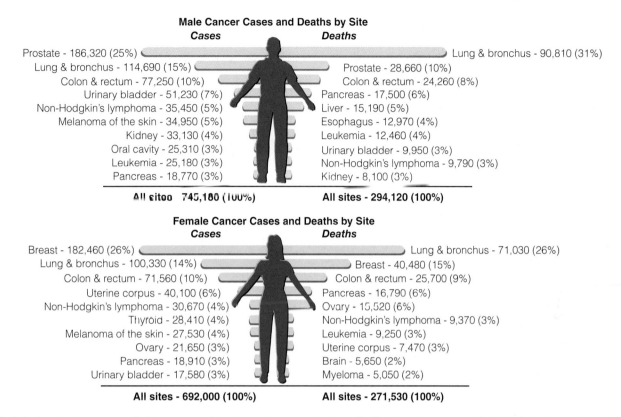

**Male Cancer Cases and Deaths by Site**

*Cases* — *Deaths*

Prostate - 186,320 (25%)
Lung & bronchus - 114,690 (15%)
Colon & rectum - 77,250 (10%)
Urinary bladder - 51,230 (7%)
Non-Hodgkin's lymphoma - 35,450 (5%)
Melanoma of the skin - 34,950 (5%)
Kidney - 33,130 (4%)
Oral cavity - 25,310 (3%)
Leukemia - 25,180 (3%)
Pancreas - 18,770 (3%)

Lung & bronchus - 90,810 (31%)
Prostate - 28,660 (10%)
Colon & rectum - 24,260 (8%)
Pancreas - 17,500 (6%)
Liver - 15,190 (5%)
Esophagus - 12,970 (4%)
Leukemia - 12,460 (4%)
Urinary bladder - 9,950 (3%)
Non-Hodgkin's lymphoma - 9,790 (3%)
Kidney - 8,100 (3%)

All sites - 745,180 (100%)  All sites - 294,120 (100%)

**Female Cancer Cases and Deaths by Site**

*Cases* — *Deaths*

Breast - 182,460 (26%)
Lung & bronchus - 100,330 (14%)
Colon & rectum - 71,560 (10%)
Uterine corpus - 40,100 (6%)
Non-Hodgkin's lymphoma - 30,670 (4%)
Thyroid - 28,410 (4%)
Melanoma of the skin - 27,530 (4%)
Ovary - 21,650 (3%)
Pancreas - 18,910 (3%)
Urinary bladder - 17,580 (3%)

Lung & bronchus - 71,030 (26%)
Breast - 40,480 (15%)
Colon & rectum - 25,700 (9%)
Pancreas - 16,790 (6%)
Ovary - 15,520 (6%)
Non-Hodgkin's lymphoma - 9,370 (3%)
Leukemia - 9,250 (3%)
Uterine corpus - 7,470 (3%)
Brain - 5,650 (2%)
Myeloma - 5,050 (2%)

**All sites - 692,000 (100%)**   **All sites - 271,530 (100%)**

*Excludes basal and squamous cell skin cancers and in situ carcinoma except urinary bladder. Percentages may not total 100% due to rounding.
**Source:** American Cancer Society, *Cancer Facts and Figures 2008.* Atlanta: American Cancer Society, Inc. Reprinted by permission.

Cancer will develop in approximately one of every two men and one of every three women in the United States, striking approximately three of every four families. About 565,650 Americans died from cancer in 2008, and approximately 1,437,180 new cases were diagnosed that same year.[1] The incidence of cancer is higher in African Americans than in any other racial or ethnic group. Statistical estimates of the incidence of cancer and deaths by sex and site for 2008 are given in Figure 12.6. These estimates exclude **nonmelanoma skin cancer** and carcinoma in situ.

## Critical Thinking

Have you ever had, or do you now have, any family members with cancer? Can you identify lifestyle or environmental factors as possible contributors to the disease? If not, are you concerned about your genetic predisposition, and, if so, are you making lifestyle changes to decrease your risk?

Like coronary heart disease, cancer is largely preventable. As much as 80 percent of all human cancer is related to lifestyle or environmental factors (including diet and obesity, tobacco use, sedentary lifestyle, excessive use of alcohol, and exposure to occupational hazards—see Figure 12.7). Most of these cancers could be prevented through positive lifestyle habits.

Research sponsored by the American Cancer Society and the National Cancer Institute showed that individuals who have a healthy lifestyle have some of the lowest cancer mortality rates ever reported in scientific studies. In a landmark study, a group of about 10,000 members of the Church of Jesus Christ of Latter-day Saints (commonly referred to as the Mormon church) in California was reported to have only about one-third (men) to one-half (women) the rate of cancer mortality of the general white population[2] (Figure 12.8). In this study, the investigators looked at three general health habits in the participants: lifetime abstinence from smoking, regular physical activity, and sufficient sleep. In addition, healthy lifestyle guidelines (encouraged by the church since 1833)

**Nonmelanoma skin cancer** Cancer that spreads or grows at the original site but does not metastasize to other regions of the body.

FIGURE 12.7 Estimates of the relative role of the major cancer-causing factors.

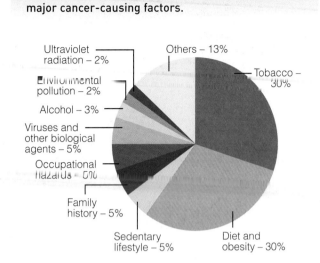

*Source:* Harvard Center for Cancer Prevention. *Causes of Human Cancer, Harvard Report on Cancer Prevention,* 1 (1996).

FIGURE 12.8 Effects of a healthy lifestyle on cancer mortality rate.

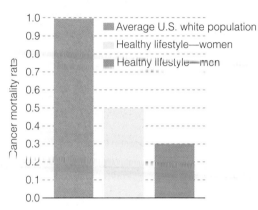
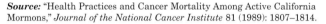

*Source:* "Health Practices and Cancer Mortality Among Active California Mormons," *Journal of the National Cancer Institute* 81 (1989): 1807–1814.

include abstaining from all forms of tobacco, alcohol, and drugs and adhering to a well-balanced diet based on grains, fruits, and vegetables, and moderate amounts of poultry and red meat. The conclusion is that lifestyle is definitely an important factor in the risk for cancer.

Equally important is that approximately 10.8 million Americans with a history of cancer were alive in 2008. Currently, 6 in 10 people diagnosed with cancer are expected to be alive five years after their initial diagnosis.[3]

# Guidelines for Preventing Cancer

The biggest factor in fighting cancer today is health education. People need to be informed about the risk factors for cancer and the guidelines for early detection. The most effective way to protect against cancer is to change negative lifestyle habits and behaviors. Following are some guidelines for preventing cancer. For most Americans who do not use tobacco, increased physical activity and dietary choices are the most important modifiable risk factors.

**Dietary Changes** The American Cancer Society estimates that one-third of all cancer in the United States is related to poor nutrition and lack of physical activity. A healthy diet, therefore, is crucial to decrease the risk for cancer. The diet should be predominantly vegetarian, high in fiber, and low in fat (particularly from animal sources). **Cruciferous vegetables**, tea, soy products, calcium, and omega-3 fats are encouraged. Protein intake should be kept within the recommended nutrient guidelines. If alcohol is used, it should be in moderation. Obesity should be avoided.

Green and dark yellow vegetables, cruciferous vegetables (cauliflower, broccoli, cabbage, Brussels sprouts, and kohlrabi), and beans (legumes) seem to protect against cancer. Folate—found naturally in dark green leafy vegetables, dried beans, and orange juice—may reduce the risk for colon and cervical cancers. Brightly colored fruits and vegetables also contain **carotenoids** and vitamin C. Lycopene, one of the many carotenoids (a phytonutrient—see the following discussion), has been linked to lower risk for cancers of the prostate, colon, and cervix. Lycopene is especially abundant in cooked tomato products.

The evidence for vitamin D in protecting against cancer continues to mount each day. Vitamin D is the most powerful regulator of cell growth and keeps cells from becoming malignant. The protective effect of vitamin D appears to be strongest against breast, colon, and prostate cancers and possibly lung and digestive cancers. You should strive for "safe sun" exposure, that is, up to 15 minutes of unprotected sun exposure, on most days of the week between the hours of 10:00 a.m. and 4:00 p.m. For people living in the northern United States and Canada, with limited sun exposure during the winter months, a vitamin $D_3$ supplement of up to 2,000 international units (IU) per day is strongly recommended. Additional cancer-protective benefits of this vitamin have already been discussed in Chapter 3 (see "Vitamin D," page 97).

Some researchers believe that the antioxidant effect of vitamins and the mineral selenium help to protect the body. During normal metabolism, most of the oxygen in the human body is converted into stable forms of carbon dioxide and water. A small amount, however, ends up in an unstable form known as oxygen free radicals, which are thought to attack and damage the cell membrane and DNA, leading to the formation of cancers. Antioxidants are thought to absorb free radicals before they can cause damage and also interrupt the sequence of reactions once

## Behavior Modification Planning

### TIPS FOR A HEALTHY CANCER-FIGHTING DIET

Increase intake of phytonutrients, fiber, cruciferous vegetables, and more antioxidants by

I PLAN TO | I DID IT

- ☐ ☐ Eating a predominantly vegetarian diet
- ☐ ☐ Eating more fruits and vegetables every day (six to eight servings per day maximize anti-cancer benefits)
- ☐ ☐ Increasing the consumption of broccoli, cauliflower, kale, turnips, cabbage, kohlrabi, Brussels sprouts, hot chili peppers, red and green peppers, carrots, sweet potatoes, winter squash, spinach, garlic, onions, strawberries, tomatoes, pineapple, and citrus fruits in your regular diet
- ☐ ☐ Eating vegetables raw or quickly cooked by steaming or stir-frying
- ☐ ☐ Substituting tea and fruit and vegetable juices for coffee and soda
- ☐ ☐ Eating whole-grain breads
- ☐ ☐ Including calcium in the diet (or from a supplement)
- ☐ ☐ Including soy products in the diet
- ☐ ☐ Using whole-wheat flour instead of refined white flour in baking
- ☐ ☐ Using brown (unpolished) rice instead of white (polished) rice

Decrease daily fat intake to 20 percent of total caloric intake by

- ☐ ☐ Limiting consumption of beef, poultry, or fish to no more than 3 to 6 ounces (about the size of a deck of cards) once or twice a week
- ☐ ☐ Trimming all visible fat from meat and removing skin from poultry prior to cooking
- ☐ ☐ Decreasing the amount of fat and oils used in cooking
- ☐ ☐ Substituting low-fat for high-fat dairy products
- ☐ ☐ Using salad dressings sparingly
- ☐ ☐ Using only half to three-quarters of the amount of fat required in baking recipes
- ☐ ☐ Limiting fat intake to mostly monounsaturated (olive oil, canola oil, nuts, and seeds) and omega-3 fats (fish, flaxseed, and flaxseed oil)
- ☐ ☐ Eating fish once or twice a week
- ☐ ☐ Including flaxseed oil in the diet

## Try It

Make a copy of these "Cancer-Fighting Diet" tips and each week incorporate into your lifestyle two additional dietary behaviors from the above list.

---

damage has begun. Research is still required in this area because a clear link has not been established.

**Phytonutrients** **Phytonutrients** are compounds found in abundance in fruits, vegetables, beans, nuts, and seeds. These nutrients may prevent cancer by blocking the formation of cancerous tumors and perhaps even disrupting the process once it has started. Each plant contains hundreds of phytonutrients. Examples of these nutrients and their effects are found in Table 12.1. To obtain the best possible protection, a minimum of five servings of a variety of fruits and vegetables should be consumed each day. Fruits and vegetables should be consumed several times a day (instead of in one meal) to maintain phytonutrients at effective levels throughout the day. Phytonutrient blood levels drop within 3 hours of consuming foods containing these nutrients.

**Fiber** Although not 100 percent conclusive, studies have linked low intake of fiber to increased risk for colon cancer. Fiber binds to bile acids in the intestine for excretion from the body in the stools. The interaction of bile acids

---

**Cruciferous vegetables** Plants that produce cross-shaped leaves (cauliflower, broccoli, cabbage, Brussels sprouts, kohlrabi), which seem to have a protective effect against cancer.

**Carotenoids** Pigment substances in plants that are often precursors to vitamin A. More than 600 carotenoids are found in nature, about 50 of which are precursors to vitamin A, the most potent one being beta-carotene.

**Phytonutrients** Compounds found in fruits and vegetables that block formation of cancerous tumors and disrupt the progress of cancer.

PRINCIPLES AND LABS

**TABLE 12.1** Selected Phytonutrients: Their Effects and Sources

| Phytochemical | Effect | Good Sources |
|---|---|---|
| Sulforaphane | Removes carcinogens from cells | Broccoli |
| PEITC | Keeps carcinogens from binding to DNA | Broccoli |
| Genistein | Prevents small tumors from accessing capillaries to get oxygen and nutrients | Soybeans |
| Flavonoids | Helps keep cancer-causing hormones from locking onto cells | Most fruits and vegetables |
| p-Coumaric and chlorogenic acids | Disrupts the chemical combination of cell molecules that can produce carcinogens | Strawberries, green peppers, tomatoes, pineapple |
| Capsaicin | Keeps carcinogens from binding to DNA | Hot chili peppers |

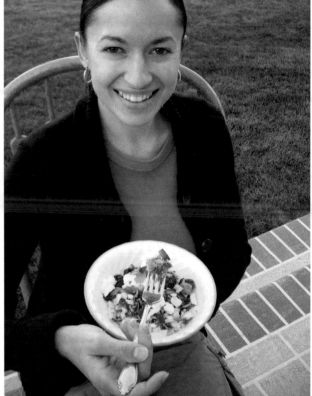

© Fitness & Wellness, Inc.

Cruciferous vegetables are recommended in a cancer-prevention diet.

with intestinal bacteria releases carcinogenic by-products. The production of bile acid increases with higher fat content in the small intestine (created, of course, by higher fat content in the diet).

Daily consumption of 25 (women) to 38 (men) grams of fiber is recommended. Whole grains are high in fiber and contain vitamins and minerals—folate, selenium, and calcium—which seem to decrease the risk for colon cancer. Selenium protects against prostate cancer and, possibly, lung cancer. Calcium may protect against colon cancer by preventing the rapid growth of cells in the colon, especially in people with colon polyps.

**Tea** Polyphenols (a group of phytonutrients) are potent cancer-fighting antioxidants found in fresh fruits and vegetables and many grains. A prime source is tea. Green, black, and red tea all seem to provide protection. Evidence also points to certain components in tea that can block the spread of cancers to other parts of the body. Polyphenols are known to block the formation of **nitrosamines** and quell the activation of **carcinogens**. Polyphenols also are thought to fight cancer by shutting off the formation of cancer cells, turning up the body's natural detoxification defenses, and thereby suppressing progression of the disease. Different types of tea contain different mixtures of polyphenols. White tea appears to have the highest amount, followed by green and black tea. Herbal teas do not provide the same benefits as regular tea.

Observational data on tea-drinking habits in China showed that people who regularly drank green tea had about half the risk for chronic gastritis and stomach cancer, and the risk decreased further as the number of years

of drinking green tea increased.[4] In Japan, where people drink green tea regularly but smoke twice as much as people in the United States, the incidence of lung cancer is half that of the United States.

The antioxidant effect of one of the polyphenols in green tea, epigallocatechin gallate, or EGCG, is at least 25 times more effective than vitamin E and 100 times more effective than vitamin C at protecting cells and DNA from damage believed to cause cancer, heart disease, and other diseases associated with free radicals.[5] EGCG also is twice as strong as the red wine antioxidant resveratrol in helping to prevent heart disease.

Many of the benefits of regular tea consumption warrant further investigation. Optimistic results in animal studies are still unclear in humans. Drinking two or more cups of tea daily, preferably white or green, in place of popular high-sugar/nutrient-deficient sodas is encouraged.

**Spices** Although still in the early stages, research is uncovering cancer-fighting phytonutrients in many traditional spices. These phytonutrients may alter damaging carcinogenic pathways, provide antioxidant effects, promote cancer-fighting enzymes, decrease inflammation, stimulate the immune system, and suppress the development of tumors.[6] Ginger, oregano, curry, pepper, cloves, fennel, rosemary, and turmeric are all encouraged for use in cooking and at the table.

**Sugar** New evidence indicates that frequent consumption of sugar and high-sugar foods may be associated with greater risk for pancreatic cancer, one of the most deadly forms of cancer.[7] Sugar is rapidly absorbed into the blood, quickly raising glucose and insulin levels. Researchers theorize that excessive glucose poisons and kills pancreatic cells, increasing cancer risk. Excessive insulin results in insulin-like growth factor, believed to increase cell proliferation and cancer.

The data showed that people who consumed the most sugar, including creamed fruit, syrup-based drinks, soft drinks, and foods such as coffee, tea, and cereal to which sugar is added had almost a 70 percent higher risk of developing pancreatic cancer compared with those with the lowest sugar consumption. Individuals who drank more than two soft drinks a day almost doubled the risk for pancreatic cancer.

**Dietary Fat** High intake of fat may promote cancer and excessive weight. Some experts recommend that total fat intake be limited to less than 20 percent of total daily calories.[8] Fat intake should consist of primarily monounsaturated omega-3 fats (found in flaxseed and several types of cold-water fish), which seem to offer protection against colorectal, pancreatic, breast, oral, esophageal, and stomach cancers. Omega-3 fats block the synthesis of prostaglandins, bodily compounds that promote growth of tumors.

**Processed Meat and Protein** Salt-cured, smoked, and nitrite-cured foods have been associated with cancers of the esophagus, stomach, colon, and rectum. Processed meats (hot dogs, ham, bacon, sausage, and lunch meats) should be consumed sparingly and always with vitamin C–rich foods such as orange juice, as vitamin C seems to discourage the formation of nitrosamines. These potentially cancer-causing compounds are formed when nitrites and nitrates, which are used to prevent the growth of harmful bacteria in processed meats, combine with other chemicals in the stomach.

The combination of the heme protein with iron, both found abundantly in red meat (but not poultry and fish), also contributes to the formation of nitrosamines in the large intestine, increasing the risk for colorectal cancer.

Further, nutritional guidelines discourage the excessive intake of protein. Too much animal protein appears to decrease blood enzymes that prevent precancerous cells from developing into tumors. According to the National Cancer Institute, eating substantial amounts of red meat may increase the risk for colorectal, pancreatic, breast, prostate, and renal cancer. Cooking protein at high temperature should be avoided or done only occasionally. The data suggest that grilling, broiling, or frying meat, poultry, or fish at high temperatures to "medium well" or "well done" leads to the formation of carcinogenic substances known as heterocyclic amines (HCAs) and polycyclic aromatic hydrocarbons (PAHs). Individuals who prefer their meat medium well or well done have a much higher risk for colorectal and stomach cancers.

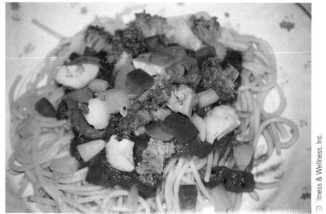

Nutrition guidelines for a cancer-prevention program include a diet low in fat and high in fiber, with ample amounts of fruits and vegetables.

Cooking proteins at high temperatures changes amino acids into HCAs that collect on the surface of meats. Charring meat increases their formation to an even greater extent. PAHs are formed when fat drips onto the rocks or coals of the grill. The subsequent fire flare-up releases smoke that coats the food with PAHs.

An electric contact grill such as a George Foreman grill is preferable when cooking meats because cooking temperatures are easily controlled. When cooking on an outdoor grill, line the grill with foil to keep the drippings off the rocks or coals. Microwaving the meat for a couple of minutes before barbecuing also decreases the risk, as long as the fluid released by the meat is discarded. Most of the potential carcinogens collect in this solution. For an occasional outdoor barbecue, trim off excess fat to avoid flare-ups and turn meats over frequently to decrease HCA formation. Removing the skin before serving and cooking at lower heat to medium also lowers the risk.

**Soy** Soy protein seems to decrease the formation of carcinogens during cooking of meats. Soy foods may help because soy contains chemicals that prevent cancer. Although further research is merited, isoflavones (phytonutrients) found in soy are structurally similar to estrogen and may prevent breast, prostate, lung, and colon cancers. Isoflavones, frequently referred to as "phytoestrogens" or "plant estrogens," also block angiogenesis. Presently, it is not known whether the health benefits of soy are derived from isoflavones by themselves or in combination with other nutrients found in soy.

**Nitrosamines** Potentially cancer-causing compounds formed when nitrites and nitrates, which prevent the growth of harmful bacteria in processed meats, combine with other chemicals in the stomach.

**Carcinogens** Substances that contribute to the formation of cancers.

One drawback of soy was found in studies in which animals with tumors were given large amounts of soy. The estrogen-like activity of soy isoflavones actually led to the growth of estrogen-dependent tumors. Experts, therefore, caution women with breast cancer or a history of this disease to limit their soy intake because it could stimulate cancer cells by closely imitating the actions of estrogen. No specific recommendations are presently available as to the recommended amount of daily soy protein intake to prevent cancer.

Based on the traditional diets of people (including children) in China and Japan who consume soy foods regularly, there doesn't seem to be an unsafe natural level of consumption. Soy protein powder supplementation, however, may elevate intake of soy protein to an unnatural (and perhaps unsafe) level.

**Alcohol Consumption** People should consume alcohol in moderation, because too much alcohol raises the risk for developing certain cancers, especially when it is combined with tobacco (smoking or smokeless). In combination, these substances significantly increase the risk for cancers of the mouth, larynx, throat, esophagus, and liver. Approximately 17,000 deaths from cancer yearly are attributed to excessive use of alcohol, often in combination with smoking. The combined action of heavy alcohol and tobacco use can increase the odds of developing cancer of the oral cavity fifteenfold.

## Excessive Body Weight

Maintaining recommended body weight is encouraged. Based on estimates, excess weight accounts for 14 to 20 percent of deaths from cancer.[9] Furthermore, obese men and women have a more than 50 percent increased risk for dying from any form of cancer.[10] Adult weight gain increases the risk for many cancers, including those of the breast, colon/rectum, endometrium, and kidney. Obesity may also increase the risk for pancreatic, gallbladder, ovarian, thyroid, and cervical cancers. Investigators theorize that excess weight raises hormone levels in the body that stimulate tumor growth.

## Abstaining from Tobacco

Cigarette smoking by itself is a major health hazard. If we include all related deaths, smoking is responsible for more than 440,000 unnecessary deaths in the United States each year. The World Health Organization estimates that smoking causes 5 million deaths worldwide annually. The average life expectancy for a chronic smoker is about 15 years shorter than for a nonsmoker.[11]

The biggest carcinogenic exposure in the workplace is to cigarette smoke. Of all cancers, at least 30 percent are tied to smoking, and 87 percent of lung cancers are linked to smoking. Use of smokeless tobacco can also lead to nicotine addiction and dependence, as well as increased risk for cancers of the mouth, larynx, throat, and esophagus.

## Avoiding Excessive Exposure to Sun

"Safe sun" exposure, up to 15 minutes of unprotected exposure per day, is beneficial to health; but too much exposure to ultraviolet radiation is a major contributor to skin cancer.

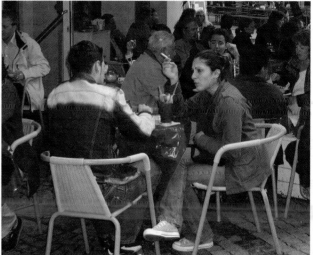

Heavy drinking and smoking greatly increase the risk of oral cancer.

The most common sites of skin cancer are the areas exposed to the sun most often (face, neck, and back of the hands). Ultraviolet (UV) rays are strongest when the sun is high in the sky. Therefore, you should avoid prolonged sun exposure between 10:00 a.m. and 4:00 p.m. Take the shadow test: If your shadow is shorter than you, the UV rays are at their strongest.

The three types of skin cancer are:

1. Basal cell carcinoma
2. Squamous cell carcinoma
3. Malignant melanoma

Nearly 90 percent of the almost 1 million cases of basal cell or squamous cell skin cancers reported yearly in the United States could have been prevented by protecting the skin from the sun's rays. **Melanoma**, the most deadly type, caused approximately 8,420 deaths in 2008. One in every six Americans eventually will develop some type of skin cancer.

One to two blistering sunburns can double the lifetime risk for melanoma, even more so if the sunburn takes place prior to age 18, when cells divide at a much faster rate than later in life. Furthermore, nothing is healthy about a "healthy tan." Tanning of the skin is the body's natural reaction to permanent and irreversible damage from too much exposure to the sun. Even small doses of sunlight add up to a greater risk for skin cancer and premature aging. The tan fades at the end of the summer season, but the underlying skin damage does not disappear.

The stinging sunburn comes from **ultraviolet B (UVB) rays,** which are also thought to be the main cause of premature wrinkling and skin aging, roughened/leathery/sagging skin, and skin cancer. Unfortunately, the damage may not become evident until up to 20 years later. By comparison, skin that has not been overexposed to the sun remains smooth and unblemished and, over time, shows less evidence of aging.

Sun lamps and tanning parlors provide mainly **ultraviolet A (UVA) rays.** Once thought to be safe, they too are now known to be damaging and have been linked to melanoma. As little as 15 to 30 minutes of exposure to UVA rays can be as dangerous as a day spent in the sun. Similar to regular exposure to sun, short-term exposure to recreational tanning at a salon causes DNA alterations that can lead to skin cancer.[12]

Sunscreen lotion should be applied about 30 minutes before lengthy exposure to the sun because the skin takes that long to absorb the protective ingredients. You should select sunscreens labeled "broad spectrum," as these products block both UVA and UVB rays. A **sun protection factor (SPF)** of at least 15 is recommended. SPF 15 means that the skin takes 15 times longer to burn than it would with no lotion. If you ordinarily get a mild sunburn after 20 minutes of noonday sun, an SPF 15 allows you to remain in the sun about 300 minutes before burning. Sunscreens with stronger SPF factors are not necessarily better. They should be applied just as often, and they block only an additional 3 to 4 percent of UV rays. An SPF 15 is adequate for most people. When swimming or sweating, you should reapply waterproof sunscreens more often, because all sunscreens lose strength when they are diluted.

Even better than sunscreen is wearing protective clothing, including long-sleeved shirts, long pants, and a hat with a two- to three-inch brim all the way around. This sun-protection strategy is even more critical for fair-skinned individuals who burn readily or turn red after only a few minutes of unprotected sun exposure, have a large number of moles, or have a personal or family history of skin cancer risk. Sun-protective fabrics, such as manufactured by Coolibar® or Sun Precautions®, offer additional protection. You can also use RIT Sun Guard, a laundry additive that when used in washing penetrates the fibers and subsequently absorbs UV rays during sun exposure. The additive blocks up to 96 percent of UVA and UVB rays.

## Monitoring Estrogen, Radiation Exposure, and Potential Occupational Hazards

Although intake of estrogen has been linked to endometrial cancer in some studies, other evidence contradicts those findings. As to exposure to radiation, although it increases the risk for cancer, the benefits of X-rays may outweigh the risk involved, and most medical facilities use the lowest dose possible to keep the risk to a minimum. Occupational hazards—such as exposure to asbestos fibers, nickel and uranium dusts, chromium compounds, vinyl chloride, and bischloromethyl ether—increase the risk for cancer. Cigarette smoking magnifies the risk from occupational hazards.

## Physical Activity

An active lifestyle has been shown to have a protective effect against cancer. Although the mechanism is not clear, physical fitness and cancer mortality in men and women may have a graded and consistent inverse relationship (Figure 12.9). A daily 30-minute, moderate-intensity exercise program lowers the risk for colon cancer and may lower the risk for cancers of the

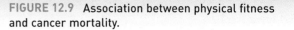

**FIGURE 12.9** Association between physical fitness and cancer mortality.

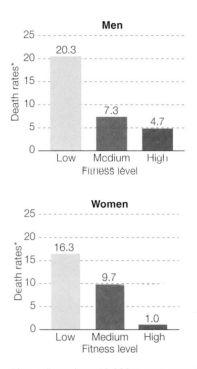

*Age-adjusted per 10,000 person-year at follow-up

***Source:*** S. N. Blair, H. W. Kohl III, R. S. Paffenbarger, Jr., D. G. Clark, D. H. Cooper, and L. W. Gibbons, "Physical Fitness and All-Cause Mortality: A Prospective Study of Healthy Men and Women," *Journal of the American Medical Association* 262 (1989): 2395–2401. Reprinted with permission.

breast and reproductive system. Growing evidence suggests that the body's autoimmune system may play a role in preventing cancer and that moderate exercise improves the autoimmune system.

New research among 38,410 men followed for an average period of 17.2 years indicated a strong inverse relationship between cardiorespiratory fitness and cancer mortality; that is, the lower-fit men had greater cancer death rates than the higher-fit men.[13] Other data suggest that in men 65 or older, exercising vigorously at least three times per week decreases the risk for advanced or fatal prostate cancer by 70 percent.[14]

Data on women indicate that regular exercise lowers the risk for breast cancer by up to 30 percent. And women who are active throughout life cut their risk for endome-

**Melanoma** The most virulent, rapidly spreading form of skin cancer.

**Ultraviolet B (UVB) rays** Portion of sunlight that causes sunburn and encourages skin cancers.

**Ultraviolet A (UVA) rays** Light rays provided by sun lamps and tanning parlors known to damage skin and promote skin cancers.

**Sun protection factor (SPF)** Degree of protection offered by ingredients in sunscreen lotion; at least SPF 15 is recommended.

## Behavior Modification Planning

### CANCER PROMOTERS

Do you currently avoid the following cancer promoters?

I PLAN TO

I DID IT

- ☐ ☐ Physical inactivity
- ☐ ☐ Being more than 10 pounds overweight
- ☐ ☐ Frequent consumption of red meat
- ☐ ☐ A diet high in fat
- ☐ ☐ Charred/burned foods
- ☐ ☐ Frequent consumption of nitrate-/nitrite-cured, salt-cured, or smoked foods
- ☐ ☐ Alcohol consumption
- ☐ ☐ Excessive sun exposure
- ☐ ☐ Estrogens
- ☐ ☐ Methyleugenol (flavoring agent in packaged foods)
- ☐ ☐ Radon
- ☐ ☐ Wood dust (high levels)

### Try It

In your Online Journal or class notebook, make a list of cancer promoters around you and note whether you take necessary actions to avoid them. If you do not, note what it would take for you to do so.

trial cancer by about 40 percent. Those who started exercise in adulthood cut their risk by about 25 percent.[15] Among women diagnosed with breast cancer, those who walk 2 to 3 miles per hour one to three times per week are 20 percent less likely to die of the disease. Those who walk three to five times per week cut their risk in half.[16] Researchers believe that the decreased levels of circulating ovarian hormones through physical activity decrease breast cancer risk.

**Early Detection** Fortunately, many cancers can be controlled or cured through early detection. The real problem comes when cancerous cells spread, because they become more difficult to destroy. Therefore, effective prevention, or at least early detection, is crucial. Herein lies the importance of periodic screening. Once a month, women should practice breast self-examination (BSE); and men, testicular self-examination (TSE). Men should pick a regular day each month (for example, the first day of each

month) to practice TSE, and women should perform BSE two or three days after the menstrual period is over.

**Other Factors** The contributions of many of the other much-publicized factors are not as significant as those just pointed out. Intentional food additives, saccharin, processing agents, pesticides, and packaging materials currently used in the United States and other developed countries seem to have minimal consequences. High levels of tension and stress and poor coping may affect the autoimmune system negatively and render the body less effective in dealing with the various cancers. In the workplace, the biggest carcinogenic exposure is to cigarette smoke.

Genetics plays a role in susceptibility in about 10 percent of all cancers. Most of the effect is seen in the early childhood years. Some cancers are a combination of genetic and environmental liability; genetics may add to the environmental risk of certain types of cancers. "Environment" means more than pollution and smoke. It incorporates diet, lifestyle-related events, viruses, and physical agents such as X-rays and exposure to the sun.

# Warning Signals of Cancer

Everyone should become familiar with the following seven warning signals of cancer and bring any that are present to a physician's attention:

1. Change in bowel or bladder habits
2. Sore that does not heal
3. Unusual bleeding or discharge
4. Thickening or lump in the breast or elsewhere
5. Indigestion or difficulty in swallowing
6. Obvious change in wart or mole
7. Nagging cough or hoarseness

The recommendations for early detection of cancer in asymptomatic people by the American Cancer Society, outlined in Table 12.2, should be heeded in regular physical examinations as part of a cancer-prevention program. In Lab 12.1, you will be able to determine how well you are doing in terms of a cancer-prevention program. Lab 12.2 provides a questionnaire developed by the American Medical Association to alert people to symptoms that may indicate a serious health problem. Although in most cases nothing serious will be found, any symptom calls for a physician's attention as soon as possible. Scientific evidence and testing procedures for the prevention and early detection of cancer do change. Studies continue to provide new information. The intent of cancer-prevention programs is to educate and guide people toward a lifestyle that will help prevent cancer and enable early detection of malignancy.

Treatment of cancer should always be left to specialized physicians and cancer clinics. Current treatment modalities include surgery, radiation, radioactive substances, chemotherapy, hormones, and immunotherapy.

**TABLE 12.2  Screening Guidelines for the Early Detection of Cancer in Asymptomatic People**

| Site | Recommendation |
|------|----------------|
| BREAST | • Yearly mammograms are recommended starting at age 40. The age at which screening should be stopped should be individualized by considering the potential risks and benefits of screening in the context of overall health status and longevity.<br>• Clinical breast exam should be part of a periodic health exam, about every 3 years for women in their 20s and 30s, and every year for women 40 and older.<br>• Women should know how their breasts normally feel and report any breast change promptly to their health care providers. Breast self-exam is an option for women starting in their 20s.<br>• Screening MRI is recommended for women with an approximately 20%–25% or greater lifetime risk of breast cancer, including women with a strong family history of breast or ovarian cancer and women who were treated for Hodgkin's disease. |
| COLON & RECTUM | Beginning at age 50, men and women should follow one of the examination schedules below:<br>• A fecal occult blood test (FOBT) or fecal immunochemical test (FIT) every year<br>• A flexible sigmoidoscopy (FSIG) every 5 years<br>• Annual FOBT or FIT and flexible sigmoidoscopy every 5 years*<br>• A double-contrast barium enema every 5 years<br>• A colonoscopy every 10 years |
| PROSTATE | The PSA test and the digital rectal exam should be offered annually, beginning at age 50, to men who have a life expectancy of at least 10 years. Men at high risk (African American men and men with a strong family history of one or more first-degree relatives diagnosed with prostate cancer at an early age) should begin testing at age 45. For both men at average risk and high risk, information should be provided about what is known and what is uncertain about the benefits and limitations of early detection and treatment of prostate cancer so that they can make an informed decision about testing. |
| UTERUS | **Cervix:** Screening should begin approximately 3 years after a woman begins having vaginal intercourse, but no later than 21 years of age. Screening should be done every year with regular Pap tests or every 2 years using liquid-based tests. At or after age 30, women who have had 3 normal test results in a row may get screened every 2 to 3 years. Alternatively, cervical cancer screening with HPV DNA testing and conventional or liquid-based cytology could be performed every 3 years. However, doctors may suggest a woman get screened more often if she has certain risk factors, such as HIV infection or a weak immune system. Women 70 years and older who have had 3 or more consecutive normal Pap tests in the last 10 years may choose to stop cervical cancer screening. Screening after total hysterectomy (with removal of the cervix) is not necessary unless the surgery was done as a treatment for cervical cancer.<br><br>**Endometrium:** The American Cancer Society recommends that at the time of menopause all women should be informed about the risks and symptoms of endometrial cancer and strongly encouraged to report any unexpected bleeding or spotting to their physicians. Annual screening for endometrial cancer with endometrial biopsy beginning at age 35 should be offered to women with or at risk for hereditary nonpolyposis colon cancer (HNPCC). |
| CANCER-RELATED CHECKUP | For individuals undergoing periodic health examinations, a cancer-related checkup should include health counseling and, depending on a person's age and gender, might include examinations for cancers of the thyroid, oral cavity, skin, lymph nodes, testes, and ovaries, as well as for some nonmalignant diseases. |

*Combined testing is preferred over either annual FOBT or FIT, or FSIG every 5 years, alone. People who are at moderate or high risk for colorectal cancer should talk with a doctor about a different testing schedule.
**Source:** American Cancer Society, *Cancer Facts & Figures 2008* (Atlanta: American Cancer Society, Inc.). Reprinted by permission.

# Cancer: Assessing Your Risks

Figure 12.10 provides a self-testing questionnaire to help you assess your cancer risk. The factors listed in the questionnaire are the major risk factors for specific cancer sites and by no means represent the only ones that might be involved. Check your status against the factors contained in this questionnaire. Based on the number of risk factors that apply to you, rate yourself on a scale from 1 to 3 (1 = low risk, 2 = moderate risk, and 3 = high risk) for each cancer site. Explanations of the risk factors for each type of cancer follow. If you are at higher risk, you are advised to discuss the results with your physician. Record your risk level totals for each cancer site in Lab 12C.

**FIGURE 12.10  Cancer Questionnaire: Assessing Your Risks.**

Name:_____ Date:_____

Course_____ Section:_____ Gender:_____ Age:_____

### Assessing Your Risks for Cancer

Read each question concerning each site and its specific risk factors. Be honest in your responses. Your risk increases as you move beyond item 1 for each factor. For example, the risk for lung cancer increases progressively as you age. If none of the answers apply, skip to the next question. Based on the number of risk factors that apply to you, rate yourself on a scale from 1 to 3 (1 for low risk, 2 for moderate risk, and 3 for high risk) for each cancer site. Record your results in Lab 12C.

### Lung Cancer

■ Gender
1. Female
2. Male

■ Age
1. 40 or less
2. 41–50
3. 51–60
4. >60

■ Smoking status
1. Non-smoker
2. Smoker

■ Type of smoking
1. Ex-cigarette smoker
2. Pipe and/or cigar, but not cigarettes
3. Cigarettes or little cigars

■ Amount of cigarettes smoked per day
1. 0 cigarettes
2. Less than 1 pack per day
3. 1 pack
4. 1–2 packs
5. 2+ packs

■ Type of cigarette
1. Non-smoker
2. Low tar/nicotine
3. Medium tar/nicotine
4. High tar/nicotine

■ Duration of smoking
1. Never smoked
2. Ex-smoker
3. Up to 15 years
4. 15–25 years
5. 25+ years

■ Type of industrial work
1. Mining
2. Uranium and radioactive products
3. Asbestos

### Colon/Rectum Cancer

■ Age
1. 40 or less
2. 41–60
3. >60

■ Has anyone in your immediate family ever had
1. One or more polyps of the colon
2. Colon cancer

■ Have you ever had
1. Cancer of the breast or uterus
2. Ulcerative colitis
3. One or more polyps of the colon
4. Colon cancer

■ Bleeding from the rectum (other than obvious hemorrhoids or piles)
1. No
2. Yes

■ Are you physically active?
1. Yes
2. No

### Skin Cancer

■ Frequent work or play in the sun:
1. No
2. Yes

■ Work in mines, around coal tars, or around radioactivity:
1. No
2. Yes

■ Complexion—fair and/or light skin:
1. No
2. Yes

### Breast Cancer

■ Age group
1. 35 or less
2. 36–50
3. >75

■ Race group
1. Asian American
2. Hispanic American
3. African American
4. White

■ Family history
1. None
2. Mother, sister, aunt, or grandmother with breast cancer

■ Your history
1. No breast disease
2. Previous lumps or cysts
3. Previous breast cancer

■ Maternity
1. First pregnancy before 25
2. First pregnancy after 25
3. No pregnancies

■ Are you physically active?
1. Yes
2. No

■ Hormone replacement therapy (HRT)
1. Never used or more than 5 years off HRT
2. Less than 5 years off HRT
3. Short-term use
4. Long-term use (several years)

■ Alcohol
1. Less than 1 drink per day
2. 2–5 drinks per day
3. More than 5 drinks per day

■ Obesity
1. Pre-menopausal
2. Post-menopausal

### Cervical Cancer
(Lower portion of uterus. These questions do not apply to a woman who has had a total hysterectomy.)

■ Age group
1. 25 or less
2. 26–40
3. 41–55
4. >55

■ Race
1. White
2. Oriental
3. Hispanic American
4. Puerto Rican
5. African American

■ Number of pregnancies
1. 0
2. 1–3
3. 4 and over

■ Viral infections
1. Never
2. Herpes and other viral infections or ulcer formations on the vagina

■ Age at first intercourse
1. Never
2. 25 and over
3. 20–24
4. 15–19
5. Before 15

■ Bleeding between periods or after intercourse
1. No
2. Yes

**FIGURE 12.10 Cancer Questionnaire: Assessing Your Risks.** *(continued)*

## Endometrial Cancer

(Body of uterus. These questions do not apply to a woman who has had a total hysterectomy.)

■ Age group
1. 40 or less
2. 41–50
3. >50

■ Race
1. African American
2. Hispanic American
3. Asian American
4. White

■ Births
1. 5 or more
2. 1 to 4
3. None

■ Weight
1. Normal
2. Underweight for height
3. 20–49 pounds overweight
4. 50 or more pounds overweight

■ Diabetes (elevated blood sugar)
1. No
2. Yes

■ Estrogen hormone intake
1. None
2. Yes, occasionally
3. Yes, regularly

■ Abnormal uterine bleeding
1. No
2. Yes

■ Hypertension (high blood pressure)
1. No
2. Yes

■ Are you physically active?
1. Yes
2. No

## Prostate Cancer (men)

■ Age
1. 50–65
2. >65

■ Family history
1. No
2. Yes

■ Are you African American or of African-American descent?
1. No
2. Yes

■ Is your diet high in saturated fat?
1. No
2. Yes

■ Are you physically active?
1. Yes
2. No

## Testicular Cancer (men)

■ Did you have an undescended testicle not corrected before age 6?
1. No
2. Yes

■ Did you suffer from testicular atrophy following mumps or a virus infection?
1. No
2. Yes

■ Family history
1. No
2. Yes

■ Have you suffered recurring injuries to the testicle(s)?
1. No
2. Yes

■ Do you suffer from abnormalities of the endocrine system (e.g., high hormone levels of pituitary gonadotropin or androgens)?
1. No
2. Yes

■ Have you been diagnosed with incomplete testicular development?
1. No
2. Yes

## Pancreatic Cancer

■ Age
1. <35
2. 35–55
3. 56–70
4. >70

■ Tobacco use
1. Non-user
2. Ex-user
3. Pipe, cigar, or smokeless tobacco
4. Cigarettes

■ Sugar
1. Limited sugar consumption
2. Moderate sugar consumption
3. Excessive sugar consumption

■ Weight
1. Normal
2. 10 to 50 pounds overweight
3. 50 or more pounds overweight

■ Are you physically active?
1. Yes
2. No

■ Have you been diagnosed with chronic pancreatitis?
1. No
2. Yes

■ Have you been diagnosed with cirrhosis?
1. No
2. Yes

■ Are you diabetic?
1. No
2. Yes

■ Do you consume a high-fat diet?
1. No
2. Yes

■ Race
1. Non–African American
2. African American

## Kidney and Bladder Cancer

■ Smoking history
1. Non-smoker
2. Ex-smoker
3. Cigarette smoker

■ Were you diagnosed with congenital (inborn) abnormalities of the kidneys or bladder?
1. No
2. Yes

■ Have you been exposed to aniline dyes, naphthalenes, or benzidines?
1. No
2. Yes

■ Do you have a history of schistosomiasis (a parasitic bladder infection)?
1. No
2. Yes

■ Do you suffer from frequent urinary tract infections?
1. No
2. Yes
3. Yes, mainly after age 50

## Oral Cancer

■ Tobacco use
1. Non-user
2. Ex-user
3. Pipe, cigar, or smokeless tobacco
4. Cigarettes

■ Alcohol use
1. Do not drink alcohol
2. Less than 1 drink per day/women or 2 drinks per day/men
3. More than 1 drink per day/women or 2 drinks per day/men

## Esophageal and Stomach Cancer

■ How many servings of fruits and vegetables do you consume daily?
1. >8
2. 5–8
3. 3–5
4. <3

■ How often do you consume salt-cured, smoked, or nitrate-cured foods?
1. Rarely
2. Less than once per week
3. 1–3 times per week
4. >3 times per week

(continued)

PRINCIPLES AND LABS

**FIGURE 12.10  Cancer Questionnaire: Assessing Your Risks. *(continued)***

■ Have you been told that you have an imbalance in stomach acid?
1. No
2. Yes

■ Do you have a history of pernicious anemia?
1. No
2. Yes

■ Have you been diagnosed with chronic gastritis or gastric polyps?
1. No
2. Yes

■ Family history of esophageal or stomach cancer?
1. No
2. Yes

**Ovarian Cancer (Women)**

■ Age
1. <50
2. 51–60
3. 61–70
4. >70

■ Do you have a personal history of ovarian problems?
1. No
2. Yes

■ Have you had estrogen post-menopausal hormone therapy?
1. No
2. Yes

■ Do you have an extensive history of menstrual irregularities?
1. No
2. Yes

■ Family history
1. None
2. Breast cancer
3. Ovarian cancer

■ Do you have a personal history of breast cancer?
1. No
2. Yes

■ Have you had a child?
1. Yes
2. No

■ Body weight
1. Normal
2. 10 to 50 pounds overweight
3. 50 or more pounds overweight

■ Do you have a family history of non-polyposis colon cancer?
1. No
2. Yes

**Thyroid Cancer**

■ Age
1. <35
2. 35–55
3. 56–70
4. >70

■ Did you receive radiation therapy to the head and neck region in childhood or adolescence?
1. No
2. Yes

■ Do you have a family history of thyroid cancer?
1. No
2. Yes

**Liver Cancer**

■ Do you have a personal history of cirrhosis of the liver?
1. No
2. Yes

■ Do you have a personal history of hepatitis B virus?
1. No
2. Yes

■ Have you been exposed to vinyl chloride (industrial gas used in plastics manufacturing)?
1. No
2. Yes

■ Have you been exposed to aflatoxin (natural food contaminant)?
1. No
2. Yes

**Leukemia**

■ Family history
1. No
2. Yes

■ Do you suffer from Down syndrome or other genetic abnormalities?
1. No
2. Yes

■ Have you had excessive exposure to ionizing radiation?
1. No
2. Yes

■ Are you exposed to environmental chemicals?
1. No
2. Yes

**Lymphomas**

■ Are you physically active?
1. Yes
2. No

■ Do you have a family history of lymphomas?
1. No
2. Yes

■ Are you exposed to
1. Herbicides
2. Organic solvents

■ Have you had an organ transplant?
1. No
2. Yes

■ Have you been diagnosed with any the following?
1. Epstein-Barr virus
2. HIV
3. Human T-cell leukemia/lymphoma virus-I (HTLV-I) virus

# Common Sites of Cancer

## Lung Cancer

### Risk Factors

1. **Gender.** Men have a higher risk for developing lung cancer than do women, when type (cigarette, cigar, pipe), amount, and duration of smoking are equal. Because more women are smoking cigarettes for a longer duration than previously, however, their incidence of lung and upper respiratory tract (mouth, tongue, and larynx) cancer is increasing. By type of cancer, lung cancer is now number one in mortality for women.

2. **Age.** The occurrence of lung and upper respiratory tract cancers increases with age.

3. **Smoking status.** Cigarette smokers have 20 times or even greater risk than nonsmokers. The rates for ex-smokers who have not smoked for 10 years, however, approach those for nonsmokers.

4. **Type of smoking.** Pipe and cigar smokers are at higher risk for lung cancer than nonsmokers. Cigarette smokers are at much higher risk than nonsmokers or pipe and cigar smokers. All forms of tobacco, including chewing, markedly increase the user's risk for developing cancer of the mouth.

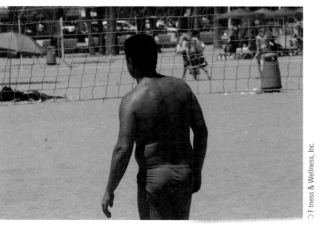

Tanning poses a risk for skin cancer from overexposure to ultraviolet rays. Tanned skin is the body's natural reaction to permanent and irreversible damage—a precursor to severe or fatal skin cancer.

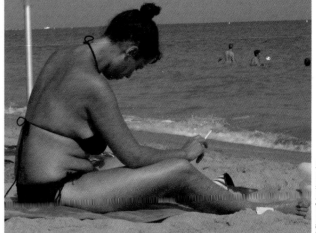

Excessive sun exposure, cigarette smoking, and excessive body weight are major risk factors for cancer.

5. Number of cigarettes smoked per day. Males who smoke less than half a pack per day have rates of lung cancer 5 times higher than nonsmokers. Males who smoke one to two packs per day have 15 times higher lung cancer rates than nonsmokers. Males who smoke more than two packs per day are 20 times more likely than nonsmokers to develop lung cancer.

6. Type of cigarette. Smokers of cigarettes low in tar and nicotine have slightly lower rates of lung cancer.

7. Duration of smoking. The frequency of lung and upper respiratory tract cancers increases with the length of time people have smoked.

8. Type of industrial work. Exposure to certain mining materials, uranium and radioactive products, or asbestos has been demonstrated to be associated with lung cancer. Exposure to materials in other industries also carries a higher risk. Smokers who work in these industries have greatly increased risks. Exposure to arsenic, radon, radiation from occupational/medical/environmental sources, and air pollution increase the risk for lung cancer.

### Colon/Rectal Cancer
**Risk Factors**

1. Age. Colon cancer occurs more frequently after 50 years of age.

2. Family predisposition. Colon cancer is more common in families that have a previous history of this disease.

3. Personal history. Polyps and bowel diseases are associated with colon cancer.

4. Rectal bleeding. Rectal bleeding may be a sign of colorectal cancer.

5. Physical inactivity. Strong scientific evidence points to a higher risk for colorectal cancer in physically inactive individuals.

In addition to the previously mentioned risk factors, smoking, alcohol consumption, a diet high in saturated fat and/or red meat, a diet low in fiber, inadequate consumption of fruits and vegetables, a history of breast or endometrial cancer, and inflammatory bowel disease increase the risk for colon or rectal cancer.

### Skin Cancer
**Risk Factors**

1. Complexion. Risk factors vary for different types of skin. Individuals with light complexions, natural blonde or red hair, and those who burn easily are at greater risk.

2. Personal and family history of melanoma and moles. Of particular note are large or unusual moles or a large number of moles.

3. Sun exposure. Excessive UV light is a culprit in skin cancer. Protect yourself with a sunscreen medication.

4. Work environment. Working in mines or around coal tar or radioactive materials can cause cancer of the skin.

Risks for skin cancer are difficult to state. For instance, a person with a dark complexion can work longer in the sun and be less likely to develop cancer than a light-skinned person. Furthermore, a person wearing a long-sleeved shirt and a wide-brimmed hat who spends hours working in the sun has less risk than a person wearing a swimsuit who sunbathes for only a short time. The risk increases greatly with age, and family history also plays a role.

### Critical Thinking

What significance does a "healthy tan" have in your social life? Are you a "sun worshiper," or are you concerned about skin damage, premature aging, and potential skin cancer in your future?

If any of the previous risk factors apply to you, you need to protect your skin from the sun or any other toxic material. Changes in moles, warts, or skin sores are important and should be evaluated by your doctor (Figure 12.11).

Skin Self-Exam. One of the easiest and quickest self-exams is a brief survey to detect possible skin cancers (Figure 12.12). Simple skin self-exams can reduce deaths from melanoma by as much as 63 percent, saving as many as 4,500 lives in the United States each year.

- Make a drawing of yourself. Include a full frontal view, a full back view, and close up views of your head (both sides), the soles of your feet, the tops of your feet, and the backs of your hands.
- After you get out of the bath or shower, examine yourself closely in a full-length mirror. On your sketch, make note of any moles, warts, or other skin marks you find anywhere on your body. Pay particular attention to areas that are exposed to the sun constantly, such as your face, the tops of your ears, and your hands.
- Briefly describe each mark on your sketch—its size, color, texture, and so on.
- Repeat the exam about once a month. Watch for changes in the size, texture, or color of moles, warts, or other skin marks. If you notice any difference, contact your physician. You also should contact a doctor if you have a sore that does not heal.

## Breast Cancer
### Risk Factors

1. Age. The risk for breast cancer increases significantly after 50 years of age.

2. Race. Breast cancer occurs more frequently in white women than any other group.

3. Family history. The risk for breast cancer is higher in women with a family history of it. The risk is even higher if more than one family member has developed breast cancer, and is further enhanced by the closeness

**FIGURE 12.11  Warning signs of melanoma: ABCD Rule.**

**A.** *Asymmetry:* One half of a mole or lesion doesn't look like the other half.

**B.** *Border:* A mole has an irregular, scalloped, or not clearly defined border.

**C.** *Color:* The color varies or is not uniform from one area of a mole or lesion to another, whether the color is tan, brown, black, white, red, or blue.

**D.** *Diameter:* The lesion is larger than 6 millimeters (¼ inch) or larger than a pencil eraser.

1/4"

Adapted from *FDA Consumer,* May 1991.

**FIGURE 12.12  Self exam for skin cancer.**

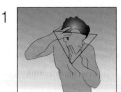

1  Examine your face, especially the nose, lips, mouth, and ears —front and back. Use one or both mirrors to get a clear view.

2  Thoroughly inspect your scalp, using a blow dryer and mirror to expose each section to view. Get a friend or family member to help, if you can.

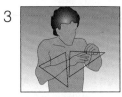

3  Check your hands carefully: palms and backs, between the fingers, and under the fingernails. Continue up the wrists to examine both front and back of your forearms.

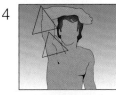

4  Standing in front of a full-length mirror, begin at the elbows and scan all sides of your upper arms. Don't forget the underarms.

5  Next focus on the neck, chest, and torso. Women should lift breasts to view the underside.

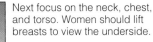

6  With your back to the full-length mirror, use the hand mirror to inspect the back of your neck, shoulders, upper back, and any part of the back of your upper arms you could not view in step 4.

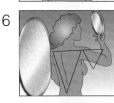

7  Still using both mirrors, scan your lower back, buttocks, and backs of both legs.

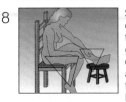

8  Sit down; prop each leg in turn on another stool or chair. Use the hand mirror to examine the genitals. Check front and sides of both legs, thigh to shin; ankles, tops of feet, between toes, and under toenails. Examine soles of feet and heels.

Reprinted with permission from *Family Practice Recertification* 14, no. 3 (March 1992).

**FIGURE 12.13** Breast self-examination.

**Looking**

Stand in front of a mirror with your upper body unclothed. Look for changes in the shape and size of the breast, and for dimpling of the skin or "pulling in" of the nipples. Any changes in the breast may be made more noticeable by a change in position of the body or arms. Look for any of the above signs or for changes in shape from one breast to the other.

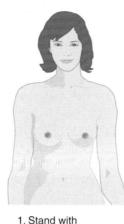
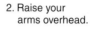
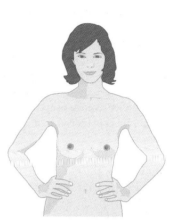

1. Stand with your arms down.

2. Raise your arms overhead.

3. Place your hands on your hips and tighten your chest and arm muscles by pressing firmly.

**Feeling**

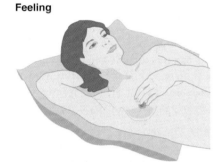
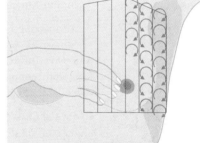
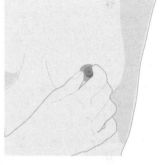

1. Lie flat on your back. Place a pillow or towel under one shoulder, and raise that arm over your head. With the opposite hand, you'll feel with the pads, not the fingertips, of the three middle fingers, for lumps or any change in the texture of the breast or skin.

2. The area you'll examine is from your collarbone to your bra line and from your breastbone to the center of your armpit. Imagine the area divided into vertical strips. Using small circular motions (the size of a dime), move your fingers up and down the strips. Apply light, medium, and deep pressure to examine each spot. Repeat this same process for your other breast.

3. Gently squeeze the nipple of each breast between your thumb and index finger. Any discharge, clear or bloody, should be reported to your doctor immediately.

*Source:* From *An Invitation to Health,* 11th edition, by Dianne Hales. ©2005. Reprinted with permission of Wadsworth, a division of Thomson Learning, Inc.

of the relationship (e.g., a mother or sister with breast cancer indicates a higher risk than a cousin with breast cancer).

4. **Personal history.** A previous history of breast or ovarian cancer indicates a higher risk.

5. **Maternity.** The risk is higher in women who have never had children and in women who bear children after 30 years of age.

6. **Physical inactivity.** Physically inactive women are at higher risk.

7. **Hormone replacement therapy (HRT).** Long-term use of a combination of progesterone and estrogen increases the risk. The risk seems to apply to current and recent users.

8. **Alcohol.** Two or more alcoholic drinks per day clearly enhance breast cancer risk.

9. **Obesity.** Adipose tissue increases estrogen levels. Higher estrogen levels, particularly following menopause, increase the risk.

Women with low to moderate risk should practice monthly BSE (Figure 12.13) and have their breasts examined by a doctor as a part of a cancer-related checkup. Periodic **mammograms** should be included as recom-

**Mammogram** Low-dose X-rays of the breasts used as a screening technique for the early detection of breast cancer.

mended. Women at high risk should practice monthly BSE and have their breasts examined regularly by a doctor. See your doctor for the recommended examinations (including mammograms and physical exam of breasts).

Clinical breast exams by a physician are recommended every 3 years for women between ages 20 and 40 and every year for women over age 40. The American Cancer Society also recommends an annual mammogram for women over age 40. The latter is still an area of debate among health care practitioners, and personal risk factors should be considered to determine the frequency of mammograms.

Other possible risk factors for breast cancer that are not listed in the questionnaire are high breast tissue density (a mammographic measure of the amount of glandular breast tissue relative to fatty breast tissue), a long menstrual history (onset of menstruation prior to age 13 and ending later in life), postmenopausal hormone therapy, recent use of oral contraceptives or post-menopausal estrogens, excessive caloric intake, high saturated fat intake, refined carbohydrates, drinking two or more alcoholic beverages per day, chronic cystic disease, and ionizing radiation. To decrease the risk, increase fiber, folic acid, monounsaturated fat, and vegetable consumption, and increase daily physical activity.

## Cervical Cancer (Women)
### Risk Factors

1. Age. The highest occurrence is in the 40-and-over age group. The scoring numbers in the questionnaire represent the relative rates of cancer for different age groups—that is, a 45-year-old woman has a risk three times greater than a 20-year-old.

2. Race. Puerto Ricans and other Hispanic Americans and African Americans have higher rates of cervical cancer.

3. Number of pregnancies. Women who have delivered several children have a higher occurrence.

4. Viral infections. Viral infections of the cervix and vagina are associated with cervical cancer.

5. Age at first intercourse. Women with earlier intercourse and with more sexual partners are at higher risk.

6. Bleeding. Irregular vaginal bleeding may be a sign of uterine cancer.

Early detection through a Pap test during a pelvic exam should be performed annually in women who are or have been sexually active or who have reached the age of 18. Following three normal tests during three consecutive years, the Pap test may be done less frequently, at the discretion of the physician.

## Endometrial Cancer (Women)
### Risk Factors

1. Age. Endometrial cancer is seen in older age groups. The scoring numbers by age group represent relative rates of endometrial cancer at different ages—for ex-

ample, a 50-year-old woman has a risk 12 times higher than that of a 35-year-old woman.

2. Race. White women have a higher occurrence.

3. Births. The fewer children the woman has delivered, the higher is the risk for endometrial cancer.

4. Weight. Women who are overweight are at higher risk.

5. Diabetes. Cancer of the endometrium is associated with diabetes.

6. Estrogen use. Cancer of the endometrium is associated with high cumulative exposure to estrogen. Obesity and hormone replacement therapy increase estrogen exposure. You should consult your physician before starting or stopping any estrogen therapy.

7. Abnormal bleeding. Women who do not have cyclic menstrual periods are at greater risk.

8. Hypertension. Cancer of the endometrium is associated with high blood pressure.

9. Physical inactivity. The risk for endometrial cancer is higher among physically inactive women.

Additional risk factors that may be associated with endometrial cancer but are not included in the questionnaire are infertility, a prolonged history of failure to ovulate, and menopause occurring after age 55. Women over age 40 should have a yearly pelvic exam by a physician.

## Prostate Cancer (Men)
The prostate gland is actually a cluster of smaller glands that encircle the top section of the urethra (urinary channel) at the point where it leaves the bladder. Although the function of the prostate is not entirely clear, the muscles of these small glands help squeeze prostatic secretions into the urethra.

### Risk Factors

1. Advancing age. The highest incidence of prostate cancer is found in men over age 65 (more than 70 percent of cases).

2. Family history

3. Race. African American men and Jamaican men of African American descent have the highest rates in the world.

4. Diet. A diet high in saturated fat.

5. Physical inactivity. The risk is greater in physically inactive men.

Prostate cancer is difficult to detect and control because the causes are not known. Death rates can be lowered through early detection and awareness of the warning signals. Detection is done by a digital rectal exam of the gland and a prostate-specific antigen (PSA) blood test once a year after the age of 50. Possible warning signals include difficulties in urination (especially at night), painful urination, blood in the urine, and constant pain in the lower back or hip area. Factors that decrease the risk include increasing the consumption of selenium-rich foods (up to 200 micrograms per day), including consumption of tomato-rich foods and fatty fish in the diet two or three times per week; avoiding a high-fat (especially animal fat) diet; increasing daily consumption of produce and grains; taking a daily supplement of vitamin E (preferably mixed tocopherols); and maintaining recommended vitamin D intake (found in multivitamins and fortified milk and manufactured by the body when exposed to sunlight).

**Testicular Cancer (Men)** Testicular cancer accounts for only 1 percent of all male cancers, but it is the most common type of cancer seen in men between ages 25 and 35. The incidence is slightly higher in Caucasians than in African Americans, and it is rarely seen in middle-aged and older men. The malignancy rate of testicular tumors is 96 percent, but if it is diagnosed early, this type of cancer is highly curable.

### Risk Factors

1. Undescended testicle not corrected before age 6

2. Atrophy of the testicle following mumps or virus infection

3. Family history of testicular cancer

4. Recurring injury to the testicle

5. Abnormalities of the endocrine system (e.g., high hormone levels of pituitary gonadotropin or androgens)

6. Incomplete testicular development

The incidence of testicular cancer is quite high in males born with an undescended testicle. Therefore, this condition should be corrected early in life. Parents of infant males should make sure that the child is checked by a physician to ensure that the testes have descended into the scrotum.

Some of the warning signals associated with testicular cancer are a small lump on the testicle, slight enlargement (usually painless) and change in consistency of the testis, sudden buildup of blood or fluid in the scrotum, pain in the groin and lower abdomen or discomfort accompanied by a sensation of dragging and heaviness, breast enlargement or tenderness, and enlarged lymph glands.

Early diagnosis of testicular cancer is essential, because this type of cancer spreads rapidly to other parts of the body. Because in most cases no early symptoms or pain is associated with testicular cancer, most people do not see a physician for months after discovering a lump or a slightly enlarged testis. Unfortunately, this delay allows almost 90 percent of testicular cancer to metastasize (spread) before a diagnosis is made. TSE once a month following a warm bath or shower (when the scrotal skin is relaxed) is recommended. Guidelines for performing a TSE are given in Figure 12.14.

**Pancreatic Cancer** The pancreas is a thin gland that lies behind the stomach. This gland releases insulin and pancreatic juice. Insulin regulates blood sugar, and pancreatic juice contains enzymes that aid in digesting food.

**FIGURE 12.14 Testicular self-examination.**

#### How to Examine the Testicles

You can increase your chances of early detection of testicular cancer by regularly performing a testicular self-examination (TSE). The following procedure is recommended:

■ Perform the self-exam once a month. Select an easy day to remember such as the first day or first Sunday of the month.

■ Learn how your testicle feels normally so that it will be easier to identify changes. A normal testicle should feel oval, smooth, and uniformly firm, like a hard-boiled egg.

■ Perform TSE following a warm shower or bath, when the scrotum is relaxed.

■ Gently roll each testicle between your thumb and the first three fingers until you have felt the entire surface. Pay particular attention to any lumps, change in size or texture, pain, or a dragging or heavy sensation since your last self-exam. Do not confuse the epididymis at the rear of the testicle for an abnormality.

■ Bring any changes to the attention of your physician. A change does not necessarily indicate a malignancy, but only a physician is able to determine that.

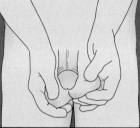

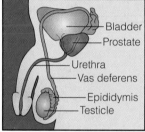

Bladder
Prostate
Urethra
Vas deferens
Epididymis
Testicle

### Possible Risk Factors

1. Increased incidence between ages 35 and 70, but significantly higher around age 55

2. Cigarette and cigar smoking, which may account for up to 30 percent of pancreatic cancer cases

3. Excessive sugar intake, which may increase the risk of developing pancreatic cancer by 70 percent

4. Obesity

5. Physical inactivity

6. Chronic pancreatitis

7. Cirrhosis

8. Diabetes

9. High-fat diet

10. African-American race

Detection of pancreatic cancer is difficult because (a) no symptoms are apparent in the early stages and (b) advanced disease symptoms are similar to those of other diseases. Only a biopsy can provide a definite diagnosis, but because pancreatic cancer is primarily a "silent" disease, the need for a biopsy is apparent only when the disease is already in an advanced stage.

Warning signals that may be related to pancreatic cancer include pain in the abdomen or lower back; jaundice; loss of weight and appetite; nausea; weakness, weariness, and loss of energy; agitated depression; dizziness; chills; muscle spasms; double vision; and coma.

**Kidney and Bladder Cancer** The kidneys are the organs that filter the urine, and the bladder stores and empties the urine. Most of these two types of cancer are caused by environmental factors. Bladder cancer occurs most frequently between the ages of 50 and 70. Of all bladder cancers, 80 percent are seen in men, and the incidence among Caucasian males is twice that among African-American males.

**Possible Risk Factors**
1. Heavy cigarette smoking, responsible for almost half of all deaths from bladder cancer in men and one-third of deaths from bladder cancer in women
2. Congenital abnormalities of either organ, detectable by a physician
3. Exposure to certain chemical compounds, such as aniline dyes, naphthalenes, or benzidines
4. History of schistosomiasis, a parasitic bladder infection
5. Frequent urinary-tract infections, particularly after age 50

Avoiding cigarette smoking and occupational exposure to cancer-causing chemicals is important to decrease the risk. Bloody urine, especially in repeated occurrences, is always a warning sign and requires immediate evaluation. Bladder cancer is diagnosed through urine analysis and examination of the bladder with a cystoscope (a small tube that is inserted into the tract through the urethra).

**Oral Cancer** Oral cancer affects the mouth, lips, tongue, salivary glands, pharynx, larynx, and floor of the mouth. Most of these cancers seem to be related to cigarette smoking and excessive consumption of alcohol.

**Risk Factors**
1. Heavy use of tobacco (cigarette, cigar, pipe, or smokeless)
2. Excessive alcohol consumption

Regular examinations and good dental hygiene help in prevention and early detection of oral cancer. Warning signals include a sore that doesn't heal or a white patch in the mouth, a lump, problems with chewing and swallowing, or a constant feeling of having "something" in the throat. A person with any of these conditions should be evaluated by a physician or a dentist. A tissue biopsy normally is conducted to diagnose the presence of cancer.

**Esophageal and Stomach Cancer** The incidence of gastric cancer in the United States has dropped about 40 percent in the last 30 years. Cancer experts attribute this drastic decrease to changes in dietary habits and refrigeration. This type of cancer is more common in men, and the incidence is higher in African-American males than in Caucasian males.

**Risk Factors**
1. A diet low in fresh fruits and vegetables
2. High consumption of salt-cured, smoked, and nitrate-cured foods
3. Imbalance in stomach acid
4. History of pernicious anemia
5. Chronic gastritis or gastric polyps
6. Family history of these types of cancer

Prevention is accomplished primarily by increasing dietary intake of complex carbohydrates and fiber and decreasing the intake of salt-cured, smoked, and nitrate-cured foods. In addition, regular guaiac testing for occult blood (hemoccult test) is recommended. Warning signals for this type of cancer include indigestion for 2 weeks or longer, blood in the stools, vomiting, and rapid weight loss.

**Ovarian Cancer (Women)** The ovaries are part of the female reproductive system that produces and releases the egg and the hormone estrogen. Ovarian cancer develops more frequently after menopause, and the highest incidence is seen between ages 55 and 64.

**Risk Factors**
1. Higher risk with age
2. History of ovarian problems
3. Estrogen post-menopausal hormone therapy
4. Extensive history of menstrual irregularities
5. Family history of breast or ovarian cancer
6. Personal history of breast cancer
7. Nulliparity (no pregnancies)
8. Excessive body weight
9. Hereditary nonpolyposis colon cancer

In most cases, ovarian cancer has no signs or symptoms. Therefore, regular pelvic examinations to detect signs of enlargement or other abnormalities are highly recommended. Some warning signals may be an enlarged abdomen, abnormal vaginal bleeding, unexplained digestive disturbances in women over age 40, and "normal"-size (premenopause-size) ovaries after menopause. Mutations to the BRCA1 and BRCA2 genes are also a risk factor. These are tumor suppressor genes located on chromosomes 17 and 13. Mutations to these genes increase cancer risk.

**Thyroid Cancer** The thyroid gland, located in the lower portion of the front of the neck, helps regulate growth and metabolism. Thyroid cancer occurs almost twice as often in women as in men. The incidence also is higher in Caucasians than African Americans.

**Risk Factors**
1. Age
2. Radiation therapy of the head and neck region received in childhood or adolescence
3. Family history of thyroid cancer

Regular inspection for thyroid tumors is done by palpating the gland and surrounding areas during a physical examination. Thyroid cancer is slow-growing; therefore, it is highly treatable. Nevertheless, any unusual lumps in front of the neck should be reported promptly to a physician. Although thyroid cancer does not have many warning signals (besides a lump), these may include difficulty swallowing, choking, labored breathing, and persistent hoarseness.

**Liver Cancer** The incidence of liver cancer in the United States is low. Men are more prone than women, and the disease is more common after age 60.

### Risk Factors

1. History of cirrhosis of the liver

2. History of hepatitis B virus

3. Exposure to vinyl chloride (industrial gas used in plastics manufacturing) and aflatoxin (a natural food contaminant)

Prevention consists primarily of avoiding the risk factors and being aware of warning signals. Possible signs and symptoms are a lump or pain in the upper right abdomen (which may radiate into the back and the shoulder), fever, nausea, rapidly deteriorating health, jaundice, and tenderness of the liver.

**Leukemia** Leukemia is a type of cancer that interferes with blood-forming tissues (bone marrow, lymph nodes, and spleen) by producing too many immature white blood cells. People who have leukemia cannot fight infection very well. The causes of leukemia are mostly unknown, although suspected risk factors have been identified.

### Possible Risk Factors

1. Inherited susceptibility, but not transmitted directly from parent to child

2. Greater incidence in individuals with Down syndrome (mongolism) and a few other genetic abnormalities

3. Excessive exposure to ionizing radiation

4. Environmental exposure to chemicals such as benzene, found in gasoline and cigarette smoke

Detection is not easy because early symptoms can be associated with other serious ailments. When leukemia is suspected, the diagnosis is made through blood tests and a bone marrow biopsy.

Early warning signals include fatigue, pallor, weight loss, easy bruising, nosebleeds, loss of appetite, repeated infections, hemorrhages, night sweats, bone and joint pain, and fever. At a more advanced stage, fatigue increases, hemorrhages become more severe, pain and high fever continue, the gums swell, and various skin disorders occur.

**Lymphoma** Lymphomas are cancers of the lymphatic system. The lymphatic system consists of lymph nodes found throughout the body and a network of vessels that link these nodes. The lymphatic system participates in the

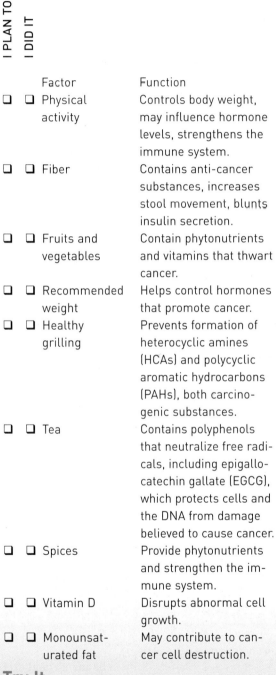

## Behavior Modification Planning

### LIFESTYLE FACTORS THAT DECREASE CANCER RISK

Do you have these healthy lifestyle factors working in your favor?

| I PLAN TO | I DID IT | Factor | Function |
|-----------|----------|--------|----------|
| ❏ | ❏ | Physical activity | Controls body weight, may influence hormone levels, strengthens the immune system. |
| ❏ | ❏ | Fiber | Contains anti-cancer substances, increases stool movement, blunts insulin secretion. |
| ❏ | ❏ | Fruits and vegetables | Contain phytonutrients and vitamins that thwart cancer. |
| ❏ | ❏ | Recommended weight | Helps control hormones that promote cancer. |
| ❏ | ❏ | Healthy grilling | Prevents formation of heterocyclic amines (HCAs) and polycyclic aromatic hydrocarbons (PAHs), both carcinogenic substances. |
| ❏ | ❏ | Tea | Contains polyphenols that neutralize free radicals, including epigallocatechin gallate (EGCG), which protects cells and the DNA from damage believed to cause cancer. |
| ❏ | ❏ | Spices | Provide phytonutrients and strengthen the immune system. |
| ❏ | ❏ | Vitamin D | Disrupts abnormal cell growth. |
| ❏ | ❏ | Monounsaturated fat | May contribute to cancer cell destruction. |

### Try It

In your Online Journal or class notebook, note ways you can incorporate all of these factors into your everyday lifestyle.

body's immune reaction to foreign cells, substances, and infectious agents.

**Possible Risk Factors**

As with leukemia, the causes of lymphomas are unknown. Individuals who have received organ transplants are at higher risk. Some researchers suspect that a form of herpes virus (called Epstein-Barr virus) is active in the initial stages of lymphosarcomas. Risk of non-Hodgkin's lymphoma is higher in people who carry the human immunodeficiency virus (HIV) and human T-cell leukemia/lymphoma virus I (HTLV-I). A family history increases the risk as well.

Other researchers suggest that certain external factors may alter the immune system, making it more susceptible to the development and multiplication of cancer cells. Exposure to herbicides, organic solvents, and other chemicals may also increase risk, as may poor diet and insufficient physical inactivity.

Prevention of lymphoma is limited because little is known about its causes. Enlargement of a lymph node or a cluster of lymph nodes is the first sign of lymphoma. Other signs and symptoms are an enlarged spleen or liver, weakness, fever, back or abdominal pain, nausea/vomiting, unexplained weight loss, unexplained itching and sweating, and fever at night that lasts for a long time.

## Critical Thinking

You have learned about many of the risk factors for major cancer sites. How will this information affect your health choices in the future? Will it be valuable to you, or will you quickly forget all you have learned and remain in a Contemplation stage at the end of this course?

# What Can You Do?

If you are at high risk for any form of cancer, you are advised to discuss this with your physician. An ounce of prevention is worth a pound of cure. Although cardiovascular disease is the number one killer in the United States, cancer is the number one fear. Of all cancers, 60 to 80 percent are preventable, and about 50 percent are curable. Most cancers are lifestyle related, so being aware of the risk factors and following the screening guidelines (see Table 12.2) and basic recommendations for preventing cancer will greatly decrease your risk for developing it.

# ASSESS YOUR BEHAVIOR

Log on to http://www.cengage.com/sso/ to take the cancer risk self-assessment and to modify your Behavior Change Planner if you wish.

1. Are you physically active on most days of the week?

2. Does your diet include ample amounts of colorful fruits and vegetables and of fiber, and is it low in red and processed meats?

3. Are you aware of your family history of cancer?

4. Do you practice monthly breast self-examination (women) or testicular self-examination (men)?

5. Do you respect the sun's rays? Do you use sunscreen lotion or wear protective clothing when you are in the sun for extended periods of time? Do you perform regular skin self-examinations?

6. Are you familiar with the seven warning signals of cancer and the cancer-screening guidelines?

# ASSESS YOUR KNOWLEDGE

Log on to http://www.cengage.com/sso/ to assess your understanding of this chapter's topics by taking the Student Practice Test and exploring the modules recommended in your Personalized Study Plan.

1. Cancer can be defined as
   a. a process whereby some cells invade and destroy the immune system.
   b. uncontrolled growth and spread of abnormal cells.
   c. the spread of benign tumors throughout the body.
   d. interference of normal body functions through blood-flow disruption caused by angiogenesis.
   e. All are correct choices.

2. Cancer treatment becomes more difficult when
   a. cancer cells metastasize.
   b. angiogenesis is disrupted.
   c. a tumor is encapsulated.
   d. cells are deficient in telomerase.
   e. cell division has stopped.

3. The leading cause of deaths from cancer in women is
   a. lung cancer.
   b. breast cancer.
   c. ovarian cancer.
   d. skin cancer.
   e. endometrial cancer.

4. Cancer
   a. is primarily a preventable disease.
   b. is often related to tobacco use.
   c. has been linked to dietary habits.
   d. has risk that increases with obesity.
   e. All are correct choices.

5. About 60 percent of cancers are related to
   a. genetics.
   b. environmental pollutants.
   c. viruses and other biological agents.
   d. ultraviolet radiation.
   e. diet, obesity, and tobacco use.

6. A cancer-prevention diet should include
   a. ample amounts of fruits and vegetables.
   b. cruciferous vegetables.
   c. phytonutrients.
   d. soy products.
   e. all of the above.

7. The biggest carcinogenic exposure in the workplace is to
   a. asbestos fibers.
   b. cigarette smoke.
   c. biological agents.
   d. nitrosamines.
   e. pesticides.

8. Which of the following is *not* a warning signal of cancer?
   a. Change in bowel or bladder habits
   b. Nagging cough or hoarseness
   c. A sore that does not heal
   d. Indigestion or difficulty in swallowing
   e. All of the above are warning signals of cancer.

9. The risk for breast cancer is higher in
   a. women under age 50.
   b. women with more than one family member with a history of breast cancer.
   c. minority groups than white women.
   d. women who had children prior to age 30.
   e. all of the above groups.

10. The risk for prostate cancer can be decreased by
    a. consuming selenium-rich foods.
    b. adding fatty fish to the diet.
    c. avoiding a high-fat diet.
    d. including tomato-rich foods in the diet.
    e. all of the above.

Correct answers can be found at the back of the book.

# MEDIA MENU

You can find the links below at the book companion site: www.cengage.com/health/hoeger/plfw10e

- Assess your risk for cancer.
- Check how well you understand the chapter's concepts.

## Internet Connections

- American Cancer Society. This comprehensive site features fact sheets and information on a variety of cancer types. The site explores treatment options, including alternative or complementary therapies. It features the popular cancer profiler for personalized cancer-treatment information, the cancer survivors' network, and a search engine for local resources. *http://www.cancer.org*

- National Cancer Institute. This government site, from the National Institutes of Health, provides statistics, frequently asked questions, and information on research and support resources. It includes links to Web pages with information about specific cancers. *http://www.nci.nih.gov*

- Susan G. Komen Breast Cancer Foundation. This site provides a wealth of breast cancer information, including a video showing the correct way to perform a breast self-exam, and the Komen NetQuiz, which allows you to test your knowledge of breast cancer. *http://www.komen.org/bci*

# NOTES

1. American Cancer Society, *Cancer Facts & Figures 2008* (New York: ACS, 2008).

2. J. E. Enstrom, "Health Practices and Cancer Mortality Among Active California Mormons," *Journal of the National Cancer Institute* 81 (1989): 1807–1814.

3. See note 1.

4. V. W. Setiawan, et al., "Protective Effect of Green Tea on the Risks of Chronic Gastritis and Stomach Cancer," *International Journal of Cancer* 92 (2001): 600–604.

5. L. Mitscher and V. Dolby, *The Green Tea Book—China's Fountain of Youth* (New York: Avery Press, 1997).

6. "Curbing Cancer's Reach: Little Things That Might Make a Big Difference," *Environmental Nutrition* 29, no. 6 (2006): 1, 6.

7. S. C. Larsson, L. Bergkvist, and A. Wolk, "Consumption of Sugar-Sweetened Foods and the Risk of Pancreatic in a Prospective Study," *American Journal of Clinical Nutrition* 84 (2006): 1171–1176.

8. J. H. Weisburger and G. M. Williams, "Causes of Cancer," *American Cancer Society Textbook of Clinical Oncology* (Atlanta: ACS, 1995): 10–39.

9. See note 1.

10. E. E. Calle, C. Rodriguez, K. Walker-Thurmond, and M. J. Thun, "Overweight, Obesity, and Mortality from Cancer in a Prospectively Studied Cohort of U.S. Adults," *New England Journal of Medicine* 348 (2003): 1625–1638.

11. American Cancer Society, *1995 Cancer Facts & Figures* (New York: ACS, 1995).

12. S. E. Whitmore, W. L. Morison, C. S. Potten, and C. Chadwick, "Tanning Salon Exposure and Molecular Alterations," *Journal of the American Academy of Dermatology* 44 (2001): 775–780.

13. S. W. Farrell, et al., "Cardiorespiratory Fitness, Different Measures of Adiposity, and Cancer Mortality in Men," *Obesity* 15 (2007): 3140–3149.

14. E. L. Giovannucci, "A Prospective Study of Physical Activity and Incident and Fatal Prostate Cancer," *Archives of Internal Medicine* 165 (2005): 1005–1010.

15. C. W. Matthews, et al., "Physical Activity and Risk of Endometrial Cancer: A Report from the Shanghai Endometrial Cancer Study," *Cancer Epidemiology Biomarkers & Prevention* 14 (2005): 779–785.

16. M. D. Holmes, et al., "Physical Activity and Survival After Breast Cancer Diagnosis," *Journal of the American Medical Association* 293 (2005): 2479–2486.

# SUGGESTED READINGS

American Cancer Society. *Cancer Facts & Figures 2008*. New York: ACS, 2008.

American Cancer Society. "Causes of Cancer." *Textbook of Clinical Oncology*. Atlanta: ACS, 1995.

American Heart Association and American Cancer Society. *Living Well, Staying Well*. New York: Random House, 1999.

American Institute for Cancer Research. *Stopping Cancer Before It Starts*. New York: Griffin, 2000.

"Eating to Beat Cancer." Special supplement to the *Tufts University Health & Nutrition Letter* 25, no. 3 (May 2007).

# LAB 12A: Cancer Prevention Guidelines

Name _____   Date _____   Grade _____

Instructor _____   Course _____   Section _____

**Necessary Lab Equipment**
None required.

**Objective**
To encourage healthy lifestyle practices that will help decrease the risk for cancer.

### I. Cancer Prevention: Are You Taking Control?

Today, scientists think most cancers may be related to lifestyle and environment—what you eat and drink, whether you smoke, and where you work and play. The good news, then, is that you can help reduce your own cancer risk by taking control of things in your daily life.

**12 Steps to a Healthier Life and Reduced Cancer Risk**                                    Yes   No

1. **Are you eating more cabbage-family vegetables?**
   They include broccoli, cauliflower, Brussels sprouts, all cabbages, and kale.                ☐    ☐

2. **Does your diet include high-fiber foods?**
   Fiber is found in whole grains, fruits, and vegetables including peaches, strawberries,
   potatoes, spinach, tomatoes, wheat and bran cereals, rice, popcorn, and whole-wheat bread.    ☐    ☐

3. **Do you choose foods with vitamin A?**
   Fresh foods with beta-carotene, including carrots, peaches, apricots, squash, and
   broccoli, are the best source—not vitamin pills.                                             ☐    ☐

4. **Is vitamin C included in your diet?**
   You'll find it naturally in lots of fresh fruits and vegetables, including grapefruit, cantaloupe,
   oranges, strawberries, red and green peppers, broccoli, and tomatoes.                         ☐    ☐

5. **Are you physically active and do you monitor calorie intake to avoid weight gain?**

   Total number of daily steps: ⬚⬚⬚⬚⬚⬚   Total minutes of daily physical activity: ⬚⬚⬚⬚⬚⬚   ☐    ☐

6. **Are you cutting overall fat intake?**
   This is done by eating lean meat, fish, skinned poultry, and low-fat dairy products.          ☐    ☐

7. **Do you limit salt-cured, smoked, nitrite-cured foods?**
   Choose bacon, ham, hot dogs or salt-cured fish only occasionally if you like them a lot.      ☐    ☐

8. **If you smoke, have you tried quitting?**                                                    ☐    ☐

9. **If you drink alcohol, is your intake moderate (no more than two drinks per day for
   men and one per day for women)?**                                                            ☐    ☐

10. **Do you get almost daily "safe sun" exposure, and yet respect the sun's rays?**
    "Safe sun" exposure means up to 15 minutes of unprotected sun exposure (without sunscreen) to
    the face, arms, and hands during peak daylight hours on most days of the week. If not, do you
    take a daily vitamin $D_3$ supplement?                                                       ☐    ☐

    Do you protect yourself with sunscreen (at least SPF 15) and wear long sleeves and a hat,
    especially during midday hours (10 a.m. to 4 p.m.) if you are going to be exposed to the sun for
    a prolonged period?                                                                          ☐    ☐

11. **Do you have a family history of any type of cancer? If so, have you brought this to the
    attention of your personal physician?**                                                     ☐    ☐

12. **Are you familiar with the seven warning signals for cancer?**                             ☐    ☐

If you answered "yes" to most of these questions, **congratulations.** You are taking control of simple lifestyle factors that will help you feel better and reduce your risk for cancer.

---

Adapted from the American Cancer Society, Texas Division.

# LAB 12B: Recognizing Early Signs of Illness

Name _____ Date _____ Grade _____

Instructor _____ Course _____ Section _____

**Necessary Lab Equipment**
None required.

**Objective**
To encourage early recognition of symptoms to improve the chances for cure or control.

Many serious illnesses begin with apparently minor or localized symptoms that, if recognized early, can alert you to act in time for the disease to be cured or controlled. In most cases, nothing is seriously wrong. **If you experience any of the following symptoms, discuss the problem with your physician without delay.** Check only conditions that apply.

☐ 1. Rapid loss of weight—more than about 4 kg (10 lbs) in 10 weeks—without apparent cause.

☐ 2. A sore, scab, or ulcer, either in the mouth or on the body, that fails to heal within about 3 weeks.

☐ 3. A skin blemish or mole that begins to bleed or itch or that changes color, size, or shape.

☐ 4. Severe headaches that develop for no obvious reason.

☐ 5. Sudden attacks of vomiting, without preceding nausea.

☐ 6. Fainting spells for no apparent reason.

☐ 7. Visual problems such as seeing "haloes" around lights or intermittently blurred vision, especially in dim light.

☐ 8. Increasing difficulty with swallowing.

☐ 9. Hoarseness without apparent cause that lasts for a week or more.

☐ 10. A "smoker's cough" or any other nagging cough that has been getting worse.

☐ 11. Blood in coughed-up phlegm, or sputum.

☐ 12. Constantly swollen ankles.

☐ 13. A bluish tinge to the lips, the insides of the eyelids, or the nailbeds.

☐ 14. Extreme shortness of breath for no apparent reason.

☐ 15. Vomiting of blood or a substance that resembles coffee grounds.

☐ 16. Persistent indigestion or abdominal pain.

☐ 17. A marked change in normal bowel habits, such as alternating attacks of diarrhea and constipation.

☐ 18. Bowel movements that look black and tarry.

☐ 19. Rectal bleeding.

☐ 20. Unusually cloudy, pink, red, or smoky-looking urine.

☐ 21. In men, discomfort or difficulty when urinating.

☐ 22. In men, discharge from the tip of the penis.

☐ 23. In women, a lump or unusual thickening of a breast or any alteration in breast shape such as flattening, bulging, or puckering of skin.

☐ 24. In women, bleeding or unusual discharge from the nipple.

☐ 25. In women, vaginal bleeding or "spotting" that occurs between usual menstrual periods or after menopause.

# LAB 12C: Cancer Risk Profile

Name _____    Date _____    Grade _____

Instructor _____    Course _____    Section _____

### Necessary Lab Equipment
None required.

### Objective
To determine your risk for selected cancer sites.

### I. Cancer Risk Profile

**Instructions**—Read the section "Cancer: Assessing Your Risks" (beginning on page 435) and complete the Cancer Questionnaire: Assessing Your Risks in Figure 12.10 (pages 436–438). Rate yourself on a scale from 1 to 3 (1 = low risk, 2 = moderate risk, 3 = high risk) according to the risk factors provided for each site and write the scores and risk categories in the blanks provided below.

| Cancer Site | Total Points Men | Total Points Women | Risk Category |
|---|---|---|---|
| Lung | ☐ | ☐ | ☐ |
| Colon-Rectum | ☐ | ☐ | ☐ |
| Skin | ☐ | ☐ | ☐ |
| Breast | | ☐ | ☐ |
| Cervical | | ☐ | ☐ |
| Endometrial | | ☐ | ☐ |
| Prostate | ☐ | | |
| Testicular | ☐ | | |
| Pancreatic | ☐ | ☐ | ☐ |
| Kidney and Bladder | ☐ | ☐ | ☐ |
| Oral | ☐ | ☐ | ☐ |
| Esophageal and Stomach | ☐ | ☐ | ☐ |
| Ovarian | | ☐ | |
| Thyroid | ☐ | ☐ | ☐ |
| Liver | ☐ | ☐ | ☐ |
| Leukemia | ☐ | ☐ | ☐ |
| Lymphomas | ☐ | ☐ | ☐ |

## II. Stage of Change for Cancer Prevention

Using Figure 2.5 (page 57) and Table 2.3 (page 57), identify your current stage of change for participation in a cancer-prevention program:

## III. Personal Interpretation

In the space provided below, discuss your results for the various cancer sites. State your feelings about cancer and comment on any experiences that you may have had with cancer patients.

_____

_____

_____

_____

_____

_____

_____

_____

_____

## IV. Cancer Prevention

Discuss lifestyle habits that you should eliminate and habits that you need to adopt to reduce your own risk of cancer. Also indicate how you can best implement and adhere to these changes.

_____

_____

_____

_____

_____

_____

_____

_____

_____

# Addictive Behavior

**13**

Sze Fei Wong/istockphoto.com

## Objectives

- Address the detrimental effects of addictive substances, including marijuana, cocaine, methamphetamine, MDMA, heroin, and alcohol
- List the detrimental health effects of tobacco use in general
- Recognize cigarette smoking as the largest preventable cause of premature illness and death in the United States
- Enumerate the reasons people smoke
- Explain the benefits and the significance of a smoking-cessation program
- Learn how to implement a smoking-cessation program, to help yourself (if you smoke) or someone else go through the quitting process
- Find out if you're prone to addictive behavior. Plan for a smoke-free future.

**CENGAGENOW**

Check your understanding of the chapter contents by logging on to CengageNOW and accessing the pre-test, personalized learning plan, and post-test for this chapter.

# FAQ

## What is drug addiction and how quickly can someone become addicted to drugs?

Drug addiction (addictive behavior, substance abuse, or chemical dependency) is a complex brain disease characterized by compulsive and uncontrollable drug cravings even at the peril of serious negative consequences. How quickly addictive behavior develops cannot be predicted. There are vast individual differences in sensitivity to different drugs among people.

Psychological and physiologic factors, as well as the type of drug used itself, influence a person's response to the drug and subsequent addiction to it. Whereas one individual may use a certain drug several times without harmful effects, someone else may seriously overdose the first time that this same drug is used. All drugs have potentially damaging effects, and some have life-threatening consequences. One single moment of weakness, or caving in to peer pressure, can easily result in a lifetime nightmare, not just for users, but for everyone around them as well.

## How can I tell if someone is addicted to drugs?

People with addictive behavior compulsively seek and use drugs despite potential serious repercussions, such as physical and family problems, loss of a job, or problems with the law. Some individuals realize that they need to cut down on their drinking/drug use, or they are told to do so by others. At times they crave alcohol or drugs when they first get up in the morning and they feel bad or guilty about their addictive behavior. If you see any of these signs in someone you know, that person is most likely addicted to drugs.

## How is drug addiction treated?

In the early stages of substance abuse, most people believe that they can stop using the drug(s) on their own. Most of these attempts, however, fail to achieve long-term abstinence. Long-term drug use results in altered brain functions that linger on long after the person stops using drugs. Effective treatment of drug addiction is rarely accomplished without professional help. Treatment modalities are behavioral-based therapies, oftentimes combined with medication to help the body detoxify and effectively manage symptoms of withdrawal. Responses to these therapies vary among individuals, and several courses of rehab may be necessary to overcome the problem. For some individuals, it becomes a lifetime battle, and relapses are possible even after prolonged periods of abstinence.

Substance abuse remains one of the most serious health problems afflicting society. Chemical dependency is extremely destructive, having ruined and ended millions of lives. When addictive behaviors are at issue, education is vital—more, perhaps, than with any other unhealthy behavior. Education concerning these subjects may assist in the search for answers, treatment, and a more productive and better life. The information in this chapter will help you make informed decisions. The time to make healthy choices is now.

# Addiction

When most people think of **addiction,** they probably think of dark and dirty alleys, an addict shooting drugs into a vein, or a wino passed out next to a garbage can after having spent an evening drinking alcohol. Psychotherapists have described addiction as a problem of imbalance or unease within the body and mind.

Almost anything can be addicting. Of the many types of addiction, some addictive behaviors are more detrimental than others. The most serious form is chemical dependency on drugs such as tobacco, alcohol, cocaine, methamphetamine, MDMA (Ecstasy), heroin, marijuana, or prescription drugs. Less serious are addictions to work, coffee, shopping, and even exercise.

People who are addicted to food eat to release stress or boredom or to reward themselves for every small personal achievement. Many people are addicted to television and the Internet. Others become so addicted to their jobs that all they think about is work. It may start out as enjoyable, but when it totally consumes a person's life, work can become an unhealthy behavior. If you find that you are readily irritated, moody, grouchy, constantly tired, not as alert as you used to be, or making more mistakes than usual, you may be becoming a workaholic and need to slow down or take time off work.

Even though exercise has enhanced the health and quality of life of millions of people, a relatively small number become obsessed with exercise, which has the potential for overuse and addiction. Compulsive exercisers feel guilty and uncomfortable when they miss a day's workout. Often, they continue to exercise even when they have injuries and sicknesses that require proper rest for adequate recovery. People who exceed the recommended guidelines to develop and maintain fitness (see Chapters 6, 7, 8, and 9) are exercising for reasons other than health—including addictive behavior.

Addiction to caffeine can have undesirable side effects. In some individuals, caffeine doses as low as 200 mg can produce an abnormally rapid heart rate, abnormal heart rhythms, higher blood pressure, and increased secretion of gastric acids, leading to stomach problems and possible birth defects in offspring. It also may induce symptoms of anxiety, depression, nervousness, and dizziness.

The caffeine content of drinks varies according to the product. In 6 ounces of coffee, for example, the content varies from 65 mg in instant coffee to as high as 180 mg in drip coffee. Soft drinks, mainly colas, range in caffeine content from about 30 to 70 mg per 12-ounce can.

Energy drinks on the market, such as Red Bull, Full Throttle, Jolt, Rockstar, and Adrenaline Rush, usually have an even higher caffeine content: somewhere in the range of 70 to 140 mg in an 8- to 12-ounce drink. The U.S. Food and Drug Administration (FDA) requires that caffeine be listed on the labels of all energy drinks, but it does not mandate that the amount be specified. Most health experts agree that moderate caffeine consumption, about 300 mg per day, is safe for most adults.

Unknown to most consumers, however, caffeine is now added to a variety of other food items such as energy bars, candy, gum, and even oatmeal. Individuals who are caffeine sensitive should read all food labels for potential caffeine in those items.

Although the previous examples may be the first addictions you think of, they are by no means the only forms. Other addictions can be to gambling, pornography, sex, people, places, and on and on.

According to the 2006 National Survey on Drug Use and Health (NSDUH) by the U.S. Department of Health and Human Services,[1] the illicit drug category with the largest number of new users is the illegal use of prescription pain relievers. About 2.2 million people used pain relievers nonmedically for the first time within the past year. The average age of these new users was 21.9 years. Marijuana use followed a close second, with 2.1 million new users the same year.

**Risk Factors for Addiction** Although addictive behaviors cover a wide spectrum, they have factors in common that predispose people to addiction. Among these factors are the following:[2]

- The behavior is reinforced.
- The addiction is an attempt to meet basic human needs, such as physical needs, the need to feel safe, the need to belong, the need to feel important, or the need to reach one's potential.
- The addiction seems to relieve stress temporarily.
- The addiction results from peer pressure.
- The addiction can be present within the person's value system (a person whose values wouldn't let him or her shoot heroin may be able to rationalize compulsive eating or obsessive playing of computer games, for example).
- A serious physical illness is present, and the addiction may provide escape from pain or the fear of disfigurement.
- The addict feels pressured to perform or succeed.
- The addict has self-hate.
- A genetic link is present. Heredity might dictate susceptibility to some addictions.
- Society allows addiction. Advertising even encourages it (you can sleep better with a pill; snacking helps you enjoy life more fully; parties and sports are more fun with alcohol; shop 'til you drop; and so on).

The same general traits and behaviors are involved in all kinds of addictions, whether they involve food, sex, gambling, shopping, or drugs.

Most people with addictions deny their problem. Even when the addiction is clear to people around them, addicts continue to deny that they are addicted. Instead, they tend to get angry when someone tries to talk about the behavior and are likely to make excuses for their actions. Many addicts also blame others for their problem. In some cases, an addict admits the problem but fails to take any steps to change.

Recognizing that all forms of addiction are unhealthy, this chapter focuses on some of the most self-destructive addictive substances in our society: marijuana, cocaine, methamphetamine, MDMA, heroin, alcohol, and tobacco. More than half a million Americans die each year from tobacco, alcohol, and illegal drug use.

# Drugs and Dependence

A drug is any substance that alters the user's ability to function. Drugs encompass over-the-counter drugs, prescription medications, and illegal substances. Many drugs lead to physical and psychological dependence.

Any drug can be misused and abused. "Drug misuse" implies the intentional and inappropriate use of over-the-counter or prescribed medications.[3] Examples include

---

**Addiction** Compulsive and uncontrollable behavior(s) or use of substance(s).

taking more medication than prescribed, mixing drugs, not following prescription instructions, or discontinuing a drug prior to a physician's approval. "Drug abuse" is the intentional and inappropriate use of a drug resulting in physical, emotional, financial, intellectual, social, spiritual, or occupational consequences of the abuse.[4] Many substances, if used in the wrong manner, can be abused.

When drugs are used regularly, they integrate into the body's chemistry, increasing the user's tolerance to the drug and forcing the user to increase the dosage constantly to obtain similar results. Drug abuse leads to serious health problems, and more than half of all adolescent suicides are drug related. Often, drug abuse opens the gate to other illegal activities. According to the U.S. Department of Justice, the majority of convicted criminals—about 80 percent of federal and state inmates—have abused drugs.

Approximately 60 percent of the world's production of illegal drugs is consumed in the United States. An estimated 35 million people in the United States used illegal drugs within the past year, and 112 million people, or 45 percent of the population, have used them at least once in their lives. Each year, Americans spend more than $65 billion on illegal drugs.

According to the U.S. Department of Education, today's drugs are stronger and more addictive, and they pose a greater risk than ever before. If you are uncertain about addictive behavior(s) in your life, the Addictive Behavior Questionnaire in Lab 13A can help you identify a potential problem. Some of the most commonly abused drugs in our society are discussed next.

## Nonmedical Use of Prescription Drugs

Based on a 2006 NSDUH report, 20 percent of the population aged 12 or older, or almost 50 million Americans, reported nonmedical use of psychotherapeutic drugs at some point in their lifetime. Psychotherapeutic drugs include any prescription pain reliever, tranquilizer, stimulant, or sedative (but not over-the-counter drugs). The most commonly abused prescription medications are:

- Opioids, commonly prescribed to treat pain. These include codeine and morphine.
- Central nervous system depressants, used to treat anxiety and sleep disorders. Examples include Mebaral, Nembutal, Valium, and Xanax.
- Stimulants, prescribed to treat the sleep disorder narcolepsy, attention-deficit hyperactivity disorder (ADHD), and obesity. Examples include Dexedrine, Adderall, Ritalin, and Concerta.

As with illegal drugs, abuse of prescription drugs presents serious health consequences. The risks associated with psychotherapy drug misuse or abuse vary depending on the drug. Some of the risks include respiratory depression or cessation, decreased or irregular heart rate, high body temperature, seizures, and cardiovascular failure. Abuse of prescription drugs, or using them in a manner other than exactly as prescribed, can lead to addictive behavior.

## Marijuana

**Marijuana** (pot, grass, or weed, as it is commonly called) is the most widely used illegal drug in the United States. Estimates by the Office of National Drug Control Policy indicate that 40 percent of Americans have smoked marijuana. Approximately 25 million people in the United States use marijuana regularly. Most users smoke loose marijuana that has been rolled into a joint or packed into a pipe. A few users bake it into foods such as brownies or use it to brew a tea. Marijuana cigarettes are often laced with other drugs such as crack cocaine.

In small doses, marijuana has a sedative effect. Larger doses produce physical and psychological changes. Studies in the 1960s indicated that the potential effects of marijuana were exaggerated and that the drug was relatively harmless. The drug as it is used today, however, is as much as 10 times stronger than when the initial studies were conducted. Most of the research today shows marijuana to be dangerous and harmful.

The main, and most active, psychoactive and mind-altering ingredient in marijuana is thought to be delta-9-tetrahydrocannabinol (THC). In the 1960s, THC content in marijuana ranged from .02 to 2 percent. Users called the latter "real good grass." Today's THC content averages 4 to 6 percent, although it has been reported as high as 27 percent. The THC content in sinsemilla, a variety of high-potency marijuana grown from the seedless female cannabis plant, averages 12 percent.

THC reaches the brain within a few seconds after marijuana smoke is inhaled, and the psychic and physical changes reach their peak in about 2 or 3 minutes. THC then is metabolized in the liver to waste metabolites, but

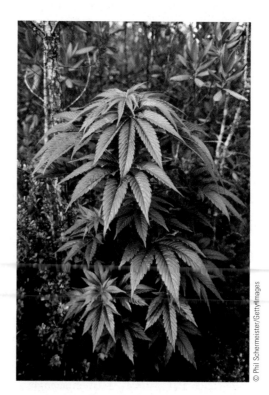

Cannabis sativa.

30 percent of it remains in the body a week after the marijuana was smoked. THC is not completely eliminated until 30 days or more after an initial dose of the drug. The drug always remains in the system of regular users.

Some of the short-term effects of marijuana are **tachycardia**, dryness of the mouth, reddened eyes, stronger appetite, decrease in coordination and tracking (the eyes' ability to follow a moving stimulus), difficulty in concentration, intermittent confusion, impairment of short-term memory and continuity of speech, interference with the physical and mental learning process during periods of intoxication, and increased risk for heart attack for a full day after smoking the drug. Another common effect is the **amotivational syndrome**. This syndrome persists after periods of intoxication but usually disappears a few weeks after the individual stops using the drug.

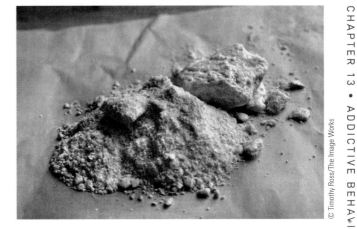

Powdered cocaine.

## Critical Thinking

The legalization of marijuana for medical purposes is being heatedly debated across the United States. Do you think this decision should rest with the government, medical personnel, or the individuals themselves?

Long-term harmful effects include atrophy of the brain (leading to irreversible brain damage), less resistance to infectious diseases, chronic bronchitis, lung cancer (marijuana smoke may contain as much as 50 to 70 percent more cancer-producing hydrocarbons than cigarette smoke), and possible sterility and impotence.

One of the most common myths about marijuana use is that it is not addictive. Lobbyists work to convince the federal government to legalize marijuana for medicinal purposes. Ample scientific evidence clearly shows that regular users of marijuana do develop physical and psychological dependence. As with cigarette smokers, when regular users go without the drug, they crave the substance, go through mood changes, are irritable and nervous, and develop an obsession to get more.

Cocaine  Similar to marijuana, **cocaine** was thought for many years to be relatively harmless. This misconception came to an abrupt halt in the mid-1980s when two well-known athletes—Len Bias (basketball) and Don Rogers (football)—died suddenly following cocaine overdoses. Currently, there are an estimated 2.4 million chronic cocaine users and 6 million occasional cocaine users in the United States. In 2006, almost 1 million people tried the drug for the first time. Over the years, cocaine has been given several different names, including, among others, coke, C, snow, blow, nose candy, toot, flake, Peruvian lady,

white girl, and happy dust. This drug can be sniffed or snorted, smoked, or injected.

When cocaine is snorted, it is absorbed quickly through the mucous membranes of the nose into the bloodstream. The drug is usually arranged in fine powder lines 1 to 2 inches long. Each line stimulates the autonomic nervous system for about 30 minutes. When cocaine is injected intravenously, larger amounts can enter the body in a shorter time. The popularity of cocaine is based on the almost universal guarantee that users will find themselves in an immediate state of euphoria and well-being. It is an expensive drug—$400 to $1,800 per ounce for powdered cocaine. The addiction begins with a desire to get high, often at social gatherings, and usually with the assurance that "occasional use is harmless." At least 25 percent of these first-time users will become addicted in four years, and for many it is the beginning of a lifetime nightmare.

Animal research with cocaine has shown that all laboratory animals can become compulsive cocaine users. Animals work more persistently at pressing a bar for cocaine than bars for other drugs, including opiates. In one instance, an addicted monkey pressed the bar almost 13,000 times until it finally got a dose of cocaine. People respond in a similar way. Cocaine addicts prefer drug usage to any other activity and use the drug until the supply or the user is exhausted.

Cocaine users also exhibit unusual behaviors compared with their previous conduct, even to the point where a user has been known to sell a child to obtain more cocaine. Educated people are not immune to cocaine addiction.

**Marijuana** A psychoactive drug prepared from a mixture of crushed leaves, flowers, small branches, stems, and seeds from the hemp plant *cannabis sativa*.

**Tachycardia** Faster-than-normal heart rate.

**Amotivational syndrome** A condition characterized by loss of motivation, dullness, apathy, and no interest in the future.

**Cocaine** 2-beta-carbomethoxy-3-beta-benzoxytropane, the primary psychoactive ingredient derived from coca plant leaves.

Some, including lawyers, physicians, and athletes, have daily habits that cost them hundreds to thousands of dollars, with binges in the $20,000–$50,000 range. Cocaine addiction can lead to loss of a job and profession, loss of family, bankruptcy, and death.

Increasingly more popular is crack cocaine, a smokable form of cocaine. It is many times more potent than cocaine and is highly addictive. Two-thirds of users in the United States who are addicted to cocaine use crack. Because it is so potent, crack doses are smaller and, therefore, less expensive, at $5 to $40 each, although users still spend hundreds of dollars a day to support their addiction.

Crack typically is made by boiling cocaine hydrochloride in a solution of baking soda, then letting the solution dry. The residue then is broken up, to be smoked in a pipe. The high from crack comes within seconds, faster than the high from injected cocaine. The crack high lasts about 12 minutes, which is shorter than the high from snorted or injected cocaine. Choosing to use cocaine in this form heightens the risk for emphysema and heart attack.

Cocaine seems to alleviate fatigue and raise energy levels, as well as lessen the need for food and sleep. Following the high comes a "crash," a state of physiologic and psychological depression, often leaving the user with the desire to get more. This can produce a constant craving for the drug. Similar to alcoholics, cocaine users recover only by abstaining completely from the drug. A single "backslide" can result in renewed addiction.

Light to moderate cocaine use is typically associated with feelings of pleasure and well-being. Sustained cocaine snorting can lead to a constant runny nose, nasal congestion and inflammation, and perforation of the nasal septum. Long-term consequences of cocaine use include loss of appetite, digestive disorders, weight loss, malnutrition, insomnia, confusion, anxiety, and cocaine psychosis, characterized by paranoia and hallucinations. In one type of hallucination, referred to as formication, or "coke bugs," the chronic user perceives imaginary insects or snakes crawling on or underneath the skin.

High doses of cocaine can cause nervousness, dizziness, blurred vision, vomiting, tremors, seizures, strokes, angina, cardiac arrhythmias, and high blood pressure. As with smoking marijuana, there is an increased risk for heart attack following cocaine use. The user's risk may be 24 times higher than normal for up to three hours following cocaine use. Almost one-third of cocaine users who incurred a heart attack had no symptoms of heart disease prior to taking cocaine. In addition, intravenous users are at risk for hepatitis, HIV, and other infectious diseases.

Large overdoses of cocaine can precipitate sudden death from respiratory paralysis, cardiac arrhythmias, and severe convulsions. If individuals lack an enzyme used in metabolizing cocaine, as few as two to three lines of cocaine may be fatal.

Chronic users who constantly crave the drug often turn to crime, including murder, to sustain their habit. Some users view suicide as the only solution to this sad syndrome.

## Methamphetamine

**Methamphetamine**, or "meth," is a more potent form of amphetamine and has become the fastest-growing drug threat in the United States. **Amphetamines** in general are part of a large group of synthetic agents used to stimulate the central nervous system. Amphetamines were widely given to soldiers during World War II to help them overcome fatigue, improve endurance, enhance battlefield ferocity, heighten mood, and keep them going. During the Vietnam War, U.S. soldiers used more amphetamines than did soldiers from all countries combined during World War II.

A powerfully addictive drug, methamphetamine falls under the same category of psychostimulant drugs as amphetamines and cocaine. It is also known as a "club drug," a group of illegal substances used at dance clubs, rock concerts, and raves (all-night dance parties). Other club drugs include MDMA, LSD, GHB, Rohypnol, and ketamine.

Methamphetamine typically is a white, odorless, bitter-tasting powder that dissolves readily in water or alcohol. The drug is a potent central nervous system stimulant that produces a general feeling of well-being, decreases appetite, increases motor activity, and decreases fatigue and the need for sleep.

Based on the 2006 NSDUH, an estimated 14 million Americans age 12 and older have tried methamphetamine. Unlike most other drugs, methamphetamine reaches rural and urban populations alike. Young people especially prefer methamphetamine because of its low cost and long-lasting effects—up to 12 hours following use.

Methamphetamine was easily manufactured in clandestine "meth labs" using over-the-counter pseudoephedrine, typically found in cold medications. Because of the ease of accessibility to methamphetamine ingredients, in March 2006 the federal Combat Meth Act of 2005 was signed into law. This law requires retailers to keep cold medications behind the counter, and consumers are limited as to the amount they can purchase.

Methamphetamine labs can be set up almost anywhere, including garages, basements, or hotel rooms. The abundance of potential meth lab sites makes it difficult for drug enforcement agencies to locate many of these facilities. The risk of injury in a meth lab, however, is high, because potentially explosive environmental contaminants are discarded during production of the drug.

U.S. production of methamphetamine is now limited and will likely remain at low levels in the near future. Production in Canada, however, has increased significantly, primarily by Canadian-based Asian drug trafficking organizations. These organizations run large-capacity super labs. All Canadian labs combined are believed to produce more than 2 million tablets per week. Mexico is also coming into prominence as a source of meth supply.

Methamphetamine can be snorted, swallowed, smoked, or injected. It is commonly referred to as "speed" or "crystal" when snorted or taken orally, "ice" or "glass" when smoked, and "crank" when injected. Depending on how it is taken, methamphetamine affects the body differently. Smoked or injected methamphetamine provides an immediate intense, pleasurable rush that lasts only a few minutes. Negative effects, nonetheless, can continue for several hours. When the drug is snorted or taken orally, the user does not experience a rush but develops a feeling of euphoria that lasts up to 16 hours.

Users of methamphetamine experience increases in body temperature, blood pressure, heart rate, and breathing rate; a decrease in appetite; hyperactivity; tremors; and violent behavior. High doses produce irritability, paranoia, irreversible damage to blood vessels in the brain (causing strokes), and risk for sudden death from hypothermia and convulsions if not treated at once.

Chronic abusers experience insomnia, confusion, hallucinations, inflammation of the heart lining, schizophrenia-like mental disorder, and brain cell damage similar to that caused by a stroke. Physical changes to the brain may last months or perhaps become permanent. Over time, methamphetamine use may reduce brain levels of **dopamine**, which can lead to symptoms similar to those of Parkinson's disease. In addition, users frequently are involved in violent crime, homicide, and suicide. Using methamphetamine during pregnancy may cause prenatal complications, premature delivery, and abnormal physical and emotional development of the child.

Similar to other stimulants, methamphetamine is often used in a binge cycle. Addiction takes hold quickly because the person develops tolerance to methamphetamine within minutes of using it. The "high" disappears long before blood levels of the drug drop significantly. The user then attempts to maintain the pleasurable feelings by taking in more of the drug, and a binge cycle ensues.

The binge cycle, which can last for a couple of weeks, consists of several stages. The initial rush lasts 5 to 30 minutes. During this stage, heart rate, blood pressure, and metabolism increase and the user receives a great sense of pleasure. The high follows, lasting up to 16 hours. During this stage, users become arrogant and more argumentative. The binge stage sets in next and lasts between

2 and 14 days. Addicts continue to use the drug in an attempt to maintain the high for as long as possible.

When addicts no longer can achieve a satisfying high, they enter the "tweaking stage," the most dangerous stage in the cycle. At this point, users may have gone without food for several days and without sleep anywhere from 3 to 15 days. They become paranoid, irritable, and violent. Tweakers crave more of the drug, but no amount of amphetamines will restore the pleasurable, euphoric feelings they achieved during the high. Thus, the addicts become increasingly frustrated, unpredictable, and dangerous to those around them (including police officers and medical personnel) and to themselves. Once they finally crash, they are no longer dangerous. The users now become lethargic and sleep for 1 to 3 days.

Following the crash, addicts fall into a 1- to 3-month period of withdrawal. During this stage, they can be paranoid, aggressive, fatigued, depressed, suicidal, and filled with an intense craving for another high. Reuse of the drug relieves these feelings. Therefore, the incidence of relapse in users who seek treatment is high.

### MDMA (Ecstasy)

**MDMA**, also known as Ecstasy, became popular among teenagers and young adults in the United States in the mid-1980s, when it evolved into the most common "club drug." Although its use already constituted a serious drug problem in Europe, MDMA was not illegal in the United States until 1985. Prior to 1985, few Americans abused this drug. In the 1970s, some therapists used MDMA as a tool to help patients open up and feel at ease. MDMA is named for its chemical structure: 3,4-methylenedioxymethamphetamine. Street names for the drug are X-TC, E, Adam, and love drug.

More than 12.3 million persons aged 12 and older reported using Ecstasy at least once in their lifetime. The number of users (people who had used the drug within the last 30 days) in 2006 was 528,000. More than 1 in 44 eighth graders have tried MDMA at least once, and more than 1 in 16 high school seniors have used the drug.

MDMA use, once popular primarily among Hispanic Americans and Caucasians, has now spread to a wide range of demographic subgroups. Typically, dealers push the drug as a way to increase energy, pleasure, and self-confidence. MDMA is now available in numerous settings,

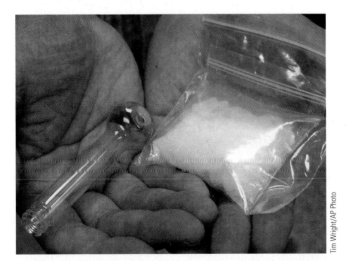

Tim Wright/AP Photo

"Ice," so named for its appearance, is a smokable form of methamphetamine.

**Methamphetamine** A potent form of amphetamine.

**Amphetamines** A class of powerful central nervous system stimulants.

**Dopamine** A neurotransmitter that affects emotional, mental, and motor functions.

**MDMA** A synthetic hallucinogen drug with a chemical structure that closely resembles MDA and methamphetamine; also known as Ecstasy.

including high schools, private homes, malls, and other popular gathering places for teenagers and young adults.

The trafficking of MDMA is increasing at an alarming rate, and multiple agencies have reported large seizures of the drug. Between 2004 and 2006, the amount of MDMA seized by federal law enforcement increased from 1.42 to 5.5 million dosage units.

Although MDMA usually is swallowed in the form of one or two pills in doses of up to 120 mg per pill, it can also be smoked, snorted, or, occasionally, injected. Because the drug often is prepared with other substances, users have no way of knowing the exact potency of the drug or additional substances found in each pill. Further, many users combine MDMA with alcohol, marijuana, or other drugs, which makes it even more dangerous to use.

MDMA shares characteristics with stimulants and hallucinogens. Its chemical structure closely parallels the hallucinogen **MDA** (methylenedioxyamphetamine) and methamphetamine, both manmade stimulants that damage the brain. The addictive properties of MDMA and stimulation of hyperactivity have been compared to stimulants such as amphetamines and cocaine. The chemical structure of MDMA and its appeal, however, are similar to hallucinogens, but with milder psychedelic effects.

Among young people, MDMA has a reputation for being fun and harmless as long as it is used sensibly. But it is not a harmless drug. Research is uncovering many negative side effects. The pleasurable effects peak about an hour after a pill is swallowed and last for 2 to 6 hours. Users claim to feel enlightened and introspective, accepting of themselves and trustful of others. Because they tend to act and feel closer to, or more intimate with, the people around them, some believe this drug to be an aphrodisiac, even though MDMA actually hampers sexual ability. MDMA also acts as a stimulant by increasing brain activity and making users feel more energetic.

Like most addictive drugs, the effects of MDMA are said to diminish with each use. MDMA users may experience rapid eye movement, faintness, blurred vision, chills, sweating, nausea, muscle tension, and teeth-grinding. Users often bring infant pacifiers to raves to combat the latter side effect. Individuals with heart, liver, or kidney disease or high blood pressure are especially at risk because MDMA increases blood pressure, heart rate, and body temperature. Thus, its use may lead to seizures, kidney failure, a heart attack, or a stroke. The hot, crowded atmosphere at raves and dance clubs also heightens the risk to the user. Deaths are more likely when water is unavailable because the crowded atmosphere, combined with the stimulant effects of MDMA, causes dehydration (bottled water is often sold at inflated prices at raves). Other evidence suggests that a pregnant woman using MDMA may find long-term learning and memory difficulties in her child.

The damaging effects of the drug can be long-lasting and are possible after only a few uses. Long-term side effects, lasting for weeks after use, include confusion, depression, sleep disorders, anxiety, aggression, paranoia, and impulsive behavior. Questions still remain about other potential long-term effects. Verbal and visual memory may be significantly impaired for years after prolonged use. Researchers are focusing on these lasting side effects, which may be the result of depleted serotonin, a neurotransmitter that is released with each dose of MDMA. The short-term effect of serotonin release is increased brain activity. Serotonin helps to regulate sleep cycles, pain, emotion, and appetite. Because MDMA may damage the neurons that release serotonin, long-term effects could be dangerous.

Advocates of MDMA are attempting to get approval to study medical uses of the drug. For example, MDMA could relieve suffering in terminally ill cancer patients. It also could help people in therapy for marital problems by encouraging introspection and conversation. Because MDMA is heralded as an instant antidepressant, it may help people who are in mourning. Opponents, meanwhile, question the value of MDMA as an effective treatment modality because its effects diminish with continued use.

## Heroin

For the first time in decades, **heroin** use is on the increase, and it is again being publicized by pop culture. Heroin started to make a comeback in 1991 and became increasingly stylish in 1995 following the arrests and deaths of prominent rock stars who abused the drug. According to the 2006 NSDUH, about 3.8 million Americans ages 12 and older (1.5 percent) reported trying heroin at least once. Approximately 560,000 reported heroin use during the past year, and 338,000 reported heroin use during the past month. Although the most common users are suburban, middle-class people and lower-income populations, its use is starting to appear in more affluent communities as well.

Common nicknames for heroin include diesel, dope, dynamite, white death, nasty boy, china white, H. Harry, gumball, junk, brown sugar, smack, tootsie roll, black tar, and chasing the dragon. Heroin is classified as a narcotic drug. It is synthesized from morphine, a natural substance found in the seedpod of several types of poppy plants. In its purest form, heroin is a white powder, but on the streets it is typically available in yellow or brown powders. The latter colors are attained when pure heroin is combined with other drugs or substances such as sugar, cornstarch, chalk, brick dust, or laundry soap. Heroin also is sold in a hardened or solid form (black tar), which usually is dissolved with other liquids for use in injectable form. Many users combine heroin with cocaine, a risky process commonly called "speedballing."

Today's heroin is more pure, powerful, and affordable than ever before. Highly dangerous, heroin is a significant health threat to users, who have no way of determining the strength of the drug purchased on the street, which places them at a constant risk for overdose and death. The 2006 report from the Drug Abuse Warning Network indicated that approximately 12 percent of all drug-related cases seen in hospital emergency rooms that year involved heroin use.

Heroin can be injected intravenously or intramuscularly, sniffed/snorted, or smoked. Although injection is the predominant method of heroin use, users are turning away from intravenous injections because of the risk for HIV infection. The availability of relatively low priced, high-purity heroin further contributes to the number of people who smoke or snort the drug. Some users have the misconception that heroin is less addictive when it is snorted or smoked. Whether injected, snorted, or smoked, heroin is an extremely addictive drug, and both physical and psychological dependence develop rapidly. Drug tolerance sets in quickly, and each time the drug is used, a higher dose is required to produce the same effects. Use of heroin induces a state of euphoria that comes within seconds of intravenous injection or within 5 to 15 minutes with other methods of administration. Because the drug is a sedative, during the initial rush the person has a sense of relaxation and does not feel any pain. In users who inhale the drug, however, the rush may be accompanied by nausea, vomiting, intense itching, and at times severe asthma attacks. As the rush wears off, users experience drowsiness, confusion, slowed cardiac function, and decreased breathing rate.

A heroin overdose can cause convulsions, coma, and death. During an overdose, heart rate, breathing, blood pressure, and body temperature drop dramatically. These physiologic responses can induce vomiting and tight muscles and cause breathing to stop. Death is often the result of lack of oxygen or choking to death on vomit.

About 4 to 5 hours after taking the drug, withdrawal sets in. Heroin withdrawal is painful and usually lasts up to 2 weeks—but could go on for several months. Symptoms of short-term use include red/raw nostrils, bone and muscle pains, muscle spasms and cramps, sweating, hot and cold flashes, runny nose and eyes, drowsiness, sluggishness, slurred speech, loss of appetite, nausea, diarrhea, restlessness, and violent yawning. Heroin use can also kill a developing fetus or cause a spontaneous abortion.

Symptoms of long-term use of heroin include hallucinations, nightmares, constipation, sexual difficulties, impaired vision, reduced fertility, boils, collapsed veins, and a significantly elevated risk for lung, liver, and cardiovascular diseases, including bacterial infections in blood vessels and heart valves. The additives used in street heroin can clog vital blood vessels because these additives do not dissolve in the body, leading to infections and death of cells in vital organs. Sudden infant death syndrome (SIDS) also is seen more frequently in children born to addicted mothers.

Heroin addiction is treated with behavioral therapies and pharmaceutical agents. Medication suppresses withdrawal symptoms, which makes it easier for patients to stop using heroin. The combination of these two treatment modalities helps the individual learn to lead a more stable, productive, and drug-free lifestyle.

## Alcohol

Drinking **alcohol** has been a socially acceptable behavior for centuries. Alcohol is an accepted accompaniment at parties, ceremonies, dinners, sport contests,

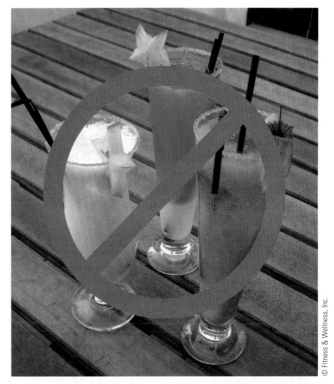

The sale of alcohol was illegal in the United States between 1920 and 1933.

the establishment of kingdoms or governments, and the signing of treaties between nations. Alcohol also has been used for medical reasons as a mild sedative or as a painkiller for surgery.

For a short period of 14 years, from 1920 to 1933, by constitutional amendment, the sale and use of alcohol were declared illegal in the United States. This amendment was repealed because drinkers and nondrinkers alike questioned the right of government to pass judgment on individual moral standards. In addition, organized crime activities to smuggle and sell alcohol illegally expanded enormously during this period.

Alcohol is the cause of one of the most significant health-related drug problems in the United States today. Based on the 2006 NSDUH, more than 125 million people 12 years and older (50.9 percent) used alcohol within a month of the survey, and 57 million (23 percent) participated in binge drinking at least once in the 30 days prior to the survey. About 17 million (6.9 percent) were heavy drinkers; and 1 in 8 drove under the influence of alcohol at least once in the 12 months prior to the interview. The

**MDA** A hallucinogenic drug that is structurally similar to amphetamines.

**Heroin** A potent drug that is a derivative of opium.

**Alcohol (ethyl alcohol)** A depressant drug that affects the brain and slows down central nervous system activity; has strong addictive properties.

highest prevalence was among 21 to 25 year olds, with almost 70 percent of this age group using alcohol within a month of the survey.

The number of adults who abuse alcohol or are alcohol dependent has risen from 13.8 million in 1991–92 to approximately 10 million in 2006. Among younger people, ages 12 to 20, 10.8 million (28.3 percent) used alcohol in the month leading up to the survey. Alcohol drinkers are also more likely to misuse other drugs. Over half of lifetime drinkers have used one or more illicit drugs at some time in their lives, compared with only 8 percent of lifetime nondrinkers.

In young people between the ages of 12 and 17, among those who drank heavily during the past month, 57.6 percent of them also used illicit drugs during that time frame. Among nondrinkers in that same age group, only 4.8 percent used illicit drugs during those same 30 days.

Although some health benefits are derived from moderate alcohol consumption, the media have extensively exaggerated these benefits. They like to discuss this topic because it seems to be "a vice that's good for you." Research supports the assertion that consuming no more than two alcoholic beverages a day for men and one for women provides modest benefits in decreasing the risk for cardiovascular disease. Not reported in the media, however, is that these modest health benefits do not always apply to African Americans.

The benefits of modest alcohol use can be equated to those obtained through a small daily dose of aspirin (about 81 mg per day, or the equivalent of a baby aspirin) or eating a few nuts each day. Aspirin or a few nuts do not lead to impaired judgment or actions that you may later regret or have to live with for the rest of your life.

**Consequences of Drinking Alcohol** Alcohol is not for everyone. **Alcoholism** seems to have both a genetic and an environmental component. The reasons some people can drink for years without becoming addicted, whereas others follow the downward spiral of alcoholism, are not understood. The addiction to alcohol develops slowly. Most

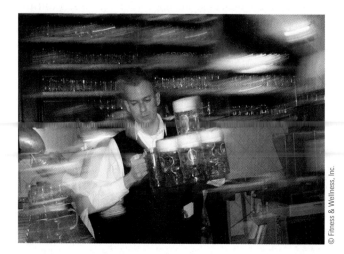

Approximately 14 million people in the U.S. will develop a drinking problem during their lifetime.

people think they are in control of their drinking habits and do not realize they have a problem until they become alcoholics, when they find themselves physically and emotionally dependent on the drug. This addiction is characterized by excessive use of, and constant preoccupation with, drinking. Alcohol abuse, in turn, leads to mental, emotional, physical, and social problems.

The effects of alcohol intake include impaired peripheral vision, decreased visual and hearing acuity, slower reaction time, reduced concentration and motor performance (including increased swaying), and impaired judgment of distance and speed of moving objects. Further, alcohol alleviates fear, increases risk-taking, stimulates urination, and induces sleep. A single large dose of alcohol also may decrease sexual function. Two of the most serious consequences of alcohol abuse are increased risks for accidents and violent behavior. Excessive drinking has been linked to more than half of all deaths from car accidents. The risk for rape, domestic violence, child abuse, suicide, and murder also increases with alcohol abuse.

One of the most unpleasant, dangerous, and life-threatening effects of drinking is the **synergistic action** of alcohol when combined with other drugs, particularly central nervous system depressants. Each person reacts to a combination of alcohol and other drugs in a different way. The effects range from loss of consciousness to death.

Long-term effects of alcohol abuse are serious and often life-threatening (Figure 13.1). Some of these detrimental effects are lower resistance to disease; **cirrhosis** of the liver; higher risk for oral, esophageal, stomach, and liver cancer; **cardiomyopathy**; irregular heartbeat; elevated blood pressure; greater risk for stroke; inflammation of the esophagus, stomach, small intestine, and pancreas; stomach ulcers; sexual impotence; birth defects; malnutrition; damage to brain cells leading to loss of memory; depression; psychosis; and hallucinations.

**Social Consequences of Alcohol Abuse** Alcohol abuse further leads to social problems that include loss of friends and jobs, separation of family members, child abuse, domestic violence, divorce, and problems with the law. Heavy drinking further contributes to decreased performance at work and school because drinkers are more likely to arrive late, make more mistakes, leave assignments incomplete, encounter problems with fellow workers or students, get lower grades and job evaluations, and flunk out of school or lose jobs. Alcohol abuse also worsens financial concerns because drinkers have less money for needed items such as food and clothing, fail to pay bills, and may have additional medical expenses, insurance premiums, and fines to pay.

**Alcohol on Campus** Alcohol is the number-one drug problem among college students. According to national surveys, about 66 percent of full-time college students reported using alcohol within the past month, and 45 percent had engaged in binge drinking (consumed five or more drinks in a row). Alcohol is a factor in about 28 percent of all college dropouts.

FIGURE 13.1 Long-term risks associated with alcohol abuse.

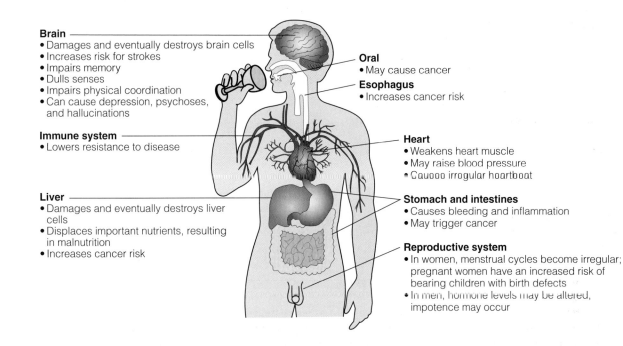

**Brain**
• Damages and eventually destroys brain cells
• Increases risk for strokes
• Impairs memory
• Dulls senses
• Impairs physical coordination
• Can cause depression, psychoses, and hallucinations

**Immune system**
• Lowers resistance to disease

**Liver**
• Damages and eventually destroys liver cells
• Displaces important nutrients, resulting in malnutrition
• Increases cancer risk

**Oral**
• May cause cancer

**Esophagus**
• Increases cancer risk

**Heart**
• Weakens heart muscle
• May raise blood pressure
• Causes irregular heartbeat

**Stomach and intestines**
• Causes bleeding and inflammation
• May trigger cancer

**Reproductive system**
• In women, menstrual cycles become irregular; pregnant women have an increased risk of bearing children with birth defects
• In men, hormone levels may be altered, impotence may occur

FIGURE 13.2 Average number of drinks by college students per week by GPA.

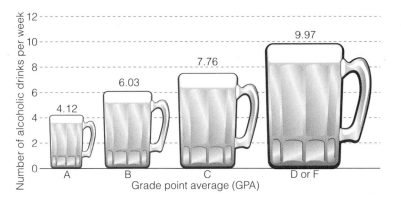

*Source:* C. A. Presley, J. S. Leichliter, and P. W. Meilman, *Alcohol and Drugs on American College Campuses: Findings from 1995, 1996, and 1997 (A Report to College Presidents)* (Carbondale, IL: Southern Illinois University, 1999).

The statistics are sobering. For college students between the ages of 18 and 24,[5]

• 1,700 died from alcohol-related unintentional injuries.
• Almost 700,000 were assaulted by another student who had been drinking.
• 599,000 were unintentionally injured under the influence of alcohol.
• More than 150,000 developed alcohol-related health problems.
• More than 97,000 were victims of alcohol-related sexual assault or date rape.
• 400,000 had unprotected sex.
• More than 100,000 were too intoxicated to know if they'd consented to having sex.
• 2.1 million drove under the influence of alcohol in the past year.

In terms of academic work, a national survey involving about 94,000 college students from 197 colleges and universities conducted over three years showed that grade point average (GPA) was related to average number of drinks per week (Figure 13.2).[6] Students with a "D" or "F" GPA reported a weekly consumption of almost ten drinks. Students with "A" GPAs consumed about four drinks per

**Alcoholism** Disease in which an individual loses control over drinking alcoholic beverages.

**Synergistic action** The effect of mixing two or more drugs, which can be much greater than the sum of two or more drugs acting by themselves.

**Cirrhosis** A disease characterized by scarring of the liver.

**Cardiomyopathy** A disease affecting the heart muscle.

week. Of significant concern, young adults ages 18 to 22 enrolled full time in college are more likely than their peers (part-time students and those not enrolled in college) to use alcohol, binge-drink, and drink heavily.

In another national survey of almost 55,000 undergraduate students from 131 colleges, close to 25 percent of students said that their academic problems resulted from alcohol abuse. Of greater concern, 29 percent of the surveyed students admitted driving while intoxicated. Of the 16 million college students in the United States, between 2 and 3 percent eventually will die from alcohol-related causes. This represents more students than those who will receive advanced degrees (master's and doctorate degrees combined).

Another major concern is that more than half of college students participate in games that involve heavy drinking (consuming five or more drinks in one sitting). Often, students take part because of peer pressure and fear of rejection. About 45 percent reported binge drinking at least once during the month prior to the survey. Excessive drinking can precipitate unplanned and unprotected sex (risking HIV infection), date rape, and alcohol poisoning. When some young people turn 21, they "celebrate" by having 21 drinks. Unaware of the risks of excessive alcohol intake in a relatively short period of time, drinking friends then try to let them "sleep it off," only to

find out that they never wake up, but rather suffer death from alcohol poisoning.

**How to Cut Down on Drinking** To find out if drinking is a problem in your life, refer to the questionnaire in Lab 13A, developed by the American Medical Association. If you respond "yes" twice or more on this questionnaire, you may be jeopardizing your health.

If a person is determined to control the problem, it is not that difficult. The first and most important step is to want to cut down. If you want to do this but you cannot seem to do so, you had better accept the probability that alcohol is becoming a serious problem for you, and you should seek guidance from your physician or from an organization such as Alcoholics Anonymous. The next few suggestions also may help you cut down your alcohol intake.

- Set reasonable limits for yourself. Decide not to exceed a certain number of drinks on a given occasion, and stick to your decision. No more than two beers or two cocktails a day is a reasonable limit for men and only one for women. If you set a target such as this and consistently do not exceed it, you have proven to yourself that you can control your drinking.
- Learn to say no. Many people have "just one more" drink because others in the group are doing this or because someone puts pressure on them, not because they really want a drink. When you reach the sensible limit you have set for yourself, politely but firmly refuse to exceed it. If you are being the generous host, pour yourself a glass of water or juice "on the rocks." Nobody will notice the difference.
- Drink slowly. Don't gulp down a drink. Choose your drinks for their flavor, not their "kick," and savor the taste of each sip.
- Dilute your drinks. If you prefer cocktails to beer, try tall drinks: Instead of downing gin or whiskey straight or nearly so, drink it diluted with a mixer such as tonic water or soda water in a tall glass. That way you can enjoy both the flavor and the act of drinking, but you will take longer to finish each drink. Also, you can make your two- or one-drink limit last all evening or switch to the mixer by itself.
- Do not drink on your own. Confine your drinking to social gatherings. You may have a hard time resisting the urge to pour yourself a relaxing drink at the end of a hard day, but many formerly heavy drinkers have found that a soft drink satisfies the need as well as alcohol did. What may help you really unwind, even with no drink at all, is a comfortable chair, loosened clothing, and perhaps a soothing audiotape, television program, good book to read, or even some low- to moderate-intensity physical activity.

## Behavior Modification Planning

### WHEN YOUR DATE DRINKS . . .

- **Don't** make excuses for his/her behavior, no matter how embarrassing.
- **Don't** allow embarrassment to put you in a situation with which you are uncomfortable.
- **Do** be sure that body language and tone of voice match verbal messages you send.
- **Do** leave as quickly as you can, without your date. Don't stop to argue. Intoxicated people can't listen to reason.
- **Do** call a cab, a friend, or your parents. **Don't** ride home with your date.

For women:

- **Do** make your position clear. "No!" is much more effective than "Please stop!" or "Don't!"
- **Do** make it clear that you will call the police if rape is attempted.

"Sexuality Under the Influence of Alcohol," *Human Sexuality Supplement to Current Health 2* (October 1990): p. 3.

### Try It

In your Online Journal or class notebook, write down strategies you can incorporate today to ensure your health and wellness.

# Treatment of Addictions

Recovery from any addiction is more likely to be successful with professional guidance and support. The first step is to recognize the reality of the problem. The Addictive

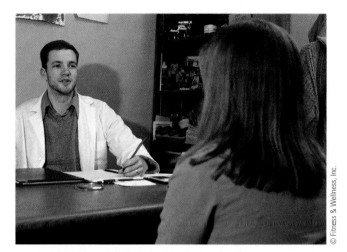

The sooner treatment for addiction is started, the longer the user stays in treatment, the better the chances for recovery and a more productive life.

Behavior Questionnaire in Lab 13A will help you recognize possible addictive behavior in yourself or someone you know. If the answers to more than half of these questions are positive, you may have a problem, in which case you should contact a physician, your institution's counseling center, or the local mental health clinic for a referral (see the Yellow Pages in your phone book).

You also may contact the Substance Abuse and Mental Health Services Administration (SAMHSA) at 1-800-662-HELP (1-800-662-4357) for referral to 24-hour substance abuse treatment centers in your local area. All information discussed during a phone call to this center is kept strictly confidential. Information also is available on the Internet at http://www.samhsa.gov. The national center provides printed information on drug abuse and addictive behavior.

About 4 million Americans received treatment for addictive behavior in 2006. An additional 21.1 million people were estimated to need treatment for illicit drug or alcohol abuse, but did not receive such treatment at any specialty facility.[7]

Among intervention and treatment programs for addiction are psychotherapy, medical care, and behavior modification. If addiction is a problem in your life, you need to act upon it without delay. Addicts do not have to resign themselves to a lifetime of addiction. The sooner you start, and the longer you stay in treatment, the better are your chances to recover and lead a healthier and more productive life.

# Tobacco Use

People throughout the world have used tobacco for hundreds of years. Before the 18th century, they smoked tobacco primarily in pipes or as cigars. Cigarette smoking did not become popular until the mid-1800s, and its use started to increase dramatically in the 20th century.

In 1900, people in the United States consumed 2.5 billion cigarettes, compared with 640 billion in 1981. This figure dropped to 487 billion in 1995. Per capita consumption of cigarettes by Americans over the age of 18 dropped from 4,345 cigarettes in 1963 to 1,691 in 2006.[8] Nonetheless, more than 60 million Americans still smoke cigarettes.

When tobacco leaves are burned, hot air and gases containing **tar** (chemical compounds) and **nicotine** are released in the smoke. More than 4,000 toxic chemicals have been found in tobacco smoke, and at least 69 are proven carcinogens. The harmful effects of cigarette smoking and tobacco use in general were not exactly known until the early 1960s, when research began to show a link between tobacco use and disease.

In 1964, the U.S. Surgeon General issued the first major report presenting scientific evidence that cigarettes were indeed a major health hazard in our society. More than 42 percent of the U.S. adult population smoked cigarettes at the time. In 2006, 21 percent of adults and 20 percent of high school seniors smoked cigarettes (Figure 13.3). Young people who smoke are also more likely to abuse other illicit drugs. Smokers between the ages of 12 and 17 are nine times more likely to use drugs than nonsmokers in this same age group (47.8 percent versus 5.4 percent).

**Morbidity and Mortality** Tobacco use in all its forms is considered a significant threat to life. World Health Organization estimates indicate that 10 percent of the 6 billion people presently living will die as a result of smoking-related illnesses, which kill approximately 5.4 million people each year. At the present rate of escalation, this figure is expected to climb to 8 million deaths annually by 2030. A total of 100 million tobacco-related deaths occurred in the 20th century, and based on estimates, there will be one billion deaths in the 21st century.

To gain some perspective on the seriousness of the tobacco problem, American Cancer Society statistics indicate that overdoses of illegal drugs kill about 17,000 people per year in the United States, and drug felonies and drug-related murders kill another 1,600 people each year. This brings drug-related deaths to a grand total of 18,600 annually. By comparison, tobacco, a legal drug, kills about 23 times as many people as all illegal drugs combined.

## Critical Thinking

Do you think the government should outlaw the use of tobacco in all forms? Or does the individual have the right to engage in self-destructive behavior?

**Tar** Chemical compound that forms during the burning of tobacco leaves.

**Nicotine** Addictive compound found in tobacco leaves.

**FIGURE 13.3** Trends in cigarette smoking by high school students and adults, United States, 1965–2006.

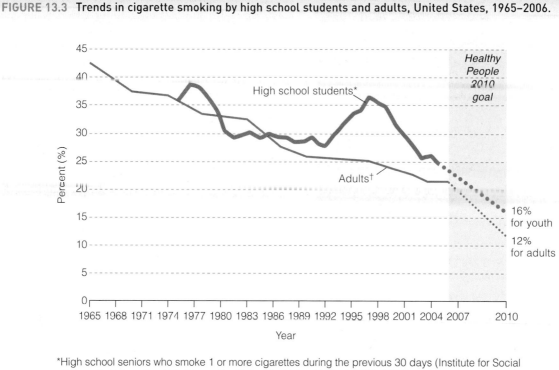

*High school seniors who smoke 1 or more cigarettes during the previous 30 days (Institute for Social Research, University of Michigan, Monitoring the Future Project, 1975–2004).
†Total population of adults who are current cigarette smokers (National Health Interview Surveys, 1965–2003).

*Source:* Centers for Disease Control and Prevention, Atlanta, 2008. Downloaded from http://www.cdc.gov/nccdphp/publications/aag/osh.htm, August 20, 2008.

Cigarette smoking is the largest preventable cause of illness and premature death in the United States. Death rates from heart disease, cancer, stroke, aortic aneurysm, chronic bronchitis, emphysema, and peptic ulcers all increase with cigarette smoking.

In pregnant women, cigarette smoking has been linked to retarded fetal growth, higher risk for spontaneous abortion (miscarriage), and prenatal death. Smoking is also the most prevalent cause of injury and death from fire. The average life expectancy for a chronic smoker is 13 to 14 years shorter than for a nonsmoker, and the death rate among chronic smokers during their most productive years of life, between ages 25 and 65, is twice the national average. The American Cancer Society estimates that if we consider all related deaths, smoking is responsible for more than 440,000 unnecessary deaths each year—enough deaths to wipe out the entire population of Miami and Miami Beach in a single year. For every tobacco-related death, there are 20 others, or 8.8 million people in the United States, who suffer from at least one serious illness associated with cigarette smoking.

Based on a report by U.S. government physicians, each cigarette shortens life by 7 minutes. This figure represents 5.5 million years of potential life that Americans lose to smoking each year.

### Effects on Cardiovascular System
Estimates by the American Heart Association indicate that more than 30 percent of fatal heart attacks—or 120,000 in the

United States annually—result from smoking. The risk for heart attack is 50 to 100 percent higher for smokers than for nonsmokers. The mortality rate following heart attacks also is higher for smokers, because their attacks usually are more severe and their risk for deadly arrhythmias is much greater.

Cigarette smoking affects the cardiovascular system by increasing heart rate, blood pressure, and susceptibility to atherosclerosis, blood clots, coronary artery spasm, cardiac arrhythmia, and arteriosclerotic peripheral vascular disease. Evidence also indicates that smoking decreases high-density lipoprotein (HDL) cholesterol, the "good" cholesterol that lowers the risk for heart disease. Smoking further increases the amount of fatty acids, glucose, and various hormones in the blood. The carbon monoxide in smoke hinders the capacity of the blood to carry oxygen to body tissues. Both carbon monoxide and nicotine can damage the inner walls of the arteries and thereby encourage the buildup of fat on them. Smoking also causes increased adhesiveness and clustering of platelets in the blood, decreases platelet survival and clotting time, and increases blood thickness. Any of these effects can precipitate a heart attack.

### Smoking and Cancer
The American Cancer Society reports that 87 percent of lung cancer is attributable to smoking. Lung cancer is the leading cancer killer, accounting for approximately 161,840 deaths in the United States in 2008, or about 30 percent of all deaths from can-

**FIGURE 13.4** Normal and diseased alveoli in lungs.

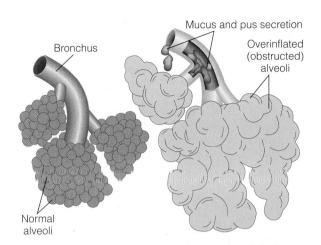

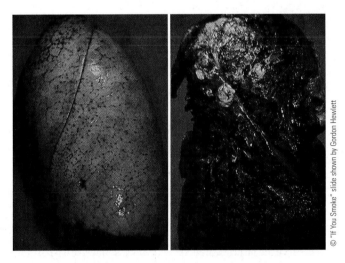

Normal lung (left) is contrasted with diseased lung (right). The white growth near the top of the diseased lung is cancer; the dark appearance on the bottom half is emphysema.

cer.[9] Cigarette smoking also leads to chronic lower respiratory disease, the third leading cause of death in the United States (see also Chapter 1). Figure 13.4 illustrates normal and diseased **alveoli**.

The most common carcinogenic exposure in the workplace is cigarette smoke. Both fatal and nonfatal cardiac events are increased greatly in people who are exposed to passive smoke. About 50,000 additional deaths result each year in the United States from secondhand smoke (also known as environmental tobacco smoke, or ETS), including 40,000 from cardiovascular diseases, 3,400 from lung cancer, and 430 from SIDS.[10] Furthermore, almost 22 million children between the ages of 3 and 11 are exposed to secondhand smoke, and approximately 30 percent of the indoor workforce is not protected by smoke-free workplace policies. According to the U.S. Surgeon General, the evidence clearly shows that there is no risk-free level of exposure to ETS, prompting Dr. Richard Carmona, former

## Adverse Effects of Secondhand Smoke

- A 30 percent increase in coronary heart disease risk (some adverse effects begin within minutes to hours of exposure).
- Increases blood clotting, enhancing the risk of heart attacks and strokes.
- Lowers HDL (good) cholesterol.
- Increases oxidation of LDL cholesterol, enhancing atherosclerosis.
- Increases oxygen-free radicals.
- Decreases levels of antioxidants.
- Increases chronic inflammation.
- Increases insulin resistance, leading to higher blood sugar levels and risk for diabetes.
- Increases lung and overall cancer risk.
- Increases risk for pulmonary diseases.
- Increases risk for adverse effects during pregnancy.
- Increases sudden infant death syndrome (SIDS) risk.

U.S. Surgeon General (2002–2006), to state: "Based on the science, I wouldn't allow anyone in my family to stand in a room with someone smoking."

Although half of all cancers are now curable, the five-year survival rate for lung cancer is less than 13 percent. Furthermore, cigarette smoking is responsible for most cancers of the oral cavity, larynx, and esophagus (Figure 13.5). Tobacco use is also related to the development of and deaths from bladder, pancreas, kidney, and cervical cancers.

## Critical Thinking

You are in a designated nonsmoking area and the person next to you lights up a cigarette. What can you say to this person to protect your right to clean air?

**Alveoli** Air sacs in the lungs where gas exchange (oxygen and carbon dioxide) takes place.

**FIGURE 13.5** The health effects of smoking.

**Stroke**
tobacco smoke estimated to cause
1/3 of strokes

**Cancer of larynx**
more frequent in smokers

**Lung cancer**
risks greatly elevated (90% due to
smoking in men, 79% in women)

**Heart attacks**
smoking more than doubles risks

**Peptic (stomach) ulcers**
smokers more vulnerable

**Pancreatic cancer**
30% linked to smoking

**Cervical cancer**
smoking may increase risk of this disease
in women

**Unborn babies**
at risk for premature birth, low birthweight, stunted
development, and infant death if mother smokes

**Mouth (oral) cancer**
smoking increases risk 3–4 times

**Esophageal cancer**
risk much higher in smokers

**Chronic lung diseases**
(bronchitis and emphysema)
most are due to smoking

**Circulatory disease**
risks increased

**Bladder and kidney cancer**
elevated risks in smokers

**Other Forms of Tobacco** Many tobacco users are aware of the health consequences of cigarette smoking but may fail to realize the risk of pipe smoking, cigar smoking, and tobacco chewing. As a group, pipe and cigar smokers have lower risks for heart disease and lung cancer than cigarette smokers. Nevertheless, blood nicotine levels in pipe and cigar smokers have been shown to approach those of cigarette smokers, because nicotine is still absorbed through the membranes of the mouth. Therefore, these tobacco users still have a higher risk for heart disease than nonsmokers do.

Cigarette smokers who substitute pipe or cigar smoking for cigarettes usually continue to inhale the smoke, which actually results in more nicotine and tar being brought into their lungs. Consequently, the risk for disease is even higher if pipe or cigar smoke is inhaled. The risk and mortality rates for lip, mouth, and larynx cancer for pipe smoking, cigar smoking, and tobacco chewing are actually higher than for cigarette smoking.

**Smokeless Tobacco** Smokeless tobacco has been promoted in the past as a safe alternative to cigarette smoking. The Advisory Committee to the U.S. Surgeon General has stated that smokeless tobacco represents a significant health risk and is just as addictive as cigarette smoking.

Unlike smoking, the use of smokeless tobacco has increased during the last 15 years. Currently, some 15 million Americans use tobacco in this form. The greatest concern is the increase in the use of "spit" tobacco, especially by young people. More than 2 million people under age 25 use spit tobacco, including 13.2 percent of high school males. The average starting age for smokeless tobacco use is 10 years old. One million three hundred thousand individuals 12 years and older started using smokeless tobacco in 2006, up 30 percent from 2002.

Using smokeless tobacco can lead to gingivitis and periodontitis. It carries a fourfold increase in oral cancer, and in some cases even premature death. People who chew or dip also have a higher rate of cavities, sore gums, bad breath, and stained teeth. Their senses of smell and taste diminish; consequently, they tend to add more sugar and salt to food. These practices alone increase the risk for being overweight and having high blood pressure. Nicotine addiction and its related health risks also hold true for smokeless tobacco users. Nicotine blood levels ap-

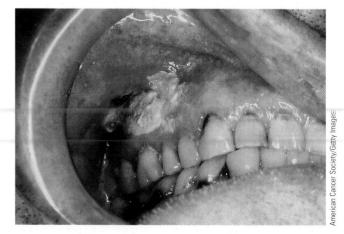

Smokeless tobacco can lead to gum and teeth damage as well as oral cancer (pictured).

proach those of cigarette smokers, increasing the risk for diseases of the cardiovascular system. Further, research has revealed changes in heart rate and blood pressure similar to those of cigarette smokers.

Using tobacco in any form can be addictive and poses a serious threat to health and well-being. Completely eliminating its use is the single most important lifestyle change a tobacco user can make to improve health, quality of life, and longevity.

## Health Care Costs of Tobacco Use
Heavy smokers use the health care system, especially hospitals, twice as much as nonsmokers do. The yearly cost to a given company has been estimated to be up to $5,000 per smoking employee. These costs include employee health care, absenteeism, additional health insurance, morbidity/disability and early mortality, on-the-job time lost, property damage/maintenance and depreciation, worker compensation, and the impact of secondhand smoke.

If every smoker were to give up cigarettes, in 1 year alone sick time would drop by approximately 90 million days, heart conditions would decrease by 280,000, chronic bronchitis and emphysema would number 1 million fewer cases, and total death rates from cardiovascular disease, cancer, and peptic ulcers would fall off drastically.

Every day more than 1,200 Americans die from smoking-related illnesses. That is the equivalent of three fully loaded jumbo jets crashing every day with no survivors.[11] Imagine what the coverage and concern would be if 440,000 people each year were to die in the United States alone because of airplane accidents! People would not even consider flying anymore. Most people would think of it as a form of suicide.

Smoking kills more Americans in a single year than died in battle during World War II and the Vietnam War combined. Think of the public outrage if 440,000 Americans were to die annually in a meaningless war. What if a single nonprescription drug were to cause more than 138,000 deaths from cancer and 120,000 fatal heart attacks each year? The U.S. public would not tolerate these situations. We would mount an intense fight to prevent the deaths.

Yet, are we not committing slow suicide by smoking cigarettes? Isn't tobacco a nonprescription drug available to almost anyone who wishes to smoke, killing more than 440,000 people each year? If cigarettes were invented today, the tobacco industry would be put on trial for mass murder.

## Trends
The fight against all forms of tobacco use has been gaining momentum. This was not always the case. It has been difficult to fight an industry that wields such enormous financial and political influence as does the tobacco industry in the United States. Tobacco is the sixth-largest cash crop in the United States, producing 2.5 percent of the gross national product. The tobacco industry has influenced elections cleverly by emphasizing the individual's right to smoke, avoiding the fact that so many people die because of it.

Philip Morris, one of the largest tobacco-producing companies in the world, receives nearly 70 percent of its profits from the sale of cigarettes. Philip Morris has donated millions of dollars to prominent organizations, so they no longer question the detrimental effects of tobacco use. Among the organizations that have received donations from Philip Morris are United Way, YMCA, Salvation Army, Pediatric AIDS Foundation, Red Cross, Cystic Fibrosis Foundation, March of Dimes, Easter Seals, Muscular Dystrophy Association, Multiple Sclerosis Society, Hemophilia Foundation, United Cerebral Palsy, American Civil Liberties Union, American Bar Association, Task Force for Battered Women, Boy Scouts, Boys and Girls Club, and Big Brothers and Big Sisters. We call Colombian drug runners unprincipled scum (responsible for about 19,100 illegal drug–related deaths per year), yet we welcome Philip Morris with glee and we call it civic pride.[12]

Tobacco was socially accepted for many years. Cigarette smoking, however, is no longer acceptable in most social circles. Smoking is prohibited in most public places as a result of nonsmokers and ex-smokers alike fighting for their rights to clean air and health.

Many smokers are unaware of, or simply do not care to realize, how much cigarette smoke bothers nonsmokers. Smokers sometimes think that blowing the smoke off to the side is enough to get it out of the way. As a matter of fact, it is not enough. Smokers do not comprehend this until they quit and later find themselves in that situation. Suddenly they realize why cigarette smoke is so unpleasant and undesirable to most people.

The FDA Drug Abuse Advisory Committee has taken a strong stance against the use of all forms of tobacco products. Although the American Heart Association (AHA) commends the work initiated by the FDA, the AHA has further stated that the FDA and the federal government have an obligation to take regulatory action against the national problem of nicotine addiction and abuse of cigarettes and tobacco products in general. In a statement before the FDA Drug Abuse Advisory Committee, the AHA indicated that "it is a national health travesty that a product (tobacco), which accounts for over 440,000 deaths in the U.S. each year, has escaped regulation under every major health and safety law enacted by Congress to protect the public health."[13] A U.S. Surgeon General's report for the year 2000 on reducing tobacco use stated that health education combined with social, economic, and regulatory approaches is imperative to offset the tobacco industry's marketing and promotion and to promote nonsmoking environments.[14]

# Why People Smoke

People typically begin to smoke without realizing its detrimental effects on their health and life in general. Although people start to smoke for many different reasons, the three fundamental instigators are peer pressure, the desire to appear "grown up," and rebellion against authority. Smoking only three packs of cigarettes can lead to physiologic addiction, turning smoking into a nasty habit that has become the most widespread example of drug dependency in the United States.

## Smoking Addiction and Dependency

The drug nicotine has strong addictive properties. Within seconds of inhalation, nicotine affects the central nervous system and can act simultaneously as a tranquilizer and a stimulant. The stimulating effect produces strong physiologic and psychological dependency. The physical addiction to nicotine is six to eight times more powerful than the addiction to alcohol, and most likely greater than that of some of the hard drugs currently used.

Psychological dependency develops over a longer time. People smoke to help themselves relax, and they also gain a certain amount of pleasure from the ritual of smoking. Smokers automatically associate many activities of daily life with cigarettes—coffee drinking, alcohol drinking, being part of a social gathering, relaxing after a meal, talking on the telephone, driving, reading, and watching television. In many cases, the social rituals of smoking are the most difficult to eliminate. The dependency is so strong that years after people have stopped smoking, they may still crave cigarettes when they engage in certain social activities.

Most of the remaining information in this chapter is written directly to smokers. Nonsmokers, however, will gain a better understanding of smokers by reading it. The following material also provides valuable information so you can help others implement a smoking-cessation program.

## "Why Do You Smoke?" Test

Most people smoke for a variety of reasons. To find out why people smoke, the National Clearinghouse for Smoking and Health developed the simple "Why Do You Smoke?" Test. This test, contained in Lab 13B, lists some statements by smokers describing what they get out of smoking cigarettes. Smokers are asked to indicate how often they have the feelings described in each statement when they are smoking.

The scores obtained on this test assess smokers for each of six factors that describe individuals' feelings when they smoke. The first three highlight the positive feelings that people derive from smoking. The fourth factor relates to reducing tension and relaxing. The fifth reveals the extent of dependence on cigarettes. The sixth factor differentiates habit smoking and purely automatic smoking. Each of the remaining factors fits one of the six reasons for smoking discussed next. A score of 11 or above on any factor indicates that smoking is an important source of satisfaction for you. The higher you score (15 is the highest), the more important a given factor is in your smoking, and the more useful a discussion of that factor can be in your attempt to quit.

If you do not score high on any of the six factors, chances are that you do not smoke much or have not been smoking for long. If so, giving up smoking, and staying off, should be fairly easy.

1. **Stimulation.** If you score high or fairly high on the stimulation factor, you are one of those smokers who is stimulated by the cigarette. You think it helps wake you up, organize your energies, and keep you going. If you try to give up smoking, you may want a safe substitute—a brisk walk or moderate exercise, for example—whenever you feel the urge to smoke.

2. *Handling.* Handling things can be satisfying, but you can keep your hands busy in many ways without lighting up or playing with a cigarette. Why not toy with a pen or pencil? Try doodling. Play with a coin, a piece of jewelry, or some other harmless object.

3. *Pleasure / Pleasurable Relaxation.* Finding out whether you use the cigarette to feel good—you get real, honest pleasure from smoking—or to keep from feeling bad (Factor 4) is not always easy. About two-thirds of smokers score high or fairly high on accentuation of pleasure, and about half of those also score as high or higher on reduction of negative feelings. Those who do get real pleasure from smoking often find that honest consideration of the harmful effects of their habit is enough to help them quit. They substitute social and physical activities and find that they do not seriously miss cigarettes.

4. *Crutch: Tension Reduction.* Many smokers use cigarettes as a crutch during moments of stress or discomfort. Ironically, the heavy smoker—the person who tries to handle severe personal problems by smoking many times a day—is apt to discover that cigarettes do not help deal with problems effectively. This kind of smoker may stop smoking readily when everything is going well but may be tempted to start again in a time of crisis. Again, physical exertion or social activity may be a useful substitute for cigarettes, especially in times of tension.

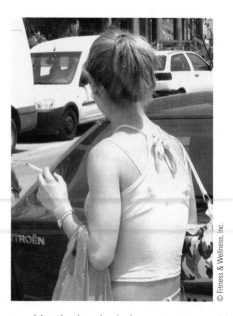

Cigarette smoking is the single largest preventable cause of illness and premature death in the United States.

5. *Craving: Psychological Addiction.* Quitting smoking is difficult for people who score high on this factor. The craving for a cigarette begins to build the moment the previous cigarette is put out, so tapering off is not likely to work. This smoker must go **cold turkey**. If you are dependent on cigarettes, you might try smoking more than usual for a day or two to spoil your taste for cigarettes, then isolating yourself completely from cigarettes until the craving is gone.

6. *Habit.* If you are smoking from habit, you no longer get much satisfaction from cigarettes. You light them frequently without even realizing you are doing it. You may have an easy time quitting and staying off if you can break the habitual patterns you have built up. Cutting down gradually may be effective if you change the way you smoke cigarettes and the conditions under which you smoke them. The key to success is to become aware of each cigarette you smoke. You can do this by asking yourself, "Do I really want this cigarette?" You might be surprised at how many you do not want.

# Smoking Cessation

If you are contemplating a smoking-cessation program or are preparing to stop cigarette smoking, you need to know that quitting smoking is not easy. Annually, only about 20 percent of smokers who try to quit the first time succeed. The addictive properties of nicotine and smoke make quitting difficult.

The American Psychiatric Association and the National Institute on Drug Abuse have indicated that nicotine is perhaps the most addictive drug known to humans. The U.S. Surgeon General has concluded that:[15]

- Cigarettes and other forms of tobacco are addicting.
- Nicotine is the drug responsible for the addictive behavior.
- Pharmacological and behavioral traits that determine addiction to tobacco are similar to those that determine addiction to drugs such as heroin and cocaine.

Smokers develop a tolerance to nicotine and tobacco smoke. They become dependent on both and get physical and psychological withdrawal symptoms when they stop smoking. Even though giving up smoking can be extremely difficult, it is by no means impossible, as attested by the many people who have quit.

During the last four decades, cigarette smoking in the United States had declined gradually among smokers of all ages. Of concern, the latest data indicate that the rate of people who smoke has leveled off since 2003.

Surveys have shown that between 75 and 90 percent of all smokers would like to quit. In 1964 (when the U.S. Surgeon General first reported the link between smoking and increased risk for disease and mortality), 40 percent of the adult population—53 percent of men and 32 percent of women—smoked. In 2006, only 23.5 percent of adult men and 18.1 percent of adult women smoked. More than 45 million Americans have given up cigarettes. More than 49 percent of all adults who have ever smoked have quit since 1964.

Further, more than 91 percent of successful ex-smokers have been able to do it on their own, either by quitting cold turkey or by using self-help kits available from organizations such as the American Cancer Society, the American Heart Association, and the American Lung Association. Only 6.8 percent of ex-smokers have done so as a result of formal cessation programs. Smokers' information and treatment centers are listed in the Yellow Pages of the telephone book.

**"Do You Want to Quit?" Test** The most important factor in quitting cigarette smoking is the person's sincere desire to do so. Although a few smokers can simply quit, this usually is not the case. Those who can quit easily are primarily light or casual smokers. They realize that the pleasure of an occasional cigarette is not worth the added risk for disease and premature death. For heavy smokers, quitting most likely will be a difficult battle. Even though many do not succeed the first time around, the odds of quitting are much better for those who repeatedly try to stop.

If you are a smoker and want to find your readiness to quit, the "Do You Want to Quit?" Test, developed by the National Clearinghouse for Smoking and Health, contained in Lab 13B, will measure your attitude toward the four primary reasons you want to quit smoking. The results indicate whether you are ready to start the program. On this test, the higher you score in any category, say, the Health category, the more important that reason is to you. A score of 9 or above in one of these categories indicates that this is one of the most important reasons you may want to quit.

1. Health. Knowing the harmful consequences of cigarettes, many people have stopped smoking and many others are considering doing so. If your score on the Health factor is 9 or above, the health hazards of smoking may be enough to make you want to quit now. If your score on this factor is low (6 or below), consider the hazards of smoking. You may be lacking important information or may even have incorrect information. If so, health considerations are not playing the role they should in your decision to keep smoking or to quit.

2. Example. Some people stop smoking because they want to set a good example for others. Parents quit to make it easier for their children to resist starting to smoke. Doctors quit so they can be role models for their patients. Teachers quit to discourage their students from smoking. Sports stars want to set an example for their young fans. Husbands quit to influence their wives to quit, and vice versa. Examples have a significant influ-

---

**Cold turkey** Eliminating a negative behavior all at once.

ence on our behavior. Surveys show that almost twice as many high school students smoke if both parents are smokers, compared with those whose parents are non-smokers or former smokers. If your score is low (6 or lower), you might not be interested in giving up smoking to set an example for others. Perhaps you do not realize how important your example could be.

3. Aesthetics. People who score high (9 or above) in this category recognize and are disturbed by some of the unpleasant aspects of smoking. The smell of stale smoke on their clothing, bad breath, and stains on their fingers and teeth might be reason enough to consider quitting.

4. Mastery. If you score 9 or above on this factor, you are bothered by knowing that you cannot control your desire to smoke. You are not your own master. Awareness of this challenge to your self-control may make you want to quit.

### Breaking the Habit

The following seven-step plan has been developed as a guide to help you quit smoking. You should complete the total program in 4 weeks or less. Steps One through Four combined should take no longer than 2 weeks. A maximum of 2 additional weeks is allowed for the rest of the program.

**Step One** Decide positively that you want to quit. Avoid negative thoughts of how difficult this can be. Think positive. You can do it.

Now prepare a list of the reasons you smoke and why you want to quit (Lab 13B). Make several copies of the list and keep them in places where you commonly smoke. Frequently review the reasons for quitting, because this will motivate and prepare you psychologically to quit.

When the reasons for quitting outweigh the reasons for smoking, you will have an easier time quitting. Read as much information as possible on the detrimental effects of tobacco and the benefits of quitting.

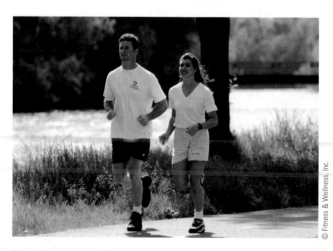

Starting an exercise program prior to giving up cigarettes encourages cessation and helps with weight control during the process.

**Step Two** Initiate a personal diet and exercise program. About one-third of the people who quit smoking gain weight. This could be caused by one or a combination of the following reasons:

1. Food becomes a substitute for cigarettes.
2. Appetite increases.
3. Basal metabolism may slow down.

If you start an exercise and weight-control program prior to quitting smoking, weight gain should not be a problem. If anything, exercise and lower body weight create more awareness of healthy living and strengthen the motivation for giving up cigarettes.

Even if you gain some weight, the harmful effects of cigarette smoking are much more detrimental to human health than a few extra pounds of body weight. Experts have indicated that as far as the extra load on the heart is concerned, giving up one pack of cigarettes a day is the equivalent of losing between 50 and 75 pounds of excess body fat!

**Step Three** Decide on the approach you will use to stop smoking. You may quit cold turkey or gradually cut down the number of cigarettes you smoke daily. Base your decision on your scores obtained on the "Why Do You Smoke?" Test. If you score 11 points or higher in either the "Crutch: Tension Reduction" or the "Craving: Psychological Addiction" categories, your best chance for success is quitting cold turkey. If your highest scores occur in any of the other four categories, you may choose either approach.

People still argue about which approach is more effective. Quitting cold turkey may cause fewer withdrawal symptoms than tapering off gradually. When you are cutting down slowly, the fewer cigarettes you smoke, the more important each one becomes. Therefore, you have a greater chance for relapse and returning to the original number of cigarettes you smoked. But when the cutting-down approach is accompanied by a definite target date for quitting, the technique has been shown to be quite effective. Smokers who taper off without a target date for quitting are the most likely to relapse.

**Step Four** Keep a daily log of your smoking habit for a few days. This will help you understand the situations in which you smoke. To assist you in doing this, make copies of Lab 13B, or develop your own form. Keep this form with you, and every time you smoke, record the required information. Keep track of the number of cigarettes you smoke, times of day you smoke them, events associated with smoking, amount of each cigarette smoked, and a rating of how badly you needed that cigarette. Rate each cigarette from 1 to 3:

   1 = desperately needed
   2 = moderately needed
   3 = no real need
This daily log will assist you in three ways:

1. You will get to know your habit.
2. It will help you eliminate cigarettes you do not crave.

**3.** It will help you find positive substitutes for situations that trigger your desire to smoke.

**Step Five** Set the target date for quitting. If you are going to taper off gradually, read the instructions under the "Cutting Down Gradually" discussion before you proceed to Step Six. When you set the target date, choose a special date to add a little extra incentive. An upcoming birthday, anniversary, vacation, graduation, family reunion—all are examples of good dates to free yourself from smoking. Dates when you are going to be away from events and environments that trigger your desire to smoke may be especially helpful. Once you have set the date, do not change it. Do not let anyone or anything interfere with this date.

Let your friends and relatives know of your intentions and ask for their support. Consider asking someone else to quit with you. That way, you can support each other in your efforts to stop. Avoid anyone who will not support you in your effort to quit. When you are attempting to quit, other people can be a prime obstacle. Many smokers are intolerable when they first stop smoking, so some friends and relatives prefer that the person continue to smoke.

**Step Six** Stock up on low-calorie foods—carrots, broccoli, cauliflower, celery, popcorn (butter- and salt-free), fruits, sunflower seeds (in the shell), sugarless gum—and drink plenty of water. Keep the food handy on the day you stop and the first few days following cessation. Substitute this food for a cigarette when you want one.

**Step Seven** On your quit day and the first few days thereafter, do not keep cigarettes handy. Stay away from friends and events that trigger your desire to smoke, and drink a lot of water and fruit juices. To replace the old behavior with new behavior, replace smoking time with new, positive substitutes that will make smoking difficult or impossible.

When you want a cigarette, take a few deep breaths and then occupy yourself by doing any of a number of things, such as talking to someone else, washing your hands, brushing your teeth, eating a healthy snack, chewing on a straw, doing dishes, playing sports, going for a walk or a bike ride, going swimming, and so on. Engage in activities that require the use of your hands. Try gardening, sewing, writing letters, drawing, doing household chores, or washing the car. Visit nonsmoking places such as libraries, museums, stores, and theaters. Plan an outing or a trip away from home. Any of these activities can keep your mind off cigarettes. Record your choice of activity or substitute under the Remarks/Substitutes column in Lab 13B.

### Quitting Cold Turkey
Many people have found that quitting all at once is the easiest way to do it. Most smokers have tried this approach at least once. Even though it might not work the first time, they don't allow themselves to get discouraged, and they eventually succeed. Many times, after several attempts, all of a sudden they are able to overcome smoking without too much difficulty.

On the average, as few as three smokeless days are sufficient to break the physiologic addiction to nicotine. The psychological addiction may linger for years but will get weaker as time goes by.

### Cutting Down Gradually
Tapering off cigarettes can be done in several ways:

**1.** Eliminate cigarettes you do not strongly crave (those ranked numbers 3 and 2 on your daily log).

**2.** Switch to a brand lower in nicotine/tar every few days.

**3.** Smoke less of each cigarette.

**4.** Smoke fewer cigarettes each day.

Most people prefer a combination of these four suggestions.

Before you start cutting down, set a target date for quitting. Once the date is set, don't change it. The total time until your quit date should be no longer than 2 weeks. Reduce the total number of cigarettes you smoke each day by 10 to 25 percent. As you smoke less, be careful not to take more puffs or inhale more deeply as you smoke, because this would offset the principle of cutting down.

As an aid in tapering off, make several copies of Lab 13B. (By now you should have already completed the first daily log of your smoking habit—see Step Four under "Breaking the Habit" on the opposite page.) Start a new daily log and every night review your data and set goals for the following day.

Decide and record which cigarettes will be easiest to give up, what brand you will smoke, the total number of cigarettes to be smoked, and how much of each you will smoke. Log any comments or situations you want to avoid, as well as any substitutes you could use to help you in the program. For example, if you always smoke while drinking coffee, substitute juice for coffee. If you smoke while driving, arrange for a ride or take a bus to work. If you smoke with a certain friend at lunch, avoid having lunch with that friend for a week or so. Continue using this log until you have stopped smoking completely.

### Nicotine-Substitution Products
Nicotine-substitution drug products such as nicotine transdermal patches and nicotine gum were developed to help people kick the tobacco habit. These products are most effective when they are used in a physician-supervised cessation program. As with tapering off, these products gradually decrease the amount of nicotine used until the person no longer craves the drug.

Nicotine patches supply a steady dose of nicotine through the skin. The patches are more effective when used in conjunction with exercise.[16] About eight out of ten smokers who use this therapy successfully quit smoking. Only about half of those who use patches alone are able to quit.

Nicotine-replacement patches are available in various doses, delivering anywhere from about 5 to 21 mg of nicotine in a 24-hour period. A typical program lasts between

# Behavior Modification Planning

## TIPS TO HELP STOP SMOKING

Check the suggestions that may work for you and in corporate them into your own retraining program.

**I PLAN TO**

**I DID IT**

### Preparing to Quit

☐ ☐ Create a personal list of reasons to quit. Keep the list handy, review it frequently, and add to it as needed.

☐ ☐ Know what to expect. Information is available from government sources, health organizations, doctors, hospitals, or on the Web. Talk with people who have quit or contact a local group or a hotline.

☐ ☐ Review any past attempts to quit. Determine what worked and what didn't work for you.

☐ ☐ Get a physical examination and discuss your desire to quit smoking with your doctor. Ask whether medication may help you quit.

☐ ☐ Create a stop-smoking plan customized to your personality, preferences, and schedule. If you are tapering off, set intermediate goals. Make sure to plan for times of intense desire for a cigarette. Be prepared and determine what you can use as a substitute for that cigarette. Is there anyone you can call for assistance or to help you distract your mind? Do not forget to include rewards for your success. Sign a contract and ask a friend to sign it as a witness.

☐ ☐ Determine your quit day. Choose a special day, such as a birthday, an anniversary, or a holiday. Select a day on which you will not feel a strong temptation to smoke—for instance, a stressful work day. Once you pick a date, do not alter this date.

☐ ☐ Enlist the support of friends, loved ones, team members, co-workers—as many people as you can. Ask others not to smoke around you or leave cigarettes in view. If you can, find someone else who wants to quit with you.

☐ ☐ Inquire about counseling. Individual, group, and telephone counseling can improve your chances of success.

☐ ☐ Consider starting a weight loss and exercise program before you quit. Such positive action will increase your confidence in your ability to quit and can keep you from gaining weight when you stop smoking.

☐ ☐ Stage a farewell activity to cigarettes and smoking; perhaps by overindulging so the idea of smoking is no longer appealing, or with a ceremony to destroy all cigarettes, lighters, and ashtrays.

☐ ☐ Change your environment. Clean your room or house, clothes, and car to remove the scent of tobacco smoke. Rearrange the furniture, paint the walls a different color, open windows to freshen the air, and buy plants or flowers.

☐ ☐ Plan changes in your routine. Reschedule regular activities, use different routes to get to places you normally go, go to bed earlier and get up earlier, avoid being rushed.

☐ ☐ Start a new hobby or other activity; for example, dancing, making videos, painting, acting, or learning to cook ethnic foods—something enjoyable that you've wanted to do for a long time.

☐ ☐ Stock up on healthy, low-calorie snacks.

### While Tapering Off

☐ ☐ Keep cigarettes as hard to get as possible. Leave them with someone else, lock them up, wrap them up like gifts with lots of tape or ribbon.

☐ ☐ Don't store cigarettes—wait until one pack is finished before buying another.

☐ ☐ Never carry matches or a lighter.

☐ ☐ Each time you want to smoke, write down what you are doing and feeling and how important the cigarette is to you—before you light up.

☐ ☐ Smoke only in uninteresting or uncomfortable places.

☐ ☐ Put off the first cigarette of the day for as long as possible.

☐ ☐ Smoke just half a cigarette.

After Quitting

- ❏ ❏ To help prevent relapse, rather than saying "I quit smoking," say "I don't want to smoke."
- ❏ ❏ Get plenty of sleep.
- ❏ ❏ Eat regular, healthy, appetizing meals; pay attention to the flavors and textures of the foods.
- ❏ ❏ Be mindful of negative thoughts and replace them with positive actions—from "I can't stand this" to "What else can I do right now to keep my mind off cigarettes?" for example.
- ❏ ❏ Spend time in places where smoking is not allowed—libraries, museums, churches, malls, movie theaters.
- ❏ ❏ Tune in to the sights and scents around you.
- ❏ ❏ Drink plenty of water and other low-calorie drinks (but avoid caffeine).
- ❏ ❏ Deal with one minute, one hour, and one day at a time.
- ❏ ❏ Plan something that will bring you pleasure every day.
- ❏ ❏ Be aware of life stressors and plan a variety of ways to relax without cigarettes.
- ❏ ❏ Avoid situations in which you used to smoke, including being with people who smoke.
- ❏ ❏ Be wary of alcohol: Drinking lowers your chances of success.
- ❏ ❏ Use your lungs more by increasing daily physical activity and sports participation. Try to notice how clean the air feels flowing in and out of your lungs.
- ❏ ❏ Celebrate and reward yourself for each success.
- ❏ ❏ Visit your dentist and have your teeth cleaned and whitened.
- ❏ ❏ Calculate how much money you are saving and use this money to reward yourself or someone else with a small luxury.
- ❏ ❏ Consult your doctor if you are concerned about your physical or emotional feelings.
- ❏ ❏ If you gain weight, don't attempt to lose the weight until after you get over the craving for cigarettes.

Instead of Smoking a Cigarette

- ❏ ❏ Take several deep breaths, focusing on your breathing and the fresh air that you are inhaling.
- ❏ ❏ Tell yourself to wait three minutes; redirect your thoughts by visualizing a serene landscape or planning a dream vacation or weekend away from home.
- ❏ ❏ Go for a walk. If you have a dog, take the dog for a walk.
- ❏ ❏ Chew gum or suck on hard, sugarless candy—always carry some with you.
- ❏ ❏ Talk to someone you can easily reach for support.
- ❏ ❏ Munch on carrots, celery sticks, or other healthy snacks.
- ❏ ❏ Use your hands: Wash dishes, sweep the floor, brush your teeth, write in a journal, sketch a cartoon, play a musical instrument.
- ❏ ❏ Go swimming or take a shower.

If You Relapse

- ❏ ❏ Don't be discouraged—most people try several times before they are finally able to kick the habit.
- ❏ ❏ Instead of berating yourself, remember your successes and recommit to quitting.
- ❏ ❏ Re-evaluate your smoking-cessation plan and modify it as necessary.
- ❏ ❏ Remember that relapse doesn't mean failure. Failure comes to those who give up. Instead, learn from your mistake and reach once more for your goal.

## Try It

Nicotine is believed to be the most addictive drug we know. Smokers who are trying to kick the habit need behavioral change strategies to enhance their rate of success. From the above strategies, prepare a list of those that may work for you. On a daily basis, conduct nightly audits on how well you have done that day. Every third day, review all of the above strategies and make changes to your list as necessary.

3 and 10 weeks, with an average weekly cost to the consumer of about $50.

Public safety concerns regarding the use of nicotine patches, including indications, precautions, warnings, contraindications, potential abuse, and marketing and labeling issues are monitored and regulated by the FDA. People contemplating their use should pay careful attention to contraindications and potential side effects. Pregnant and lactating women and people with heart disease or high blood pressure or who have had a recent heart attack should check with their physician prior to using nicotine-substitution products. Skin redness, swelling, or rashes are sometimes associated with the use of nicotine patches. Other undesirable side effects are listed on the label and should be monitored closely.

## Critical Thinking

If you ever smoked or now smoke cigarettes, discuss your perceptions of how others accepted your behavior. If you smoked and have quit, how did you accomplish the task, and has it changed the way others view you? If you never smoked, how do you perceive smokers?

# Life After Cigarettes

When you first quit smoking, you can expect a series of withdrawal symptoms for a few days; among them are lower heart rate and blood pressure, headaches, gastrointestinal discomfort, mood changes, irritability, aggressiveness, and difficulty sleeping.

The physiologic addiction to nicotine is broken only 3 days following your last cigarette. Thereafter, you should not crave cigarettes as much. For the habitual smoker, the psychological dependency could be the most difficult to break. The first few days probably will not be as difficult as the first few months. Any of the activities of daily life that you have associated with smoking—either stress or relaxation, joy or unhappiness—may trigger a relapse even months, or at times years, after quitting.

Ex-smokers should realize that even though some harm may have been done already, it is never too late to quit. The greatest early benefit is a lower risk for sudden death. Furthermore, the risk for illness starts to decrease the moment you stop smoking. You will have fewer sore throats and sores in the mouth, less hoarseness, no more cigarette cough, and lower risk for peptic ulcers.

Circulation to the hands and feet will improve, as will gastrointestinal and kidney and bladder functions. Everything will taste and smell better. You will have more energy, and you will gain a sense of freedom, pride, and well-being. You no longer will have to worry whether you have enough cigarettes to last through a day, a party, a meeting, a weekend, or a trip.

When you first quit and you think how tough it is and how miserable you feel because you cannot have a cigarette, try the opposite: Think of the benefits and how great it is not to smoke! The ex-smoker's risk for heart disease approaches that of a lifetime nonsmoker 10 years following cessation; and for cancer, 15 years after quitting.

If you have been successful and stopped smoking, a lot of events can still trigger your urge to smoke. When confronted with these events, some people rationalize and think, "One cigarette won't hurt. I've been off for months (years in some cases)" or "I can handle it. I'll smoke just today." It won't work! Before you know it, you will be back to the regular nasty habit. Be prepared to take action in those situations by finding substitutes such as those provided in the "Tips to Help Stop Smoking" box that begins on page 474.

Start thinking of yourself as a nonsmoker—no "butts" about it. Remind yourself how difficult it has been and how long it has taken you to get to this point. If you have come this far, you certainly can resist brief moments of temptation. It will get easier rather than harder as time goes on.

The simple pleasures of life, such as taste and smell, improve with smoking cessation.

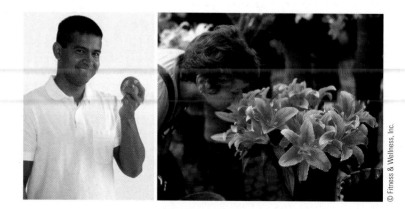

## ASSESS YOUR BEHAVIOR

 Log on to http://www.cengage.com/sso/ to take the Wellness Profile assessment and gauge your level of risk in the area of addictive behavior.

1. Is your life free of addictive behavior? If not, will you commit right now to seek professional help at your institution's counseling center? Addictive behavior destroys health and lives—don't let it waste yours.

2. Are you prepared to walk away, even at the peril of losing close friendships and relationships, if you are put in a situation where you are pressured to drink, smoke, or engage in any other form of drug (legal or illegal) abuse?

## ASSESS YOUR KNOWLEDGE

 Log on to http://www.cengage.com/sso/ to assess your understanding of this chapter's topics by taking the Student Practice Test and exploring the modules recommended in your Personalized Study Plan.

1. The following substance is not an object of chemical dependency.
   a. Ecstasy
   b. Alcohol
   c. Cocaine
   d. Heroin
   e. All are objects of chemical dependency.

2. The most widely used illegal drug in the United States is
   a. marijuana.
   b. alcohol.
   c. cocaine.
   d. heroin
   e. Ecstasy.

3. Cocaine use
   a. causes lung cancer.
   b. leads to atrophy of the brain.
   c. can lead to sudden death.
   d. causes amotivational syndrome.
   e. All these things are possible.

4. Methamphetamine
   a. is less potent than amphetamine.
   b. increases fatigue.
   c. helps a person relax.
   d. is a central nervous system stimulant.
   e. increases the need for sleep.

5. Ecstasy
   a. is popular among middle-age people.
   b. is a relatively harmless drug.
   c. is used primarily by African-American males.
   d. increases heart rate and blood pressure.
   e. All are correct choices

6. Treatment of chemical dependency is
   a. accomplished primarily by the individual alone.
   b. most successful when there is peer pressure to stop.
   c. best achieved with the help of family members.
   d. seldom accomplished without professional guidance.
   e. usually done with the help of friends.

7. Cigarette smoking is responsible for about _____ unnecessary deaths in the United States each year.
   a. 10,000
   b. 80,000
   c. 250,000
   d. 440,000
   e. 1,000,000

8. Cigarette smoking increases death rates from
   a. heart disease.
   b. cancer.
   c. stroke.
   d. aortic aneurysm.
   e. all of the above.

9. The percentage of lung cancer attributed to cigarette smoking is
   a. 25 percent.
   b. 43 percent.
   c. 58 percent.
   d. 64 percent.
   e. 87 percent.

10. Smoking cessation results in
    a. a decrease in sore throats.
    b. improved gastrointestinal function.
    c. a decrease in risk for sudden death.
    d. better tasting of foods.
    e. All of these changes occur.

Correct answers can be found at the back of the book.

# MEDIA MENU

You can find the links below at the book companion site: www.cengage.com/health/hoeger/plfw10e

- Take a self-assessment to see if you are prone to addictive behavior.
- Check how well you understand the chapter's concepts.

## Internet Connections

- National Institute on Alcohol Abuse and Alcoholism. This site, sponsored by the U.S. government, features information on research and education related to alcohol use and abuse. *http://www.niaaa.nih.gov*
- CDC Page on Smoking and Health: Tobacco Information and Prevention Source. A comprehensive site featuring educational information, research, reports from the U.S. Surgeon General, tips on how to quit, and much more. *http://www.cdc.gov/tobacco*

- NIDA Drug Pages from the National Institute on Drug Abuse. This site features information about a comprehensive list of drugs, including alcohol, nicotine, marijuana, cocaine, Ecstasy, amphetamines, steroids, prescription medications, and more. The site also features an excellent chart listing the common drugs of abuse according to category and examples of commercial and street names, as well as intoxication effects and potential health consequences. *http://www.nida.nih.gov*
- Drugpages Facts on Tap: Alcohol and Your College Experience. This outstanding site is geared to college students, featuring links to the following topics and more: Risky Relationship: Alcohol and Sex, College Experience: Alcohol and Student Life, The Naked Truth: Alcohol and Your Body, and When Someone Else's Drinking Gives You a Hangover. *http://www.factsontap.org*

# NOTES

1. U.S. Department of Health & Human Services, Office of Applied Studies, "Results from the 2006 National Survey on Drug Use and Health: National Findings," http://oas.samhsa.gov/nsduh/2k6nsduh/2k6Results.cfm#TOC (downloaded July 22, 2008).

2. W. W. K. Hoeger, L. W. Turner, and B. Q. Hafen, *Wellness: Guidelines for a Healthy Lifestyle* (Belmont, CA: Wadsworth/Thomson Learning, 2007).

3. R. Goldberg, *Drugs Across the Spectrum* (Belmont, CA: Wadsworth/Thomson Learning, 2006).

4. See note 3.

5. R. Hingson, et al., "Magnitude of Alcohol-Related Mortality and Morbidity Among U.S. College Students Ages 18–24: Changes from 1998 to 2001," *Annual Review of Public Health* 26 (2005): 259–279.

6. C. A. Presley, J. S. Leichliter, and P. W. Meilman, *Alcohol and Drugs on American College Campuses: Findings from 1995, 1996, and 1997 (A Report to Col-*

*lege Presidents)* (Carbondale: Southern Illinois University, 1999).

7. See note 1.

8. U.S. Department of Agriculture, *Tobacco Outlook Report* (Washington DC: U.S. Department of Agriculture, Market and Trade Economics Division, Economic Research Service, 2007).

9. American Cancer Society, *Cancer Facts & Figures 2008* (New York: ACS, 2008).

10. U.S. Public Health Service, *The Health Consequences of Involuntary Exposure to Tobacco Smoke: A Report of the Surgeon General—Executive Summary* (Rockville, MD: U.S. Department of Health and Human Services, 2006).

11. "Wellness Facts," *University of California Berkeley Wellness Letter* 14 (1998): 1.

12. American Cancer Society, *World Smoking & Health* (Atlanta: ACS, 1993).

13. American Heart Association, *AHA Public Affairs/Coalition on Smoking: Health Position* (Dallas: AHA, 1996).

14. U.S. Department of Health and Human Services, *Reducing Tobacco Use: A Report of the Surgeon General* (Atlanta: U.S. Department of Health and Human Services, Centers for Disease Control and Prevention, National Center for Chronic Disease Prevention and Health Promotion, Office on Smoking and Health, 2000).

15. U.S. Department of Health and Human Services, *Nicotine Addiction, A Report of the Surgeon General* (Atlanta: U.S. Department of Health and Human Services, Centers for Disease Control and Prevention, National Center for Chronic Disease Prevention and Health Promotion, 1988).

16. R. H. Zwick, et al., "Exercise in Addition to Nicotine Replacement Therapy Improves Success Rates in Smoking Cessation," *Chest* 130, no. 4 (2006): 145S

# SUGGESTED READINGS

American Cancer Society. *2009 Cancer Facts & Figures.* New York: ACS, 2009.

Doweiko, H. E. *Concepts of Chemical Dependency.* Belmont, CA: Wadsworth/Thomson Learning, 2006.

Goldberg, R. *Drugs Across the Spectrum.* Belmont, CA: Wadsworth/Thomson Learning, 2006.

U.S. Office on Smoking and Health. *Smoking and Health: A Report of the Surgeon General.* Washington, DC: U.S. Department of Health, Education and Welfare, 1979.

U.S. Public Health Service. *The Health Consequences of Involuntary Exposure to Tobacco Smoke: A Report of the Surgeon General—Executive Summary.* Rockville, MD: U.S. Department of Health and Human Services, 2006.

# LAB 13A: Addictive Behavior Questionnaires

Name _____  Date _____  Grade _____

Instructor _____  Course _____  Section _____

## Necessary Lab Equipment
None required.

## Objective
To determine possible addictive behavior.

## Instruction
The following questionnaires are for your own personal information. Answer all questions on a separate sheet of paper and keep that sheet for yourself. Turn in only this page to your instructor as proof that you have read and completed the questionnaire. If you wish to do so, you may personally discuss the results of these questionnaires with your course instructor.

## I. Stage of Change for Addictive Behavior
If chemical dependency is a problem in your life, use Figure 2.5 (page 57) and Table 2.3 (page 57) to identify your current stage of change for participation in a treatment program for addictive behavior.

## II. Recognizing Addictive Behavior
The following questionnaire has been designed to identify possible addictive behavior (chemical dependency). This test is not designed to determine if you have an addictive disease, but rather to help recognize potential addictive behavior in yourself or the people around you. The term "drug" may imply illicit substances or drugs (such as marijuana, cocaine, heroin, ecstasy, or methamphetamine), misuse of prescription drugs (painkillers, sleeping pills), or alcohol abuse.

1. Are you a compulsive person?

2. Are you a person of excesses?

3. Do you depend heavily on others or are you completely independent of others?

4. Do you spend a lot of time thinking about a drug(s)?

5. Do you use drugs other than for medical reasons?

6. Do you misuse prescription drugs?

7. Are you unable to stop using drugs or limit their use to required situations only?

8. Can you get through a week without misusing drugs?

9. Do friends or relatives sense or mention that you have a drug problem?

10. Has drug misuse ever created a problem between you and friends or relatives?

11. Have family members or friends ever sought help for problems associated with your misuse of drugs?

12. Have you ever sought help for drug misuse?

13. Do you deny or lie about the misuse of drugs?

14. Do you tend to associate with people who exhibit the same behaviors or take the same drugs you do?

15. Do you get angry at people who try to keep you from getting the drugs you desire?

16. Do you have a difficult time stopping the use of a drug when you start misusing it?

17. Do you experience withdrawal symptoms if you do not take the drugs you wish to have?

18. Has the misuse of drugs affected the way you function in life (school, work, recreation)?

19. Have you put yourself or others at risk by your actions while misusing drugs?

20. Have you unsuccessfully tried to cut back or stop the misuse of drugs?

## Interpretation
If you answered "yes" to five or more of these questions, you may have an addictive behavior and should seek further evaluation by a physician, your institution's counseling center, or contact the local mental health clinic for a referral (see the Yellow Pages in your local phone book). You may also contact the National Center for Substance Abuse Treatment at 1-800-662-4357 for 24-hour substance abuse treatment centers in your area. Depending on the question (for example, 7, 8, 12, 15, 16, 17, 18, 20), note that even fewer than five "yes" answers may already be indicative of chemical dependency.

## III. Alcohol Abuse: Are You Drinking Too Much?

Using a separate sheet of paper, specifically indicate the steps that you are going to take to correct addictive behavior(s) and identify people or organizations that you will contact to help you get started.

1. When you are holding an empty glass at a party, do you always actively look for a refill instead of waiting to be offered one?

2. If given the chance, do you frequently pour out a more generous drink for yourself than seems to be the "going" amount for others?

3. Do you often have a drink or two when you are alone, either at home or in a bar?

4. Is your drinking ever the direct cause of a family quarrel, or do quarrels often seem to occur, if only by coincidence, after you have had a drink or two?

5. Do you feel that you must have a drink at a specific time every day—right after work, for instance?

6. When worried or under unusual stress, do you almost automatically take a stiff drink to "settle your nerves"?

7. Are you untruthful about how much you have had to drink when questioned on the subject?

8. Does drinking ever cause you to take time off work or to miss scheduled meetings or appointments?

9. Do you feel physically deprived if you cannot have at least one drink every day?

10. Do you sometimes crave a drink in the morning?

11. Do you sometimes have "mornings after" when you cannot remember what happened the night before?

### How to Score

You should regard a "yes" answer to any one of the above questions as a warning sign. Do not increase your consumption of alcohol. Two "yes" answers suggest that you already may be becoming dependent on alcohol. Three or more "yes" answers indicate that you may have a serious problem and you should get professional help. Also refer to page 464 for general guidelines to cut down your drinking.

From *American Medical Association Family Medical Guide* by The American Medical Association. Copyright © 1982 by The American Medical Association. Used by permission of Random House, Inc.

## IV. Changing Addictive Behavior

Using a separate sheet of paper, specifically indicate the steps that you are going to take to correct addictive behavior(s) and identify people or organizations that you will contact to help you get started.

# LAB 13B: Smoking Cessation Questionnaires

Name _____     Date _____     Grade _____

Instructor _____     Course _____     Section _____

**Necessary Lab Equipment**
None required.

**Objective**
To develop a smoking cessation program either for your-self or for friends and relatives.

## I. Introduction

The forms provided in this lab have been designed to help smokers identify reasons why they smoke and their readiness to initiate a smoking cessation program. These forms should be filled out prior to initiating a smoking cessation program. Interpretation of the results are given in this chapter ("Why Do You Smoke?" Test, pages 470–471). The daily cigarette smoking log, Part V of this lab, has been developed to help smokers get to know their habit, cut down on cigarettes not really needed, and find positive substitutes when confronted with situations that trigger their desire to smoke.

## II. "Why Do You Smoke?" Test

| | Always | Fre-quently | Occa-sionally | Seldom | Never |
|---|---|---|---|---|---|
| A. I smoke cigarettes to keep myself from slowing down. | 5 | 4 | 3 | 2 | 1 |
| B Handling a cigarette is part of the enjoyment of smoking it. | 5 | 4 | 3 | 2 | 1 |
| C. Smoking cigarettes is pleasant and relaxing. | 5 | 4 | 3 | 2 | 1 |
| D. I light up a cigarette when I feel angry about something. | 5 | 4 | 3 | 2 | 1 |
| E. When I have run out of cigarettes, I find it almost unbearable until I can get them. | 5 | 4 | 3 | 2 | 1 |
| F. I smoke cigarettes automatically without even being aware of it. | 5 | 4 | 3 | 2 | 1 |
| G. I smoke cigarettes for stimulation, to perk myself up. | 5 | 4 | 3 | 2 | 1 |
| H. Part of the enjoyment of smoking a cigarette comes from the steps I take to light up. | 5 | 4 | 3 | 2 | 1 |
| I. I find cigarettes pleasurable. | 5 | 4 | 3 | 2 | 1 |
| J. When I feel uncomfortable or upset about something, I light up a cigarette. | 5 | 4 | 3 | 2 | 1 |
| K. I am very much aware of the fact when I am not smoking a cigarette. | 5 | 4 | 3 | 2 | 1 |
| L. I light up a cigarette without realizing I still have one burning in the ashtray. | 5 | 4 | 3 | 2 | 1 |
| M. I smoke cigarettes to give me a "lift." | 5 | 4 | 3 | 2 | 1 |
| N. When I smoke a cigarette, part of the enjoyment is watching the smoke as I exhale it. | 5 | 4 | 3 | 2 | 1 |
| O. I want a cigarette most when I am comfortable and relaxed. | 5 | 4 | 3 | 2 | 1 |
| P. When I feel "blue" or want to take my mind off cares and worries, I smoke cigarettes. | 5 | 4 | 3 | 2 | 1 |
| Q. I get a real gnawing hunger for a cigarette when I haven't smoked for a while. | 5 | 4 | 3 | 2 | 1 |
| R. I've found a cigarette in my mouth and didn't remember putting it there. | 5 | 4 | 3 | 2 | 1 |

**How to Score:** (See pages 470–471 to interpret your test results.)

Enter the numbers you have circled on the test questions in the spaces provided below, putting the number you have circled to question A on line A, to question B on line B, and so on. Add the three scores on each line to get a total for each factor. For example, the sum of your scores over lines A, G, and M gives you your score on "Stimulation"; lines B, H, and N give the score on "Handling." Scores can vary from 3 to 15. Any score 11 and above is high; any score 7 and below is low.

| | | | | |
|---|---|---|---|---|
| A _____ | + G _____ | + M _____ | = _____ | Stimulation |
| B _____ | + H _____ | + N _____ | = _____ | Handling |
| C _____ | + I _____ | + O _____ | = _____ | Pleasure/Relaxation |
| D _____ | + J _____ | + P _____ | = _____ | Crutch: Tension Reduction |
| E _____ | + K _____ | + Q _____ | = _____ | Craving: Psychological Addiction |
| F _____ | + L _____ | + R _____ | = _____ | Habit |

From *A Self-Test for Smokers*, U.S. Department of Health and Human Services, 1983.

## III. "Do You Want to Quit?" Test

| | Strongly Agree | Mildly Agree | Mildly Disagree | Strongly Disagree |
|---|---|---|---|---|
| A. Cigarette smoking might give me a serious illness. | 4 | 3 | 2 | 1 |
| B. My cigarette smoking sets a bad example for others. | 4 | 3 | 2 | 1 |
| C. I find cigarette smoking to be a messy kind of habit. | 4 | 3 | 2 | 1 |
| D. Controlling my cigarette smoking is a challenge to me. | 4 | 3 | 2 | 1 |
| E. Smoking causes shortness of breath. | 4 | 3 | 2 | 1 |
| F. If I quit smoking cigarettes, it might influence others to stop. | 4 | 3 | 2 | 1 |
| G. Cigarettes cause damage to clothing and other personal property. | 4 | 3 | 2 | 1 |
| H. Quitting smoking would show that I have willpower. | 4 | 3 | 2 | 1 |
| I. My cigarette smoking will have a harmful effect on my health. | 4 | 3 | 2 | 1 |
| J. My cigarette smoking influences others close to me to take up or continue smoking. | 4 | 3 | 2 | 1 |
| K. If I quit smoking, my sense of taste or smell will improve. | 4 | 3 | 2 | 1 |
| L. I do not like the idea of feeling dependent on smoking. | 4 | 3 | 2 | 1 |

**How to Score:** (See page 471, "Do You Want to Quit" Test, to interpret your results.)

Write the number you have circled after each statement on the test in the corresponding space to the right. Add the scores on each line to get your totals. For example, the sum of your scores A, E, and I gives you your score for the Health factor. Scores can vary from 3 to 12. Any score of 9 or over is high; any score 6 or under is low.

A [＿＿＿] + E [＿＿＿] + I [＿＿＿] = [＿＿＿] Health
B [＿＿＿] + F [＿＿＿] + J [＿＿＿] = [＿＿＿] Example
C [＿＿＿] + G [＿＿＿] + K [＿＿＿] = [＿＿＿] Aesthetics
D [＿＿＿] + H [＿＿＿] + L [＿＿＿] = [＿＿＿] Mastery

From *A Self-Test for Smokers,* U.S. Department of Health and Human Services, 1983.

## IV. Reasons to Smoke, Reasons to Quit

Reasons to Smoke Cigarettes

1. ＿＿＿＿＿＿＿＿＿＿＿＿＿＿＿＿＿＿＿＿＿＿＿＿＿＿＿＿＿＿＿＿＿＿＿＿＿＿＿＿＿＿＿＿＿＿＿＿＿＿
2. ＿＿＿＿＿＿＿＿＿＿＿＿＿＿＿＿＿＿＿＿＿＿＿＿＿＿＿＿＿＿＿＿＿＿＿＿＿＿＿＿＿＿＿＿＿＿＿＿＿＿
3. ＿＿＿＿＿＿＿＿＿＿＿＿＿＿＿＿＿＿＿＿＿＿＿＿＿＿＿＿＿＿＿＿＿＿＿＿＿＿＿＿＿＿＿＿＿＿＿＿＿＿
4. ＿＿＿＿＿＿＿＿＿＿＿＿＿＿＿＿＿＿＿＿＿＿＿＿＿＿＿＿＿＿＿＿＿＿＿＿＿＿＿＿＿＿＿＿＿＿＿＿＿＿
5. ＿＿＿＿＿＿＿＿＿＿＿＿＿＿＿＿＿＿＿＿＿＿＿＿＿＿＿＿＿＿＿＿＿＿＿＿＿＿＿＿＿＿＿＿＿＿＿＿＿＿

Reasons to Quit Cigarette Smoking

1. ＿＿＿＿＿＿＿＿＿＿＿＿＿＿＿＿＿＿＿＿＿＿＿＿＿＿＿＿＿＿＿＿＿＿＿＿＿＿＿＿＿＿＿＿＿＿＿＿＿＿
2. ＿＿＿＿＿＿＿＿＿＿＿＿＿＿＿＿＿＿＿＿＿＿＿＿＿＿＿＿＿＿＿＿＿＿＿＿＿＿＿＿＿＿＿＿＿＿＿＿＿＿
3. ＿＿＿＿＿＿＿＿＿＿＿＿＿＿＿＿＿＿＿＿＿＿＿＿＿＿＿＿＿＿＿＿＿＿＿＿＿＿＿＿＿＿＿＿＿＿＿＿＿＿
4. ＿＿＿＿＿＿＿＿＿＿＿＿＿＿＿＿＿＿＿＿＿＿＿＿＿＿＿＿＿＿＿＿＿＿＿＿＿＿＿＿＿＿＿＿＿＿＿＿＿＿
5. ＿＿＿＿＿＿＿＿＿＿＿＿＿＿＿＿＿＿＿＿＿＿＿＿＿＿＿＿＿＿＿＿＿＿＿＿＿＿＿＿＿＿＿＿＿＿＿＿＿＿

## V. Daily Cigarette Smoking Log

Today's Date: _____ Quit Date: _____ Decision Date: _____

Cigarettes to be smoked today: _____ Brand: _____

| No. | Time | Activity | Rating[a] | Amount Smoked[b] | Remarks/Substitutes |
|-----|------|----------|-----------|------------------|---------------------|
| 1. | | | | | |
| 2. | | | | | |
| 3. | | | | | |
| 4. | | | | | |
| 5. | | | | | |
| 6. | | | | | |
| 7. | | | | | |
| 8. | | | | | |
| 9. | | | | | |
| 10. | | | | | |
| 11. | | | | | |
| 12. | | | | | |
| 13. | | | | | |
| 14. | | | | | |
| 15. | | | | | |
| 16. | | | | | |
| 17. | | | | | |
| 18. | | | | | |
| 19. | | | | | |
| 20. | | | | | |

[a]Rating:  1 = desperately needed,  2 = moderately needed,  3 = no real need
[b]Amount Smoked: entire cigarette, two thirds, half, etc.

Additional Comments, list of friends and/or activities to avoid.

_____

_____

_____

_____

_____

## VI. Conclusion

In a few sentences, indicate your feelings about cigarette smoking and what you have learned from the previous questionnaires.

_____

_____

_____

_____

_____

_____

_____

_____

_____

_____

_____

_____

_____

# Preventing Sexually Transmitted Infections

14

© Fitness & Wellness, Inc.

## Objectives

- Name and describe the most common sexually transmitted infections
- Outline the health consequences of sexually transmitted infections
- Define the difference between HIV and AIDS
- Explain the seriousness of the AIDS epidemic in the United States and worldwide
- Describe ways to prevent acquiring sexually transmitted infections
- Evaluate your risk of HIV/AIDS.

CENGAGENOW™

Check your understanding of the chapter contents by logging on to CengageNOW and accessing the pre-test, personalized learning plan, and post-test for this chapter.

# FAQ

**What is the difference between a sexually transmitted infection (STI) and a sexually transmitted disease (STD)?**

Health experts have replaced the term "STD" with "STI." The concept of disease implies a clear medical condition that manifests itself through signs or symptoms that define a specific disease. In terms of STIs, once infected, a person may or may not develop signs or symptoms indicative of disease. The unfortunate reality is that in the early stages of infection, many individuals with STIs exhibit no signs or symptoms, or such that are so mild that they are often ignored.

**What is "safe sex"?**

Safe sex means taking precautions during sexual intercourse or other form of sexual contact, designed to prevent the exchange of blood, semen, vaginal fluids, or breast milk that can keep you or your partner from getting a sexually transmitted infection (STI). These infections include chlamydia, gonorrhea, pelvic inflammatory disease, genital warts, genital herpes, syphilis, and HIV, among others. When unsure about your partner, use a lubricated latex condom from start to finish for each sexual act. If you think your partner should use a condom but refuses to do so, say no to sex with that person. While a condom definitely reduces the risk for infection, you need to realize that even with condom use, you may acquire an STI. Condoms may not totally cover surrounding infected areas, and sometimes they rupture.

**How does HIV damage the immune system?**

Upon HIV infection, the virus attacks and starts killing CD4 cells in the immune system. CD4 cells are a special type of white blood cell that fights off infections (viral, fungal, and parasitic). Initially, the body can make more CD4 cells to replace the cells damaged by HIV. Eventually, however, the body is unable to replace all damaged cells. As the number of CD4 cells decreases, the immune system weakens and the person is more susceptible to sickness, illness, and infections, including the development of AIDS.

**Am I at risk for contracting HIV in a medical or dental office?**

HIV transmission in a health care setting is extremely rare. The implementation of strict infection control procedures protects both the patient and the health care provider. Only one such case, of patients having been infected by a Florida dentist in 1990, has been reported by the CDC. Data on more than 22,000 patients treated by 63 HIV-infected health care providers reveal no cases of transmission from provider to patient in a health care setting.

Based on estimates by the World Health Organization, 1 million people worldwide are infected daily with **sexually transmitted infections (STIs)**, not including human immunodeficiency virus (HIV). STIs have also reached epidemic proportions in the United States. Of the more than 25 known STIs, some are still incurable. According to the American Social Health Association, more than half of all Americans will acquire at least one STI in their lifetime.

Each year, more than 19 million people in the United States are newly infected with STIs, almost half of which are seen in young people between the ages of 15 and 24.[1] Currently, the United States has the highest rate of sexually transmitted diseases of any country in the industrialized world. Following are brief descriptions of the leading STIs, their symptoms, and their treatments (if any).

# Chlamydia

**Chlamydia** is the most prevalent STI in the United States. It is a bacterial infection that spreads during vaginal, anal, or oral sex, or from the vagina to a newborn baby during childbirth. Chlamydia can damage the reproductive system seriously. This infection is considered to be a major factor in male and female infertility. Because symptoms are usually mild or absent, three of four people with the infection don't know they're ill until the infection has become quite serious. Infertility often occurs "silently"

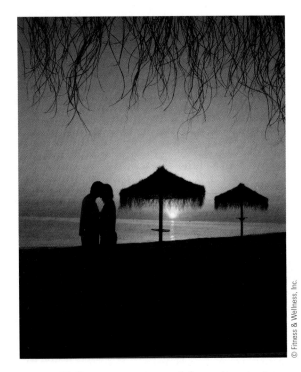

More than 25 diseases are spread through sexual contact. About 1 in 4 adults in the United States has a sexually transmitted disease.

because the individual is unaware of the infection until it is too late to prevent the irreversible damage.

Each year there are about 2.3 million cases of chlamydia in the United States.[2] Almost 80 percent of these cases are reported in women between the ages of 15 and 24. Only about 1 million cases are reported each year because most people are not aware of their infection. Testing is also frequently skipped because patients are mistreated for symptoms that mimic other STIs. Women are frequently reinfected if their sex partners are not treated.

Symptoms of serious infection include abdominal pain, fever, nausea, vaginal bleeding, and arthritis. Although chlamydia can be treated successfully with oral antibiotics, its damage to the reproductive system is irreversible. Regular testing for chlamydia is recommended for all sexually active women under the age of 25, for older women with multiple sexual partners and/or previous STIs, and for those who do not regularly use condoms.

## Gonorrhea

One of the oldest STIs, **gonorrhea** is caused by a bacterial infection. Gonorrhea is transmitted through contact with the vagina, penis, anus, or mouth of an infected person. According to the Centers for Disease Control and Prevention (CDC), approximately 700,000 individuals get new gonorrheal infections each year in the United States, but only about one half of the cases are reported.[3]

Typical symptoms in men include a pus-like secretion from the penis and painful urination. Infected women may have discharge and painful urination as well. Up to 80 percent of infected women, however, don't experience any symptoms until the infection has become fairly serious. At this stage, women develop fever, severe abdominal pain, and pelvic inflammatory disease (discussed next).

If untreated, gonorrhea can produce widespread bacterial infection, infertility, heart damage, and arthritis in men and women, and blindness in children born to infected women. Gonorrhea is treated successfully with penicillin and other antibiotics.

## Pelvic Inflammatory Disease

Estimates indicate that each year in the United States more than 1 million women experience an acute episode of a condition known by the umbrella term **pelvic inflammatory disease (PID)**.[4] PID is not truly an STI but, rather, refers to complications resulting from STIs, especially chlamydia and gonorrhea. PID often develops when the STI spreads to the fallopian tubes, uterus, and ovaries. Sexually active women, especially those under age 25, are at higher risk for developing PID. These women are at higher risk because the cervix is not yet fully matured, increasing the risk for STIs that lead to PID. The more sex partners a woman has, the greater the risk for PID.

Complications associated with PID typically include scarring and obstruction of the fallopian tubes (which may lead to infertility), ectopic pregnancies, and chronic pelvic pain. If a woman with PID becomes pregnant, she could have an ectopic (tubal) pregnancy, which destroys the embryo and can kill the woman. More than 100,000 women in the United States become infertile as a result of PID.

Typical symptoms of PID are fever, nausea, vomiting, chills, spotting between menstrual periods, heavy bleeding during periods, and pain in the lower abdomen during sexual intercourse, between menstrual periods, or during urination. Many times, however, women do not know they have PID because these symptoms are not always present.

PID is treated with antibiotics, bed rest, and sexual abstinence. Further, surgery may be required to remove infected or scarred tissue or to repair or remove the fallopian tubes or uterus.

**Sexually transmitted infections (STIs)** Communicable diseases spread through sexual contact.

**Chlamydia** A sexually transmitted disease, caused by a bacterial infection, that can cause significant damage to the reproductive system.

**Gonorrhea** A sexually transmitted disease caused by a bacterial infection.

**Pelvic inflammatory disease (PID)** An overall designation referring to the effects of other STIs, primarily chlamydia and gonorrhea.

# Human Papillomavirus and Genital Warts

**Human papillomavirus (HPV)** is one of the most common causes of sexually transmitted infection. There are over 100 strains of HPV, and more than 30 are sexually transmitted. Most HPVs are harmless; infected people have no signs or symptoms, and the infection clears up without any form of treatment. Some strains of HPV infect the genital area, including the skin of the penis, the vulva, anus, lining of the vagina, cervix, and rectum, and can cause **genital warts.** Others are known as "high risk" types and in rare cases may lead to cancers of the cervix, vulva, vagina, anus, or penis.

Approximately 6.2 million new cases of HPV are reported each year, and at least 20 million Americans are infected.[5] At least half of sexually active people acquire genital HPV infection during their lifetime. At least 80 percent of women will acquire genital HPV infection by age 50. Most women are diagnosed with HPV through an abnormal Pap test. Infection is spread through genital or oral contact, and from the vagina to a newborn baby. Because most people have no signs or symptoms, they are unaware of the infection and can transmit the virus to a sex partner.

Genital warts show up anywhere from 1 to 8 months after exposure. These warts may be flat or raised and usually are found on the penis or around the vulva and the vagina. They also can appear in the mouth, throat, or rectum, on the cervix, or around the anus. Based on data from the CDC, as many as 1 million new cases of genital warts are diagnosed yearly in the United States. In some cities, nearly half of all sexually active teenagers have genital warts.

Health problems associated with genital warts include increased risk for cancers of the cervix, vulva, vagina, anus, or penis, and enlargement and spread of the warts, leading to obstruction of the urethra, vagina, and anus. Because babies born to infected mothers commonly develop warts over their bodies, cesarean section is recommended for childbirth.

Treatment requires completely removing all warts. This can be done by freezing them with liquid nitrogen, dissolving them with chemicals, or removing them through electrosurgery or laser surgery. Infected patients may have to be treated more than once, because genital warts can recur.

Prevention of HPV infection is best accomplished through a mutually monogamous sexual relationship with an uninfected partner. It is difficult to know, however, if a person who has been sexually active in the past is currently infected.

In 2006, the U.S. Food and Drug Administration (FDA) approved the use of the first vaccine, Gardasil, developed to prevent cervical cancer and other HPV-caused diseases in women. The Gardasil vaccine protects against four HPV types that cause 70 percent of cervical cancers and 90 percent of genital warts. The vaccine has been approved for use in girls and women between the ages of 9 and 26. To get the full benefits of the vaccine, women should get the vaccine before they become sexually active. Gardasil is most effective in women who have not been infected with any of the four HPV types covered by the vaccine. Few women, however, are infected with all four HPV types, thus vaccination will still offer protection against those viruses that have not been acquired. The vaccine has not been widely tested in women over 26. Licensing for this group of women may become available if the vaccine proves to be safe and effective for the older age group as well.

# Genital Herpes

One of the most common STIs, **genital herpes** is caused by the herpes simplex virus (HSV). There are several types of HSV that produce different ailments, including genital herpes, oral herpes, shingles, and chicken pox. The two most common forms of HSV are types 1 and 2. In type 1—the HSV most often known to cause oral herpes—cold sores or fever blisters appear on the lips and mouth. HSV 2 is better known as the virus that causes genital herpes.

Approximately 50 percent of Americans, or 135 million people over the age of 12, are infected with HSV 1. Most of these individuals acquired the virus as children. By age 50, more than 80 percent of the population has been exposed to HSV 1. Another 45 million people, or about 20 percent of the population over the age of 12, are infected with the type 2 virus.[6] One in four women, one in five men, and one in five adolescents are currently infected with genital herpes (HSV 2).

HSV is a highly contagious virus. Victims are most contagious during an outbreak, and HSV most often spreads by contact with an active lesion or sore. The infection also can be spread through virus-containing secretions from the vagina or penis. A few days following infection, a tingling sensation and lesions appear on the infected areas, most notably the mouth, genitals, and rectum, but can also surface on other parts of the body. Lesions can be somewhat painful.

Individuals infected with oral HSV 1 may shed the virus in saliva about 5 percent of the time, when they have no other symptoms of infection or visible lesions. In the

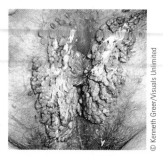

An advanced case of genital warts on the female.

first year of infection, genital HSV 2–infected individuals can shed the virus up to 10 days when they show no symptoms, but the frequency decreases over time.

In conjunction with the lesions, victims usually have mild fever, swollen glands, and headaches. The symptoms disappear within a few weeks, causing some people to believe they are cured. Presently, though, herpes is incurable and its victims remain infected.

The fundamental difference between the two main types of HSV lies in their preferred "site of residence." The HSV 1 virus typically establishes latency in a collection of nerve cells near the ear known as the trigeminal ganglion. HSV 2 usually establishes latency at the base of the spine in the sacral ganglion. The virus can remain dormant for a long time, but repeated outbreaks are common. The number of outbreaks tends to decrease over the years. New outbreaks can be precipitated by excessive fatigue, stress, cold, wind, wetness, heat, sun, sweating, rubbing/chafing/friction, lack of sleep, illness, and restrictive clothing. Diet also plays a role, as foods such as popcorn, coffee, peanuts, chocolate, and alcohol may trigger outbreaks.

Our society has typically labeled HSV 1 infection (cold sores) an "acceptable" viral infection, whereas infection with HSV 2 is viewed as a "bad" infection. The social stigma and emotional perspective of genital herpes make it difficult to objectively compare it with an oral infection, labeled as "just a cold sore" and acceptable to most people. HSV types 1 and 2, nonetheless, both cause oral and genital herpes. People who have an outbreak of oral herpes should not touch their own or someone else's genitals after touching the oral cold sores. Doing so can lead to a herpes infection of the genitals (genital HSV 1 infection). Oral sex can also result in transmission of HSV from the lips to the genitals. Thirty percent of all new cases of genital herpes result from HSV 1 infection. The opposite is true as well: Oral sex with a genital HSV 2–infected person can cause oral HSV 2 infection (although there seems to be some degree of immunity against oral HSV 2 in people already infected with oral HSV 1). People with oral or genital sores should take care not to touch them. Following hand contact with cold or herpes sores, individuals should carefully wash themselves with soap. Avoid touching the eyes as well, as this can cause vision damage.

During an outbreak, genital lesions may appear in areas that can be covered by a latex condom, but they can also appear in areas that cannot be covered. Use of a latex condom may protect against genital herpes only when the infected area is completely covered. Condoms, however, may not cover all infected areas. Thus genital herpes infections still occur. Individuals with HSV infection should abstain from sexual activity when lesions or other herpes symptoms are present. Sex partners of infected individuals should always be informed that they may become infected even if no lesions or symptoms are present. The best preventive approach is a mutually monogamous sexual relationship with an uninfected partner. Blood tests are available to determine HSV infection.

# Syphilis

Another common type of STI, also caused by bacterial infection, is **syphilis**. It is referred to as "the great imitator" because signs and symptoms are often indistinguishable from other diseases. More than 36,000 new cases are reported each year.[7] The incidence is highest in women between 20 and 24 years of age and men between 30 and 39.

Syphilis is transmitted through direct contact with a syphilis sore during vaginal, anal, or oral sex. In the primary stage, between 10 and 90 days following infection (average 21 days), a painless sore appears where the bacteria entered the body (sometimes multiple sores appear). A sore also can appear on the lips or in the mouth. This sore disappears on its own in 3 to 6 weeks. If untreated, the infection progresses to the secondary stage.

During the secondary stage, as the initial sore is healing, or several weeks thereafter, skin rashes and mucous membrane lesions appear. A rough/reddish-brown rash can be seen on the palms of the hands and the bottoms of the feet, although different types of rashes can appear on other parts of the body. Additional sores may also appear within 6 months of the initial outbreak. Signs and symptoms of the secondary stage will disappear with or without treatment. Untreated, the infection will progress into the latent stage.

A latent stage, during which the victim is not contagious, may last up to 30 years, lulling victims into thinking they are healed. During the last stage of the infection, some people develop paralysis, crippling, gradual blindness, heart disease, brain and organ damage, or dementia, or die as a direct result of the infection.

Syphilis is diagnosed by microscopic examination of material from a sore or through a simple blood test. One of the oldest known STIs, syphilis once killed its victims, but now penicillin and other antibiotics are used to treat it. A single injection of penicillin will cure individuals who have been infected for less than a year. Additional treatments are necessary for people infected longer than a year. Antibiotics are also available for individuals allergic to penicillin. People infected with syphilis must abstain from sexual activity until all syphilis sores have completely disappeared. Sexual partners must also be informed of potential infection so that they can seek treatment if necessary.

---

**Human papillomavirus (HPV)** A group of viruses that can cause sexually transmitted diseases.

**Genital warts** A sexually transmitted disease caused by a viral infection.

**Genital herpes** A sexually transmitted disease caused by a viral infection of the herpes simplex virus types I and II. The virus can attack different areas of the body but typically causes blisters on the genitals.

**Syphilis** A sexually transmitted disease caused by a bacterial infection.

**VANESSA WAS IN A FATAL CAR ACCIDENT LAST NIGHT. ONLY SHE DOESN'T KNOW IT YET.**

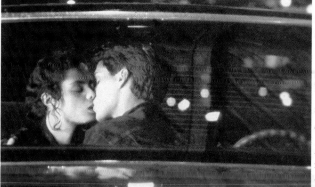

National Institute on Drug Abuse, U.S. Department of Health & Human Services

Drug and alcohol use can make people more willing to have unplanned and unprotected sex, thereby risking HIV infection.

# HIV and AIDS

Of all sexually transmitted infections, **HIV** is the most frightening because in many cases it is fatal, and it has no known cure. **AIDS** is the end stage of infection by HIV. In Lab 14A, you will have the opportunity to evaluate your basic understanding of HIV and AIDS.

HIV is a chronic infectious disease that is passed from one person to another through blood-to-blood and sexual contact. The virus spreads most commonly among individuals who engage in risky behavior such as having unprotected sex or sharing hypodermic needles. When a person becomes infected with HIV, the virus multiplies and attacks and destroys white blood cells. These cells are part of the immune system, and their function is to fight off infections and diseases in the body.

As the number of white blood cells that are killed increases, the body's immune system gradually breaks down or may be destroyed completely. Without an immune system, a person becomes susceptible to various **opportunistic infections** and to cancers.

HIV is a progressive infection. At first, people who become infected with HIV might not know they are infected. An incubation period of weeks, months, or years may pass during which no symptoms appear. The virus may live in the body 10 years or longer before symptoms emerge. HIV infection can produce neurological abnormalities, leading to depression, memory loss, slower mental and physical response time, and sluggishness in limb movements that may progress to a severe disorder known as HIV dementia.

When the infection progresses to a point at which certain diseases develop, the person is said to have AIDS. HIV itself doesn't kill. Nor do people die from AIDS. "AIDS" is the term designating the final stage of HIV infection, and death is the result of a weakened immune system that is unable to fight off opportunistic infections.

Earliest symptoms of AIDS include unexplained weight loss, constant fatigue, mild fever, swollen lymph glands, diarrhea, and sore throat. Advanced symptoms include loss of appetite, skin diseases, night sweats, and deterioration of mucous membranes.

Most of the illnesses that AIDS patients develop are harmless and rare in the general population but are fatal to AIDS victims. The two most common fatal conditions in

AIDS patients are *Pneumocystis carinii* pneumonia (a parasitic infection of the lungs) and Kaposi's sarcoma (a type of skin cancer). The AIDS virus also may attack the nervous system, causing damage to the brain and spinal cord. An unsettling finding is that brain damage is seen even in patients who are on drug therapy. The brain appears to provide a haven for HIV where drugs cannot follow, leading to a selective destruction pattern of brain regions that control motor, language, and sensory functions. This finding may explain why individuals often display slower reflexes and disruption of balance and gait in the early stages of AIDS. Patients also frequently exhibit mild vocabulary loss, judgment problems, and difficulty planning.

The only means to determine whether someone has HIV is through an HIV antibody test. Being HIV-positive does not necessarily mean that the person has AIDS. Several years can go by before the person develops the diseases that fit the case definition of AIDS.

Upon becoming infected, the immune system forms antibodies that bind to the virus. According to the CDC, most infected individuals will show these antibodies within 3 months of infection, the average being 20 days. In rare cases, they are not detectable until after 6 months or longer.

If HIV infection is suspected, a person should wait at least 3 months to be tested. If the test is negative and the person still suspects infection, the test should be repeated 3 months later. During this time, and from then on, individuals should refrain from further endangering themselves and others through risky behaviors. Some people are tested to reassure themselves that their risky behaviors are acceptable. Even if the test turns up negative for HIV, this does not represent a "license" to continue risky behaviors.

No one has to become infected with HIV. At present, once infected, a person cannot become uninfected. There is no second chance. Everyone must protect themselves against this chronic infection. If people do not—and are so

**FIGURE 14.1** Proportion of HIV/AIDS cases among adults and adolescents, by transmission category, United States (33 states), 2003–2006.

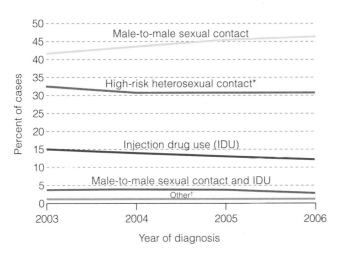

Note: Data include persons with a diagnosis of HIV infection regardless of their AIDS status at diagnosis. Data from 33 areas with confidential name-based HIV infection reporting since at least 2003. Data have been adjusted for reporting delays, and cases without risk factor information were proportionally redistributed.
*Heterosexual contact with a person known to have or be at high risk for HIV infection.
†Includes hemophilia, blood transfusion, perinatal exposure, and risk factor not reported or not identified.

**Source:** http://www.cdc.gov/hiv/topics/surveillance/resources/slides/general/index.htm (downloaded August 20, 2008).

**FIGURE 14.2** Proportion of HIV/AIDS cases among adults and adolescents, by gender and transmission category, United States (33 states), 2006.

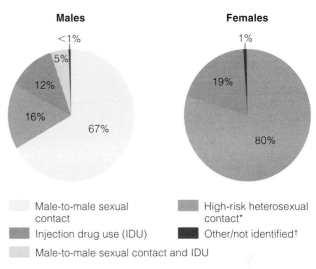

Note: Data include persons with a diagnosis of HIV infection regardless of their AIDS status at diagnosis. Data from 33 states with confidential name-based HIV infection reporting since at least 2003. Data have been adjusted for reporting delays, and cases without risk factor information were proportionally redistributed.
*Heterosexual contact with a person known to have or be at high risk for HIV infection.
†Includes hemophilia, blood transfusion, perinatal exposure, and risk factor not reported or not identified.

**Source:** Centers for Disease Control and Prevention. Adapted from http://www.cdc.gov/hiv/topics/surveillance/resources/slides/general/index.htm (downloaded August 20, 2008).

ignorant as to believe it cannot happen to them—they are putting themselves and their partners at risk.

New therapies are preventing AIDS from developing in a growing number of HIV-infected individuals. Professionals, however, disagree as to how many HIV carriers actually will develop AIDS. Even if individuals have not developed AIDS, they can pass on the virus to others, who then could easily develop AIDS.

## Transmission of HIV
HIV is transmitted by the exchange of cellular body fluids, including blood and other body fluids containing blood; semen; vaginal secretions; and maternal milk. These fluids can be exchanged:

- During sexual intercourse
- By using hypodermic needles that infected individuals have used previously
- Between a pregnant woman and her developing fetus
- By infection of a baby from the mother during childbirth
- During breastfeeding (less frequently)
- From a blood transfusion or organ transplant (rarely)

The primary modes of HIV transmission cases in the United States are presented in Figures 14.1 and 14.2. A total of 35,314 new infections were reported in 2006. Of all new infections, 50 percent were reported in men who had

sex with men, 33 percent in men and women through high-risk heterosexual sex, 13 percent by injection drug use, 3 percent in male-to-male sexual contact and injection drug use combined, and 1 percent in other unidentified categories.

The proportion of AIDS cases by race/ethnicity is given in Figure 14.3. Currently, about 49 percent of HIV infections occur in African Americans, followed by Caucasians (30 percent), and Hispanics (18 percent). Asians/Pacific Islanders and American Indians/Alaska Natives each account for 1 percent or less of diagnoses.

Today, the risk of being infected with HIV from a blood transfusion is slight. Prior to 1985, several cases of HIV infection came from blood transfusions because the blood had been donated by HIV-infected individuals. Now, all

**HIV (human immunodeficiency virus)** Virus that leads to acquired immunodeficiency syndrome (AIDS).

**AIDS (acquired immunodeficiency syndrome)** Any of a number of diseases that arise when the body's immune system is compromised by HIV; the final stage of HIV infection.

**Opportunistic infections** Infections that arise in the absence of a healthy immune system, which would fight them off in healthy people.

**FIGURE 14.3** Estimated Number of Persons Living with HIV/AIDS, by race/ethnicity, United States (33 states), 2003–2006.

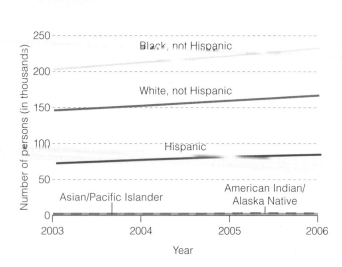

Note: Data include persons with a diagnosis of HIV infection regardless of their AIDS status at diagnosis. Data from 33 states with confidential name-based HIV infection reporting since at least 2003. Data have been adjusted for reporting delays.

*Source:* http://www.cdc.gov/hiv/topics/surveillance/resources/slides/race-ethnicity/index.htm (downloaded August 20, 2008).

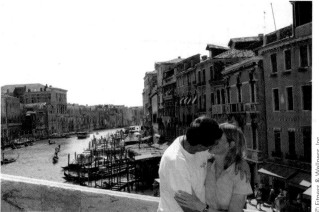

A monogamous sexual relationship almost completely removes people from risking HIV infection and the danger of developing other sexually transmitted diseases.

individuals who donate blood are first tested for HIV. To be absolutely safe, people who are planning to have surgery might consider storing their own blood in advance, so safe blood will be available if a transfusion becomes necessary.

A myth regarding HIV is that it can be transmitted by donating blood. People cannot get HIV from giving blood. Health professionals use brand-new needles every time they withdraw blood from a person. They use these needles only once and destroy them immediately after each person has donated blood.

People do not get HIV because of who they are but, rather, because of what they do. HIV and AIDS can threaten anyone, anywhere: men, women, children, teenagers, young people, older adults, Caucasians, African Americans, Hispanic Americans, Asian Americans, Native Americans, Africans, Europeans, homosexuals, heterosexuals, bisexuals, drug users. Nobody is immune to HIV. HIV can be transmitted between males, between females, from male to female, or from female to male. Although HIV and AIDS are preventable, nearly all of the people who get HIV do so because they engage in risky behaviors.

**Risky Behaviors** You cannot tell if people are infected with HIV or have AIDS by simply looking at them or taking their word. Not you, not a nurse, not even a doctor can tell without an HIV antibody test. Therefore, every time you engage in risky behavior, you run the risk of contracting HIV. The two most basic risky behaviors are:

1. *Having unprotected vaginal, anal, or oral sex with an HIV-infected person.* Unprotected sex means having sex without using a condom properly. A person should select only latex (rubber or prophylactic) condoms that state "disease prevention" on the package. Although you might have unprotected sex with an infected person and not get the virus, you can get it by having unprotected sex only once with an infected individual.

Rubbing during sexual intercourse often damages mucous membranes and causes unseen bleeding (even in the mouth). During vaginal, anal, or oral sexual contact, infected blood, semen, or vaginal fluids can penetrate the mucous membranes that line the vagina, the penis, the rectum, the mouth, or the throat. From the membrane, HIV then travels into the previously uninfected person's blood.

Health experts believe that unprotected anal sex is the riskiest type of sex. Even though bleeding is not visible in most cases, anal sex almost always causes tiny tears and bleeding in the rectum. This happens because the rectum does not stretch easily, the mucous membrane is quite thin, and small blood vessels lie directly beneath the membrane. Condoms also are more likely to break during anal intercourse because more friction is produced in a smaller cavity. All of these factors greatly enhance the risk for transmitting HIV.

Although latex condoms, if used correctly, provide for "safer" sex, they are not 100 percent foolproof. Abstaining from sex is the only 100 percent sure way to protect yourself from HIV infection and other STIs.

2. *Sharing hypodermic needles or other drug paraphernalia with someone who is infected.* Following an injection, a small amount of blood remains in the needle, and sometimes in the syringe itself. If the person who used the syringe is infected with HIV and someone else uses that same syringe to shoot up, regardless of the drug used (legal or illegal), that small amount of blood is sufficient to spread the virus. All used syringes should be destroyed and disposed of immediately.

In addition, a person must be cautious when getting acupuncture, getting a tattoo, or having the ears or other body parts pierced. If the needle had been used previously on an HIV-infected person and was not disinfected properly, the person risks getting HIV.

Otherwise-prudent people often act irrationally and engage in risky behaviors when they are under the influence of drugs. Getting high can make you willing to have sex when you really didn't plan to—thereby running the risk of contracting HIV.

Small concentrations of the virus have been found in saliva and teardrops. In principle, if both people have open cuts on the lips or in the mouth or gums, HIV could be transmitted through open-mouth kissing. Prolonged open-mouth kissing can damage the mouth or lips and allow HIV to be transmitted from an infected person to a partner through cuts or sores in the mouth. These cases, however, are rare.

### Myths About HIV Transmission

The HIV virus cannot be transmitted through perspiration. Sporting activities with no physical contact pose no risk to uninfected individuals unless blood from an open wound of an infected player comes in direct contact with the open wound of an uninfected player. The skin is an excellent line of defense against HIV. Blood from an infected person cannot penetrate the skin except through an opening in the skin. As an extra precaution, a person should use vinyl or latex gloves when performing work that requires direct contact with someone else's blood or open wound.

HIV is not transmitted through casual contact. HIV cannot be caught by spending time with, shaking hands with, or hugging an infected person; using a toilet seat, dishes, or silverware used by an HIV patient; or sharing a drink, food, a towel, or clothes with a person who has HIV.

Some people fear getting HIV from health care professionals. The chances of getting infected during physical or medical procedures are practically nil. Health care workers take extra care to protect themselves and their patients from HIV.

Another myth regarding HIV transmission is that you can get it from insects or animals. The H in HIV stands for "human." You cannot catch HIV from insects or animals. Animals do not contract HIV.

### Wise Dating

With the advent of the Internet, people now search for sex partners online. Use of the Internet to find sexual partners may further increase the risk for contracting an STI. A study reported in the *Journal of the American Medical Association* showed that those who seek sex partners over the Internet are at greater risk. These people also are more likely to have characteristics that increase their chances of transmitting STIs.[8]

Dating and getting to know other people are normal aspects of life. Dating, however, does not mean the same thing as having sex. Sexual intercourse as a part of dating can be risky, and one of the risks is AIDS. You can't tell if someone you are dating or would like to date has been exposed to HIV. The good news is that as long as you avoid

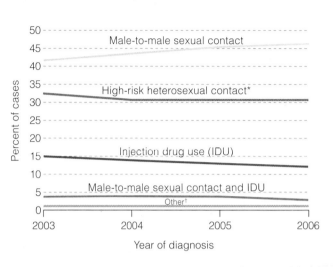

**FIGURE 14.4** Estimated number of AIDS cases, deaths, and persons living with AIDS, United States and dependent areas, 1985–2006.

Note: Data include persons with a diagnosis of HIV infection regardless of their AIDS status at diagnosis. Data from 33 areas with confidential name-based HIV infection reporting since at least 2003. Data have been adjusted for reporting delays, and cases without risk factor information were proportionally redistributed.
*Heterosexual contact with a person known to have or be at high risk for HIV infection.
†Includes hemophilia, blood transfusion, perinatal exposure, and risk factor not reported or not identified.

***Source:*** http://www.cdc.gov/hiv/topics/surveillance/resources/slides/epidemiology/index.htm (downloaded August 20, 2008).

sexual activity and don't share drug needles, you are not at risk for contracting HIV.

### Trends in HIV Infection and AIDS

As of 2007, estimates indicate that about 33 million people worldwide are infected with HIV, and more than 25 million have died from AIDS since the epidemic began in 1981. Close to 2.5 million new worldwide infections were reported in 2007. And women are becoming increasingly affected, with 15.4 million women now living with HIV.[9]

About 1.2 million people in the United States are infected with HIV. About 25 percent of them are unaware of the infection. One in every 300 Americans is infected, and about 26 percent of the newly reported cases are women.

Through the end of 2006, an estimated cumulative number of 982,498 AIDS cases were diagnosed in the United States (Figure 14.4), and an estimated 545,805 people died from the diseases caused by HIV. About 70 percent of the people who died are in the 25- to 44-year-old age group.

Although initially more than half of all AIDS cases in the United States occurred in homosexual or bisexual men, HIV infection also spreads among heterosexuals. Many heterosexuals practice unprotected sex because they don't believe it can happen to their segment of the population. HIV is an epidemic that does not discriminate by sexual orientation.

As with any other serious illness, HIV-infected people and AIDS patients deserve respect, understanding, and support. Rejection and discrimination are traits of immature, hateful, and ignorant people. Education, knowledge, and responsible behaviors are the best ways to minimize fear and discrimination.

## HIV Testing

A person can be tested for HIV in several ways. You may look up your local Public Health Department or AIDS Information Service (or related names) in the phone book. Testing results are kept confidential.

Many states also conduct anonymous testing. Your name is never recorded. You can call several toll-free hotlines or access the CDC website (www.cdc.gov/hiv) for more information on anonymous testing, treatment programs, support services, and information about HIV, AIDS, and STIs in general. All information discussed during a phone call to these hotlines is kept strictly confidential. The numbers to call are:

- National AIDS Hotline: 1-800-CDC-INFO (1-800-232-4636) in English and Spanish
- National AIDS Hotline for the hearing impaired (TTY): 1-888-232-6348
- STI Hotline: 1-800-227-8922
- Information on local testing facilities is also available online at www.hivtest.org.

In 2006, the CDC released revised recommendations for HIV testing. All patients ages 13 to 64 in health care settings should be tested, including pregnant women during the routine panel of prenatal screening tests. The recommendations further include annual screening for persons at high risk for infection. Consent for HIV testing is now included in the general consent form for medical care. Patients, however, can decline testing if they choose to do so.

## HIV Treatment

Even though several drugs are being tested to treat and slow the infection process, AIDS has no known cure. At least 40 different approaches to an AIDS vaccine are being explored. The best advice at this point is to take a preventive approach.

Antiretroviral drugs are available that delay the progress of infection, allow HIV-infected patients to live healthier and longer, and even keep some people from developing AIDS. These drugs do not cure HIV infection or AIDS. They may suppress the virus (decrease your viral load), even to undetectable levels, but they do not completely eliminate the virus. The sooner the treatment is initiated, the better is the prognosis for a longer life.

For HIV-infected individuals, viral load tests are available to detect the amount of virus present in the blood. These tests measure HIV RNA, the part of HIV that knows how to make more virus. Following drug therapy, undetectable viral load does not mean the person is cured. It means that the amount of HIV in the blood is so low that it cannot be detected. As there is no known cure, the person is still infected with HIV and can infect others. Although undetectable in the blood, the virus is still present in other body tissues and the lymph system.

Developing a vaccine to prevent HIV infection or AIDS seems highly unlikely in the near future. People should not expect a medical breakthrough. Treatment modalities, however, continue to improve and allow HIV-infected individuals and AIDS patients to live longer and more productive lives.

Several AIDS clinical trials are available in the United States. These projects are cosponsored by the CDC, the

## Behavior Modification Planning

### PROTECTING YOURSELF AND OTHERS FROM STIs

Are you sexually active? If you are not, read the following items to better educate yourself regarding intimacy. If you are sexually active, continue through all the questions below.

- Do you plan ahead before you get into a sexual situation?
- Do you know whether your partner now has or has ever had an STI? Are you comfortable asking your partner this question?
- Are you in a mutually monogamous sexual relationship and you know that your partner does not have an STI?
- Do you have multiple sexual partners? If so, do you *always* practice safe sex?
- Do you avoid alcohol and drugs in situations where you may end up having planned or unplanned sex?
- Do you abstain from sexual activity if you know or suspect that you have an STI? Do you seek medical care and advice as to when you can safely resume sexual activity?

### Try It

Taking chances during sexual contact is not worth the risk of an STI. Sex lasts a few minutes; the STI can last a lifetime, with potentially fatal consequences. Think ahead, know the facts, and don't place yourself in a situation where you may no longer be able to or have the desire to say no. Keep in mind that more than half of all Americans will acquire at least one STI in their lifetime. A few minutes of sexual pleasure can easily have consequences that you may regret for the rest of your life.

FDA, the National Institute of Allergy and Infectious Diseases, the National Library of Medicine, and the National Institutes of Health. The purpose of AIDS clinical trials is to evaluate experimental drugs and various therapies for people at all stages of HIV infection. Interested individuals can call 1-800-TRIALS-A. As with all HIV testing, calls are completely confidential. Eligibility to participate in an AIDS clinical trial varies, and all applicants are evaluated individually. By calling the telephone number given, an interested person will receive information on the purpose and location of the trials (studies) that are open, eligibility requirements and exclusion criteria, and names and telephone numbers of persons to contact.

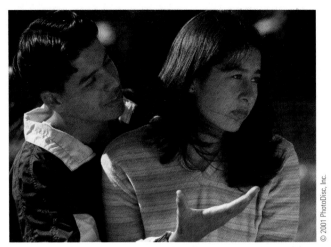

If someone does not respect your choice to wait, he or she certainly does not deserve your friendship or, for that matter, anything else.

# Guidelines for Preventing Sexually Transmitted Infections

The good news is that you can do things to prevent the spread of STIs and take precautions to keep yourself from becoming a victim. The facts are in: The best prevention technique is a mutually **monogamous** sexual relationship. This one behavior will remove you almost completely from any risk for developing an STI.

Unfortunately, in today's society, trust is elusive. You may be led to believe that you are in a safe, monogamous relationship when your partner actually (a) may cheat on you and get infected, (b) has a one-night stand with someone who is infected, (c) got the virus several years ago before the current relationship and still doesn't know about the infection, (d) may choose not to tell you about the infection, or (e) shoots up drugs and becomes infected. In any of these cases, HIV can be passed on to you.

Because your future and your life are at stake, and because you may never know if your partner is infected, you should give serious and careful consideration to postponing sex until you believe you have found an uninfected person with whom you can have a lifetime monogamous relationship. In doing so, you will not have to live with the fear of catching HIV or other STIs or deal with an unplanned pregnancy.

As strange as this may seem to some, many people postpone sexual activity until they are married. This is the best guarantee against HIV and other STIs. Young people should understand that married life will provide plenty of time for fulfilling and rewarding sex.

If you choose to delay sex, don't let peers pressure you into having sex. Some people would have you believe that you aren't a "real" man or woman if you don't have sex. Manhood and womanhood are not proven during sexual intercourse but, instead, through mature, responsible, and healthy choices.

Other people lead you to believe that love doesn't exist without sex. Sex in the early stages of a relationship is not the product of love. It is simply the fulfillment of a physical, and often selfish, drive. A loving relationship develops over a long time with mutual respect.

Then there are those who enjoy bragging about their sexual conquests and mock people who choose to wait. Many of these conquests are only fantasies expounded in an attempt to gain popularity with peers.

Teenagers are especially susceptible to peer pressure leading to premature sexual intercourse. The result? More than 750,000 teen pregnancies per year and a 31 percent pregnancy rate for all girls at least once as a teenager. Presently, the U.S. teen pregnancy rate is one of the highest of the industrialized nations. Too many young people wish they had postponed sex and silently admire those who do. Sex lasts only a few minutes. The consequences of irresponsible sex may last a lifetime. And in some cases, they are fatal!

Sexual promiscuity never leads to a trusting, loving, and lasting relationship. Mature people respect others' choices. If someone doesn't respect your choice to wait, he or she certainly doesn't deserve your friendship or, for that matter, anything else.

There is no greater sex than that between two loving and responsible individuals who mutually trust, admire, and love each other. Contrary to many beliefs, these relationships are possible. They are built upon unselfish attitudes and behaviors.

As you look around, you will find that many people hold these values. Seek them out and build your friendships and future around people who respect you for who you are and what you believe. You don't have to compromise your choices or values. In the end, you will reap the greater rewards of a lasting relationship free of HIV and other STIs.

**Monogamous** Describes a sexual relationship in which two people have sexual relations with only each other.

Also, be prepared so you will know your course of action before you get into an intimate situation. Look for common interests and work together toward them. Express your feelings openly: "I'm not ready for sex; I just want to have fun, and kissing is fine with me." If your friend doesn't accept your answer and isn't willing to stop the advances, be prepared with a strong response. Statements like, "Please stop" or "Don't!" are for the most part ineffective. Use a firm statement such as, "No, I'm not willing to have sex" or "I've already thought about this and I'm not going to have sex." If this still doesn't work, label the behavior as rape and say, "This is rape, and I'm going to call the police."

## Critical Thinking

Discuss how the information presented in this chapter has affected your feelings and perceptions about sex. What impact will this information have on your wellness lifestyle?

## Reducing the Risk for STIs and HIV Infection

Based upon recommendations from health experts, observing the following precautions can reduce your risk for STIs, including HIV infection and, subsequently, AIDS:

1. Postpone sex until you and your uninfected partner are prepared to enter into a lifetime monogamous relationship.

2. Unless you are in a monogamous relationship and you know your partner isn't infected (which you may never know for sure), practice safer sex every time you have sex and don't have sexual contact with anyone who doesn't practice safe sex. This means you should use a latex condom from start to finish for each sexual act. If your partner refuses to use a condom, say no to sex with that person.

3. Use "barrier" methods of contraception to help prevent the infection from spreading. Condoms, diaphragms, and spermicidal suppositories, foams, and jellies can all deter the spread of certain STIs. Spermicidal agents may act as a disinfectant as well. Young people are especially susceptible. Traditionally, teenagers have not used birth-control methods at all and therefore remain at high risk for STIs and unwanted pregnancies. At this time, take a few minutes and list at least three ways you might bring up the subject of condoms with your partner. Also, think of ways you might convince a person to use a condom. If your partner refuses to use a condom, your answer should be quite simple: "No condom, no sex."

4. Know your partner and limit your sexual relationships. The days are gone when safe sex resulted from anonymous encounters at a bathhouse or a singles bar. Having only one partner lowers your chances of becoming infected. Although you can still become infected by having unprotected sex with one person only, the more partners you have, the greater are your chances for infection.

5. Don't have sex with prostitutes.

6. Determine the conditions under which you will allow sex. Ask yourself: "Am I willing to have sex with this person?" If you decide to have sex, practice safer sex. There is no reason to accept anything else. You will feel better about yourself.

7. Plan before you get into a sexual situation. Discuss STIs with the person you are contemplating having sex with before you do so. Even though talking about STIs might be awkward, the short-lived embarrassment of addressing intimate questions can keep you from contracting or spreading infection. If you don't know the person well enough to address this issue or you are uncertain about the answers, don't have sex with this individual.

8. Negotiate safer sex. Focus on the problem and not the person. Describe your feelings about the problem, using "I" instead of "you." For example, you might say, "I'm feeling awkward and uncomfortable. The only way I can feel comfortable is by using a condom." You also can offer options and provide alternative solutions. You might indicate to your partner, "We can work this out together. Let's go for a drive and get a condom. We'll feel better about what we're doing."

9. If you are sexually promiscuous, have periodic physical checkups. You can easily get exposed to an STI from a person who does not have any symptoms and who is unaware of the infection. Sexually promiscuous men and women between ages 15 and 35 are a particularly high-risk group for developing STIs.

10. Avoid sexual contact with anyone who has had sex with one or more individuals at risk for getting HIV, even if they are now practicing safer sex.

11. If you do have sex with someone who might be infected with HIV or whose history is unknown to you, avoid exchanging body fluids.

12. Don't share toothbrushes, razors, or other implements that could become contaminated with blood with anyone who is, or who might be, infected with HIV.

13. If you suspect that your partner is infected with an STI, ask. He or she may not even be aware of the infection, so look for signs, such as sores, redness, inflammation, a rash, growths, warts, or a discharge. If you are unsure, abstain.

14. If you know you have an infection, be responsible enough to abstain from sexual activity. Go to a physician or a clinic for treatment and ask your doctor when

you can safely resume sexual activity. Abstain until it is safe. Just as you want to be protected in a sexual relationship, you should want to protect your partner as well. If you are diagnosed with an STI and you believe you know the person who gave it to you, think of ways you might bring up the subject of STIs with this person. You need to take responsibility and discuss this matter with your partner. As a result of your conversation, medical treatment can be initiated and other people can be protected from infection as well.

15. Wear loose-fitting clothes made from natural fibers. Tight-fitting clothing made from synthetic fibers (especially underwear and nylon pantyhose) can create conditions that encourage the growth of bacteria and can actually aggravate STIs.

16. Consider abstaining from sexual relations if you have any kind of an illness or disease, even a common cold. Any kind of illness makes you more susceptible to other illnesses, and lower immunity can make you more vulnerable to STIs. The same holds true for times when you are under extreme stress, when you are fatigued, and when you are overworked. Drugs and alcohol also can lower your resistance to infection.

17. Thoroughly wash immediately after sexual activity. Although washing with hot, soapy water will not guarantee safety against STIs, it can prevent you from spreading certain germs on your fingers and might wash away bacteria and viruses that have not entered the body yet.

18. Be cautious regarding procedures (such as acupuncture, tattooing, and ear piercing) in which needles or other nonsterile instruments may be used again and again to pierce the skin or mucous membranes. These procedures are safe if proper sterilization methods are followed or disposable needles are used. Before undergoing the procedure, ask what precautions are being taken.

19. If you are planning to undergo artificial insemination, insist that frozen sperm be obtained from a laboratory that tests all donors for infection with HIV. Donors should be tested twice before the lab accepts the sperm—once at the time of donation and again a few months later.

20. If you know you will be having surgery in the near future, and if you are able, consider donating blood for your own use. This will eliminate completely the already small risk of contracting HIV through a blood transfusion. It also will eliminate the more substantial risk for contracting other bloodborne diseases, such as hepatitis, from a transfusion.

Avoiding risky behaviors that destroy quality of life and life itself is crucial to a healthy lifestyle. Learning the facts and acting upon your personal values so you can make responsible choices can protect you and those around you from painful, embarrassing, startling, unexpected, or fatal conditions.

# ASSESS YOUR BEHAVIOR

 Log on to http://www.cengage.com/sso/ to take the Wellness Profile assessment and gauge your level of risk in the area of sexual behavior.

1. Do you believe that a mutually monogamous sexual relationship is the best way to prevent STIs? If not, do you always take precautions to practice safer sex?

2. If you are not prepared to have a sexual relationship, are you prepared to say so? Have you prepared exactly what to say if you are asked to have sex?

3. Have you carefully considered the consequences of engaging in a sexual relationship, including the risk for STIs, HIV infection, your partner being untruthful about his/her sexual history and STIs, and the potential for an unplanned pregnancy?

4. Are you capable of discussing your and your partner's sexual history prior to engaging in a sexual relationship?

5. If you have an STI or a history of STIs, are you sufficiently responsible to have an open and honest discussion with a potential partner about the risk for infection and consequences thereof?

# ASSESS YOUR KNOWLEDGE

Log on to http://www.cengage.com/sso/ to assess your understanding of this chapter's topics by taking the Student Practice Test and exploring the modules recommended in your Personalized Study Plan.

1. What percentage of Americans will develop at least one STI in their lifetime?
   a. 30 percent
   b. 17 percent
   c. 25 percent
   d. 15 percent
   e. 20 percent

2. Which of the following sexually transmitted infections is *not* caused by a bacterial infection?
   a. Chlamydia
   b. Genital warts
   c. Syphilis
   d. Gonorrhea
   e. All of the above are caused by bacterial infections.

3. Chlamydia
   a. can cause damage to the reproductive system that cannot be reversed by treatment, even if successful.
   b. can cause infertility.
   c. may occur without symptoms.
   d. may cause arthritis.
   e. All of the choices are correct.

4. Gonorrhea can cause
   a. widespread bacterial infection.
   b. infertility.
   c. heart damage.
   d. arthritis.
   e. all of the above.

5. Treatment of genital warts is done by
   a. dissolving the warts with chemicals.
   b. electrosurgery.
   c. freezing the warts with liquid nitrogen.
   d. All of the above choices apply.
   e. None of the above choices is correct.

6. Herpes
   a. is incurable.
   b. causes sores that are treated with electrosurgery.

   c. requires antibiotics for successful treatment and cure.
   d. is caused by a bacterial infection.
   e. is not a serious STI because the person becomes uninfected once the sores heal.

7. Cold sores
   a. can cause genital herpes.
   b. are not highly contagious.
   c. are treatable if caused by bacterial infection.
   d. All of the above choices are correct.
   e. None of the above choices is correct.

8. The only way to determine whether someone is infected with HIV is through
   a. an AIDS outbreak.
   b. a physical exam by a physician.
   c. a bacterial culture test.
   d. an HIV antibody test.
   e. All of the choices are correct.

9. HIV
   a. attacks and destroys white blood cells.
   b. readily multiplies in the human body.
   c. breaks down the immune system.
   d. increases the likelihood of developing opportunistic infections and cancers.
   e. All of the above are correct.

10. The best way to protect yourself against STIs is
   a. through the use of condoms for all sexual acts.
   b. by knowing about the people who have previously had sex with your partner.
   c. through a mutually monogamous sexual relationship.
   d. by having sex only with an individual who has no symptoms of STIs.
   e. All of the above choices provide equal protection against STIs.

Correct answers can be found at the back of the book.

# MEDIA MENU

You can find the links below at the book companion site: www.cengage.com/health/hoeger/plfw10e

- Take a self-assessment to see how healthy you are in the area of sexual behavior.
- Check how well you understand the chapter's concepts.

## Internet Connections

- Sexuality Information from Columbia University Health Education Department "Go Ask Alice." This site presents a series of frank questions and answers about sex, organized into several categorics, including sexual intercourse, abstinence, and kissing. *http://www .goaskalice.columbia.edu*
- The Body: Safer Sex and Prevention. This site features information for consumers, gay men, and health care professionals on a variety of prevention issues, including safer sex and general prevention measures, con-

doms, sexual communication skills, sexual and nonsexual prevention, effective educational programs, treatment, and research. *http://www.thebody.com/ safesex.html*

- American Social Health Association (ASHA). This site features information on a variety of sexually transmitted infections, a comprehensive section of frequently asked questions, and information about STI hotlines. It also features a link to iwannaknow.org, the ASHA STI prevention Web site for teens. *http://www.ashastd .org*
- CDC National Center for HIV, STI, and TB Prevention. This comprehensive site features a variety of links to information regarding HIV/AIDS prevention, including the latest statistics. *http://www.cdc.gov/hiv/dhap .htm*

# NOTES

1. Centers for Disease Control and Prevention, "Sexually Transmitted Diseases," http://www.cdc.gov/std/default .htm (downloaded July 23, 2008).

2. See note 1.

3. See note 1.

4. See note 1.

5. See note 1.

6. See note 1.

7. See note 1.

8. M. McFarlane, S. S. Bull, and C. A. Rietmeijer, "The Internet as a Newly Emerging Risk Environment for Sexually Transmitted Diseases," *Journal of the American Medical Association* 284 (2000): 443–446.

9. Avert International AIDS Charity, "Worldwide HIV & AIDS Statistics," http://www.avert.org/worldstats.htm (downloaded July 23, 2008).

# SUGGESTED READINGS

Blona, R., and J. Levitan. *Healthy Sexuality.* Belmont, CA: Wadsworth/Thomson Learning, 2006.

Centers for Disease Control and Prevention. "Sexually Transmitted Diseases Guidelines 2006." *Morbidity and Mortality Weekly Report* 55 (August 4, 2006) No. RR-11.

Hoeger, W. W. K., L. W. Turner, and B. Q. Hafen. *Wellness: Guidelines for a Healthy Lifestyle.* Belmont, CA: Wadsworth/ Thomson Learning, 2007.

# LAB 14A: Self-Quiz on HIV and AIDS

Name _____  Date _____  Grade _____

Instructor _____  Course _____  Section _____

**Necessary Lab Equipment**
None required.

**Objective**
To evaluate basic understanding of HIV and AIDS.

**Instruction**
Please answer all of the following questions.

Indicate whether the following statements are true or false, then turn the page to see how well you understand HIV and AIDS.

|  | True | False |
|---|---|---|
| 1. AIDS—acquired immunodeficiency syndrome—is the end stage of infection caused by the human immunodeficiency virus, HIV. | ☐ | ☐ |
| 2. HIV is a chronic infectious disease that spreads among individuals who choose to engage in risky behavior such as unprotected sex or the sharing of hypodermic needles. | ☐ | ☐ |
| 3. AIDS is curable. | ☐ | ☐ |
| 4. Abstaining from sex is the only 100 percent sure way to protect yourself from HIV infection. | ☐ | ☐ |
| 5. A person infected with HIV can look and feel healthy. | ☐ | ☐ |
| 6. Condoms are 100 percent effective in protecting you against HIV infection. | ☐ | ☐ |
| 7. Using drugs and alcohol makes a person less likely to use a condom and use it correctly. | ☐ | ☐ |
| 8. If you're sexually active, latex condoms provide the best protection against HIV infection. | ☐ | ☐ |
| 9. Using drugs and alcohol can make you more likely to have unplanned and unprotected sex. | ☐ | ☐ |
| 10. A pregnant woman who has HIV can transmit the virus to her baby during childbirth. | ☐ | ☐ |
| 11. You can become HIV-infected by donating blood. | ☐ | ☐ |
| 12. HIV can be transmitted by spending time with or through casual contact (shaking hands, hugging) with an infected person. | ☐ | ☐ |
| 13. The only means to determine whether someone has HIV is through an HIV antibody test. | ☐ | ☐ |
| 14. HIV can completely destroy the immune system. | ☐ | ☐ |
| 15. The HIV virus may live in the body 10 years or longer before AIDS symptoms develop. | ☐ | ☐ |
| 16. People infected with HIV have AIDS. | ☐ | ☐ |
| 17. Once infected with HIV, a person never becomes uninfected. | ☐ | ☐ |
| 18. HIV infection is preventable. | ☐ | ☐ |
| 19. Drugs are now available that can lengthen the life of an HIV-infected person. | ☐ | ☐ |
| 20. Early treatment can reduce the symptoms of HIV-infected people. | ☐ | ☐ |

*(continued)*

Selected items on this questionnaire are adapted from *Test Your Survival Smarts: Self-Quiz on Drugs and AIDS,* National Institute on Drug Abuse, U. S. Department of Health & Human Services.

Answers:

1. True. AIDS is the term used to define the manifestation of opportunistic diseases and cancers that occur as a result of HIV infection (also referred to as "HIV disease").

2. True. People do not get HIV because of who they are, but because of what they do. Almost all of the people who get HIV do so because they choose to engage in risky behaviors.

3. False. There is no cure for AIDS, and none seems forthcoming.

4. True. Abstinence will protect you from HIV infection. But you may still get the disease by sharing hypodermic needles.

5. True. The symptoms of HIV are often not noticeable until several years after a person has been infected. That's why—no matter who your partner is—it is important to always protect yourself against HIV and the risk of developing AIDS, either by abstaining from sex or by *always* practicing safe sex.

6. False. Only abstaining from sex gives you 100 percent protection, but condoms, if used correctly, are effective in protecting against HIV infection.

7. True. Teens who are drunk or high are less likely to use condoms because, under the influence, they forget or believe that nothing "bad" can happen.

8. True. Proper use, however, is necessary to minimize the risk of infection.

9. True. Otherwise-prudent people often act irrationally and engage in risky behaviors when they are under the influence of drugs and alcohol.

10. True. HIV transmission can occur between a pregnant woman and her baby during childbirth. A baby can also be infected through breastfeeding, although this occurs less frequently.

11. False. A myth regarding HIV is that it can be transmitted by donating blood. People cannot get HIV from giving blood. A brand-new needle is used by health professionals every time they draw blood. These needles are used only once and are destroyed and thrown away immediately after each individual has donated blood.

12. False. HIV is transmitted by the exchange of cellular body fluids, including blood and other body fluids containing blood, semen, vaginal secretions, and maternal milk. These fluids are most often exchanged during sexual intercourse, by using hypodermic needles previously used by infected individuuals, or by contact with open wounds, cuts, or sores.

13. True. Not you, not a nurse, not even a doctor, can tell without an HIV antibody test. Upon HIV infection, the immune system's line of defense against the virus is the formation of antibodies that bind to the virus. On the average it takes 3 months for the body to manufacture enough antibodies to show positive in an HIV antibody test. Sometimes it takes 6 months or longer.

14. True. The virus multiplies, then attacks and destroys white blood cells. These cells are part of the immune system, and their function is to fight off infections and diseases in the body. As the number of white blood cells killed increases, the body's immune system gradually breaks down or may be completely destroyed.

15. True. Ten years or longer may go by before the person develops AIDS.

16. False. Being HIV-positive does not necessarily mean that the person has AIDS. It may be 10 years or longer following infection before the individual develops the symptoms that fit the case definition of AIDS. From that point on, the person may live another 2 to 3 years. In essence, from the point of infection, the individual may endure a chronic disease for about 12 or more years.

17. True. There is no second chance. Everyone must protect himself or herself against HIV infection.

18. True. The best prevention technique is abstaining from sex until the time comes for a mutually monogamous sexual relationship (two people having a sexual relationship only with each other). That one behavior will almost completely remove you from any risk of HIV infection or developing any other sexually transmitted disease.

19. True. Available antiretroviral drugs can delay the progress of infection, allow HIV-infected individuals to live healthier and longer lives, and even keep some people from developing AIDS. However, these drugs do not cure HIV infection or AIDS.

20. True. The sooner treatment is initiated, the better the prognosis is for a longer life.

# Lifetime Fitness and Wellness

**15**

## Objectives

- Understand the effects of a healthy lifestyle on longevity
- Learn to differentiate between physiologic and chronological age
- Estimate your life expectancy and determine your real physiologic age
- Learn about complementary and alternative medicine practices
- Learn guidelines for preventing consumer fraud
- Understand factors to consider when selecting a health/fitness club
- Know how to select appropriate exercise equipment
- Review health/fitness accomplishments and chart a wellness program for the future
- Discover how you've changed and plan for a healthy future.

Check your understanding of the chapter contents by logging on to CengageNOW and accessing the pre-test, personalized learning plan, and post-test for this chapter.

# FAQ

### How does regular physical activity affect chronological versus physiologic age?

Chronological age is your actual age—that is, how old you are. Physiologic age is used in reference to your functional capacity to perform physical work at any stage of your life. Data on individuals who have taken part in systematic physical activity throughout life indicate that these people maintain a higher level of functional capacity and do not experience the declines typical in later years. From a functional point of view, typical sedentary people in the United States are about 25 years older than their chronological age indicates. Thus, an active 60-year-old person can have a physical capacity similar to that of an inactive 35-year-old person. Similarly, a sedentary 20-year-old college student most likely has the physical capacity of a 45-year-old active individual

### What is the difference between conventional medicine, complementary and alternative medicine, and integrative medicine?

Conventional medicine implies the practice of traditional medicine by medical doctors, osteopaths, and allied health professionals such as registered nurses, physical therapists, and psychologists.

Complementary and alternative medicine is a group of diverse medical and health care systems, practices, and products that are not presently considered to be part of conventional medicine. The safety and effectiveness of many of these practices have not been rigorously tested through well-designed scientific studies. Integrative medicine uses a combination of conventional medicine and complementary and alternative medicine treatments for which there is some scientific evidence of safety and effectiveness.

### What is the greatest benefit of a lifetime wellness lifestyle?

There are many benefits derived from an active wellness lifestyle, including greater functional capacity, good health, less sickness, lower health care expenses and time under medical supervision, and a longer and more productive life. Without question, these benefits altogether translate into one great benefit: an optimum quality of life. That is, the freedom to live life to its fullest without functional and health limitations. Most people go through life wishing that they could live without these limitations. The power, nevertheless, is within each of us to do so. And it is accomplished only by taking action today and living a wellness way of life for the rest of our lives.

Better health, higher quality of life, and longevity are the three most important benefits derived from a lifetime fitness and wellness program. You have learned that physical fitness in itself does not always lower the risk for chronic diseases and ensure better health. Thus implementation of healthy behaviors is the only way to attain your highest potential for well-being. The real challenge will come now that you are about to finish this course: maintaining your own lifetime commitment to fitness and wellness. Adhering to a program in a structured setting is a lot easier, but from now on, you will be on your own.

In this chapter you will have an opportunity to evaluate how well you are adhering to health-promoting behaviors and how these behaviors will affect your **physiologic age** and length of life. You will also learn how to chart a personal wellness program for the future.

Research data indicate that healthy (and unhealthy) lifestyle actions you take today will have an impact on health and quality of life in middle and advanced age. Whereas most young people don't seem to worry much about health and longevity, you may want to take a closer look at the quality of life of your parents or other middle-aged and older friends and relatives that you know. Though you may have a difficult time envisioning yourself at that age, their health status and **functional capacity** may help you determine how you would like to live when you reach your fourth, fifth, and subsequent decades of life.

Although previous research has documented declines in physiologic function and motor capacity as a result of aging, no hard evidence at present proves that large declines in physical work capacity are related primarily to aging alone. Lack of physical activity—a common phe-

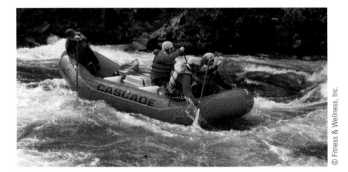

Good physical fitness provides freedom to enjoy many of life's recreational and leisure activities without limitations.

© Fitness & Wellness, Inc.

**FIGURE 15.1** Relationships between physical work capacity, aging, and lifestyle habits.

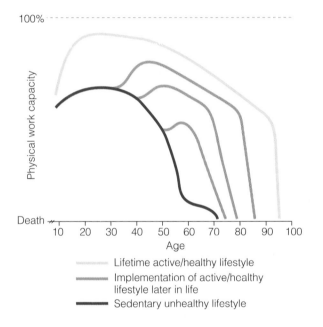

# Life Expectancy and Physiologic Age

Aging is a natural process, but some people seem to age better than others. Most likely you know someone who looks much younger than his or her **chronological age** indicates—and vice versa: someone who appears much older than his or her chronological age indicates. For example, you may have an instructor who you would have guessed was about 40, but in reality is 52 years old. On the other hand, you may have a relative who looks 60 but is actually 50 years old. Why the differences?

During the aging process, natural biological changes occur within the body. Although no one measurement can predict how long you will live, the rate at which aging changes take place depends on a combination of genetic and lifestyle factors. Your lifestyle habits will determine to a great extent how your genes will affect your aging process. Hundreds of research studies now point to critical lifestyle behaviors that will determine your statistical chances of dying at a younger age or living a longer life. Research also shows that lifestyle behaviors have a far greater impact on health and longevity than do your genes alone.

## Critical Thinking

How long would you like to live, and are you concerned about how you will live the rest of your life?

nomenon in our society as people age—is accompanied by decreases in physical work capacity that are greater by far than the effects of aging itself.

Unhealthy behaviors precipitate premature aging. For sedentary people, any type of physical activity is seriously impaired by age 40, and productive life ends before age 60. Most of these people hope to live to be age 65 or 70 and often must cope with serious physical ailments. These people "stop living at age 60 but are buried at age 70" (see the theoretical model in Figure 15.1).

Scientists believe that a healthy lifestyle allows people to live a vibrant life—a physically, intellectually, emotionally, socially active, and functionally independent existence—to age 95. Such are the rewards of a wellness way of life. When death comes to active people, it usually is rather quick and not as a result of prolonged illness. In Figure 15.1, note the low, longer slope of the "unhealthy lifestyle" before death.

Throughout this book, you have studied many of these factors. The question that you now need to ask yourself is: Are your lifestyle habits accelerating or decelerating the rate at which your body is aging? To help you determine how long and how well you may live the rest of your life, the **Life Expectancy** and Physiologic Age Prediction questionnaire is provided in Lab 15A. By looking at 46 critical genetic and lifestyle factors, you will be able to

**Physiologic age** The biological and functional capacity of the body as it should be in relation to the person's maximal potential at any given age in the lifespan.

**Functional capacity** The ability to perform the ordinary and unusual demands of daily living without limitations and excessive fatigue or injury.

**Chronological age** Calendar age.

**Life expectancy** How many years a person is expected to live.

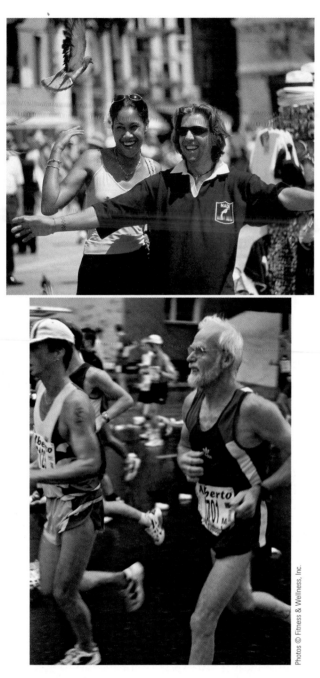

Photos © Fitness & Wellness, Inc.

A healthy lifestyle enhances functional capacity, quality of life, and longevity.

estimate your life expectancy and your real physiologic age. Of greater importance, most of these factors are under your own control, and you can do something to make them work *for* you instead of against you.

As you fill out the questionnaire, you must be completely honest with yourself. Your life expectancy and physiologic age prediction are based on your present lifestyle habits, should you continue those habits for life. Using the questionnaire, you will review factors you can modify or implement in daily living that may add years and health to your life. Please note that the questionnaire is not a precise scientific instrument, but rather an estimated life expectancy analysis according to the impact of

lifestyle factors on health and longevity. Also, the questionnaire is not intended as a substitute for advice and tests conducted by medical and health care practitioners.

# Complementary and Alternative Medicine (CAM)

**Conventional Western medicine**, also known as allopathic medicine, has seen major advances in care and treatment modalities during the last few decades. Conventional medicine is based on scientifically proven methods, wherein medical treatments are tested through rigorous scientific trials. In addition to a **primary care physician** (medical doctor), people seek advice from other practitioners of conventional medicine, including **osteopaths, dentists, oral surgeons, orthodontists, ophthalmologists, optometrists, physician assistants,** and **nurses**.

Notwithstanding modern technological and scientific advancements, many medical treatments either do not improve the patient's condition or create other ailments themselves. Only about 20 percent of conventional treatments have been proven to be clinically effective in scientific trials.[1] Thus, millions of consumers are turning to **complementary and alternative medicine**, or **CAM** (also called "unconventional," "nonallopathic," or "integrative" medicine), in search of answers to their health problems. Unconventional medicine is referred to as complementary or alternative because patients use it to either augment their regular medical care or replace conventional practices, respectively.

The reasons for seeking complementary and alternative treatments are diverse, including lack of progress in curing illnesses and disease, frustration and dissatisfaction with physicians, lack of personal attention, testimonials about the effectiveness of alternative treatments, and rising health care costs.

According to the Centers for Disease Control and Prevention, approximately 40 percent of American adults aged 18 and over use some form of CAM services on a yearly basis. This figure increases to about 60 percent when prayer is specifically included for health reasons.[2] People who use CAM tend to be more educated and believe that body, mind, and spirit all contribute to good health.

The National Center for Complementary and Alternative Medicine (NCCAM) was established under the National Institutes of Health to examine methods of healing that have previously been unexplored by science. CAM includes treatments and health care practices not widely taught in medical schools, not generally used in hospitals, and not usually reimbursed by medical insurance companies. Many physicians now endorse complementary and alternative treatments, and an ever-increasing number of medical schools are offering courses in this area.

**FIGURE 15.2** The five domains of complementary and alternative medicine.

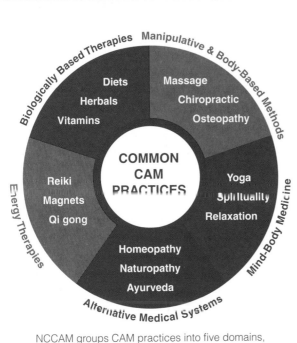

NCCAM groups CAM practices into five domains, recognizing that there can be some overlap among them. Examples of CAM practices within each domain are given above.

*Source:* http://nccam.nih.gov/news/camssurvey_fs1.htm, downloaded August 9, 2004.

The NCCAM classifies CAM therapies into five categories, or domains (see Figure 15.2):[3]

1. *Alternative medical systems.* Alternative medical systems are built upon complete systems of theory and practice. Often, these systems have evolved apart from and earlier than the conventional medical approach used in the United States. Examples of alternative medical systems that have developed in Western cultures include homeopathic medicine and naturopathic medicine. Examples of systems that have developed in non-Western cultures include traditional Chinese medicine and ayurveda.

2. *Mind/body interventions.* Mind/body medicine uses a variety of techniques designed to enhance the mind's capacity to affect bodily function and symptoms. Some techniques that were considered CAM in the past have become mainstream (for example, patient support groups and cognitive-behavioral therapy). Other mind/body techniques are still considered CAM, including meditation, prayer, mental healing, and therapies that use creative outlets such as art, music, and dance.

3. *Biologically based therapies.* Biologically based therapies in CAM use substances found in nature, such as herbs, foods, and vitamins. Some examples include dietary supplements, herbal products, and so-called natural but as yet scientifically unproven therapies (for example, using shark cartilage to treat cancer).

4. *Manipulative and body-based methods.* Manipulative and body-based methods in CAM involve manipulation and/or movement of one or more parts of the body. Some examples include chiropractic or osteopathic manipulation and massage.

5. *Energy therapies.* Energy therapies involve the use of energy fields. They are of two types:
   a. Biofield therapies are intended to affect energy fields that purportedly surround and penetrate the human body. The existence of such fields has not yet been scientifically proven. Some forms of energy therapy manipulate biofields by applying pressure and/or manipulating the body by placing the hands in, or through, these fields. Examples include qi gong, reiki, and therapeutic touch.
   b. Bioelectromagnetic-based therapies involve the unconventional use of electromagnetic fields, such as pulsed fields, magnetic fields, or alternating-current or direct-current fields.

Alternative medicine practices have not gone through the same standard scrutiny as conventional medicine. Nonallopathic treatments are often based on theories that have not been scientifically proven. This does not imply that unconventional medicine practices do not help people.

**Conventional Western medicine** Traditional medical practice based on methods that are tested through rigorous scientific trials; also called allopathic medicine.

**Primary care physician** A medical practitioner who provides routine treatment of ailments; typically, the patient's first contact for health care.

**Osteopath** A medical practitioner with specialized training in musculoskeletal problems who uses diagnostic and therapeutic methods of conventional medicine in addition to manipulative measures.

**Dentist** Practitioner who specializes in diseases of the teeth, gums, and oral cavity.

**Oral surgeon** A dentist who specializes in surgical procedures of the oral-facial complex.

**Orthodontist** A dentist who specializes in the correction and prevention of teeth irregularities.

**Ophthalmologist** Medical specialist concerned with diseases of the eye and prescription of corrective lenses.

**Optometrist** Health care practitioner who specializes in the prescription and adaptation of lenses.

**Physician assistant** Health-care practitioner trained to treat most standard cases of care.

**Nurse** Health-care practitioner who assists in the diagnosis and treatment of health problems and provides many services to patients in a variety of settings.

**Complementary and alternative medicine (CAM)** A group of diverse medical and health care systems, practices, and products that are not presently considered to be part of conventional medicine; also called unconventional, nonallopathic, or integrative medicine.

Many people have found relief from ailments or been cured through unconventional treatments. In due time, however, these theories will need to be investigated using scientific trials similar to those in conventional medicine.

CAM includes a wide range of healing philosophies, approaches, and therapies. The practices most often associated with nonallopathic medicine are **acupuncture, chiropractics, herbal medicine, homeopathy, naturopathic medicine, ayurveda, magnetic therapy,** and **massage therapy**. Each of these practices offers a different approach to treatments based on its beliefs about the body, some of which are hundreds or thousands of years old.

Many of these practitioners believe that their treatment modality aids the body as it performs its own natural healing process. Because of their approach, alternative treatments usually take longer than conventional allopathic medical care. Nonallopathic treatments are usually less harsh on the patient, and practitioners tend to avoid surgery and extensive use of medications.

Unconventional therapies are frequently viewed as "holistic," implying that the practitioner looks at all the dimensions of wellness when evaluating a person's condition. Practitioners often persuade patients to adopt healthier lifestyle habits that not only help to improve current conditions but also prevent other ailments.

CAM also allows patients to better understand treatments, and patients are often allowed to administer self-treatment.

Costs for CAM practices are typically lower than conventional medicine costs. With the exception of acupuncture and chiropractic care, most nonallopathic treatments are not covered by health insurance. Typically, patients pay directly for these services. Conservative estimates indicate that $21.2 billion a year is spent on alternative medical treatments, with at least $12.2 billion paid out-of-pocket.[4] These costs exceed the out-of-pocket expenses for all hospitalizations in the United States. If you are considering alternative medical therapies, consult with your health care insurance provider to determine which therapies are reimbursable.

CAM does have shortcomings, among them:

1. Many of the practitioners do not have the years of education given to conventional medical personnel and often know less about physiologic responses that occur in the body.

2. Some practices are completely devoid of science; hence, the practitioner can rarely explain the specific physiologic benefits of the treatment used. Much of the knowledge is based on experiences with previous patients.

3. The practice of CAM is not regulated like that of conventional medicine. The training and certification of practitioners, malpractice liability, and evaluation of tests and methods used in treatments are not routinely standardized. Many states, however, license practitioners in the areas of chiropractic services, acupuncture, naturopathy, homeopathy, herbal therapy, and massage therapy. Other therapies, however, are unmonitored.

4. Unconventional medicine lacks regulation of natural and herbal products. The word "natural" does not imply that the product is safe. Many products, including some herbs, can be toxic in large doses.

5. An estimated 15 million Americans (about one-fifth of all prescription users) combine high-dose vitamins and/or herbal supplements with prescription drugs.[5] Combinations such as these can yield undesirable side effects. Therefore, individuals should always let their health care practitioners know which medications and alternative (including vitamin and mineral) supplements are being taken in combination.

Herbal medicine has been around for centuries. Through trial and error, by design, or by accident, people have found that certain plant substances have medicinal properties. Today many of these plant substances have been replaced by products that are safer and more effective and have fewer negative side effects. Although science has found the mechanisms whereby some herbs work, much work remains to be done.

Many herbs or herbal remedies are not safe for human use and continue to meet resistance from the scientific community. One of the main concerns is that active ingredients in drug therapy must be administered in accurate dosages. With herbal medicine, the potency cannot always be adequately controlled.

Also, some herbs produce undesirable side effects. For example, ephedra (ma huang), a popular weight loss and energy supplement, can cause high blood pressure, rapid heart rate, tremor, seizures, headaches, insomnia, stroke, and even death. About 1,400 reports of adverse effects linked to herbal products containing ephedra, including 81 ephedra-related deaths, prompted its removal from the marketplace. St. John's wort, commonly taken as an antidepressant, can produce serious interactions with drugs used to treat heart disease. Ginkgo biloba impairs blood clotting, thus it can cause bleeding in people already on regular blood-thinning medication or aspirin therapy. Other herbs like yohimbe, chaparral, comfrey, and jin bu juan have been linked to adverse events.

Conventional health care providers are becoming more willing to refer you to someone who is familiar with alternative treatments, but you need to be an informed consumer. Ask your primary care physician to obtain valid information regarding the safety and effectiveness of a particular treatment. At times, nonetheless, the medical community resists and rejects unconventional therapies. If your physician is unable or unwilling to provide you with this information, medical, college, or public libraries and popular bookstores are good places to search for it. You need to educate yourself about the advantages and disadvantages of alternative treatments, risks, side effects, expected results, and length of therapy.

Information on a wide range of medical conditions or specific diseases can also be obtained by calling the National Institutes of Health (NIH) at (301) 496-4000. Ask the operator to direct you to the appropriate NIH office.

The NCCAM office also provides a Web site (nccam.nih .gov) with access to over 180,000 bibliographic records of research published on CAM during the last 35 years.

When you select a primary care physician or a nonallopathic practitioner, consult local and state medical boards, other health regulatory boards and agencies, and consumer affairs departments for information about a given practitioner's education, accreditation, and license and about complaints that may have been filed against this health care provider. Many of the unconventional medical fields also have national organizations that provide guidelines for practitioners and health consumers. These organizations can guide you to the appropriate regulatory agencies within your state where you can obtain information regarding a specific practitioner.

You may also talk to individuals who have undergone similar therapies and learn about the competence of the practitioner in question. Keep in mind, however, that patient testimonials do not adequately assess the safety and effectiveness of alternative treatments. Whenever possible, search for results of controlled scientific trials of the therapy in question and use this information in your decision process.

When undergoing any type of treatment or therapy, always disclose this information to all of your health care providers, whether conventional or unconventional. Adequate health care management requires that health care providers be informed of all concurrent therapies, so that they will have a complete picture of the treatment plan. Lack of knowledge by one health care provider regarding treatments by another provider can interfere with the healing process or even worsen a given condition.

Millions of Americans have benefited from CAM practices. You may also benefit from such services, but you need to make careful and educated decisions about the available options. By finding well-trained (and preferably licensed) practitioners, you increase your chances for recovery from ailments and disease.

## Critical Thinking

Have you or someone you know ever used complementary or alternative medicine treatments? What experiences did you have with these treatment modalities, and would you use them in the future?

# Quackery and Fraud

The rapid growth of the fitness and wellness industry during the last three decades has spurred the promotion of fraudulent products that deceive consumers into "miraculous," quick, and easy ways to achieve total well-being.

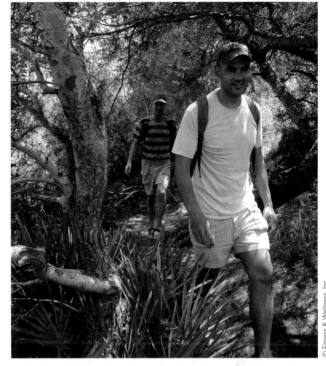

Frequent participation in recreational activities is important for health and wellness.

**Quackery/fraud** has been defined as the conscious promotion of unproven claims for profit.

Today's market is saturated with "special" foods, diets, supplements, pills, cures, equipment, books, and videos that promise quick, dramatic results. Advertisements for

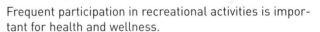

**Acupuncture** Chinese medical system that requires body piercing with fine needles during therapy to relieve pain and treat ailments and diseases.

**Chiropractics** Health care system that proposes that many diseases and ailments are related to misalignments of the vertebrae and emphasizes the manipulation of the spinal column.

**Herbal medicine** Unconventional system that uses herbs to treat ailments and disease.

**Homeopathy** System of treatment based on the use of minute quantities of remedies that in large amounts produce effects similar to the disease being treated.

**Naturopathic medicine** Unconventional system of medicine that relies exclusively on natural remedies to treat disease and ailments.

**Ayurveda** Hindu system of medicine based on herbs, diet, massage, meditation, and yoga to help the body boost its own natural healing.

**Magnetic therapy** Unconventional treatment that relies on magnetic energy to promote healing.

**Massage therapy** The rubbing or kneading of body parts to treat ailments.

**Quackery/fraud** The conscious promotion of unproven claims for profit.

these products often are based on testimonials, unproven claims, secret research, half-truths, and quick-fix statements that the uneducated consumer wants to hear. In the meantime, the organization or enterprise making the claims stands to make a large profit from the consumers' willingness to pay for astonishing and spectacular solutions to problems related to their unhealthy lifestyles.

Television, magazine, and newspaper advertisements are not necessarily reliable. For instance, one piece of equipment sold through television and newspaper advertisements promised to "bust the gut" through 5 minutes of daily exercise that appeared to target the abdominal muscle group. This piece of equipment consisted of a metal spring attached to the feet on one end and held in the hands on the other end. According to handling and shipping distributors, the equipment was "selling like hotcakes," and companies could barely keep up with consumer demands.

Three problems became apparent to the educated consumer: First, there is no such thing as spot-reducing; therefore, the claims could not be true. Second, 5 minutes of daily exercise burn hardly any calories and therefore have no effect on weight loss. Third, the intended abdominal (gut) muscles were not really involved during the exercise. The exercise engaged mostly the gluteal and lower back muscles. This piece of equipment now can be found at garage sales for about a tenth of its original cost!

Although people in the United States tend to be firm believers in the benefits of physical activity and positive lifestyle habits as a means to promote better health, most do not reap these benefits because they simply do not know how to put into practice a sound fitness and wellness program that will give them the results they want. Unfortunately, many uneducated wellness consumers are targets of deception by organizations making fraudulent claims for their products.

Deception is not limited to advertisements. Deceit is all around us: in newspaper and magazine articles, trade books, and on radio and television shows. To make a profit, popular magazines occasionally exaggerate health claims or leave out pertinent information to avoid offending advertisers. Some publishers print books on diets or self-treatment approaches that have no scientific foundation. Consumers should even be cautious about news reports of the latest medical breakthroughs. Reporters have been known to overlook important information or give certain findings greater credence than they deserve.

Precautions must also be taken when seeking health advice on the Internet. The Internet is full of both credible and dubious information. The following tips can help as you conduct a 'Net search:

- Look for credentials of the person or organization sponsoring the site.
- Check when the site was last updated. Credible sites are updated often.
- Check the appearance of the information on the site. It should be presented in a professional manner. If every sentence ends with an exclamation point, you have a good cause for suspicion.
- Exercise caution if the site's sponsor is trying to sell a product. If so, be leery of opinions posted on the site. They could be biased, given that the company's main objective is to sell a product. Credible companies trying to sell a product on the Internet usually reference their sources of health information and provide additional links that support their product.
- Compare a site's content with other credible sources. The contents should be generally similar to those of other reputable sites or publications.
- Note the address and contact information for the company. A reliable company will list more than a P.O. box, an 800 number, and the company's e-mail address. When only the latter information is provided, consumers may never be able to locate the company for questions, concerns, or refunds.
- Be on the alert for companies that claim to be innovators while criticizing competitors or the government for being closed-minded or trying to keep them from doing business.
- Watch for advertisers that use valid medical terminology in an irrelevant context or use vague pseudomedical jargon to sell their product.

Not all people who promote fraudulent products, however, know they are doing so. Some may be convinced that the product is effective. If you have questions or concerns about a health product, you may write to the National Council Against Health Fraud (NCAHF), 119 Foster Street, Peabody, MA 01960. The purpose of this organization is to provide the consumer with responsible, reliable, evidence-driven health information. The organization also monitors deceitful advertising, investigates complaints, and offers public information regarding fraudulent health claims. You may also report any type of quackery to them on their Web site at http://www.ncahf.org. The site contains an updated list of reliable and unreliable health Web sites for the consumer.

Other consumer protection organizations offer to follow up on complaints about quackery and fraud. The existence of these organizations, however, should not give the consumer a false sense of security. The overwhelming number of complaints made each year makes it impossible for these organizations to follow up on each case individually. The U.S. Food and Drug Administration's (FDA) Center for Drug Evaluation Research, for example, has developed a priority system to determine which health fraud product it should regulate first. Products are rated on how great a risk they pose to the consumer. With this in mind, you can use the following list of organizations to make an educated decision before you spend your money. You can also report consumer fraud to them:

- Food and Drug Administration. The FDA regulates safety and labeling of health products and cosmetics. You can search for the office closest to you in the federal government listings (blue pages) of the phone book.

## Behavior Modification Planning

### HEALTHY LIFESTYLE GUIDELINES

❏ I PLAN TO  ❏ I DID IT

❏ ❏ 1. Accumulate a minimum of 30 minutes of moderate-intensity physical activity at least five days per week.

❏ ❏ 2. Exercise aerobically in the proper cardiorespiratory training zone at least three times per week for a minimum of 20 minutes.

❏ ❏ 3. Accumulate at least 10,000 steps on a daily basis.

❏ ❏ 4. Strength train at least once a week using a minimum of eight exercises that involve all major muscle groups of the body.

❏ ❏ 5. Perform flexibility exercises that involve all major joints of the body two to three times per week.

❏ ❏ 6. Eat a healthy diet that is rich in whole-wheat grains, fruits, and vegetables and is low in saturated and trans fats.

❏ ❏ 7. Eat a healthy breakfast every day.

❏ ❏ 8. Do not use tobacco in any form, avoid secondhand smoke, and avoid all other forms of substance abuse.

❏ ❏ 9. Maintain healthy body weight (achieve a range between the high-physical fitness and health-fitness standards for percent body fat).

❏ ❏ 10. Get 7 to 8 hours of sleep per night.

❏ ❏ 11. Manage stress effectively.

❏ ❏ 12. Limit daily alcohol intake to two or less drinks per day if you are a man or one drink or less per day if you are a woman (or do not consume any alcohol at all).

❏ ❏ 13. Have at least one close friend or relative in whom you can confide and to whom you can express your feelings openly.

❏ ❏ 14. Be aware of your surroundings and take personal safety measures at all times.

❏ ❏ 15. Seek continued learning on a regular basis.

❏ ❏ 16. Subscribe to a reputable health/fitness/ nutrition newsletter to stay up-to-date on healthy lifestyle guidelines.

### Try It

Now that you are about to complete this course, evaluate how many of the above healthy lifestyle guidelines have become part of your personal wellness program. Prepare a list of those that you still need to work on and use Lab 15B to write SMART goals and specific objectives that will help you achieve the desired behaviors. Remember that each one of the above guidelines will lead to a longer, healthier, and happier life.

---

- Better Business Bureau (BBB). The BBB can tell you whether other customers have lodged complaints about a product, a company, or a salesperson. You can find a listing for the local office in the business section of the phone book or you can check their Web site at http://www.bbb.com.
- Consumer Product Safety Commission (CPSC). This independent federal regulatory agency targets products that threaten the safety of American families. Unsafe products can be researched and reported on their Web site at http://www.cpsc.gov.

Another way to get informed before you make your purchase is to seek the advice of a reputable professional.

Ask someone who understands the product but does not stand to profit from the transaction. As examples, a physical educator or an exercise physiologist can advise you regarding exercise equipment; a registered dietitian can provide information on nutrition and weight control programs; a physician can offer advice on nutritive supplements. Also, be alert to those who bill themselves as "experts." Look for qualifications, degrees, professional experience, certifications, and reputation.

Keep in mind that if it sounds too good to be true, it probably is. Fraudulent promotions often rely on testimonials or scare tactics and promise that their products will cure a long list of unrelated ailments; they use words like "quick fix," "time-tested," "newfound," "miraculous," "spe-

## Reliable Sources of Health, Fitness, Nutrition, and Wellness Information

| Newsletter | Approx. Yearly Issues | Annual Cost |
|---|---|---|
| *Bottom Line /Health* BottomLineSecrets.com 800-289-0409 | 12 | $29.95 |
| *Consumer Reports on Health* www.ConsumerReports.org/health 800-234-2188 | 12 | $24 |
| *Environmental Nutrition* www.environmentalnutrition.com 800-829-5384 | 12 | $30 |
| *Tufts University Health & Nutrition Letter* www.healthletter.tufts.edu 800-274-7581 | 12 | $28 |
| *University of California Berkeley Wellness Letter* www.WellnessLetter.com 386-447-6328 | 12 | $28 |

cial," "secret," "all-natural," "mail-order only," and "money-back guarantee." Deceptive companies move often, so that customers have no way of contacting the company to ask for a reimbursement.

When claims are made, ask where the claims are published. Refereed scientific journals are the most reliable sources of information. When a researcher submits information for publication in a refereed journal, at least two qualified and reputable professionals in the field conduct blind reviews of the manuscript. A blind review means the author does not know who will review the manuscript, and the reviewers do not know who submitted the manuscript. Acceptance for publication is based on this input and relevant changes.

# Deciding Your Fitness Future

Once you've decided to pursue a lifetime wellness program, you'll face several more decisions about exactly how to accomplish it. Following are a few issues you'll encounter.

**FIGURE 15.3** American College of Sports Medicine standards for health and fitness facilities.

1. A facility must have an appropriate emergency plan.
2. A facility must offer each adult member a preactivity screening that is relevant to the activities that will be performed by the member.
3. Each person who has supervisory responsibility must be professionally competent.
4. A facility must post appropriate signs in those areas of a facility that present potential increased risk.
5. A facility that offers services or programs to the youth must provide appropriate supervision.
6. A facility must conform to all relevant laws, regulations, and published standards.

Adapted from ACSM's *Health/Fitness Facility Standards and Guidelines* (Champaign, IL: Human Kinetics, 2006).

**Health/Fitness Club Memberships** You may want to consider joining a health/fitness facility. Or, if you have mastered the contents of this book and your choice of fitness activity is one you can pursue on your own (walking, jogging, cycling), you may not need to join a health club. Barring injuries, you may continue your exercise program outside the walls of a health club for the rest of your life. You also can conduct strength training and stretching programs in your own home (see Chapters 7 and 8).

To stay up-to-date on fitness and wellness developments, you probably should buy a reputable and updated fitness/wellness book every four to five years. You may subscribe to a credible health, fitness, nutrition, or wellness newsletter to stay current. You can also surf the World Wide Web, but be sure that the sites you are searching are from credible and reliable organizations.

If you are contemplating membership in a fitness facility, do all of the following:

- Make sure that the facility complies with the standards established by the American College of Sports Medicine (ACSM) for health and fitness facilities. These standards are given in Figure 15.3.
- Examine all exercise options in your community: health clubs/spas, YMCAs, gyms, colleges, schools, community centers, senior centers, and the like.
- Check to see if the facility's atmosphere is pleasurable and nonthreatening to you. Will you feel comfortable with the instructors and other people who go there? Is it clean and well kept? If the answers are no, this may not be the right place for you.
- Analyze costs versus facilities, equipment, and programs. Take a look at your personal budget. Will you really use the facility? Will you exercise there regularly? Many people obtain memberships and permit dues to be withdrawn automatically from a local bank account, yet seldom attend the fitness center.
- Find out what types of facilities are available: walking/running track, basketball/tennis/racquetball courts, aerobic exercise room, strength training room, pool,

## Reliable Health Web Sites

- American Cancer Society
  http://www.cancer.org/
- American Heart Association
  http://americanheart.org
- American College of Sports Medicine
  http://acsm.org
- Clinical Trials Listing Service
  http://www.centerwatch.com
- Healthfinder—Your Guide to Reliable Health Information
  http://www.healthfinder.gov
- HospitalWeb
  http://neuro-www.mgh.harvard.edu/hospital-web.shtml
- National Cancer Institute
  http://www.cancer.gov
- National Center for Complementary and Alternative Medicine
  http://nccam.nih.gov/
- The National Library of Medicine
  http://www.nlm.nih.gov/
- The National Institutes of Health
  http://www.nih.gov/
- The Centers for Disease Control and Prevention
  http://www.cdc.gov/
- The Medical Matrix (requires subscription)
  http://www.medmatrix.org/
- The National Council Against Health Fraud
  http://www.ncahf.org/
- The Food and Drug Administration
  http://www.fda.gov/
- WebMD
  http://webmd.com/
- World Health Organization
  http://www.who.int/en/

locker rooms, saunas, hot tubs, handicapped access, and so on.

- Check the aerobic and strength-training equipment available. Does the facility have treadmills, bicycle ergometers, stair climbers, cross-country skiing simulators, free weights, strength-training machines? Make sure the facilities and equipment meet your activity interests.
- Consider the location. Is the facility close, or do you have to travel several miles to get there? Distance often discourages participation.

- Check on times the facility is accessible. Is it open during your preferred exercise time (for example, early morning or late evening)?
- Work out at the facility several times before becoming a member. Are people standing in line to use the equipment, or is it readily available during your exercise time?
- Inquire about the instructors' qualifications. Do the fitness instructors have college degrees or professional certifications from organizations such as the ACSM or the International Dance Exercise Association (IDEA)? These organizations have rigorous standards to ensure professional preparation and quality of instruction.
- Consider the approach to fitness (including all health-related components of fitness). Is it well rounded? Do the instructors spend time with members, or do members have to seek them out constantly for help and instruction?
- Ask about supplementary services. Does the facility provide or contract out for regular health and fitness assessments (cardiovascular endurance, body composition, blood pressure, blood chemistry analysis)? Are wellness seminars (nutrition, weight control, stress management) offered? Do these have hidden costs?

**Personal Trainers** The current way of life has opened an entire new job market for personal trainers, who are presently in high demand by health and fitness participants. A **personal trainer** is a health/fitness professional who evaluates, motivates, educates, and trains clients to help them meet individualized healthy lifestyle goals. Rates typically start at $40 an hour.

Exercise sessions are usually conducted at a health/fitness facility or at the client's own home. Experience and the ability to design safe and effective programs based on the client's current fitness level, health status, and fitness goals are important. Personal trainers also recognize their limitations and refer clients to other health care professionals as necessary.

Currently, anyone who prescribes exercise can make the claim to be a personal trainer without proof of education, experience, or certification. Although good trainers need to strive to maximize their own health and fitness, a good physique and previous athletic experience do not certify a person as a personal trainer.

Because of the high demand for personal trainers, more than 200 organizations now certify fitness specialists. This has led to great confusion by clients on how to evaluate the credentials of personal trainers. "Certification" and a "certificate" are two different things. Certification implies that the individual has met educational and professional standards of performance and competence. A

---

**Personal trainer** A health/fitness professional who evaluates, motivates, educates, and trains clients to help them meet individualized healthy lifestyle goals.

certificate typically is awarded to individuals who attend a conference or workshop but are not required to meet any professional standards.

Presently, no licensing body is in place to oversee personal trainers. Thus, becoming a personal trainer is easy. At a minimum, personal trainers should have an undergraduate degree and certification from a reputable organization such as ACSM, the IDEA Health and Fitness Association, the National Strength and Conditioning Association (NSCA), or the American Council on Exercise (ACE). Undergraduate (and graduate) degrees should be conferred in a fitness-related area such as exercise science, exercise physiology, kinesiology, sports medicine, or physical education.

ACSM offers three certification levels: group exercise leader, health/fitness instructor, and health/fitness director. IDEA offers four levels: professional, advanced, elite, and master. For both ACSM and IDEA, each level of certification is progressively more difficult to obtain. The NSCA also offers a personal trainer's certification program. When looking for a personal trainer, always inquire about the trainer's education and certification credentials.

Before selecting a trainer, you must establish your program goals. Below are sample questions to ask yourself and consider when interviewing potential trainers prior to selecting one:[6]

- What are the fees? Are several sessions cheaper per session than one single session? Can individuals be trained in groups? Are there discount rates if you use company trainers? Do you have to pay a cancellation fee if you are unable to attend a given session?
- How long will you need the services of the personal trainer—one session, several times a week, periodically, indefinitely?
- Do you need a personal trainer to help you achieve certain fitness levels (cardiorespiratory, strength, flexibility) or improve health, or is losing weight your primary concern?
- What type of personality are you looking for in the trainer—a motivator, a hard-driving trainer, a gentle approach, or guidance without much pressure?

When seeking fitness advice from a health/fitness trainer via the Internet, here's a final word of caution: Be aware that certain services cannot be provided over the 'Net. An Internet trainer is not able to directly administer fitness tests, motivate, observe exercise limitations, or respond effectively in an emergency situation (e.g., spotting, administering first aid or cardiopulmonary resuscitation [CPR]) and thus is not able to design the most safe and effective exercise program for you.

Purchasing Exercise Equipment A final consideration is that of purchasing your own exercise equipment. The first question you need to ask yourself is: Do I really need this piece of equipment? Most people buy on impulse because of television advertisements or because a salesperson has convinced them it is a great piece of equipment that will do wonders for their health and fitness. Ignore claims that an exercise device or machine can provide "easy/no-sweat" results in a few minutes only. Keep in mind that the benefits of exercise are obtained only if you do exercise. With some creativity, you can implement an excellent and comprehensive exercise program with little, if any, equipment (see Chapters 6, 7, 8, and 9).

Many people buy expensive equipment only to find that they really do not enjoy that mode of activity. They do not remain regular users. Stationary bicycles (lower body only) and rowing ergometers were among the most popular pieces of equipment a few years ago. Most of them now are seldom used and have become "fitness furniture" somewhere in the basement. Furthermore, be skeptical of testimonials and before-and-after pictures from "satisfied" customers. These results may not be typical, and it doesn't mean that you will like the equipment as well.

Exercise equipment does have its value for people who prefer to exercise indoors, especially during the winter months. It supports some people's motivation and adherence to exercise. The convenience of having equipment at home also allows for flexible scheduling. You can exercise before or after work or while you watch your favorite television show.

If you are going to purchase equipment, the best recommendation is to actually try it out several times before buying it. Ask yourself several questions: Did you enjoy the workout? Is the unit comfortable? Are you too short, tall, or heavy for it? Is it stable, sturdy, and strong? Do you have to assemble the machine? If so, how difficult is it to put together? How durable is it? Ask for references—people or clubs that have used the equipment extensively. Are they satisfied? Have they enjoyed using the equipment? Talk with professionals at colleges, sports medicine clinics, or health clubs.

Another consideration is to look at used units for signs of wear and tear. Quality is important. Cheaper brands may not be durable, so your investment would be wasted.

Finally, watch out for expensive gadgets. Monitors that provide exercise heart rate, work output, caloric expenditure, speed, grade, and distance may help motivate you, but they are expensive, need repairs, and do not enhance the actual fitness benefits of the workout. Look at maintenance costs and check for service personnel in your community.

## Critical Thinking

Do you admire some people around you and would like to emulate their wellness lifestyle? What behaviors do these people exhibit that would help you adopt a healthier lifestyle? What keeps you from emulating these behaviors, and how can you overcome these barriers?

# Self-Evaluation and Behavioral Goals for the Future

The main objective of this book is to provide the information and experiences necessary to implement your personal fitness and wellness program. If you have implemented the programs in this book, including exercise, you should be convinced that a wellness lifestyle is the only way to attain a higher quality of life.

Most people who engage in a personal fitness and wellness program experience this new quality of life after only a few weeks of training and practicing healthy lifestyle patterns. In some instances, however—especially for individuals who have led a poor lifestyle for a long time—a few months may be required to establish positive habits and feelings of well-being. In the end, though, everyone who applies the principles of fitness and wellness will reap the desired benefits.

Prior to the completion of this course, you now need to identify community resources available to you that will support your path to lifetime fitness and wellness. Lab 15B will provide a road map to initiate your search for this support. You will find the process beneficial, one that will help you maintain your new wellness way of life.

## Self-Evaluation
Throughout this course you have had an opportunity to assess various fitness and wellness components and write goals to improve your quality of life. You now should take the time to evaluate how well you have achieved your own goals. Ideally, if time allows and facilities and technicians are available, reassess the health-related components of physical fitness. If you are unable to reassess these components, determine subjectively how well you accomplished your objectives. You will find a self-evaluation form in part I of Lab 15C.

## Behavioral Goals for the Future
If you have not yet achieved all of your goals during this course, or if you need to reach beyond your current achievements, a final assignment should be conducted to help you chart the future. To complete this assignment, fill out the Wellness Compass shown in part II of Lab 15C. This compass provides a list of various wellness components, each illustrating a scale from 5 to 1. A "5" indicates a low or poor rating; a "1" indicates an excellent or "wellness" rating for that component. Using the Wellness Compass, rate yourself for each component according to the following instructions:

1. Color in red a number from 5 to 1 to indicate where you stood on each component at the beginning of the semester. For example, if at the start of this course, you rated poor in cardiorespiratory endurance, color the number 5 in red.

2. Color in blue a second number from 5 to 1 to indicate where you stand on each component at the present time. If your level of cardiorespiratory endurance improved to average by the end of the semester, color the number 3 in blue. If you were not able to work on a given component, simply color in blue on top of the previous red.

3. Select one or two components you intend to work on in the next 2 months. Developing new behavioral patterns takes time, and trying to work on too many components at once most likely will lower your chances for success.

Start with components in which you think you will have a high chance for success. Next, color in yellow the intended goal (number) to accomplish by the end of the 2 months. If your goal is to achieve a "good" level of cardiorespiratory endurance, color the number 2 in yellow. When you achieve this level, you may later color the number 1, also in yellow, to indicate your next goal.

After you have completed the previous exercise, write goals and objectives for the two components you intend to work on during the next 2 months (use the form in part III of Lab 15C). As you write and work on these goals, review the SMART Goals section provided in Chapter 2, pages 55–58.

One final assignment that you should complete is to summarize your feelings about your past and present lifestyle, what you have learned in this course, and changes that you were able to successfully implement. Use part IV of Lab 15C for this evaluation and keep this summary where you can review it in months and years to come.

# The Fitness/Wellness Experience and a Challenge for the Future

Patty Neavill is a typical example of someone who often tried to change her life but was unable to do so because she did not know how to implement a sound exercise and weight control program. At age 24 and at 240 pounds, she was discouraged with her weight, level of fitness, self-image, and quality of life in general. She had struggled with her weight most of her life. Like thousands of other people, she had made many unsuccessful attempts to lose weight.

Patty put her fears aside and decided to enroll in a fitness course. As part of the course requirement, a battery of fitness tests was administered at the beginning of the semester. Patty's cardiovascular fitness and strength ratings were poor, her flexibility classification was average, and her percent body fat was 41.

Following the initial fitness assessment, Patty met with her course instructor, who prescribed an exercise and nutrition program like the one in this book. Patty fully committed to carry out the prescription. She walked/jogged five times a week. She enrolled in a weight-training course that met twice a week. Her daily caloric intake was set in the range of 1,500 to 1,700.

Determined to increase her level of activity further, Patty signed up for recreational volleyball and basketball courses. Besides being fun, these classes provided 4 additional hours of activity per week.

She took care to meet the minimum required servings from the basic food groups each day, which contributed about 1,200 calories to her diet. The remainder of the calories came primarily from complex carbohydrates.

At the end of the 16-week semester, Patty's cardiovascular fitness, strength, and flexibility ratings had all improved to the "good" category, she had lost 50 pounds, and her percent body fat had decreased to 22.5!

Patty was tall. At 190 pounds, most people would have thought she was too heavy. Her percent body fat, however, was lower than the average for college female physical education major students (about 23 percent body fat).

A thank-you note from Patty to the course instructor at the end of the semester read:

*Thank you for making me a new person. I truly appreciate the time you spent with me. Without your kindness and motivation, I would have never made it. It is great to be fit and trim. I've never had this feeling before, and I wish everyone could feel like this once in their life.*

*Thank you,*
*Your trim Patty!*

Patty had never been taught the principles governing a sound weight loss program. In her case, not only did she need this knowledge, but, like most Americans who have never experienced the process of becoming physically fit, she needed to be in a structured exercise setting to truly feel the joy of fitness.

Even more significant was that Patty maintained her aerobic and strength-training programs. A year after ending her calorie-restricted diet, her weight increased by 10 pounds, but her body fat decreased from 22.5 to 21.2 percent. As you may recall from Chapter 5, this weight increase is related mostly to changes in lean tissue, lost during the weight-reduction phase.

In spite of only a slight drop in weight during the second year following the calorie-restricted diet, the 2-year follow-up revealed a further decrease in body fat, to 19.5 percent. Patty understood the new quality of life reaped through a sound fitness program, and at the same time, she finally learned how to apply the principles that regulate weight maintenance.

If you have read and successfully completed all of the assignments set out in this book, including a regular exercise program, you should be convinced of the value of exercise and healthy lifestyle habits in achieving a new quality of life.

Perhaps this new quality of life was explained best by the late Dr. George Sheehan, when he wrote:[7]

*For every runner who tours the world running marathons, there are thousands who run to hear the leaves and listen to the rain, and look to the day when it is all suddenly as easy as a bird in flight. For them, sport is not a test but a therapy, not a trial but a reward, not a question but an answer.*

The real challenge will come now: a lifetime commitment to fitness and wellness. To make the commitment easier, enjoy yourself and have fun along the way. If you implement your program based on your interests and what you enjoy doing most, then adhering to your new lifestyle will not be difficult.

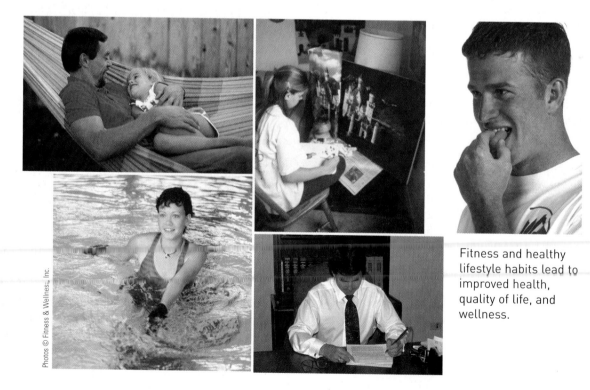

Fitness and healthy lifestyle habits lead to improved health, quality of life, and wellness.

Your activities over the last few weeks or months may have helped you develop "positive addictions" that will carry on throughout life. If you truly experience the feelings Dr. Sheehan expressed, there will be no looking back. If you don't get there, you won't know what it's like. Fitness and wellness is a process, and you need to put forth a constant and deliberate effort to achieve and maintain a higher quality of life. Improving the quality of your life, and most likely your longevity, is in your hands. Only you can take control of your lifestyle and thereby reap the benefits of wellness.

## ASSESS YOUR BEHAVIOR

Log on to http://www.cengage.com/sso/ to take the Wellness Profile assessment again and evaluate your progress.

1. Has your level of physical activity increased compared with the beginning of the term?

2. Do you participate in a regular exercise program that includes cardiorespiratory endurance, muscular strength, and muscular flexibility training?

3. Is your diet healthier now compared with a few weeks ago?

4. Are you able to take pride in the lifestyle changes that you have implemented over the last several weeks? Have you rewarded yourself for your accomplishments?

## ASSESS YOUR KNOWLEDGE

Log on to http://www.cengage.com/sso/ to assess your understanding of this chapter's topics by taking the Student Practice Test and exploring the modules recommended in your Personalized Study Plan.

1. From a functional point of view, typical sedentary people in the United States are about _____ years older than their chronological age indicates.
   a. 2
   b. 8
   c. 15
   d. 20
   e. 25

2. Which one of the following factors has the greatest impact on health and longevity?
   a. Genetics
   b. The environment
   c. Lifestyle behaviors
   d. Chronic diseases
   e. Gender

3. Your real physiologic age is determined by
   a. your birthdate.
   b. lifestyle habits.
   c. amount of physical activity.
   d. your family's health history.
   e. your ability to obtain proper medical care.

4. Complementary and alternative medicine is
   a. also known as allopathic medicine.
   b. referred to as "Western" medicine.
   c. based on scientifically proven methods.
   d. a method of unconventional medicine.
   e. All are correct choices

5. Complementary and alternative medicine health care practices and treatments are
   a. not widely taught in medical schools.
   b. endorsed by many physicians.
   c. not generally used in hospitals.
   d. not usually reimbursed by medical insurance companies.
   e. All of the above choices are correct.

6. In complementary and alternative medicine,
   a. practitioners believe that their treatment modality aids the body as it performs its own natural healing process.
   b. treatments are usually shorter than with typical medical practices.
   c. practitioners rely extensively on the use of medications.
   d. patients are often discouraged from administering self-treatment.
   e. All of the above choices are correct.

7. When the word "natural" is used with a product,
   a. it implies that the product is safe.
   b. it cannot be toxic, even when taken in large doses.
   c. it cannot yield undesirable side effects when combined with prescription drugs.
   d. there will be no negative side effects with its use.
   e. All of the choices are incorrect.

8. To protect yourself from consumer fraud when buying a new product,
   a. get as much information as you can from the salesperson.
   b. obtain details about the product from another salesperson.
   c. ask someone who understands the product but does not stand to profit from the transaction.
   d. obtain all the research information from the manufacturer.
   e. All of the choices are correct.

9. Which of the following should you consider when looking to join a health/fitness center?
   a. Location
   b. Instructor's certifications
   c. Type and amount of equipment available
   d. Verification that the facility complies with ACSM
      standards
   e. All of the choices are correct.

10. When you purchase exercise equipment, the most important factor is
    a. to try it out several times before buying it.
    b. a recommendation from an exercise specialist.
    c. cost-effectiveness.
    d. that it provides accurate exercise information.
    e. to find out how others like this piece of equipment.

Correct answers can be found at the back of the book.

# MEDIA MENU

You can find the links below at the book companion site: www.cengage.com/health/hoeger/plfw10e

- Take the Wellness Profile again to evaluate your progress.
- Check how well you understand the chapter's concepts.

### Internet Connections

- American College of Sports Medicine (ACSM). This site
  provides information on sports safety and research
  projects. The ACSM is committed to the practical application of sports medicine and exercise science to
  maintain and enhance physical fitness, health, and
  quality of life. *http://www.acsm.org*

- Getting Started with an Exercise Program. This comprehensive site, from the Department of Kinesiology
  and Health at Georgia State University, features information on the benefits of exercise, how to choose a personal trainer, exercise safety and precautions, and lots
  more. *http://www.gsu.edu/~wwwfit/getstart.html*

- RealAge. This site features diet and exercise assessment tools, such as a calculator of body mass index and
  an exercise estimator, as well as RealAge assessment
  quizzes on a variety of health topics to help determine
  your risk for disease and what you can do to reduce it.
  The main feature is an interactive online personal assessment of a variety of lifestyle behaviors that also
  gives you options for growing younger. *http://www
  .realage.com*

- National Center for Complementary and Alternative
  Medicine. This comprehensive site features information about a variety of complementary therapies geared
  for consumers, clinical practitioners, and investigators.
  The site also features a complementary medicine data-
  base, clinical trials information, and a list of resources.
  *http://nccam.nih.gov*

# NOTES

1. R. J. Donatelle, *Access to Health* (San Francisco: Benjamin Cummings, 2008).

2. U.S. Department of Health and Human Services, Centers for Disease Control and Prevention, National Center for Health Statistics, *Complementary and Alternative Medicine Use Among Adults: United States, 2002,* no. 343 (May 27, 2004).

3. National Center for Complementary and Alternative Medicine, National Institutes of Health, "Get the Facts: What Is Complementary and Alternative Medicine?" http://nccam.nih .gov/ health/whatiscam, downloaded July 15, 2008.

4. D. M. Eisenberg, et al., "Trends in Alternative Medicine Use in the United States, 1990–1997," *Journal of the American Medical Association* 280, no. 18 (1998): 1569–1575.

5. See note 4.

6. "How to Get Coaxed into Shape," *Consumer Reports on Health* 17, no. 8 (2005): 6.

7. *Dynamics of Fitness: The Body in Action* (Pleasantville, NY: Human Relations Media, 1980).

# SUGGESTED READINGS

American College of Sports Medicine. *ACSM's Health/Fitness Facility Standards and Guidelines.* Champaign, IL: Human Kinetics, 2006.

American College of Sports Medicine. *ACSM's Resources for the Personal Trainer.* Philadelphia: Lippincott Williams & Wilkins, 2007.

Bloomer, R. "Successful Attributes of a Professional Fitness Trainer." *Fitness Management* 19 (1999): 40–45.

Roizen, M. F. *Real Age: Are You As Young As You Can Be?* New York: Cliff Street Books, 1999.

# LAB 15A: Life Expectancy and Physiologic Age Prediction Questionnaire*

**Name** _____     **Date** _____     **Grade** _____

**Instructor** _____     **Course** _____     **Section** _____

**Necessary Lab Equipment**
None required.

**Objective**
To estimate the total number of years that you will live and your real physiologic age based on your present life-style habits.

**Instructions**
Circle the points to the correct answer to each question. At the end of each page, obtain a net score for that page. Be completely honest with yourself. Your age prediction is based on your lifestyle habits, should you continue those habits for life. Using this questionnaire, you will learn about factors that you can modify or implement that can add years and health to your life. The scoring system is provided at the end of the questionnaire. Please note that the questionnaire is not a precise scientific instrument, but rather an estimated life expectancy analysis according to the impact of lifestyle factors on health and longevity. This questionnaire is not intended to substitute for advice and tests conducted by medical and health-care practitioners.

## I. Questionnaire

1. What is your current health status?
   A. Excellent    +2
   B. Good    +1
   C. Average    0
   D. Fair    −1
   E. Poor    −2
   F. Bad    −3

2. How many days per week do you accumulate 30 minutes of moderate-intensity physical activity (50% to 60% of heart rate reserve—see Chapter 6)?
   A. 5 to 7    +3
   B. 3 or 4    +1
   C. 1 or 2    0
   D. Less than once per week    −3

3. How often do you participate in a vigorous-intensity cardio-respiratory exercise (over 60% of heart rate reserve) for at least 20 minutes?
   A. 3 or more times per week    +2
   B. 2 times per week    +1
   C. Once a week    −1
   D. Less than once per week    0

4. How often do you perform strength-training exercises per week (a minimum of 8 exercises using 3 to 20 repetitions to near-fatigue on each exercise)?
   A. 1–2 times    +2
   B. Less than once or less than 8 exercises with 8 to 12 reps per session    0
   C. Do not strength train    −1

5. How many times per week do you perform flexibility exercises (at least 15 minutes per stretching session)?
   A. 3 or more    +1
   B. 1 to 3 times    +.5
   C. 1 time    0
   D. Do not perform flexibility exercises    −.5

6. How many servings of fruits and vegetables do you eat on a daily basis?
   A. 9 or more    +3
   B. 6 to 8    +2
   C. 5    +1
   D. 3 or 4    0
   E. 2 or less    0

7. How many grams of fiber do you consume on an average day?
   A. 25 or over    +1
   B. Between 13 and 24    0
   C. 10 to 12 or don't know    −1
   D. Less than 10    −2

8. As a percentage of total calories, what is your average fat intake daily?
   A. 20% to 29.9%    +1
   B. 30%    0
   C. 30.1% to 35% or don't know    −1
   D. Over 35%    −2

9. As a percentage of total calories, what is your average saturated fat intake daily?
   A. 5% or less    +1
   B. More than 5% but less than 7%    0
   C. Don't know    −1
   D. Over 7%    −2

10. How many servings of red meat (3 to 6 ounces) do you consume weekly?
    A. 1 or none    +1
    B. 2 or 3    0
    C. 4 to 7    −1
    D. More than 7    −2

Page score: ☐

---

*SOURCE: Fitness & Wellness, Inc., Boise, Idaho, ©2008. Reprinted with permission.

*(continued)*

11. How many servings of fish (3 to 6 ounces) do you consume weekly?
   A. 2 or more     +1
   B. 1     0
   C. None     −1

12. As a percentage of total calories, what is your average daily trans fatty acid intake?
   A. No trans fat intake     +1
   B. Less than 1%     0
   C. 1 to 2%     −1
   D. Over 2%     −2

13. How many alcoholic drinks (a 12-ounce bottle of beer, a 4-ounce glass of wine, or a 1.5-ounce shot of 80-proof liquor) do you consume per day?
   A. Men 2 or less, women 1 or none     +1
   B. None     0
   C. Men 3–4, women 2–4     −1
   D. 5 or more     −3

14. How many milligrams of vitamin C do you get from food daily?
   A. Between 250 and 500     +1
   B. Over 90 but less than 250     +.5
   C. Less than 90     −1

15. How many micrograms of selenium do you get daily (preferably from food)?
   A. Between 100 and 200     +1
   B. Between 50 and 99     +.5
   C. Less than 50     −1

16. How many milligrams of calcium and how many international units of vitamin D do you get from food and supplements on an average day?
   A. Calcium = 1,200, vitamin D = 1,000 or more     +1
   B. Calcium = 1,200, vitamin D = 400 to 1,000     +.5
   C. Calcium = 800 to 1,200, vitamin D = less than 400     0
   D. Calcium = less than 800, vitamin D = less than 400     −1

17. How many times per week do you eat breakfast?
   A. 7     +1
   B. 5 or 6     +.5
   C. 3 or 4     0
   D. Less than 3     −.5

18. How many cigarettes do you smoke each day?
   A. Never smoked cigarettes or more than 15 years since giving up cigarettes     +2
   B. None for 5 to 14 years     +1
   C. None for 1 to 4 years     0
   D. None for 0 to 1 year     −1
   E. Smoker, less than 1 pack per day     −3
   F. Smoker, 1 pack per day     −5
   G. Smoker, up to 2 packs per day     −7
   H. Smoker, more than 2 packs per day     −10

19. Do you use tobacco products other than cigarettes?
   A. Never have     0
   B. Less than once per week     −1
   C. Once per week     −2
   D. 2 to 6 times per week     −3
   E. More than 6 times per week     −5

20. How often are you exposed to second-hand smoke or other environmental pollutants?
   A. Less than 1 hour per month     0
   B. Between 1 and 5 hours per month     −1
   C. Between 5 and 29 hours per month     −2
   D. Daily     −3

21. Do you use addictive drugs, other than tobacco or alcohol?
   A. None     0
   B. 1     −3
   C. 2 or more     −5

22. What is the age of your parents (or how long did they live)?
   A. Both over 76     +3
   B. Only one over 76     +1
   C. Both are still alive and under 70     0
   D. Only one under 76     −1
   E. Neither one lived past 76     −3

23. What is your body composition category?
   A. Excellent     +2
   B. Good     +1
   C. Average     0
   D. Overweight     −1
   E. Significantly overweight     −2

24. What is your blood pressure?
   A. 120/80 or less (both numbers)     +2
   B. 120–140 or 80–90 (either number)     −1
   C. Greater than 140/90 (either number)     −3

25. What is your HDL cholesterol?
   A. Men greater than 45, women over 55     +2
   B. Men 35 to 44, women 45 to 54     0
   C. Don't know     −1
   D. Men less than 35, women below 45     −2

26. What is your LDL cholesterol?
   A. Less than 100     +2
   B. 100 to 130     0
   C. 130 to 159     −1
   D. 160 or higher     +2
   E. Don't know     −2

27. Do you floss and brush your teeth regularly?
   A. Every day     +.5
   B. 3 to 6 days per week     0
   C. Less than 3 days per week     −.5

28. Are you a diabetic?
   A. No     0
   B. Yes, well-controlled     −1
   C. Yes, poorly or not controlled     −3

Page score: _____

29. How often do you sunbathe (tan)?
    A. Not at all     +1
    B. Between 1 and 3 times per year     −.5
    C. More than 3 times per year     −1

30. How often do you wear a seat belt?
    A. All the time     +1
    B. Most of the time     −.5
    C. Less than half the time     −1

31. How fast do you drive?
    A. Always at or below the speed limit     0
    B. Up to 5 mph over the speed limit     −.5
    C. Between 5 and 10 mph over the speed limit     −1
    D. More than 10 mph over the speed limit     −2

32. Do you drink and drive?
    A. Never     0
    B. Yes (even if only once)     −5

33. In terms of your sexual activity:
    A. I am not sexually active or I am in a monogamous sexual relationship     +1
    B. I have more than one sexual partner but I always practice safer sex     −1
    C. I have multiple sexual partners and I do not practice safer sex techniques     −3

34. What is your marital status?
    A. Happily married     +1
    B. Single and happy     0
    C. Single and unhappy     −.5
    D. Divorced     −1
    E. Widowed with a belief in life hereafter     −1
    F. Widowed     −2
    G. Married and unhappy     −2

35. On the average, how many hours of sleep do you get each night?
    A. 7 to 8     +1
    B. 7     0
    C. 6 to 7     −1
    D. Less than 6     −2

36. Your stress rating according to the Life Experiences Survey (see Lab 10A, pages 379–380) is:
    A. Excellent     +1
    B. Good     0
    C. Average     −.5
    D. Fair     −1
    E. Poor     −2

37. Your Type A behavior rating is:
    A. Low     0
    B. Medium     −1
    C. High     −2

38. When under stress (distress), how often do you practice stress management techniques?
    A. Always     +1
    B. Most of the time     +.5
    C. Not applicable (don't suffer from stress)     0
    D. Sometimes     −1
    E. Never     −2

39. Do you suffer from depression?
    A. Not at all     0
    B. Mild depression     −1
    C. Severe depression     −2

40. How often do you associate with people who have a positive attitude about life?
    A. Always     +.5
    B. Most of the time     0
    C. About half of the time     −.5
    D. Less than half the time     −1

41. Do you have close family or personal relationships whom you can trust and rely on for help in times of need?
    A. Yes     +1
    B. No     −1

42. Do you feel loved and can you routinely give affection and love?
    A. Yes     +1
    B. No     −1

43. Do you have a good sense of humor?
    A. Yes     +1
    B. No     −1

44. How satisfied are you with your school work?
    A. Satisfied     +.5
    B. It's okay     0
    C. Not satisfied     −.5

45. How do you rate your present job satisfaction?
    A. Love it     +1
    B. Like it     0
    C. It's okay     −.5
    D. Don't like it     −1
    E. Hate it     −2
    F. Not applicable     0

46. How do you rate yourself spiritually?
    A. Very spiritual     +1
    B. Spiritual     0
    C. Somewhat spiritual     −.5
    D. Not spiritual at all     −1

Page score: [＿＿＿]

Net score for all questions: [＿＿＿]

*(continued)*

### How To Score

To estimate the total number of years that you will live, (a) determine a net score by totaling the results from all 46 questions, (b) obtain an age change score by multiplying the net score by the age correction factor given below, and (c) add or subtract this number from your base life expectancy age (73 for men and 80 for women—the current life expectancies in the United States). For example, if you are a 20-year-old male and the net score from the answers to all questions was −16, your estimated life expectancy would be 68.2 years (age change score = −16 × .3 4 −4.8, life expectancy = 73 − 4.8 = 68.2).

You also can determine your real physiologic age by subtracting a positive age-change score or adding a negative age-change score to your current chronological (calendar) age. For instance, in the previous example, the real physiologic age would be 24.8 years (20 + 4.8). If the age change score had been +4.8, the real physiologic age would have been 15.2 years. Thus, a healthy lifestyle will always make your physiologic age younger than your chronological age. Your real physiologic age will have much greater significance in middle and older age, when real-age reductions of 10 to 25 years occur in people who lead healthy lifestyles. Thus a 50-year-old person could easily have a real physiologic age of 30.

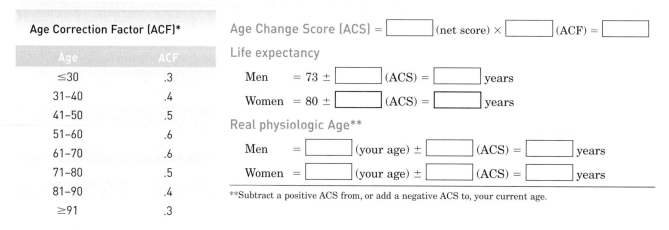

**Age Correction Factor (ACF)***

| Age | ACF |
| --- | --- |
| ≤30 | .3 |
| 31–40 | .4 |
| 41–50 | .5 |
| 51–60 | .6 |
| 61–70 | .6 |
| 71–80 | .5 |
| 81–90 | .4 |
| ≥91 | .3 |

Age Change Score (ACS) = ☐ (net score) × ☐ (ACF) = ☐

Life expectancy

Men  = 73 ± ☐ (ACS) = ☐ years

Women = 80 ± ☐ (ACS) = ☐ years

Real physiologic Age**

Men  = ☐ (your age) ± ☐ (ACS) = ☐ years

Women = ☐ (your age) ± ☐ (ACS) = ☐ years

**Subtract a positive ACS from, or add a negative ACS to, your current age.

*Adapted from M. F. Roizen, *RealAge,* (New York: Cliff Street Books, 1999).

### Behavior Modification

State your feelings about the experience of taking this questionnaire, analyze your results, and list lifestyle factors that you can work on that will positively affect your health and longevity.

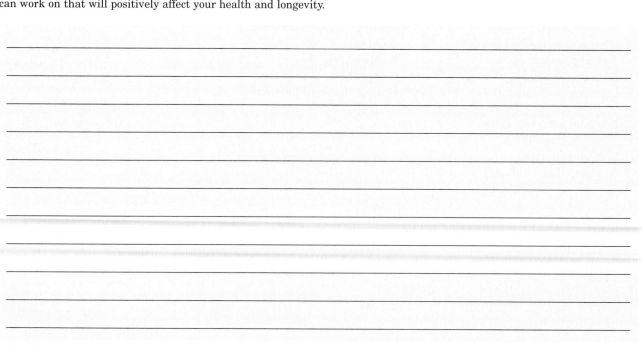

# LAB 15B: Fitness and Wellness Community Resources

Name _____  Date _____  Grade _____

Instructor _____  Course _____  Section _____

## Necessary Lab Equipment
None required.

## Objective
To identify community resources available for you to continue your path toward lifetime fitness and wellness.

## Introduction
Using a community directory, identify a minimum of three fitness, recreational, or wellness facilities that will allow you to maintain and further develop your personal fitness and wellness program. Initially, contact all three facilities by phone to obtain the pertinent information (see Item I below). Upon completion of this task, make an appointment to personally visit at least one of the facilities during a time when you would work out, and evaluate the equipment, equipment availability, personnel, and programs that would be available to you. Keep in mind that one of the options available to you may be your own campus health/fitness/recreation center. College alumni, for a fee, often have the option to continue to use such a facility.

## I. Initial Contact

|  | Facility I | Facility II | Facility III |
|---|---|---|---|
| Facility Name: | | | |
| Address: | | | |
| Distance from home: | | | |
| Mode of transportation to the facility: | | | |
| Travel time to the facility: | | | |
| Monthly fee: | | | |
| Hours of operation: | | | |
| Cardio equipment: | | | |
| Strength equipment: | | | |
| Flexibility equipment: | | | |
| Personal trainers, availability and costs: | | | |
| Personal trainers' certifications: | | | |
| Fitness tests, availability and costs: | | | |
| Exercise classes: | | | |
| Other services (nutrition, stress management, smoking cessation, cardiac profiles, etc.) | | | |
| Free trial of facility available? | | | |

## II. Facility Visit and Evaluation

1. Provide an overall impression of the facility:

_____

_____

2. Was the staff knowledgeable, accessible, and friendly?

_____

_____

3. Were you able to work out at the facility?  ___ Yes ___ No
   If so, was the equipment available and suitable to your preferences?

_____

_____

   Did you feel comfortable with other individuals using the facility (please indicate why or why not)?

_____

_____

4. Provide an overall evaluation of the locker facilities and other amenities available to you.

_____

_____

5. Overall letter grade for the facility:  A  B  C  D  E  F

## III. Ongoing educational program

1. Are there any other community resources available to you that would benefit your personal health, fitness, and wellness lifestyle program? Please list:

_____

_____

2. Contact at least one reliable health, fitness, nutrition, or wellness newsletter that you may subscribe to (see page 512) for a free copy and list the newsletter below. Also indicate if there are any other fitness/wellness materials that have provided valuable information to you.

_____

_____

3. List at least three reliable and helpful Web sites that you accessed this term and indicate why these sites were useful to you.

_____

_____

# LAB 15C: Self-Evaluation and Future Behavioral Goals

Name _____  Date _____  Grade _____

Instructor _____  Course _____  Section _____

## Necessary Lab Equipment
None required unless fitness tests are repeated.

## Objective
To conduct a self-evaluation of the goals achieved in this course and to write behavioral goals for the future.

## Lab Preparation
Review the section on SMART Goals in Chapter 2 (pages 55–58) prior to completing this lab. If time allows and technicians are available, repeat the assessments for the health-related components of fitness.

## I. Fitness Evaluation
Conduct a self-evaluation of the fitness goals you accomplished in this course. Fill in the required information on the health-related fitness components below. If you were unable to repeat your fitness assessments, subjectively determine how well you reached your goals.

1. Did you accomplish your goal for:

   Cardiorespiratory Endurance  (see Lab 6A) ☐ Yes ☐ No

   Pre-assessment $VO_{2max}$: ☐ mL/kg/min   Fitness Category: ☐

   Post-assessment $VO_{2max}$: ☐ mL/kg/min   Fitness Category: ☐

   Body Composition (see Labs 4A and 4B) ☐ Yes ☐ No

   Pre-assessment Percent Body Fat: ☐   Body Composition Category: ☐

   Post-assessment Percent Body Fat: ☐   Body Composition Category: ☐

   Muscular Strength and Endurance (see Lab 7A) ☐ Yes ☐ No

   Pre-assessment Percentile Total Points: ☐   Fitness Category: ☐

   Post-assessment Percentile Total Points: ☐   Fitness Category: ☐

   Muscular Flexibility (see Lab 8A) ☐ Yes ☐ No

   Pre-assessment Percentile Total Points: ☐   Fitness Category: ☐

   Post-assessment Percentile Total Points: ☐   Fitness Category: ☐

Current Number of Daily Steps: ☐   Activity category (see Table 1.2, page 10): ☐

II. Wellness Evaluation

Using the Wellness Compass, rate yourself for each component and plan goals for the future according to the following instructions:

1. Color in red a number from 5 to 1 to indicate where you stood on each component at the beginning of the semester (5 = poor rating, 1 = excellent or ideal rating).

2. Color in blue a second number from 5 to 1 to indicate where you stand on each component at the present time.

3. Select one or two components that you intend to work on in the next 2 months. Start with components in which you think you will have a high chance for success. Color in yellow the intended goal (number) to accomplish by the end of the 2 months. Once you achieve your goal, you later may color another number, also in yellow, to indicate your next goal.

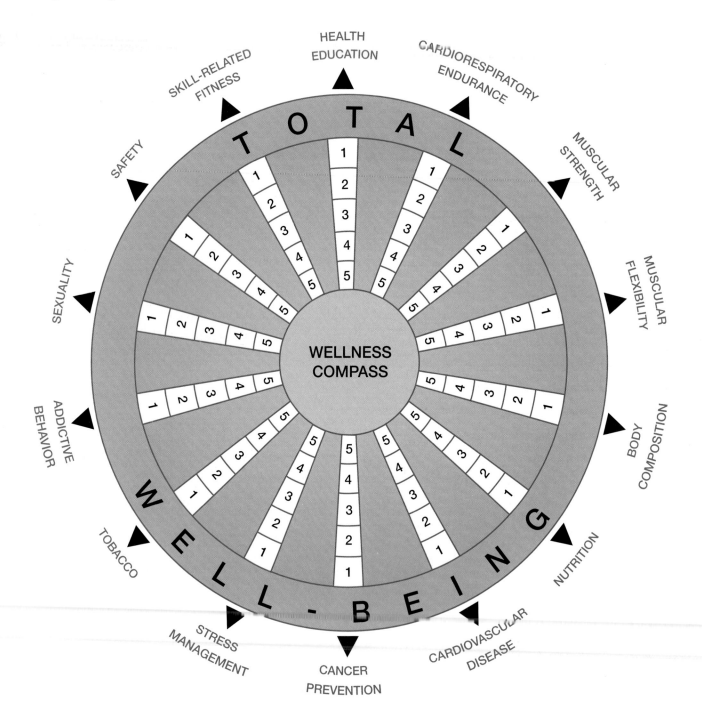

## III. Behavioral Goals for the Future

Identify one or two goals you will work on during the next couple of months and write specific objectives that you will use to accomplish each goal (you may not need six objectives; write only as many as needed).

Goal: _____

Objectives:

1. _____

2. _____

3. _____

4. _____

5. _____

6. _____

Goal: _____

Objectives:

1. _____

2. _____

3. _____

4. _____

5. _____

6. _____

## IV. This Course and Your Future Lifestyle

1. Briefly evaluate this course and its impact on your quality of life. Indicate what you feel will be needed for you to continue to adhere to an active and healthy lifestyle.

_____

_____

_____

_____

_____

_____

_____

_____

_____

2. Explain the exercise program that you implemented in this course, indicate your feelings about the outcomes of this program, and evaluate how well you accomplished your fitness goals.

_____

_____

_____

_____

_____

_____

_____

3. List nutritional or dietary changes that you were able to implement this term and the effects of these changes on your body composition and personal wellness.

_____

_____

_____

_____

_____

_____

4. List other lifestyle changes that you were able to make this term that may decrease your risk for disease. In a few sentences, explain how you feel about these changes and their impact on your overall well-being.

# APPENDIX A
# Nutritive Value of Selected Foods

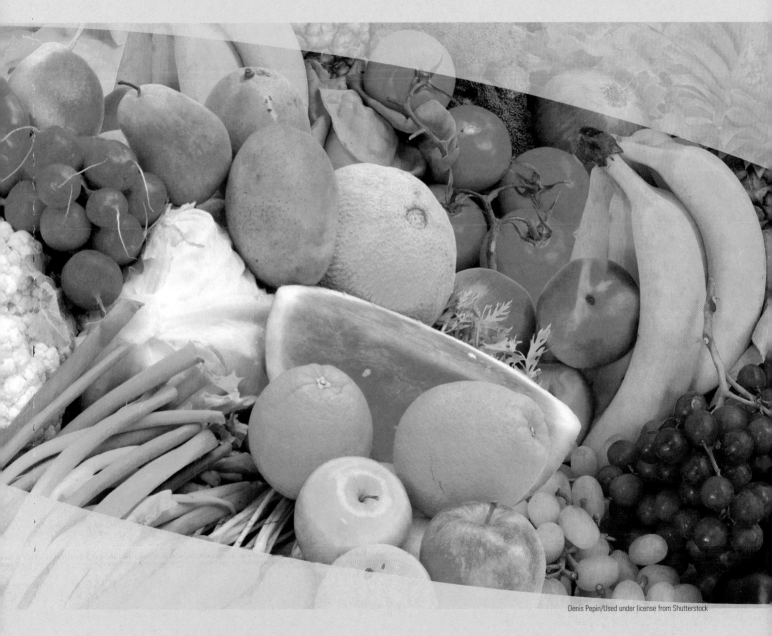

| Food Description | Qty | Measure | Wt (g) | Ener (cal) | Prot (g) | Carb (g) | Dietary Fiber (g) | Fat (g) | Sat | Mono | Poly | Trans | Chol (mg) | Calc (mg) | Iron (mg) | Sodi (mg) | Vit E (mg) | Folate (mcg) | Vit C (mg) | Selenium (mcg) |
|---|---|---|---|---|---|---|---|---|---|---|---|---|---|---|---|---|---|---|---|---|
| Almonds, dry roasted, no salt added | 1/4 | cup(s) | 35 | 206 | 8 | 7 | 4 | 18 | 1.40 | 11.61 | 4.36 | — | 0 | 92 | 1.56 | <1 | 8.97 | 11 | 0 | 1 |
| Apple juice, unsweetened, canned | 1/2 | cup(s) | 124 | 58 | <1 | 14 | <1 | <1 | 0.02 | 0.01 | 0.04 | — | 0 | 9 | 0.46 | 4 | 0.01 | 0 | 1 | <1 |
| Apples, raw medium, w/peel | 1 | item(s) | 138 | 72 | <1 | 19 | 3 | <1 | 0.04 | 0.01 | 0.07 | — | 0 | 8 | 0.17 | 4 | — | 4 | 6 | 0 |
| Applesauce, sweetened, canned | 1/2 | cup(s) | 128 | 97 | <1 | 25 | 2 | <1 | 0.04 | 0.01 | 0.07 | — | 0 | 5 | 0.45 | 4 | 0.27 | 1 | 2 | <1 |
| Apricot, fresh w/o pits | 4 | item(s) | 140 | 67 | 2 | 16 | 3 | 1 | 0.04 | 0.24 | 0.11 | — | 0 | 18 | 0.55 | 5 | 1.25 | 13 | 14 | <1 |
| Apricot, halves w/skin, canned in heavy syrup | 1/2 | cup(s) | 129 | 107 | 2 | 28 | 2 | <1 | 0.01 | 0.04 | 0.02 | — | 0 | 12 | 0.39 | 5 | 0.77 | 3 | 4 | <1 |
| Asparagus, boiled, drained | 1/2 | cup(s) | 90 | 20 | 2 | 4 | 2 | 0.19 | 0.06 | 0 | 0.12 | — | 0 | 20.7 | 0.81 | 12.6 | 1.35 | 134.1 | 6.92 | 5.48 |
| Avocado, California, whole, w/o skin or pit | 1 | item(s) | 170 | 284 | 3 | 15 | 12 | 26 | 3.59 | 16.61 | 3.42 | — | 0 | 22 | 1.00 | 14 | 3.35 | 105 | 15 | 1 |
| Bacon, cured, broiled, pan fried, or roasted | 2 | slice(s) | 13 | 68 | 5 | <1 | 0 | 5 | 1.73 | 2.33 | 0.57 | 0 | 14 | 1 | 0.18 | 291 | 0.04 | <1 | 0 | 8 |
| Bagel chips, plain | 3 | item(s) | 29 | 130 | 3 | 19 | 1 | 5 | 0.50 | — | — | — | 0 | 0 | 0.72 | 70 | — | 0 | 0 | — |
| Bagel, plain, enriched, toasted | 1 | item(s) | 66 | 195 | 7 | 38 | 2 | 1 | 0.16 | 0.09 | 0.49 | 0 | 0 | 53 | 2.52 | 379 | 0.08 | 64 | 0 | 23 |
| Banana, fresh whole, w/o peel | 1 | item(s) | 118 | 105 | 1 | 27 | 3 | <1 | 0.13 | 0.04 | 0.09 | — | 0 | 6 | 0.31 | 1 | 0.12 | 24 | 10 | 1 |
| Beans, black, boiled | 1/2 | cup(s) | 86 | 114 | 8 | 20 | 7 | <1 | 0.12 | 0.04 | 0.20 | — | 0 | 23 | 1.81 | 1 | — | 128 | 0 | 1 |
| Beans, Fordhook lima, frozen, boiled, drained | 1/2 | cup(s) | 85 | 88 | 5 | 16 | 5 | <1 | 0.07 | 0.02 | 0.14 | — | 0 | 26 | 1.55 | 59 | 0.25 | 18 | 11 | 1 |
| Beans, mung, sprouted, boiled, drained | 1/2 | cup(s) | 62 | 13 | 1 | 3 | <1 | <1 | 0.02 | 0.00 | 0.02 | — | 0 | 7 | 0.40 | 6 | 0.04 | 18 | 7 | <1 |
| Beans, red kidney, canned | 1/2 | cup(s) | 128 | 109 | 7 | 20 | 8 | <1 | 0.06 | 0.03 | 0.24 | — | 0 | 31 | 1.61 | 436 | 0.77 | 65 | 2 | 2 |
| Beans, refried, canned | 1/2 | cup(s) | 127 | 119 | 7 | 20 | 7 | 2 | 0.60 | 0.71 | 0.19 | — | 10 | 44 | 2.10 | 378 | 0.30 | 14 | 8 | 2 |
| Beans, yellow snap, string or wax, boiled, drained | 1/2 | cup(s) | 62 | 22 | 1 | 5 | 2 | <1 | 0.04 | 0.00 | 0.09 | — | 0 | 29 | 0.80 | 2 | 0.28 | 21 | 6 | <1 |
| Beef, chuck, arm pot roast, lean & fat, 1/4" fat, braised | 3 | ounce(s) | 85 | 282 | 23 | 0 | 0 | 20 | 7.97 | 8.68 | 0.77 | — | 84 | 9 | 2.64 | 51 | 0.19 | 8 | 0 | 21 |
| Beef, corned, canned | 3 | ounce(s) | 85 | 213 | 23 | 0 | 0 | 13 | 5.25 | 5.07 | 0.54 | — | 73 | 10 | 1.77 | 855 | 0.13 | 8 | 0 | 36 |
| Beef, ground, lean, broiled, well | 3 | ounce(s) | 85 | 238 | 24 | 0 | 0 | 15 | 5.89 | 6.56 | 0.56 | — | 86 | 10 | 2.08 | 76 | 0.09 | 9 | 0 | 22 |
| Beef, ground, regular, broiled, medium | 3 | ounce(s) | 85 | 246 | 20 | 0 | 0 | 18 | 6.91 | 7.70 | 0.65 | — | 77 | 9 | 2.07 | 71 | — | 8 | 0 | 16 |
| Beef, liver, pan fried | 3 | ounce(s) | 85 | 149 | 23 | 4 | 0 | 4 | 1.27 | 0.56 | 0.49 | 0.17 | 324 | 5 | 5.24 | 65 | 0.39 | 221 | 1 | 28 |
| Beef, rib steak, small end, lean, 1/4" fat, broiled | 3 | ounce(s) | 85 | 188 | 24 | 0 | 0 | 10 | 3.84 | 4.01 | 0.27 | — | 68 | 11 | 2.18 | 59 | 0.12 | 7 | 0 | 19 |
| Beef, rib, whole, lean & fat, 1/4" fat, roasted | 3 | ounce(s) | 85 | 320 | 19 | 0 | 0 | 27 | 10.71 | 11.42 | 0.94 | — | 72 | 9 | 1.96 | 54 | — | 6 | 0 | 19 |
| Beef, short loin, T-bone steak, lean, 1/4" fat, broiled | 3 | ounce(s) | 85 | 174 | 23 | 0 | 0 | 9 | 3.05 | 4.23 | 0.26 | — | 50 | 5 | 3.11 | 65 | 0.12 | 7 | 0 | 9 |
| Beer | 12 | fluid ounce(s) | 354 | 118 | 1 | 6 | <1 | <1 | 0.00 | 0.00 | 0.00 | 0 | 0 | 18 | 0.07 | 14 | 0.00 | 21 | 0 | 2 |
| Beer, light | 12 | fluid ounce(s) | 354 | 99 | 1 | 5 | 0 | 0 | 0.00 | 0.00 | 0.00 | 0 | 0 | 18 | 0.14 | 11 | 0.00 | 14 | 0 | 2 |
| Beets, sliced, canned, drained | 1/2 | cup(s) | 85 | 26 | 1 | 6 | 1 | <1 | 0.02 | 0.02 | 0.04 | 0 | 0 | 13 | 1.55 | 165 | 0.03 | 26 | 3 | <1 |
| Biscuits | 1 | item(s) | 41 | 121 | 3 | 16 | 1 | 5 | 1.40 | 1.41 | 1.82 | 0 | <1 | 33 | 1.01 | 205 | 0.01 | 26 | 0 | 7 |
| Blueberries, raw | 1/2 | cup(s) | 72 | 41 | 1 | 10 | 2 | <1 | 0.02 | 0.03 | 0.11 | — | 0 | 4 | 0.20 | 1 | 0.41 | 4 | 7 | <1 |
| Bologna, beef | 1 | slice(s) | 28 | 90 | 3 | 1 | 0 | 8 | 3.50 | 4.26 | 0.31 | — | 20 | 4 | 0.36 | 310 | — | 4 | 0 | — |
| Bologna, turkey | 1 | slice(s) | 28 | 50 | 3 | 1 | 0 | 4 | 1.00 | 1.09 | 0.98 | — | 20 | 40 | 0.36 | 270 | — | 0 | 0 | — |
| Brazil nuts, unblanched, dried | 1/4 | cup(s) | 35 | 230 | 5 | 4 | 3 | 23 | 5.30 | 8.59 | 7.20 | — | 0 | 56 | 0.85 | 1 | 2.01 | 8 | <1 | 671 |
| Bread, cracked wheat | 1 | slice(s) | 25 | 65 | 2 | 12 | 1 | 1 | 0.23 | 0.48 | 0.17 | — | 0 | 11 | 0.70 | 135 | — | 15 | 0 | 6 |
| Bread, French | 1 | slice(s) | 25 | 69 | 2 | 13 | 1 | 1 | 0.16 | 0.30 | 0.17 | — | 0 | 19 | 0.63 | 152 | 0.08 | 37 | 0 | 8 |
| Bread, mixed grain | 1 | slice(s) | 26 | 65 | 3 | 12 | 2 | 1 | 0.21 | 0.40 | 0.24 | — | 0 | 24 | 0.90 | 127 | 0.05 | 31 | <1 | 8 |
| Bread, pita | 1 | item(s) | 60 | 165 | 5 | 33 | 1 | 1 | 0.10 | 0.06 | 0.32 | — | 0 | 52 | 1.57 | 322 | 0.18 | 64 | 0 | 16 |
| Bread, pumpernickel | 1 | slice(s) | 32 | 80 | 3 | 15 | 2 | 1 | 0.14 | 0.30 | 0.40 | — | 0 | 22 | 0.92 | 215 | 0.13 | 30 | 0 | 8 |
| Bread, rye | 1 | slice(s) | 32 | 83 | 3 | 15 | 2 | 1 | 0.20 | 0.42 | 0.26 | — | 0 | 23 | 0.91 | 211 | 0.11 | 35 | <1 | 10 |
| Bread, white | 1 | slice(s) | 25 | 67 | 2 | 13 | 1 | 1 | 0.18 | 0.17 | 0.34 | — | 0 | 38 | 0.94 | 170 | 0.09 | 28 | 0 | 4 |
| Bread, whole wheat | 1 | slice(s) | 46 | 128 | 4 | 24 | 3 | 2 | 0.37 | 0.53 | 1.35 | — | 0 | 15 | 1.43 | 159 | 0.35 | 30 | 0 | 18 |
| Broccoli, chopped, boiled, drained | 1/2 | cup(s) | 78 | 27 | 2 | 6 | 3 | <1 | 0.06 | 0.03 | 0.13 | — | 0 | 31 | 0.52 | 32 | 1.13 | 84 | 51 | 1 |
| Brownie, prepared from mix | 1 | item(s) | 24 | 112 | 1 | 12 | 1 | 7 | 1.76 | 2.60 | 2.26 | — | 18 | 14 | 0.44 | 82 | 0.34 | 7 | <1 | 3 |
| Brussels sprouts, boiled, drained | 1/2 | cup(s) | 78 | 28 | 2 | 6 | 2 | <1 | 0.08 | 0.03 | 0.09 | — | 0 | 28 | 0.94 | 16 | 0.34 | 47 | 48 | 1 |
| Bulgur, cooked | 1/2 | cup(s) | 91 | 76 | 3 | 17 | 4 | <1 | 0.04 | 0.03 | 0.09 | — | 0 | 9 | 0.87 | 5 | 0.01 | 16 | 0 | 1 |
| Buns, hamburger, plain | 1 | item(s) | 43 | 120 | 4 | 21 | 1 | 2 | 0.47 | 0.48 | 0.85 | — | 0 | 59 | 1.43 | 206 | 0.03 | 48 | 0 | 8 |
| Butter | 1 | tablespoon(s) | 15 | 108 | <1 | <1 | 0 | 12 | 6.13 | 5.00 | 0.43 | — | 32 | 4 | 0.00 | 86 | 0.35 | <1 | 0 | <1 |
| Buttermilk, low fat | 1 | cup(s) | 245 | 98 | 8 | 12 | 0 | 2 | 1.34 | 0.62 | 0.08 | — | 10 | 284 | 0.12 | 257 | 0.12 | 12 | 2 | 5 |
| Cabbage, boiled, drained, no salt added | 1 | cup(s) | 150 | 33 | 2 | 7 | 3 | 1 | 0.08 | 0.05 | 0.29 | — | 0 | 47 | 0.26 | 12 | 0.18 | 30 | 30 | 1 |
| Cabbage, raw, shredded | 1 | cup(s) | 70 | 17 | 1 | 4 | 2 | <1 | 0.01 | 0.01 | 0.04 | — | 0 | 33 | 0.41 | 13 | 0.10 | 30 | 23 | 1 |

| Food | Amount | Unit | Wt (g) | Cal | Prot (g) | Carb (g) | Fiber (g) | Fat (g) | Sat (g) | Mono (g) | Poly (g) | Trans (g) | Chol (mg) | Vit A (RE) | Iron (mg) | Sod (mg) | Vit E (mg) | Calc (mg) | Vit C (mg) | Fol (μg) |
|---|---|---|---|---|---|---|---|---|---|---|---|---|---|---|---|---|---|---|---|---|
| Cake, angel food, from mix | 1 | slice(s) | 50 | 129 | 3 | 29 | <1 | <1 | 0.02 | 0.01 | 0.06 | — | 0 | 42 | 0.12 | 255 | 0.00 | 10 | 0 | 8 |
| Cake, butter pound, ready to eat commercially prepared | 1 | slice(s) | 75 | 291 | 4 | 37 | <1 | 15 | 8.67 | 4.43 | 0.80 | — | 166 | 26 | 1.04 | 299 | — | 0 | <1 | — |
| Cake, carrot, cream cheese frosting, from mix | 1 | slice(s) | 111 | 484 | 5 | 52 | 1 | 29 | 5.43 | 7.24 | 15.10 | — | 60 | 28 | 1.39 | 273 | — | 13 | 1 | — |
| Cake, chocolate, chocolate icing, commercially prepared | 1 | slice(s) | 64 | 235 | 3 | 35 | 2 | 10 | 3.05 | 5.61 | 1.18 | — | 27 | 28 | 1.41 | 214 | — | 11 | <1 | 2 |
| Cake, devil's food cupcake, chocolate frosting | 1 | item(s) | 35 | 120 | 2 | 20 | 1 | 4 | 1.80 | 1.60 | 0.60 | — | 19 | 21 | 0.70 | 92 | — | 2 | 0 | 2 |
| Cake, white, coconut frosting, from mix | 1 | slice(s) | 112 | 399 | 5 | 71 | 1 | 12 | 4.36 | 4.14 | 2.42 | — | 1 | 101 | 1.30 | 318 | 0.13 | 35 | <1 | 12 |
| Candy, Almond Joy bar | 1 | item(s) | 49 | 240 | 2 | 29 | 2 | 13 | 9.00 | 3.63 | 0.74 | 0 | 3 | 20 | 0.36 | 70 | — | 3 | 0 | — |
| Candy, Life Savers | 1 | item(s) | 2 | 8 | 0 | 2 | 0 | <1 | 0.00 | — | — | 0 | 0 | <1 | 0.04 | 1 | — | — | 0 | 0 |
| Candy, M & Ms peanut chocolate candy, small bag | 1 | item(s) | 49 | 250 | 5 | 30 | 2 | 13 | 5.00 | 5.42 | 2.07 | — | 5 | 40 | 0.36 | 25 | — | 17 | 1 | 2 |
| Candy, M & Ms plain chocolate candy, small bag | 1 | item(s) | 48 | 240 | 2 | 34 | 1 | 10 | 6.00 | 3.30 | 0.30 | — | 5 | 40 | 0.36 | 30 | — | 3 | 1 | 1 |
| Candy, milk chocolate bar | 1 | item(s) | 91 | 483 | 8 | 53 | 2 | 28 | 16.69 | 7.20 | 0.63 | — | 22 | 228 | 0.83 | 92 | — | 11 | 2 | — |
| Candy, Milky Way bar | 1 | item(s) | 58 | 270 | 2 | 41 | 1 | 10 | 5.00 | 3.50 | 0.35 | — | 5 | 60 | 0.18 | 95 | — | 6 | 1 | 3 |
| Candy, Reese's peanut butter cups | 2 | piece(s) | 45 | 250 | 5 | 25 | 1 | 14 | 5.00 | 6.17 | 2.34 | 0 | 3 | 20 | 0.36 | 140 | — | 25 | 0 | 2 |
| Candy, Special Dark chocolate bar | 1 | item(s) | 41 | 220 | 2 | 24 | 3 | 13 | 8.00 | 4.59 | 0.41 | 0 | 3 | 0 | 0.72 | 0 | — | 1 | 0 | 1 |
| Candy, Starburst fruit chews, original fruits | 1 | package | 59 | 240 | 0 | 48 | 0 | 5 | 1.00 | 2.10 | 1.83 | 0 | 0 | 10 | 0.18 | 0 | — | 0 | 30 | <1 |
| Candy, York peppermint patty | 1 | item(s) | 42 | 170 | 1 | 34 | 1 | 3 | 2.00 | 1.32 | 0.12 | 0 | 0 | 0 | 0.36 | 10 | — | 2 | 0 | — |
| Cantaloupe | ½ | cup(s) | 80 | 27 | 1 | 7 | 1 | <1 | 0.04 | 0.00 | 0.07 | — | 0 | 7 | 0.17 | 13 | 0.04 | 17 | 30 | <1 |
| Carrots, raw | ½ | cup(s) | 61 | 25 | 1 | 6 | 2 | <1 | 0.02 | 0.01 | 0.06 | 0 | 0 | 20 | 0.18 | 42 | 0.40 | 12 | 4 | <1 |
| Carrots, sliced, boiled, drained | ½ | cup(s) | 78 | 27.29 | 0.59 | 6.41 | 2.33 | 0.14 | 0.02 | 0 | 0.08 | — | 0 | 23.39 | 0.26 | 45.24 | 0.80 | 10.92 | 2.8 | 0.54 |
| Cashews, dry roasted | ¼ | cup(s) | 34 | 197 | 5 | 11 | 1 | 16 | 3.14 | 9.36 | 2.68 | — | 0 | 15 | 2.06 | 5 | 0.32 | 24 | 0 | 4 |
| Catsup/ketchup | 1 | tablespoon(s) | 15 | 14 | <1 | 4 | <1 | <1 | 0.01 | 0.01 | 0.04 | — | 0 | 3 | 0.08 | 167 | 0.22 | 2 | 2 | <1 |
| Cauliflower, boiled, drained | ½ | cup(s) | 62 | 14 | 1 | 3 | 2 | <1 | 0.04 | 0.02 | 0.13 | — | 0 | 10 | 0.20 | 9 | 0.04 | 27 | 27 | <1 |
| Celery, stalk | 2 | item(s) | 80 | 11 | 1 | 2 | 1 | <1 | 0.03 | 0.03 | 0.06 | — | 0 | 32 | 0.16 | 64 | 0.22 | 29 | 2 | <1 |
| Cereal, All-Bran | 1 | cup(s) | 62 | 160 | 8 | 46 | 20 | 2 | 0.00 | 0.00 | 1.00 | 0 | 0 | 300 | 9.00 | 160 | — | 800 | 12 | 6 |
| Cereal, All-Bran Buds | 1 | cup(s) | 91 | 212 | 6 | 73 | 42 | 3 | — | — | — | 0 | 0 | 0 | 13.64 | 606 | — | 1212 | 18 | 26 |
| Cereal, Bran Flakes, Post | 1 | cup(s) | 40 | 133 | 4 | 32 | 7 | 1 | 0.00 | 0.00 | 0.71 | — | 0 | 5 | 10.77 | 293 | — | 133 | 0 | — |
| Cereal, Cap'n Crunch | 1 | cup(s) | 36 | 144 | 2 | 30 | 1 | 2 | 0.53 | 0.39 | 0.27 | — | 0 | 5 | 6.00 | 269 | — | 133 | 0 | 7 |
| Cereal, Cheerios | 1 | cup(s) | 30 | 110 | 3 | 22 | 3 | 2 | 0.00 | 0.50 | 0.50 | — | 0 | 100 | 8.10 | 280 | — | 200 | 6 | 11 |
| Cereal, Complete wheat bran flakes | 1 | cup(s) | 39 | 120 | 4 | 31 | 7 | 1 | — | — | — | 0 | 0 | 0 | 23.94 | 279 | — | 532 | 80 | 4 |
| Cereal, Corn Flakes | 1 | cup(s) | 28 | 100 | 2 | 24 | 1 | 0 | 0.00 | 0.00 | 0.00 | 0 | 0 | 0 | 8.10 | 200 | — | 100 | 6 | 1 |
| Cereal, Corn Pops | 1 | cup(s) | 31 | 120 | 1 | 28 | 0 | 0 | 0.00 | 0.00 | 0.00 | 0 | 0 | 0 | 1.80 | 120 | — | 100 | 6 | 2 |
| Cereal, Cracklin' Oat Bran | 1 | cup(s) | 65 | 266 | 5 | 47 | 7 | 9 | 2.70 | 4.70 | 1.33 | 0 | 0 | 27 | 2.38 | 186 | — | 218 | 20 | 14 |
| Cereal, Cream of Wheat, instant, prepared | ½ | cup(s) | 121 | 61 | 2 | 13 | <1 | <1 | 0.01 | 0.01 | 0.04 | 0 | 0 | 27 | 8.60 | 1 | — | 357 | 0 | — |
| Cereal, Frosted Flakes | 1 | cup(s) | 41 | 160 | 1 | 37 | 1 | 0 | 0.00 | 0.00 | 0.00 | 0 | 0 | 0 | 5.99 | 200 | — | 133 | 8 | 2 |
| Cereal, Frosted Mini-Wheats | 5 | item(s) | 51 | 180 | 5 | 41 | 5 | 1 | 0.00 | 0.00 | 0.50 | 0 | 0 | 0 | 15.30 | 5 | — | 100 | 0 | 2 |
| Cereal, granola, prepared | ½ | cup(s) | 61 | 299 | 9 | 32 | 5 | 15 | 2.76 | 4.7 | 6.53 | — | 0 | 48 | 2.59 | 13 | 3.59 | 51 | 1 | 16.95 |
| Cereal, Kashi puffed | 1 | cup(s) | 25 | 70 | 3 | 13 | 2 | 1 | 0.00 | — | — | — | 0 | 0 | 0.72 | 0 | — | — | 0 | — |
| Cereal, Life | 1 | cup(s) | 43 | 160 | 4 | 33 | 3 | 2 | 0.35 | 0.64 | 0.61 | — | 0 | 124 | 11.92 | 218 | — | 142 | 0 | 11 |
| Cereal, Multi-Bran Chex | 1 | cup(s) | 58 | 200 | 4 | 49 | 7 | 2 | 0.00 | 0.00 | 0.00 | 0 | 0 | 100 | 16.20 | 390 | — | 100 | 6 | 5 |
| Cereal, Nutri-Grain golden wheat | 1 | cup(s) | 40 | 133 | 4 | 31 | 5 | 1 | 0.00 | 0.00 | 0.67 | — | 0 | 0 | 1.46 | 279 | — | 133 | 20 | 9 |
| Cereal, oatmeal, cooked w/water | ½ | cup(s) | 117 | 74 | 3 | 13 | 2 | 1 | 0.19 | 0.37 | 0.44 | — | 0 | 9 | 0.80 | 1 | 0.12 | 5 | 0 | 9 |
| Cereal, Product 19 | 1 | cup(s) | 30 | 100 | 2 | 25 | 1 | 0 | 0.00 | 0.00 | 0.00 | 0 | 0 | 0 | 18.00 | 210 | — | 400 | 60 | 4 |
| Cereal, Raisin Bran | 1 | cup(s) | 59 | 190 | 4 | 47 | 8 | 1 | 0.00 | 0.10 | 0.36 | — | 0 | 20 | 10.80 | 300 | — | 140 | 0 | — |
| Cereal, Rice Chex | 1 | cup(s) | 25 | 96 | 2 | 22 | <1 | 0 | 0.00 | 0.00 | 0.00 | 0 | 0 | 80 | 7.20 | 232 | — | 160 | 5 | 1 |
| Cereal, Rice Krispies | 1 | cup(s) | 26 | 96 | 2 | 23 | 0 | 0 | 0.00 | 0.00 | 0.00 | 0 | 0 | 0 | 1.44 | 256 | — | 80 | 5 | 4 |
| Cereal, Shredded Wheat | 1 | cup(s) | 25 | 88 | 3 | 20 | 3 | 1 | 0.04 | 0.01 | 0.10 | — | 0 | 10 | 1.08 | 2 | — | 12 | 0 | 1 |
| Cereal, Smacks | 1 | cup(s) | 36 | 133 | 3 | 32 | 1 | 1 | 0.00 | 0.00 | 0.00 | — | 0 | 0 | 0.48 | 67 | — | 133 | 8 | 17 |
| Cereal, Special K | 1 | cup(s) | 31 | 110 | 7 | 22 | 1 | 0 | 0.00 | 0.00 | 0.00 | 0 | 0 | 0 | 8.70 | 220 | — | 400 | 15 | 7 |
| Cereal, Total whole grain | 1 | cup(s) | 40 | 146 | 3 | 31 | 4 | 1 | 0.00 | 0.00 | 0.00 | — | 0 | 1330 | 23.94 | 253 | 31.24 | 532 | 80 | 2 |
| Cereal, Wheaties | 1 | cup(s) | 30 | 110 | 3 | 24 | 3 | 1 | 0.00 | 0.00 | 0.00 | — | 0 | 0 | 8.10 | 220 | 2.26 | 200 | 6 | 1 |
| Cheese, American, processed | 1 | ounce(s) | 28 | 106 | 6 | <1 | 0 | 9 | 5.58 | 2.54 | 0.28 | — | 27 | 156 | 0.05 | 422 | 0.08 | 2 | 0 | 4 |
| Cheese, blue, crumbled | 1 | ounce(s) | 28 | 100 | 6 | 1 | 0 | 8 | 5.29 | 2.21 | 0.23 | — | 21 | 150 | 0.09 | 395 | 0.07 | 10 | 0 | 4 |
| Cheese, cheddar, shredded | ¼ | cup(s) | 28 | 114 | 7 | <1 | 0 | 9 | 5.96 | 2.65 | 0.27 | — | 30 | 204 | 0.19 | 175 | 0.08 | 5 | 0 | 4 |
| Cheese, feta | 1 | ounce(s) | 28 | 74 | 4 | 1 | 0 | 6 | 4.18 | 1.29 | 0.17 | — | 25 | 138 | 0.18 | 312 | 0.05 | 9 | 0 | 4 |
| Cheese, Monterey jack | 1 | ounce(s) | 28 | 104 | 7 | <1 | 0 | 8 | 5.34 | 2.45 | 0.25 | — | 25 | 209 | 0.20 | 150 | 0.07 | 5 | 0 | 4 |

| Food Description | Qty | Measure | Wt (g) | Ener (cal) | Prot (g) | Carb (g) | Dietary Fiber (g) | Fat (g) | Sat | Mono | Poly | Trans | Chol (mg) | Calc (mg) | Iron (mg) | Sodi (mg) | Vit E (mg) | Folate (mcg) | Vit C (mg) | Selenium (mcg) |
|---|---|---|---|---|---|---|---|---|---|---|---|---|---|---|---|---|---|---|---|---|
| Cheese, mozzarella, part skim milk | 1 | ounce(s) | 28 | 71 | 7 | 1 | 0 | 4 | 2.83 | 1.26 | 0.13 | — | 18 | 219 | 0.06 | 173 | 0.04 | 3 | 0 | 4 |
| Cheese, Parmesan, grated | 1 | tablespoon(s) | 5 | 22 | 2 | <1 | 0 | 1 | 0.87 | 0.42 | 0.06 | — | 4 | 55 | 0.05 | 76 | 0.01 | 1 | 0 | 1 |
| Cheese, ricotta, part skim milk | 1/4 | cup(s) | 62 | 85 | 7 | 3 | 0 | 5 | 3.03 | 1.42 | 0.16 | — | 19 | 167 | 0.27 | 77 | 0.04 | 8 | 0 | 10 |
| Cheese, Swiss | 1 | ounce(s) | 28 | 106 | 8 | 2 | 0 | 8 | 4.98 | 2.04 | 0.27 | — | 26 | 221 | 0.06 | 54 | 0.11 | 2 | 0 | 5 |
| Cherries, sweet, raw | 1/2 | cup(s) | 73 | 46 | 1 | 12 | 2 | <1 | 0.03 | 0.03 | 0.04 | — | 0 | 9 | 0.26 | 0 | 0.05 | 3 | 5 | 0 |
| Chicken, broiler breast, meat & skin, flour coated, fried | 3 | ounce(s) | 85 | 189 | 27 | 1 | <1 | 8 | 2.08 | 2.98 | 1.67 | — | 76 | 14 | 1.01 | 65 | — | 5 | 0 | 20 |
| Chicken, broiler drumstick, meat & skin, flour coated, fried | 3 | ounce(s) | 85 | 208 | 23 | 1 | <1 | 12 | 3.11 | 4.61 | 2.75 | — | 77 | 10 | 1.14 | 76 | — | 9 | 0 | 16 |
| Chicken, light meat, roasted | 3 | ounce(s) | 85 | 130 | 23 | 0 | 0 | 3 | 0.92 | 1.29 | 0.79 | — | 64 | 11 | 0.92 | 43 | 0.23 | 3 | 0 | 22 |
| Chicken, roasted (meat only) | 3 | ounce(s) | 85 | 142 | 21 | 0 | 0 | 6 | 1.54 | 2.13 | 1.28 | — | 64 | 10 | 1.03 | 64 | — | 4 | 0 | 21 |
| Chickpeas or bengal gram, garbanzo beans, boiled | 1/2 | cup(s) | 82 | 134 | 7 | 22 | 6 | 2 | 0.22 | 0.48 | 0.95 | — | 0 | 40 | 2.37 | 6 | 0.29 | 141 | 1 | 3 |
| Chocolate milk, low fat | 1 | cup(s) | 250 | 158 | 8 | 26 | 1 | 3 | 1.54 | 0.75 | 0.09 | — | 8 | 288 | 0.60 | 153 | 0.05 | 13 | 2 | 5 |
| Cilantro | 1 | teaspoon(s) | 2 | <1 | <1 | <1 | <1 | <1 | 0.00 | 0.00 | 0.00 | — | 0 | 1 | 0.03 | 1 | — | 13 | 1 | <1 |
| Cocoa, hot, prepared w/milk | 1 | cup(s) | 250 | 193 | 9 | 27 | 3 | 6 | 3.58 | 1.69 | 0.09 | 0.18 | 20 | 263 | 1.20 | 110 | 0.38 | 13 | 1 | 7 |
| Coconut, dried, not sweetened | 1/4 | cup(s) | 60 | 393 | 4 | 14 | 10 | 38 | 34.06 | 1.63 | 0.42 | — | 0 | 15 | 1.98 | 22 | 0.26 | 5 | <1 | 11 |
| Cod, Atlantic cod or scrod, baked or broiled | 3 | ounce(s) | 44 | 46 | 10 | 0 | 0 | <1 | 0.07 | 0.05 | 0.13 | — | 24 | 6 | 0.22 | 35 | 0.02 | 5 | <1 | 17 |
| Coffee, brewed | 8 | fluid ounce(s) | 237 | 9 | <1 | 0 | 0 | <1 | 0.00 | 0.00 | 0.00 | — | 0 | 2 | 0.02 | 2 | 0.02 | 5 | 0 | 0 |
| Collard greens, boiled, drained | 1/2 | cup(s) | 95 | 25 | 2 | 5 | 3 | <1 | 0.04 | 0.02 | 0.16 | — | 0 | 133 | 1.10 | 15 | 0.34 | 88 | 17 | <1 |
| Cookies, animal crackers | 12 | piece(s) | 30 | 134 | 2 | 22 | <1 | 4 | 1.03 | 2.29 | 0.56 | — | 0 | 13 | 0.82 | 15 | 0.04 | 50 | 0 | 4 |
| Cookies, chocolate chip | 1 | item(s) | 30 | 140 | 2 | 16 | 1 | 8 | 2.09 | 3.26 | 2.09 | — | 13 | 11 | 0.70 | 109 | 0.54 | 16 | 0 | <1 |
| Cookies, chocolate sandwich, extra crème filling | 1 | item(s) | 13 | 65 | <1 | 9 | <1 | 3 | 0.50 | 1.39 | 1.22 | 1.10 | 0 | 3 | 0.37 | 64 | 0.25 | 6 | 0 | <1 |
| Cookies, Fig Newtons | 1 | item(s) | 16 | 55 | 1 | 10 | 1 | 1 | 0.50 | 0.50 | 0.00 | 0.50 | 0 | 5 | 0.36 | 60 | — | — | <1 | — |
| Cookies, oatmeal | 1 | item(s) | 69 | 234 | 6 | 45 | 3 | 4 | 0.70 | 1.28 | 1.85 | 0 | <1 | 26 | 1.94 | 311 | 0.23 | 30 | <1 | 17 |
| Cookies, peanut butter | 1 | item(s) | 35 | 163 | 4 | 17 | 1 | 9 | 1.65 | 4.72 | 2.43 | 0 | 13 | 28 | 0.67 | 157 | 0.74 | 21 | <1 | 5 |
| Cookies, sugar | 1 | item(s) | 16 | 61 | 1 | 7 | <1 | 3 | 0.63 | 1.27 | 0.87 | 0 | 18 | 5 | 0.32 | 50 | 0.28 | 5 | <1 | 3 |
| Corn, yellow sweet, frozen, boiled, drained | 1/2 | cup(s) | 82 | 66 | 2 | 16 | 2 | 1 | 0.08 | 0.16 | 0.26 | 0 | 0 | 2 | 0.39 | 1 | 0.06 | 29 | 3 | 1 |
| Cornbread | 1 | piece(s) | 55 | 141 | 2 | 18 | 1 | 5 | 2.09 | 1.44 | 1.50 | 0 | 21 | 88 | 1.01 | 209 | 0.33 | 36 | 2 | 6 |
| Cornmeal, yellow whole grain | 1/2 | cup(s) | 61 | 221 | 5 | 47 | 4 | 2 | 0.31 | 0.58 | 1.00 | — | 0 | 4 | 2.10 | 21 | 0.26 | 15 | 0 | 9 |
| Cottage cheese, low fat, 1% fat | 1/2 | cup(s) | 113 | 81 | 14 | 3 | 0 | 1 | 0.73 | 0.33 | 0.04 | — | 5 | 69 | 0.16 | 459 | 0.21 | 14 | 0 | 10 |
| Cottage cheese, low fat, 2% fat | 1/2 | cup(s) | 113 | 102 | 16 | 4 | 0 | 2 | 1.38 | 0.62 | 0.07 | — | 9 | 78 | 0.18 | 459 | 0.22 | 15 | 0 | 12 |
| Crab, blue, canned | 2 | ounce(s) | 57 | 56 | 12 | 0 | 0 | 1 | 0.14 | 0.12 | 0.25 | — | 50 | 57 | 0.48 | 189 | 1.04 | 24 | 2 | 18 |
| Crackers, cheese (mini) | 30 | item(s) | 30 | 151 | 3 | 17 | 1 | 8 | 2.81 | 3.63 | 0.74 | — | 4 | 45 | 1.43 | 299 | 0.56 | 46 | 0 | 3 |
| Crackers, honey graham | 4 | item(s) | 28 | 118 | 2 | 22 | 1 | 3 | 0.43 | 1.14 | 1.07 | — | 0 | 7 | 1.04 | 169 | 0.06 | 13 | 0 | 3 |
| Crackers, matzo, plain | 1 | ounce(s) | 28 | 112 | 3 | 24 | 1 | <1 | 0.06 | 0.04 | 0.17 | — | 0 | 4 | 0.90 | 1 | 0.02 | 5 | 0 | 10 |
| Crackers, Ritz | 5 | item(s) | 16 | 80 | 1 | 10 | <1 | 4 | 0.50 | 1.50 | 0.00 | — | 0 | 20 | 0.72 | 135 | — | 10 | 1 | — |
| Crackers, rye crispbread | 1 | item(s) | 10 | 37 | 1 | 8 | 2 | <1 | 0.01 | 0.02 | 0.06 | — | 0 | 3 | 0.24 | 26 | 0.08 | 5 | 0 | 4 |
| Crackers, saltine | 5 | item(s) | 15 | 65 | 1 | 11 | <1 | 2 | 0.44 | 0.96 | 0.25 | 0.54 | 0 | 18 | 0.81 | 195 | 0.15 | 19 | 0 | 2 |
| Crackers, wheat | 10 | item(s) | 30 | 142 | 3 | 19 | 1 | 6 | 1.55 | 3.43 | 0.84 | — | 0 | 15 | 1.32 | 239 | 0.15 | 35 | 0 | 2 |
| Cranberry juice cocktail | 1/2 | cup(s) | 127 | 72 | 0 | 18 | <1 | <1 | 0.01 | 0.02 | 0.06 | — | 0 | 4 | 0.19 | 3 | 0.28 | 0 | 45 | 1 |
| Cream cheese | 2 | tablespoon(s) | 29 | 101 | 2 | 1 | 0 | 10 | 6.37 | 2.85 | 0.37 | — | 32 | 23 | 0.35 | 86 | 0.00 | 4 | 0 | 1 |
| Cream, heavy whipping, liquid | 1 | tablespoon(s) | 15 | 52 | <1 | <1 | 0 | 6 | 3.45 | 1.60 | 0.21 | — | 21 | 10 | 0.00 | 6 | 0.16 | 1 | <1 | <1 |
| Cream, light whipping, liquid | 1 | tablespoon(s) | 15 | 44 | <1 | <1 | 0 | 5 | 2.90 | 1.36 | 0.13 | — | 17 | 10 | 0.00 | 5 | 0.13 | 1 | <1 | <1 |
| Croissant, butter | 1 | item(s) | 57 | 231 | 5 | 26 | 1 | 12 | 6.59 | 3.15 | 0.62 | — | 38 | 21 | 1.16 | 424 | — | 35 | <1 | 13 |
| Cucumber | 1/4 | item(s) | 75 | 11 | <1 | 3 | 1 | <1 | 0.03 | 0.00 | 0.04 | — | 0 | 12 | 0.21 | 2 | 0.02 | 5 | 2 | <1 |
| Danish pastry, nut | 1 | item(s) | 65 | 280 | 5 | 30 | 1 | 16 | 3.78 | 8.90 | 2.78 | — | 30 | 61 | 1.17 | 236 | 0.53 | 54 | 1 | 9 |
| Dates, domestic, whole | 1/4 | cup(s) | 44.5 | 126 | 1 | 33 | 4 | <1 | 0.01 | 0.01 | 0.01 | — | 0 | 17 | 0.45 | <1 | 0.02 | 5 | 0 | <1 |
| Distilled alcohol, 90 proof | 1 | fluid ounce(s) | 28 | 73 | 0 | 0 | 0 | 0 | 0.00 | 0.00 | 0.00 | — | 0 | 0 | 0.01 | <1 | 0.00 | 0 | 0 | 0 |
| Doughnut, cake | 1 | item(s) | 47 | 198 | 2 | 23 | 1 | 11 | 1.70 | 4.37 | 3.70 | — | 17 | 21 | 0.92 | 257 | — | 22 | <1 | 5 |
| Doughnut, glazed | 1 | item(s) | 60 | 242 | 4 | 27 | 1 | 14 | 3.49 | 7.72 | 1.74 | — | 4 | 26 | 0.36 | 205 | 0.00 | 13 | <1 | 5 |
| Egg substitute, Egg Beaters | 1/4 | cup(s) | 61 | 30 | 6 | <1 | 0 | 0 | 0.00 | 0.00 | 0.00 | — | 0 | 20 | 1.08 | 115 | — | 60 | 0 | 16 |
| Eggs, fried | 1 | item(s) | 46 | 92 | 6 | <1 | 0 | 7 | 1.98 | 2.92 | 1.22 | — | 210 | 27 | 0.91 | 94 | 0.56 | 23 | 0 | 16 |
| Eggs, hard boiled | 1 | item(s) | 50 | 78 | 6 | 1 | 0 | 5 | 1.63 | 2.04 | 0.71 | — | 212 | 25 | 0.60 | 62 | 0.51 | 22 | 0 | 15 |

| Food | Amt | Unit | Wt (g) | Cal | Prot (g) | Carb (g) | Fiber (g) | Fat (g) | Sat (g) | Mono (g) | Poly (g) | Trans (g) | Chol (mg) | Calc (mg) | Iron (mg) | Sodm (mg) | Zinc (mg) | Vit A | Vit C | Sel |
|---|---|---|---|---|---|---|---|---|---|---|---|---|---|---|---|---|---|---|---|---|
| Eggs, poached | 1 | item(s) | 50 | 74 | 6 | <1 | 0 | 5 | 1.54 | 1.90 | 0.68 | — | 211 | 27 | 0.92 | 147 | 0.48 | 24 | 0 | 16 |
| Eggs, raw, white | 1 | item(s) | 33 | 17 | 4 | <1 | 0 | <1 | 0.00 | 0.00 | 0.00 | — | 0 | 2 | 0.03 | 55 | 0.00 | 1 | 0 | 7 |
| Eggs, raw, whole | 1 | item(s) | 50 | 74 | 6 | <1 | 0 | 5 | 1.55 | 1.51 | 0.68 | — | 212 | 27 | 0.92 | 70 | 0.49 | 24 | 0 | 16 |
| Eggs, raw, yolk | 1 | item(s) | 17 | 53 | 3 | <1 | 0 | 4 | 1.59 | 1.55 | 0.70 | — | 205 | 21 | 0.45 | 8 | 0.43 | 24 | <1 | 9 |
| Eggs, scrambled, prepared w/milk & butter | 2 | item(s) | 122 | 203 | 14 | 3 | 0 | 15 | 4.49 | 5.82 | 2.62 | — | 429 | 87 | 1.46 | 342 | 1.04 | 37 | <1 | 27 |
| Figs, raw, medium | 2 | item(s) | 101 | 74 | 1 | 19 | 3 | <1 | 0.06 | 0.07 | 0.14 | — | 0 | 35 | 0.37 | 1 | 0.11 | — | 2 | <1 |
| Fish fillets, batter coated or breaded, fried | 3 | ounce(s) | 85 | 197.19 | 12.46 | 14.42 | 0.42 | 10.44 | 2.39 | 2.13 | 5.32 | 0 | 44 | 15.3 | 1.79 | 452.2 | — | 17 | 0 | 7.73 |
| Flounder, baked | 3 | ounce(s) | 85 | 114 | 15 | <1 | <1 | 6 | 1.15 | 2.17 | 1.44 | 0 | 44 | 19 | 0.35 | 281 | 0.41 | 7 | 3 | 34 |
| Flour, all purpose, white, bleached, enriched | 1/2 | cup(s) | 63 | 228 | 6 | 48 | 2 | 1 | 0.10 | 0.05 | 0.26 | 2 | 0 | 9 | 2.90 | 3 | 0.04 | 7 | 0 | 21 |
| Flour, whole wheat | 1/2 | cup(s) | 60 | 203 | 8 | 44 | 7 | 1 | 0.19 | 0.14 | 0.47 | 7 | 0 | 20 | 2.33 | 3 | 0.49 | 114 | 0 | 42 |
| Frankfurter, beef & pork | 1 | item(s) | 57 | 174 | 7 | 1 | 0 | 16 | 6.14 | 7.79 | 1.56 | 1 | 29 | 6 | 0.66 | 638 | 0.14 | 26 | 0 | 8 |
| Frankfurter, beef | 1 | item(s) | 45 | 149 | 5 | 2 | 0 | 13 | 5.26 | 6.44 | 0.53 | 0 | 24 | 6 | 0.68 | 513 | 0.09 | 2 | 0 | 4 |
| Frankfurter, turkey | 1 | item(s) | 45 | 102 | 6 | 1 | 0 | 8 | 2.65 | 2.50 | 2.25 | 2 | 48 | 48 | 0.83 | 642 | 0.28 | 4 | <1 | 7 |
| Frozen yogurt, chocolate, soft serve | 1/2 | cup(s) | 72 | 115 | 3 | 18 | 2 | 4 | 2.61 | 1.26 | 0.16 | — | 4 | 106 | 0.90 | 71 | — | 8 | <1 | 2 |
| Frozen yogurt, vanilla, soft serve | 1/2 | cup(s) | 72 | 117 | 3 | 17 | 0 | 4 | 2.46 | 1.10 | 0.15 | 2 | 1 | 103 | 0.22 | 63 | 0.08 | 4 | 1 | 2 |
| Fruit cocktail, canned in heavy syrup | 1/2 | cup(s) | 124 | 91 | <1 | 23 | 1 | <1 | 0.01 | 0.02 | 0.04 | 1 | 0 | 7 | 0.36 | 7 | 0.50 | 4 | 2 | 1 |
| Fruit cocktail, canned in juice | 1/2 | cup(s) | 119 | 55 | 1 | 14 | 1 | <1 | 0.00 | 0.00 | 0.00 | 1 | 0 | 9 | 0.25 | 5 | 0.47 | 3 | 1 | 1 |
| Granola bar, plain, hard | 1 | item(s) | 25 | 115 | 2 | 16 | 1 | 5 | 0.58 | 1.07 | 2.95 | 3 | 0 | 15 | 0.72 | 72 | 0.25 | 6 | <1 | 4 |
| Grape juice, sweetened, added vitamin C, from frozen concentrate | 1/2 | cup(s) | 125 | 64 | <1 | 16 | <1 | <1 | 0.04 | 0.01 | 0.03 | 0 | 0 | 5 | 0.13 | 3 | 0.00 | 1 | 30 | <1 |
| Grapefruit juice, pink, sweetened, canned | 1/2 | cup(s) | 125 | 58 | 1 | 14 | <1 | <1 | 0.02 | 0.02 | 0.03 | — | 0 | 10 | 0.45 | 3 | 0.05 | 3 | 34 | 13 |
| Grapefruit juice, white | 1/2 | cup(s) | 124 | 48 | 1 | 11 | <1 | <1 | 0.02 | 0.02 | 0.03 | — | 0 | 11 | 0.25 | 1 | 0.27 | 0 | 47 | 12 |
| Grapefruit, raw, pink or red | 1/2 | cup(s) | 115 | 48 | 1 | 12 | 2 | <1 | 0.02 | 0.02 | 0.04 | — | 0 | 25 | 0.09 | 0 | 0.09 | 2 | 36 | 2 |
| Grapes, European, red or green, adherent skin | 1/2 | cup(s) | 80 | 55 | 1 | 14 | 1 | <1 | 0.04 | 0.01 | 0.04 | — | 0 | 8 | 0.29 | 2 | 0.15 | 9 | 9 | 4 |
| Haddock, baked or broiled | 3 | ounce(s) | 44 | 50 | 11 | 0 | 0 | <1 | 0.07 | 0.01 | 0.14 | 0 | 33 | 19 | 0.60 | 39 | 0.29 | 6 | 0 | 18 |
| Halibut, Atlantic & Pacific, cooked, dry heat | 3 | ounce(s) | 85 | 119 | 23 | 0 | 0 | 2 | 0.35 | 0.82 | 0.80 | 0 | 35 | 51 | 0.91 | 59 | 0.26 | <1 | 0 | 40 |
| Ham, cured, boneless, 11% fat, roasted | 3 | ounce(s) | 85 | 151 | 19 | 0 | 0 | 8 | 2.65 | 3.77 | 1.20 | 8 | 50 | 7 | 1.14 | 1275 | — | 3 | 0 | 17 |
| Ham, deli sliced, cooked | 3 | slice(s) | 28 | 30 | 5 | 1 | 0 | 1 | 0.50 | 0.39 | 0.11 | 1 | 15 | 7 | 0.00 | 240 | — | — | 0 | — |
| Honey | 1 | tablespoon(s) | 21 | 64 | <1 | 17 | <1 | 0 | 0.00 | 0.00 | 0.00 | 0 | 0 | 1 | 0.09 | 1 | 0.00 | 0 | <1 | 1 |
| Honeydew melon | 1/2 | cup(s) | 89 | 32 | <1 | 8 | 1 | <1 | 0.03 | 0.00 | 0.05 | <1 | 0 | 5 | 0.15 | 16 | 0.02 | 16 | 16 | 16 |
| Ice cream, chocolate | 1/2 | cup(s) | 66 | 143 | 2 | 19 | 1 | 7 | 4.49 | 2.12 | 0.27 | 7 | 22 | 72 | 0.61 | 50 | 0.20 | 50 | 2 | 2 |
| Ice cream, chocolate, soft serve | 1/2 | cup(s) | 87 | 177 | 3 | 24 | 1 | 8 | 5.17 | 2.43 | 0.31 | 8 | 22 | 103 | 0.33 | 44 | 0.22 | 11 | 1 | 1 |
| Ice cream, light vanilla | 1/2 | cup(s) | 66 | 109 | 4 | 18 | <1 | 3 | 1.71 | 0.57 | 0.10 | 3 | 17 | 77 | 0.05 | 49 | 0.08 | 5 | <1 | <1 |
| Jams, jellies, preserves, all flavors | 1 | tablespoon(s) | 20 | 56 | <1 | 14 | <1 | 0 | 0.00 | 0.01 | 0.00 | <1 | 0 | 4 | 0.10 | 6 | 0.00 | 3 | 1 | 1.76 |
| Jams, jellies, preserves, all flavors, low sugar | 1 | tablespoon(s) | 18 | 25 | <1 | 6 | <1 | 0 | 0.00 | 0.01 | 0.02 | <1 | 0 | 2 | 0.05 | <1 | 0.01 | 2.20 | <1 | 4.93 |
| Kale, frozen, chopped, boiled, drained | 1/2 | cup(s) | 65 | 20 | 2 | 3 | 1 | <1 | 0.09 | 0.02 | 0.15 | 1 | 0 | 90 | 0.61 | 10 | 0.60 | 323 | 14 | 1 |
| Kiwifruit | 1 | item(s) | 77 | 46 | 1 | 11 | 3 | <1 | 0.02 | 0.03 | 0.19 | 3 | 0 | 23 | 0.38 | 2 | 0.19 | 3 | <1 | 74 |
| Lamb, chop, loin, domestic, lean & fat, 1/4" fat, broiled | 3 | ounce(s) | 85 | 269 | 21 | 0 | 0 | 20 | 8.36 | 8.25 | 1.43 | 0 | 85 | 17 | 1.54 | 65 | 0.11 | 15 | 0 | 23 |
| Lamb, leg, domestic, lean & fat, 1/4" fat, cooked | 3 | ounce(s) | 85 | 250 | 21 | 0 | 0 | 18 | 7.51 | 7.50 | 1.28 | 0 | 82 | 14 | 1.60 | 61 | 0.12 | 15 | 0 | 22 |
| Lemon juice | 1 | tablespoon(s) | 15 | 4 | <1 | 1 | <1 | 0 | 0.00 | 0.00 | 0.00 | 0 | 0 | 1 | 0.00 | <1 | 0.02 | 2 | 7 | <.1 |
| Lemonade, from frozen concentrate | 8 | fluid ounce(s) | 248 | 131 | <1 | 34 | <1 | <1 | 0.02 | 0.00 | 0.04 | <1 | 0 | 10 | 0.52 | 7 | 0.02 | 13 | <1 | 7 |
| Lentils, boiled | 1/2 | cup(s) | 99 | 115 | 9 | 20 | 8 | <1 | 0.05 | 0.06 | 0.17 | 8 | 0 | 19 | 3.30 | 2 | 0.11 | 1 | 3 | 13 |
| Lettuce, butterhead, Boston, or bibb | 1 | cup(s) | 55 | 7 | 1 | 1 | <1 | <1 | 0.04 | 0.08 | 0.06 | 17 | 0 | 19 | 0.69 | 3 | 0.10 | 40 | 2 | 13 |
| Lettuce, romaine, shredded | 1 | cup(s) | 56 | 10 | 1 | 2 | 1 | <1 | 0.02 | 0.01 | 0.09 | 2 | 0 | 19 | 0.55 | 5 | 0.07 | 77 | 14 | 2 |
| Lobster, northern, cooked, moist heat | 3 | ounce(s) | 85 | 83 | 17 | 1 | 0 | <1 | 0.09 | 0.14 | 0.08 | 1 | 61 | 52 | 0.33 | 323 | 0.85 | 9 | <1 | 14 |
| Macadamias, dry roasted, no salt added | 1/4 | cup(s) | 34 | 241 | 3 | 4 | 3 | 25 | 4.00 | 19.86 | 0.50 | 0 | 0 | 23 | 0.89 | 1 | 0.19 | 3 | <1 | 36 |
| Mayonnaise w/soybean oil | 1 | tablespoon(s) | 14 | 99 | <1 | <1 | <1 | 11 | 1.64 | 2.70 | 5.89 | 0.04 | 5 | 2 | 0.07 | 78 | 0.72 | 1 | 0 | <1 |
| Mayonnaise, low calorie | 1 | tablespoon(s) | 16 | 37 | <1 | 3 | <1 | 3 | 0.53 | 0.72 | 1.70 | — | 4 | <.1 | 0.00 | 80 | 0.32 | 0 | 3 | — |
| Milk, fat free, nonfat, or skim | 1 | cup(s) | 245 | 83 | 8 | 12 | 0 | <1 | 0.29 | 0.12 | 0.02 | — | 5 | 223 | 0.12 | 108 | 1.23 | 12 | 2 | 8 |
| Milk, fat free, nonfat, or skim, w/nonfat milk solids | 1 | cup(s) | 245 | 91 | 9 | 12 | 0 | <1 | 0.40 | 0.16 | 0.02 | — | 5 | 316 | 0.12 | 130 | 0.12 | 12 | 2 | 5 |
| Milk, low fat, 1% | 1 | cup(s) | 244 | 102 | 8 | 12 | 0 | 2 | 1.54 | 0.68 | 0.09 | — | 12 | 264 | 0.85 | 122 | 0.09 | 12 | 0 | 8 |
| Milk, low fat, 1%, w/nonfat milk solids | 1 | cup(s) | 245 | 105 | 9 | 12 | 0 | 2 | 1.48 | 0.69 | 0.09 | — | 10 | 314 | 0.12 | 127 | — | 12 | 2 | 6 |
| Milk, reduced fat, 2% | 1 | cup(s) | 244 | 122 | 8 | 11 | 0 | 5 | 2.35 | 2.04 | 0.17 | — | 20 | 271 | 0.24 | 115 | 0.07 | 12 | 2 | 6 |
| Milk, reduced fat, 2%, w/nonfat milk solids | 1 | cup(s) | 245 | 125 | 9 | 12 | 0 | 5 | 2.93 | 1.36 | 0.17 | — | 20 | 314 | 0.12 | 127 | 0.17 | 12 | 2 | 6 |
| Milk, whole, 3.3% | 1 | cup(s) | 244 | 146 | 8 | 11 | 0 | 8 | 4.55 | 1.98 | 0.48 | — | 24 | 246 | 0.07 | 105 | 0.15 | 12 | 0 | 9 |

| Food Description | Qty | Measure | Wt (g) | Ener (cal) | Prot (g) | Carb (g) | Dietary Fiber (g) | Fat (g) | Sat | Mono | Poly | Trans | Chol (mg) | Calc (mg) | Iron (mg) | Sodi (mg) | Vit E (mg) | Folate (mcg) | Vit C (mg) | Selenium (mcg) |
|---|---|---|---|---|---|---|---|---|---|---|---|---|---|---|---|---|---|---|---|---|
| | | | | | | | | | **Fat Breakdown (g)** | | | | | | | | | | | |
| Milk, whole, evaporated, canned | 2 | tablespoon(s) | 32 | 42 | 2 | 3 | 0 | 2 | 1.45 | 0.74 | 0.08 | — | 9 | 82 | 0.06 | 33 | 0.01 | 3 | 1 | 1 |
| Milkshakes, chocolate | 1 | cup(s) | 227 | 270 | 7 | 48 | 1 | 6 | 3.81 | 1.77 | 0.23 | — | 25 | 299 | 0.70 | 252 | 0.11 | 11 | 1 | 4 |
| Muffin, English, plain, enriched | 1 | item(s) | 57 | 134 | 4 | 26 | 2 | 1 | 0.15 | 0.17 | 0.51 | — | 0 | 30 | 1.43 | 264 | 0.25 | 42 | 0 | 17 |
| Muffin, English, wheat | 1 | item(s) | 57 | 127 | 5 | 26 | 3 | 1 | 0.16 | 0.16 | 0.48 | 0 | 0 | 101 | 1.64 | 218 | 0.75 | 36 | 0 | 9 |
| Muffins, blueberry | 1 | item(s) | 63 | 160 | 3 | 23 | 1 | 6 | 0.87 | 1.48 | 3.25 | — | 20 | 50 | 1.15 | 288 | 0.00 | 29 | <1 | 9 |
| Mushrooms, raw | ½ | cup(s) | 35 | 8 | 1 | 2 | <1 | <1 | 0.02 | 0.08 | 0.05 | — | 0 | 1 | 0.18 | 1 | 0.00 | 6 | 1 | 3 |
| Mustard greens, frozen, boiled drained | ½ | cup(s) | 75 | 14 | 2 | 2 | 2 | <1 | 0.01 | 0.08 | 0.04 | — | 0 | 76 | 0.84 | 19 | 1.01 | 53 | 10 | <1 |
| Oil, canola | 1 | tablespoon(s) | 14 | 120 | 0 | 0 | 0 | 14 | 0.97 | 8.01 | 4.03 | — | 0 | 0 | 0.00 | 0 | 2.33 | 0 | 0 | 0 |
| Oil, corn | 1 | tablespoon(s) | 14 | 120 | 0 | 0 | 0 | 14 | 1.73 | 3.29 | 7.98 | 0.04 | 0 | 0 | 0.00 | 0 | 1.94 | 0 | 0 | 0 |
| Oil, olive | 1 | tablespoon(s) | 14 | 119 | 0 | 0 | 0 | 14 | 1.82 | 9.98 | 1.35 | — | 0 | <1 | 0.09 | <1 | 1.94 | 0 | 0 | 0 |
| Oil, peanut | 1 | tablespoon(s) | 14 | 119 | 0 | 0 | 0 | 14 | 2.28 | 6.24 | 4.32 | — | 0 | 0 | 0.00 | 0 | 2.12 | 0 | 0 | 0 |
| Oil, safflower | 1 | tablespoon(s) | 14 | 120 | 0 | 0 | 0 | 14 | 0.84 | 10.15 | 1.95 | — | 0 | 0 | 0.00 | 0 | 4.64 | 0 | 0 | 0 |
| Oil, soybean w/cottonseed oil | 1 | tablespoon(s) | 14 | 120 | 0 | 0 | 0 | 14 | 2.45 | 4.01 | 6.54 | — | 0 | 0 | 0.00 | 0 | 1.65 | 0 | 0 | 0 |
| Okra, sliced, boiled, drained | ½ | cup(s) | 80 | 18 | 1 | 4 | 2 | <1 | 0.04 | 0.02 | 0.04 | — | 0 | 62 | 0.22 | 5 | 0.22 | 37 | 13 | <1 |
| Onions, chopped, boiled, drained | ½ | cup(s) | 106 | 47 | 1 | 11 | 2 | <1 | 0.03 | 0.03 | 0.08 | — | 0 | 23 | 0.26 | 3 | 0.02 | 16 | 6 | <1 |
| Orange juice, unsweetened, from frozen concentrate | ½ | cup(s) | 125 | 56 | 1 | 13 | <1 | <.1 | 0.01 | 0.01 | 0.01 | — | 0 | 11 | 0.12 | 1 | 0.25 | 55 | 48 | <1 |
| Orange, raw | 1 | item(s) | 131 | 62 | 1 | 15 | 3 | <1 | 0.02 | 0.03 | 0.03 | — | 0 | 52 | 0.13 | 0 | 0.24 | 39 | 70 | 1 |
| Oysters, eastern, farmed, raw | 3 | ounce(s) | 85 | 50 | 4 | 5 | 0 | 1 | 0.38 | 0.13 | 0.50 | — | 21 | 37 | 4.91 | 151 | — | 15 | 4 | 54 |
| Oysters, eastern, wild, cooked, moist heat | 3 | ounce(s) | 85 | 116 | 12 | 7 | 0 | 4 | 1.31 | 0.53 | 1.65 | — | 89 | 77 | 10.19 | 359 | — | 12 | 5 | 61 |
| Pancakes, blueberry, from recipe | 3 | item(s) | 114 | 253 | 7 | 33 | 1 | 10 | 2.26 | 2.64 | 4.74 | — | 64 | 235 | 1.96 | 470 | — | 41 | 3 | 16 |
| Pancakes, from mix w/egg & milk | 3 | item(s) | 114 | 249 | 9 | 33 | 2 | 9 | 2.33 | 2.36 | 3.33 | — | 81 | 245 | 1.48 | 576 | — | 105 | <1 | 16 |
| Papaya, raw | ½ | cup(s) | 70 | 27 | <1 | 7 | 1 | <1 | 0.03 | 0.03 | 0.02 | — | 0 | 17 | 0.07 | 2 | 0.51 | 27 | 43 | <1 |
| Pasta, egg noodles, enriched, cooked | ½ | cup(s) | 80 | 106 | 4 | 20 | 1 | 1 | 0.25 | 0.34 | 0.33 | 0.02 | 26 | 10 | 1.27 | 6 | 0.14 | 51 | 0 | 17 |
| Pasta, macaroni, enriched, cooked | ½ | cup(s) | 70 | 99 | 3 | 20 | 1 | <1 | 0.07 | 0.06 | 0.19 | — | 0 | 5 | 0.98 | 1 | 0.04 | 54 | 0 | 15 |
| Pasta, spaghetti, al dente, cooked | ½ | cup(s) | 65 | 95 | 4 | 19 | 3 | <1 | 0.05 | 0.05 | 0.15 | — | 0 | 5 | 1.00 | 1 | 0.04 | 8 | 0 | 40 |
| Pasta, spaghetti, whole wheat, cooked | ½ | cup(s) | 70 | 87 | 4 | 19 | 3 | <1 | 0.07 | 0.05 | 0.15 | — | 0 | 11 | 0.74 | 2 | 0.21 | 4 | 0 | 18 |
| Pasta, tricolor vegetable macaroni, enriched, cooked | ½ | cup(s) | 67 | 86 | 3 | 18 | 3 | <.1 | 0.01 | 0.01 | 0.03 | — | 0 | 1 | 0.33 | 4 | 0.06 | 44 | 0 | 13 |
| Peach, halves, canned in heavy syrup | ½ | cup(s) | 131 | 97 | 1 | 26 | 2 | <1 | 0.01 | 0.05 | 0.06 | — | 0 | 4 | 0.35 | 8 | 0.64 | 4 | 4 | <1 |
| Peach, halves, canned in water | ½ | cup(s) | 122 | 29 | 1 | 7 | 2 | <1 | 0.01 | 0.03 | 0.03 | — | 0 | 4 | 0.39 | 4 | 0.60 | 4 | 4 | <1 |
| Peach, raw, medium | 1 | item(s) | 98 | 38 | 1 | 9 | 1 | <1 | 0.02 | 0.07 | 0.08 | — | 0 | 6 | 0.25 | 0 | 0.72 | 4 | 6 | <.1 |
| Peanut butter, smooth | 1 | tablespoon(s) | 16 | 96 | 4 | 3 | 1 | 8 | 1.60 | 3.96 | 2.38 | — | 0 | 3 | 0.30 | 80 | 0.44 | 12 | 0 | 1 |
| Peanuts, oil roasted, salted | ¼ | cup(s) | 36 | 216 | 10 | 5 | 3 | 19 | 3.12 | 9.33 | 5.49 | — | 0 | 22 | 0.54 | 115 | 2.50 | 43 | 0 | 1 |
| Pear, halves, canned in heavy syrup | ½ | cup(s) | 133 | 98 | 1 | 25 | 2 | <1 | 0.01 | 0.04 | 0.04 | — | 0 | 7 | 0.29 | 7 | 0.11 | 1 | 1 | <1 |
| Pear, raw | 1 | item(s) | 166 | 96 | 1 | 26 | 5 | <1 | 0.01 | 0.04 | 0.05 | — | 0 | 15 | 0.28 | 2 | 0.20 | 12 | 7 | <1 |
| Peas, green, canned, drained | ½ | cup(s) | 85 | 59 | 4 | 11 | 3 | <1 | 0.05 | 0.03 | 0.14 | — | 0 | 17 | 0.81 | 214 | 0.03 | 37 | 8 | 1 |
| Peas, green, frozen, boiled, drained | ½ | cup(s) | 80 | 62 | 4 | 11 | 4 | <1 | 0.04 | 0.02 | 0.10 | — | 0 | 19 | 1.22 | 58 | 0.02 | 47 | 8 | 1 |
| Pecans, dry roasted, no salt added | ¼ | cup(s) | 57 | 403 | 5 | 8 | 5 | 42 | 3.56 | 24.92 | 11.66 | — | 0 | 21 | 1.59 | 0 | 0.74 | 9 | 0 | 2 |
| Pepperoni, beef & pork | 1 | slice(s) | 11 | 55 | 2 | <1 | <1 | 5 | 1.77 | 2.32 | 0.48 | — | 9 | 7 | 0.15 | 224 | — | <1 | 0 | 0 |
| Peppers, green bell or sweet, raw | ½ | cup(s) | 75 | 15 | <1 | 3 | 1 | <1 | 0.04 | 0.01 | 0.05 | — | 0 | 7 | 0.25 | 2 | 0.28 | 8 | 60 | <1 |
| Pickle relish, sweet | 1 | tablespoon(s) | 15 | 20 | <1 | 5 | <1 | <1 | 0.01 | 0.03 | 0.02 | — | 0 | <1 | 0.13 | 122 | 0.06 | <1 | <1 | <1 |
| Pickle, dill | 1 | ounce(s) | 28 | 5 | <1 | 1 | <1 | <1 | 0.01 | 0.00 | 0.02 | — | 0 | 3 | 0.15 | 363 | 0.03 | <1 | 1 | <1 |
| Pie crust, frozen, ready to bake, enriched, baked | 1 | slice(s) | 16 | 82 | 1 | 8 | <1 | 5 | 1.69 | 2.51 | 0.65 | — | 0 | 3 | 0.36 | 104 | 0.42 | 9 | 0 | 1 |
| Pie crust, prepared w/water, baked | 1 | slice(s) | 20 | 100 | 1 | 10 | <1 | 6 | 1.54 | 3.46 | 0.77 | — | 0 | 2 | 0.43 | 146 | — | 20 | 0 | <1 |
| Pie, apple, from home recipe | 1 | slice(s) | 155 | 411 | 4 | 58 | 2 | 19 | 4.73 | 8.36 | 5.17 | — | 0 | 1 | 1.74 | 327 | — | 37 | 3 | 12 |
| Pie, pecan, from home recipe | 1 | slice(s) | 122 | 503 | 6 | 64 | 0 | 27 | 4.87 | 13.64 | 6.97 | — | 106 | 39 | 1.81 | 320 | — | 32 | 0 | 15 |
| Pie, pumpkin, from home recipe | 1 | slice(s) | 155 | 316 | 7 | 41 | 0 | 14 | 4.92 | 5.73 | 2.81 | — | 65 | 146 | 1.97 | 349 | — | 33 | 3 | 11 |
| Pineapple, canned in extra heavy syrup | ½ | cup(s) | 130 | 108 | <1 | 28 | 1 | <1 | 0.01 | 0.02 | 0.05 | — | 0 | 18 | 0.49 | 1 | 0.01 | 7 | 9 | <1 |
| Pineapple, canned in juice | ½ | cup(s) | 125 | 75 | 1 | 20 | 1 | <1 | 0.01 | 0.01 | 0.04 | — | 0 | 17 | 0.35 | 1 | 0.01 | 6 | 12 | <1 |
| Pineapple, raw, diced | ½ | cup(s) | 78 | 37 | <1 | 10 | 1 | <1 | 0.01 | 0.01 | 0.03 | — | 0 | 10 | 0.22 | 1 | 0.02 | 12 | 28 | <.1 |
| Pinto beans, boiled, drained, no salt added | ½ | cup(s) | 114 | 117 | 2 | 5 | 0 | <1 | 0.04 | 0.03 | 0.21 | — | 0 | 17 | 0.75 | 58 | — | 146 | 7 | <.1 |
| Pomegranate | 1 | item(s) | 154 | 105 | 1 | 26 | 1 | <1 | 0.06 | 0.07 | 0.10 | — | 0 | 5 | 0.46 | 5 | 0.92 | 9 | 9 | 1 |

| Food | Amount | Unit | Wt (g) | Cal | Prot (g) | Carb (g) | Fiber (g) | Fat (g) | Sat (g) | Mono (g) | Poly (g) | Trans (g) | Chol (mg) | Calcium (mg) | Iron (mg) | Sodium (mg) |
|---|---|---|---|---|---|---|---|---|---|---|---|---|---|---|---|---|
| Popcorn, air popped | 1 | cup(s) | 8 | 31 | 1 | 6 | 1 | <1 | 0.05 | 0.09 | 0.15 | — | 0 | 1 | 0.22 | <1 |
| Popcorn, popped in oil | 1 | cup(s) | 33 | 165 | 3 | 19 | 3 | 9 | 1.61 | 2.70 | 4.43 | — | 0 | 3 | 0.92 | 292 |
| Pork, ribs, loin, country style, lean & fat, roasted | 3 | ounce(s) | 85 | 279 | 20 | 0 | 0 | 22 | 7.83 | 9.36 | 1.71 | — | 78 | 21 | 0.90 | 44 |
| Potato chips, salted | 20 | item(s) | 28 | 152 | 2 | 15 | 1 | 10 | 3.11 | 2.78 | 3.46 | — | 0 | 7 | 0.46 | 169 |
| Potatoes, au gratin mix, prepared w/water, whole milk, & butter | ½ | cup(s) | 114 | 106 | 3 | 15 | 1 | 5 | 2.94 | 1.34 | 0.15 | — | 17 | 94 | 0.36 | 499 |
| Potatoes, baked, flesh & skin | 1 | item(s) | 202 | 220 | 5 | 51 | 4 | <1 | 0.05 | 0.00 | 0.09 | — | 0 | 20 | 2.75 | 16 |
| Potatoes, baked, flesh only | ½ | cup(s) | 61 | 57 | 1 | 13 | 1 | <1 | 0.02 | 0.00 | 0.03 | — | 0 | 3 | 0.21 | 3 |
| Potatoes, hashed brown | ½ | cup(s) | 78 | 207 | 2 | 27 | 2 | 10 | 1.11 | 3.13 | 2.78 | — | 0 | 11 | 0.43 | 267 |
| Potatoes, mashed, from dehydrated granules w/milk, water, & margarine | ½ | cup(s) | 105 | 122 | 2 | 17 | 2 | 5 | 1.27 | 2.05 | 1.41 | — | 2 | 34 | 0.22 | 181 |
| Pretzels, plain, hard, twists | 5 | item(s) | 30 | 114 | 3 | 24 | 1 | 1 | 0.23 | 0.41 | 0.37 | — | 0 | 11 | 1.30 | 515 |
| Prune juice, canned | 1 | cup(s) | 256 | 182 | 2 | 45 | 3 | <1 | 0.01 | 0.05 | 0.02 | — | 0 | 31 | 3.02 | 10 |
| Prunes, dried | 2 | item(s) | 17 | 40 | <1 | 11 | 1 | <1 | 0.01 | 0.06 | 0.02 | — | 0 | 9 | 0.42 | 1 |
| Pudding, chocolate | ½ | cup(s) | 144 | 154 | 5 | 23 | 1 | 5 | 2.78 | 1.94 | 0.23 | 0 | 35 | 138 | 1.04 | 135 |
| Pudding, tapioca, ready to eat | 1 | item(s) | 142 | 169 | 3 | 28 | <1 | 5 | 0.85 | 2.24 | 1.93 | — | 1 | 119 | 0.33 | 226 |
| Pudding, vanilla | ½ | cup(s) | 136 | 116 | 5 | 17 | <1 | 3 | 1.31 | 1.21 | 0.16 | 0 | 35 | 133 | 0.25 | 134 |
| Quinoa, dry | ½ | cup(s) | 85 | 318 | 11 | 59 | 5 | 5 | 0.50 | 1.30 | 1.99 | — | 0 | 51 | 7.86 | 18 |
| Raisins, seeded, packed | ¼ | cup(s) | 41 | 122 | 1 | 32 | 2 | <1 | 0.07 | 0.01 | 0.07 | — | 0 | 12 | 1.07 | 12 |
| Raspberries, raw | ½ | cup(s) | 62 | 32 | 1 | 7 | 4 | <1 | 0.01 | 0.04 | 0.23 | — | 0 | 15 | 0.42 | 1 |
| Raspberries, red, sweetened, frozen | ½ | cup(s) | 125 | 129 | 1 | 33 | 6 | <1 | 0.01 | 0.02 | 0.11 | — | 0 | 19 | 0.81 | 1 |
| Rice, brown, long grain, cooked | ½ | cup(s) | 98 | 108 | 3 | 22 | 2 | 1 | 0.18 | 0.32 | 0.31 | — | 0 | 10 | 0.41 | 5 |
| Rice, white, long grain, boiled | ½ | cup(s) | 79 | 103 | 2 | 22 | 1 | <1 | 0.06 | 0.07 | 0.06 | — | 0 | 8 | 0.95 | 1 |
| Rice, wild brown, cooked | ½ | cup(s) | 82 | 82.81 | 3.27 | 17.49 | 1.47 | 0.27 | 0.04 | 0.04 | 0.17 | — | 0 | 2.46 | 0.49 | 2.46 |
| Roll, hard | 1 | item(s) | 57 | 167 | 6 | 30 | 2 | 2 | 0.35 | 0.65 | 0.98 | — | 0 | 54 | 1.87 | 310 |
| Salad dressing, blue cheese | 2 | tablespoon(s) | 31 | 154 | 1 | 1 | 0 | 16 | 3.03 | 3.76 | 8.51 | — | 5 | 25 | 0.06 | 335 |
| Salad dressing, French | 2 | tablespoon(s) | 31 | 143 | <1 | 5 | <1 | 14 | 1.76 | 2.63 | 6.56 | — | 0 | 7 | 0.25 | 261 |
| Salad dressing, French, low fat | 2 | tablespoon(s) | 33 | 76 | <1 | 10 | <1 | 4 | 0.36 | 1.92 | 1.64 | — | 0 | 4 | 0.28 | 262 |
| Salad dressing, Italian | 2 | tablespoon(s) | 29 | 86 | <1 | 3 | 0 | 8 | 1.32 | 1.86 | 3.80 | — | 2 | 2 | 0.19 | 486 |
| Salad dressing, Italian, diet | 2 | tablespoon(s) | 30 | 23 | <1 | 1 | 0 | 2 | 0.14 | 0.66 | 0.51 | — | 2 | 3 | 0.20 | 410 |
| Salad dressing, ranch | 2 | tablespoon(s) | 30 | 146 | <1 | 2 | <1 | 16 | 2.32 | 3.85 | 8.92 | — | 8 | 4 | 0.03 | 354 |
| Salad dressing, thousand island | 2 | tablespoon(s) | 31 | 115 | <1 | 5 | <1 | 11 | 1.59 | 2.46 | 5.68 | — | 5 | 5 | 0.37 | 269 |
| Salad dressing, thousand island, low calorie | 2 | tablespoon(s) | 31 | 62 | <1 | 7 | <1 | 4 | 0.23 | 1.98 | 0.82 | — | <1 | 5 | 0.28 | 254 |
| Salami, pork, dry or hard | 1 | slice(s) | 13 | 52 | 3 | <1 | 0 | 4 | 1.52 | 2.05 | 0.48 | — | 10 | 2 | 0.17 | 289 |
| Salmon, broiled or baked w/butter | 3 | ounce(s) | 85 | 155 | 23 | 0 | 0 | 6 | 1.16 | 2.29 | 2.33 | — | 40 | 15 | 1.02 | 99 |
| Salmon, smoked chinook (lox) | 2 | ounce(s) | 57 | 66 | 10 | 0 | 0 | <1 | 0.52 | 1.14 | 0.56 | — | 13 | 6 | 0.48 | 1134 |
| Salsa | 2 | tablespoon(s) | 16 | 4 | <1 | 1 | <1 | 0 | 0.00 | 0.00 | 0.02 | — | 0 | 5 | 0.16 | 69 |
| Sardines, Atlantic, with bones, canned in oil | 2 | item(s) | 24 | 50 | 6 | 0 | 0 | 3 | 0.36 | 0.92 | 1.23 | — | 34 | 108 | 0.70 | 121 |
| Sauerkraut, canned | ½ | cup(s) | 114 | 22 | 1 | 5 | 3 | <1 | 0.04 | 0.01 | 0.07 | — | 0 | 34 | 1.67 | 751 |
| Sausage, Italian, pork, cooked | 1 | item(s) | 68 | 220 | 14 | 1 | 0 | 17 | 6.14 | 8.13 | 2.23 | — | 53 | 16 | 1.02 | 627 |
| Sausage, smoked, pork link | 1 | piece(s) | 76 | 295 | 17 | 2 | 0 | 24 | 8.58 | 11.09 | 2.85 | — | 52 | 23 | 0.88 | 1137 |
| Scallops, mixed species, breaded, fried | 3 | item(s) | 47 | 100 | 8 | 5 | <1 | 5 | 1.24 | 2.09 | 1.32 | — | 28 | 20 | 0.38 | 216 |
| Seaweed, spirulina, dried | ½ | cup(s) | 8 | 22 | 4 | 2 | 0 | <1 | 0.20 | 0.05 | 0.16 | — | 0 | 9 | 2.14 | 79 |
| Shrimp, mixed species, breaded, fried | 3 | ounce(s) | 85 | 205.69 | 18.18 | 9.74 | 0.34 | 10.43 | 1.77 | 3.24 | 4.32 | — | 150.44 | 56.95 | 1.07 | 292.39 |
| Shrimp, mixed species, cooked, moist heat | 3 | ounce(s) | 85 | 84 | 18 | 0 | 0 | 1 | 0.25 | 0.17 | 0.37 | — | 166 | 33 | 2.63 | 190 |
| Soda, Coca-Cola Classic cola | 12 | fluid ounce(s) | 360 | 146 | 0 | 41 | 0 | 0 | 0.00 | 0.00 | 0.00 | — | 0 | 11 | 0.00 | 50 |
| Soda, Coke diet cola | 12 | fluid ounce(s) | 360 | 2 | 0 | <1 | 0 | 0 | 0.00 | 0.00 | 0.00 | — | 0 | 14 | 0.00 | 42 |
| Soda, cola | 12 | fluid ounce(s) | 426 | 179 | 0 | 46 | 0 | 0 | 0.00 | 0.00 | 0.00 | — | 0 | 7 | 0.09 | 17 |
| Soda, ginger ale | 12 | fluid ounce(s) | 366 | 124 | 0 | 32 | 0 | 0 | 0.00 | 0.00 | 0.00 | — | 0 | 11 | 0.66 | 26 |
| Soda, lemon-lime | 12 | fluid ounce(s) | 368 | 147 | 0 | 38 | 0 | 0 | 0.00 | 0.00 | 0.00 | — | 0 | 5 | 0.26 | 41 |
| Soda, root beer | 12 | fluid ounce(s) | 370 | 152 | 0 | 39 | 0 | 0 | 0.00 | 0.00 | 0.00 | — | 0 | 19 | 0.18 | 48 |
| Sour cream | 2 | tablespoon(s) | 24 | 51 | 1 | 1 | 0 | 5 | 3.13 | 1.45 | 0.19 | — | 11 | 28 | 0.14 | 13 |
| Sour cream, fat free | 2 | tablespoon(s) | 32 | 24 | 1 | 5 | 0 | <1 | 0.00 | 0.00 | 0.00 | — | 3 | 40 | 0.00 | 45 |
| Soy sauce | 1 | tablespoon(s) | 18 | 10 | 1 | 2 | <1 | <1 | 0.00 | 0.00 | 0.01 | — | 0 | 3 | 0.36 | 1029 |
| Spinach, canned, drained | ½ | cup(s) | 108 | 25 | 3 | 4 | 3 | <1 | 0.09 | 0.02 | 0.23 | — | 0 | 138 | 2.49 | 29 |
| Spinach, chopped, boiled, drained | ½ | cup(s) | 90 | 21 | 3 | 3 | 2 | <1 | 0.04 | 0.01 | 0.10 | — | 0 | 122 | 3.21 | 63 |
| Spinach, raw, chopped | 1 | cup(s) | 30 | 7 | 1 | 1 | 1 | <1 | 0.02 | 0.01 | 0.05 | — | 0 | 30 | 0.81 | 24 |
| Squash, acorn, baked | ½ | cup(s) | 103 | 57 | 1 | 15 | 5 | <1 | 0.03 | 0.01 | 0.06 | — | 0 | 45 | 0.95 | 4 |

| Food Description | Qty | Measure | Wt (g) | Ener (cal) | Prot (g) | Carb (g) | Dietary Fiber (g) | Fat (g) | Fat Breakdown (g) Sat | Mono | Poly | Trans | Chol (mg) | Calc (mg) | Iron (mg) | Sodi (mg) | Vit E (mg) | Folate (mcg) | Vit C (mg) | Selenium (mcg) |
|---|---|---|---|---|---|---|---|---|---|---|---|---|---|---|---|---|---|---|---|---|
| Squash, summer, all varieties, sliced, boiled, drained | ½ | cup(s) | 90 | 18 | 1 | 4 | 1 | <1 | 0.06 | 0.02 | 0.12 | — | 0 | 24 | 0.32 | 1 | 0.13 | 18 | 5 | <1 |
| Squash, winter, all varieties, baked, mashed | ½ | cup(s) | 103 | 38 | 1 | 9 | 3 | <1 | 0.13 | 0.05 | 0.27 | — | 0 | 23 | 0.45 | 1 | 0.12 | 21 | 10 | <1 |
| Squid, mixed species, fried | 3 | ounce(s) | 85 | 149 | 15 | 7 | 0 | 6 | 1.60 | 2.34 | 1.82 | — | 221 | 33 | 0.86 | 260 | — | 12 | 4 | 44 |
| Strawberries, raw | ½ | cup(s) | 72 | 23 | <1 | 6 | 2 | <1 | 0.01 | 0.03 | 0.11 | — | 0 | 12 | 0.30 | 1 | 0.21 | 17 | 42 | <1 |
| Strawberries, sweetened, frozen, thawed | ½ | cup(s) | 128 | 99 | 1 | 27 | 2 | <1 | 0.01 | 0.02 | 0.09 | 0 | 0 | 14 | 0.60 | 1 | 0.31 | 5 | 50 | <1 |
| Sugar, brown, packed | 1 | teaspoon(s) | 5 | 17 | 0 | 4 | 0 | 0 | 0.00 | 0.00 | 0.00 | 0 | 0 | 4 | 0.09 | 2 | 0.00 | <.1 | 0 | <.1 |
| Sugar, white, granulated | 1 | teaspoon(s) | 4 | 15 | 0 | 4 | 0 | 0 | 0.00 | 0.00 | 0.00 | 0 | 0 | <.1 | 0.00 | 0 | 0.00 | 0 | 0 | <.1 |
| Sweet potatoes, baked, peeled | ½ | cup(s) | 100 | 90 | 2 | 21 | 3 | 0 | 0.03 | 0.00 | 0.06 | 0 | 0 | 38 | 0.69 | 36 | 0.71 | 6 | 20 | <1 |
| Syrup, maple | ¼ | cup(s) | 80 | 209 | 0 | 54 | <1 | <1 | 0.03 | 0.05 | 0.08 | 0 | 0 | 54 | 0.96 | 7 | 0.00 | 0 | 0 | <1 |
| Taco shell, hard | 1 | item(s) | 13 | 62 | 1 | 8 | 1 | 3 | 0.43 | 1.19 | 1.13 | — | 0 | 21 | 0.33 | 49 | 0.22 | 17 | 0 | 2 |
| Tangerine, raw | 1 | item(s) | 84 | 37 | 1 | 9 | 2 | <1 | 0.02 | 0.03 | 0.03 | — | 0 | 12 | 0.08 | 1 | 0.17 | 17 | 26 | <1 |
| Tea, decaffeinated, prepared | 8 | fluid ounce(s) | 237 | 2 | 0 | <1 | 0 | 0 | 0.00 | 0.00 | 0.01 | 0 | 0 | 7 | 0.05 | 7 | 0.00 | 12 | 0 | 0 |
| Tea, herbal, prepared | 8 | fluid ounce(s) | 237 | 2 | 0 | <1 | 0 | 0 | 0.00 | 0.00 | 0.01 | 0 | 0 | 5 | 0.19 | 2 | 0.00 | 2 | 0 | 0 |
| Tea, prepared | 8 | fluid ounce(s) | 237 | 2 | 0 | <1 | 0 | 0 | 0.00 | 0.00 | 0.01 | 0 | 0 | 0 | 0.05 | 7 | 0.00 | 12 | 0 | 0 |
| Teriyaki sauce | 1 | tablespoon(s) | 18 | 15 | 1 | 3 | <1 | 0 | 0.00 | 0.00 | 0.00 | 0 | 0 | 5 | 0.31 | 690 | 0.00 | 4 | 0 | <1 |
| Tofu, firm | 3 | ounce(s) | 79 | 80 | 8 | 3 | <1 | 4 | 0.50 | 0.87 | 2.17 | — | 0 | 60 | 1.08 | 0 | 0.03 | — | 0 | 7 |
| Tomato juice, canned | ½ | cup(s) | 122 | 21 | <1 | 5 | <1 | <1 | 0.01 | 0.01 | 0.03 | 0 | 0 | 12 | 0.52 | 328 | 0.39 | 24 | 22 | 1 |
| Tomato sauce | ½ | cup(s) | 112 | 46 | 2 | 8 | 2 | 1 | 0.18 | 0.29 | 0.72 | 0 | 0 | 21 | 1.08 | 199 | 0.39 | 15 | 15 | 1 |
| Tomatoes, fresh, ripe, red | 1 | item(s) | 123 | 22.13 | 1.08 | 4.82 | 1.47 | 0.24 | 0.05 | 0.06 | 0.16 | 0 | 0 | 12.5 | 0.33 | 6.15 | 0.66 | 18.45 | 15.62 | 0 |
| Tomatoes, stewed, canned, red | ½ | cup(s) | 128 | 33 | 1 | 8 | 2 | <1 | 0.03 | 0.04 | 0.10 | 0 | 0 | 43 | 1.70 | 282 | 1.06 | 6 | 10 | 1 |
| Tortilla chips, plain | 6 | item(s) | 28 | 142 | 2 | 18 | 2 | 7 | 1.43 | 4.39 | 1.03 | — | 0 | 44 | 0.43 | 150 | 3.07 | 3 | 0 | 2 |
| Tortillas, corn, soft | 1 | item(s) | 26 | 58 | 1 | 12 | 1 | 1 | 0.09 | 0.17 | 0.29 | 0 | 0 | 46 | 0.36 | 42 | 3.06 | 26 | 0 | 2 |
| Tortillas, flour | 1 | item(s) | 32 | 104 | 3 | 18 | 1 | 2 | 0.56 | 1.21 | 0.34 | 0 | 0 | 40 | 1.06 | 153 | 0.50 | 33 | 0 | 7 |
| Tuna, light, canned in oil, drained | 2 | ounce(s) | 57 | 113 | 17 | 0 | 0 | 5 | 0.87 | 1.68 | 1.64 | — | 10 | 7 | 0.79 | 202 | 0.19 | 3 | 0 | 43 |
| Tuna, light, canned in water, drained | 2 | ounce(s) | 57 | 66 | 14 | 0 | 0 | <1 | 0.13 | 0.09 | 0.19 | 0 | 17 | 6 | 0.87 | 192 | 0.9 | 2 | 0 | 46 |
| Turkey, breast, processed, oven roasted, fat free | 1 | slice(s) | 28 | 25 | 4 | 1 | 0 | <1 | 0.00 | 0.00 | 0.00 | 0 | 10 | 6 | 0.00 | 330 | — | — | — | — |
| Turkey, breast, processed, traditional carved | 2 | slice(s) | 45 | 40 | 9 | 0 | 0 | 1 | 0.00 | 0.07 | 0.14 | — | 20 | 0 | 0.72 | 540 | 0.54 | 8 | 0 | 35 |
| Turkey, roasted, dark meat, meat only | 3 | ounce(s) | 85 | 159 | 24 | 0 | 0 | 6 | 2.06 | 1.39 | 1.84 | — | 72 | 27 | 1.98 | 67 | 0.08 | 5 | 0 | 35 |
| Turkey, roasted, light meat, meat only | 3 | ounce(s) | 85 | 133 | 25 | 0 | 0 | 3 | 0.88 | 0.48 | 0.73 | — | 59 | 16 | 1.15 | 54 | 1.35 | 5 | 0 | 27 |
| Turnip greens, chopped, boiled, drained | ½ | cup(s) | 72 | 14 | 1 | 3 | 3 | <1 | 0.04 | 0.01 | 0.07 | 0 | 0 | 99 | 0.58 | 21 | 0.02 | 85 | 20 | <1 |
| Turnips, cubed, boiled, drained | ½ | cup(s) | 78 | 17 | 1 | 4 | 2 | <1 | 0.01 | 0.00 | 0.03 | 0 | 0 | 26 | 0.14 | 12 | 0.28 | 7 | 9 | <1 |
| Vegetables, mixed, canned, drained | ½ | cup(s) | 82 | 40 | 2 | 8 | 2 | <1 | 0.04 | 0.01 | 0.10 | 0 | 0 | 22 | 0.86 | 121 | — | 20 | 4 | <1 |
| Vinegar, balsamic | 1 | tablespoon(s) | 15 | 10 | 0 | 2 | 0 | 0 | 0.00 | 0.00 | 0.00 | 0 | 0 | 5 | 0.00 | 7 | 0.65 | 0 | — | 0 |
| Waffle, plain, frozen, toasted | 2 | item(s) | 66 | 174 | 4 | 27 | <1 | 5 | 0.95 | 2.12 | 1.84 | — | 16 | 153 | 2.95 | 519 | 0.56 | 36 | 0 | 11 |
| Walnuts, dried black, chopped | ¼ | cup(s) | 31 | 193 | 8 | 3 | 2 | 18 | 1.05 | 4.69 | 10.96 | — | 0 | 15 | 0.98 | 1 | 0.04 | 10 | 1 | 5 |
| Watermelon | ½ | cup(s) | 77 | 23 | <1 | 6 | <1 | <1 | 0.01 | 0.03 | 0.04 | 0 | 0 | 6 | 0.19 | 1 | 0.02 | 2 | 6 | <1 |
| Wheat germ, crude | 2 | tablespoon(s) | 14 | 52 | 3 | 7 | 2 | 1 | 0.24 | 0.20 | 0.86 | — | 0 | 6 | 0.90 | 2 | 0.00 | 40 | 0 | 11 |
| Wine cooler | 10 | fluid ounce(s) | 300 | 150 | <1 | 18 | <1 | <1 | 0.01 | 0.00 | 0.02 | 0 | 0 | 17 | 0.81 | 25 | 0.00 | 5 | 11 | <1 |
| Wine, red, California | 5 | fluid ounce(s) | 150 | 125 | <1 | 4 | <.1 | <1 | 0.00 | 0.00 | 0.00 | 0 | 0 | 12 | 1.43 | 15 | 0.00 | 1 | <.1 | — |
| Wine, sparkling, domestic | 5 | fluid ounce(s) | 150 | 105 | <1 | 4 | 0 | 0 | 0.00 | 0.00 | 0.00 | 0 | 0 | 12 | — | — | — | — | — | — |
| Wine, white | 5 | fluid ounce(s) | 148 | 100 | <1 | 1 | 0 | 0 | 0.00 | 0.00 | — | 0 | 0 | 13 | 0.47 | 7 | — | 0 | 0 | — |
| Yogurt, custard style, fruit flavors | 6 | ounce(s) | 170 | 190 | 7 | 32 | 0 | 4 | 2.00 | — | — | — | 15 | 200 | 0.00 | 90 | 0.05 | 0 | 0 | <1 |
| Yogurt, fruit, low fat | 1 | cup(s) | 245 | 243 | 10 | 46 | 1 | 3 | 1.82 | 0.77 | 0.08 | 0 | 12 | 335 | 0.15 | 130 | 0.05 | 22 | 1 | 7 |
| Yogurt, fruit, nonfat, sweetened w/low calorie sweetener | 1 | cup(s) | 241 | 122 | 11 | 19 | 1 | <1 | 0.21 | 0.10 | 0.04 | 0 | 3 | 370 | 0.62 | 139 | 0.17 | 26 | 1 | 7 |
| Yogurt, plain, low fat | 1 | cup(s) | 245 | 154 | 13 | 17 | 0 | 4 | 2.45 | 1.04 | 0.11 | 0 | 15 | 443 | 0.20 | 172 | 0.05 | 27 | 2 | 8 |
| **VEGETARIAN FOODS** | | | | | | | | | | | | | | | | | | | | |
| **Prepared** | | | | | | | | | | | | | | | | | | | | |
| Macaroni & cheese (lacto) | 8 | ounce(s) | 226 | 181 | 8 | 17 | <1 | 9 | 4.37 | 2.88 | 0.89 | 0 | 22 | 157 | 0.77 | 768 | 0.29 | 39 | <.1 | 16 |
| Steamed rice & vegetables (vegan) | 8 | ounce(s) | 228 | 265 | 5 | 40 | 3 | 10 | 1.84 | 3.91 | 4.07 | 0 | 0 | 41 | 1.43 | 1403 | 3.05 | 28 | 13 | 8 |
| Vegan spinach enchiladas (vegan) | 1 | piece(s) | 82 | 93 | 5 | 15 | 2 | 2 | 0.34 | 0.55 | 1.27 | 0 | 0 | 117 | 1.13 | 134 | 0.06 | 46 | 5 | 5 |
| Vegetable chow mein (vegan) | 8 | ounce(s) | 227 | 166 | 6 | 22 | 2 | 6 | 0.65 | 2.66 | 2.47 | 0 | 0 | 190 | 3.65 | 371 | 0.06 | 47 | 7 | 6 |
| Vegetable lasagna (lacto) | 8 | ounce(s) | 225 | 177 | 12 | 25 | 2 | 4 | 1.92 | 0.93 | 0.34 | 0 | 10 | 144 | 1.91 | 637 | 0.05 | 64 | 15 | 19 |

| Food | Amt | Unit | Wt (g) | Cal | | | | | | | | | | | | | | | | |
|---|---|---|---|---|---|---|---|---|---|---|---|---|---|---|---|---|---|---|---|---|
| Vegetarian chili (vegan) | 8 | ounce(s) | 227 | 116 | 6 | 21 | 7 | 2 | 0.24 | 0.29 | 0.74 | 0 | <1 | 68 | 2.42 | 383 | 0.15 | 58 | 16 | 5 |
| Vegetarian vegetable soup (vegan) | 8 | ounce(s) | 226 | 92 | 3 | 14 | 2 | 4 | 0.77 | 1.67 | 1.30 | 0 | 0 | 37 | 1.32 | 503 | 0.55 | 38 | 24 | 1 |
| **Boca burger** | | | | | | | | | | | | | | | | | | | | |
| All American flamed grilled patty | 1 | item(s) | 71 | 110 | 14 | 6 | 4 | 4 | 1.00 | — | — | 0 | 3 | 150 | 1.80 | 370 | — | — | 0 | — |
| Boca meatless ground burger | 1/2 | cup(s) | 57 | 70 | 11 | 7 | 4 | 1 | 0.00 | — | — | 0 | 0 | 80 | 1.44 | 220 | — | — | 0 | — |
| Breakfast links | 2 | item(s) | 45 | 100 | 10 | 6 | 5 | 4 | 0.00 | — | — | 0 | 0 | 60 | 1.44 | 330 | — | — | 0 | — |
| Breakfast patties | 1 | item(s) | 38 | 80 | 8 | 5 | 3 | 4 | 0.00 | — | — | 0 | 0 | 60 | 1.44 | 260 | — | — | 0 | — |
| Vegan original patty | 1 | item(s) | 71 | 90 | 13 | 4 | 0 | 1 | 0.00 | — | — | 0 | 0 | 80 | 1.80 | 350 | — | — | 1 | — |
| **Gardenburger** | | | | | | | | | | | | | | | | | | | | |
| Black bean burger | 1 | item(s) | 71 | 80 | 8 | 11 | 4 | 2 | 0.00 | — | — | 0 | 0 | 40 | 1.44 | 330 | — | — | 0 | — |
| Chik'n grill | 1 | item(s) | 71 | 100 | 13 | 5 | 3 | 3 | 0.00 | — | — | 0 | 0 | 60 | 3.60 | 360 | — | — | 0 | — |
| Meatless breakfast sausage | 1 | item(s) | 43 | 50 | 5 | 2 | 2 | 4 | 0.00 | — | — | 0 | 0 | 20 | 0.72 | 120 | — | — | 0 | — |
| Meatless meatballs | 6 | item(s) | 85 | 110 | 12 | 8 | 8 | 5 | 1.00 | — | — | 0 | 0 | 60 | 1.80 | 400 | — | — | 0 | — |
| Original | 3 | ounce(s) | 85 | 132 | 7 | 19 | 5 | 4 | 1.80 | 1.80 | 0.60 | 24 | 24 | 72 | 0.00 | 672 | — | 12 | 1 | 8 |
| **Morningstar Farms** | | | | | | | | | | | | | | | | | | | | |
| America's Original Veggie Dog links | 1 | item(s) | 57 | 80 | 11 | 6 | 1 | 1 | 0.00 | 0.00 | 0.00 | 0 | 0 | 20 | 0.72 | 580 | — | 24 | 0 | — |
| Better n Eggs egg substitute | 1/4 | cup(s) | 57 | 20 | 5 | 0 | 0 | 0 | 0.00 | 0.00 | 0.00 | 0 | — | 20 | 0.63 | 90 | — | — | 0 | — |
| Breakfast links | 2 | item(s) | 45 | 80 | 9 | 3 | 2 | 3 | 0.50 | 2.00 | 3.00 | 0 | 0 | 0 | 1.44 | 320 | — | — | 0 | — |
| Breakfast strips | 2 | item(s) | 16 | 60 | 2 | 2 | 1 | 5 | 0.50 | 1.00 | 3.00 | 0 | 0 | 0 | 1.44 | 220 | — | — | 0 | — |
| Garden veggie patties | 2 | item(s) | 67 | 100 | 10 | 9 | 4 | 3 | 0.50 | 0.50 | 1.50 | 0 | 0 | 40 | 0.72 | 350 | — | — | 0 | — |
| Spicy black bean veggie burger | 1 | item(s) | 78 | 150 | 11 | 16 | 5 | 5 | 0.50 | 1.50 | 2.50 | 0 | 0 | 40 | 1.80 | 470 | — | 12 | 1 | 8 |
| **MIXED FOODS, SOUPS, SANDWICHES** | | | | | | | | | | | | | | | | | | | | |
| **Mixed Dishes** | | | | | | | | | | | | | | | | | | | | |
| Bean burrito | 1 | item(s) | 149 | 327 | 17 | 33 | 6 | 15 | 8.30 | 4.73 | 0.85 | 0 | 38 | 331 | 2.95 | 514 | 0.01 | 115 | 4 | 18 |
| Beef & vegetable fajita | 1 | item(s) | 223 | 397 | 23 | 35 | 3 | 18 | 5.50 | 7.53 | 3.45 | 45 | 84 | 757 | 3.74 | 246 | 0.80 | 23 | 27 | — |
| Chicken & vegetables w/broccoli, onion, bamboo shoots in soy based sauce | 1 | cup(s) | 162 | 287 | 22 | 6 | 1 | 19 | 5.13 | 7.65 | 4.68 | 84 | 22 | 962 | 1.38 | 386 | 1.12 | 13 | 8 | — |
| Chicken cacciatore | 1 | cup(s) | 230 | 266 | 28 | 5 | 1 | 14 | 3.98 | 5.78 | 3.11 | 103 | 45 | 451 | 2.21 | 246 | 0.00 | 15 | 8 | 22 |
| Chicken waldorf salad | 1/2 | cup(s) | 100 | 178 | 14 | 6 | 1 | 11 | 1.76 | 3.18 | 5.05 | 42 | 20 | 246 | 0.78 | — | 0.62 | 15 | 2 | 11 |
| Fettuccine alfredo | 1 | cup(s) | 222 | 247 | 11 | 42 | 1 | 5 | 1.61 | 0.79 | 0.43 | 9 | 0 | 153 | 1.88 | 386 | 0.00 | 103 | 1 | 35 |
| Hummus | 1/2 | cup(s) | 123 | 218 | 6 | 25 | 5 | 11 | 1.38 | 6.04 | 2.56 | 0 | 68 | 222 | 1.93 | 298 | 0.92 | 73 | 10 | 3 |
| Lasagna w/ground beef | 1 | cup(s) | 237 | 288 | 18 | 22 | 2 | 11 | 7.47 | 4.84 | 0.84 | 68 | 222 | 493 | 2.33 | — | 0.22 | 50 | 10 | 22 |
| Macaroni & cheese | 1 | cup(s) | 200 | 393 | 15 | 40 | 1 | 19 | 8.18 | 6.72 | 2.66 | 30 | 323 | 800 | 2.26 | — | 0.72 | 12 | <1 | 17 |
| Meat loaf | 1 | slice(s) | 115 | 244 | 17 | 7 | <1 | 16 | 6.15 | 6.89 | 0.83 | 85 | 54 | 423 | 2.09 | 661 | 0.00 | 9 | <1 | 5 |
| Potato salad | 1/2 | cup(s) | 125 | 179 | 3 | 14 | 2 | 10 | 1.79 | 3.10 | 4.67 | 85 | 24 | 661 | 0.81 | — | — | 20 | 13 | 22 |
| Spaghetti & meatballs w/tomato sauce, prepared | 1 | cup(s) | 248 | 330 | 19 | 39 | 3 | 12 | 3.90 | 4.40 | 2.20 | 89 | 124 | 1009 | 3.70 | — | — | 44 | 22 | 22 |
| Spicy Thai noodles (pad thai) | 8 | ounce(s) | 231 | 222 | 9 | 36 | 3 | 6 | 0.83 | 3.33 | 1.83 | 37 | 32 | 598 | 1.58 | — | 0.36 | 44 | 22 | 3 |
| Sushi w/vegetables in seaweed | 6 | piece(s) | 156 | 182 | 3 | 41 | 1 | <1 | 0.10 | 0.11 | 0.11 | 0 | 20 | 153 | 1.54 | — | 0.12 | 10 | 2 | — |
| Tuna salad | 1/2 | cup(s) | 103 | 192 | 16 | 10 | 0 | 9 | 1.58 | 2.96 | 4.23 | 13 | 17 | 412 | 1.03 | — | 0.00 | 8 | 2 | 42 |
| **Soups** | | | | | | | | | | | | | | | | | | | | |
| Chicken noodle, condensed, prepared w/water | 1 | cup(s) | 241 | 75 | 4 | 9 | 1 | 2 | 0.65 | 1.11 | 0.55 | 7 | — | 17 | 0.77 | 1106 | 0.10 | 22 | <1 | 6 |
| Cream of chicken, condensed, prepared w/milk | 1 | cup(s) | 248 | 191 | 7 | 15 | <1 | 11 | 4.64 | 4.46 | 1.64 | 27 | — | 181 | 0.67 | 1047 | — | 7 | 1 | 8 |
| Cream of mushroom, condensed, prepared w/milk | 1 | cup(s) | 248 | 203 | 6 | 15 | <1 | 14 | 5.13 | 2.98 | 4.61 | 20 | — | 179 | 0.60 | 918 | 1.24 | 10 | 2 | 4 |
| Manhattan clam chowder, condensed, prepared w/water | 1 | cup(s) | 244 | 78 | 2 | 12 | 1 | 2 | 0.38 | 0.38 | 1.29 | 2 | — | 27 | 1.63 | 578 | 0.34 | 10 | 4 | 9 |
| Minestrone, condensed, prepared w/water | 1 | cup(s) | 241 | 82 | 4 | 11 | 1 | 3 | 0.55 | 0.70 | 1.11 | 2 | — | 34 | 0.92 | 911 | — | 36 | 1 | 8 |
| New England clam chowder, condensed, prepared w/milk | 1 | cup(s) | 248 | 164 | 9 | 17 | 1 | 7 | 2.95 | 2.26 | 1.09 | 22 | — | 186 | 1.49 | 992 | 0.45 | 10 | 3 | 13 |
| Split pea, condensed, prepared w/milk | 1 | cup(s) | 165 | 85 | 4 | 19 | 2 | 2 | 0.07 | 0.03 | 0.18 | 0 | — | 30 | 1.25 | 608 | 0.00 | 61 | 9 | <1 |
| Tomato, condensed, prepared w/milk | 1 | cup(s) | 248 | 161 | 6 | 22 | 3 | 6 | 2.90 | 1.61 | 1.12 | 17 | — | 159 | 1.81 | 744 | 1.24 | 17 | 68 | 2 |
| Tomato, condensed, prepared w/water | 1 | cup(s) | 244 | 85 | 2 | 17 | <1 | 2 | 0.37 | 0.44 | 0.95 | 0 | — | 12 | 1.76 | 695 | 2.32 | 15 | 66 | <1 |
| Vegetable beef, condensed, prepared w/water | 1 | cup(s) | 244 | 78 | 6 | 10 | 2 | 2 | 0.85 | 0.81 | 0.12 | 5 | — | 17 | 1.12 | 791 | 0.37 | 10 | 2 | 4 |
| Vegetarian vegetable, condensed, prepared w/water | 1 | cup(s) | 241 | 72 | 2 | 12 | 2 | 2 | 0.29 | 0.82 | 0.72 | 0 | — | 22 | 1.08 | 822 | — | 10 | 1 | 4 |

| Food Description | Qty | Measure | Wt (g) | Ener (cal) | Prot (g) | Carb (g) | Dietary Fiber (g) | Fat (g) | Fat Breakdown (g) | | | | Chol (mg) | Calc (mg) | Iron (mg) | Sodi (mg) | Vit E (mg) | Folate (mcg) | Vit C (mg) | Selenium (mcg) |
|---|---|---|---|---|---|---|---|---|---|---|---|---|---|---|---|---|---|---|---|---|
| | | | | | | | | | Sat | Mono | Poly | Trans | | | | | | | | |
| **Sandwiches** | | | | | | | | | | | | | | | | | | | | |
| Bacon, lettuce, & tomato w/mayonnaise | 1 | item(s) | 164 | 349 | 11 | 34 | 2 | 19 | 4.54 | 7.22 | 6.07 | — | 20 | 76 | 2.54 | 837 | 1.16 | 31 | 15 | — |
| Cheeseburger, large, plain | 1 | item(s) | 185 | 609 | 30 | 47 | 0 | 33 | 14.84 | 12.74 | 2.44 | — | 96 | 91 | 5.46 | 1589 | — | 74 | 0 | 39 |
| Cheeseburger, large, w/bacon, vegetables, & condiments | 1 | item(s) | 195 | 608 | 32 | 37 | 2 | 37 | 16.24 | 14.49 | 2.71 | — | 111 | 162 | 4.74 | 1043 | — | 86 | 2 | 33 |
| Club w/bacon, chicken, tomato, lettuce & mayonnaise | 1 | item(s) | 246 | 555 | 31 | 48 | 3 | 26 | 5.94 | — | — | — | 72 | 116 | 4.05 | 855 | 1.53 | 48 | 9 | — |
| Cold cut submarine w/cheese & vegetables | 1 | item(s) | 228 | 456 | 22 | 51 | 2 | 19 | 6.81 | 8.23 | 2.28 | — | 36 | 189 | 2.51 | 1651 | — | 87 | 12 | 31 |
| Egg salad | 1 | item(s) | 126 | 278 | 10 | 29 | 1 | 13 | 2.96 | 3.97 | 4.79 | — | 217 | 107 | 2.60 | 494 | 0.13 | 82 | 1 | 24 |
| Hamburger, double patty, large w/condiments & vegetables | 1 | item(s) | 226 | 540 | 34 | 40 | 0 | 27 | 10.52 | 10.33 | 2.80 | — | 122 | 102 | 5.85 | 791 | — | 77 | 1 | 26 |
| Hamburger, large, plain | 1 | item(s) | 137 | 426 | 23 | 32 | 2 | 23 | 8.38 | 9.88 | 2.14 | — | 71 | 74 | 3.58 | 474 | — | 60 | 0 | 27 |
| Hot dog w/bun, plain | 1 | item(s) | 98 | 242 | 10 | 18 | 2 | 15 | 5.11 | 6.85 | 1.71 | — | 44 | 24 | 2.31 | 670 | — | 48 | <.1 | 26 |
| Pastrami | 1 | item(s) | 134 | 331 | 14 | 27 | 2 | 18 | 6.18 | 8.74 | 1.02 | — | 51 | 68 | 2.64 | 1335 | 0.27 | 21 | 2 | — |
| Peanut butter & jelly | 1 | item(s) | 93 | 330 | 11 | 42 | 3 | 15 | 3.00 | 6.87 | 3.82 | — | 1 | 68 | 2.11 | 409 | 2.02 | 37 | <1 | — |
| **FAST FOOD** | | | | | | | | | | | | | | | | | | | | |
| **Arby's** | | | | | | | | | | | | | | | | | | | | |
| Au jus sauce | 1 | serving(s) | 85 | 5 | <1 | 1 | <.1 | <.1 | 0.02 | — | — | — | 0 | 0 | 0.00 | 386 | — | — | — | |
| Beef 'n cheddar sandwich | 1 | item(s) | 198 | 480 | 23 | 43 | 2 | 24 | 8.00 | — | — | — | 90 | 100 | 3.60 | 1240 | — | — | 1 | |
| Curly fries, medium | 1 | serving(s) | 128 | 400 | 5 | 50 | 4 | 20 | 5.00 | — | — | — | 0 | 0 | 1.80 | 990 | — | — | 15 | |
| Market Fresh grilled chicken Caesar salad w/o dressing | 1 | serving(s) | 338 | 230 | 33 | 8 | 3 | 8 | 3.50 | — | — | — | 80 | 200 | 1.80 | 920 | — | — | 42 | |
| Roast beef deluxe sandwich, light | 1 | item(s) | 182 | 296 | 18 | 33 | 6 | 10 | 3.00 | — | 2.00 | — | 42 | 130 | 4.50 | 826 | — | — | 8 | |
| Roast beef sandwich, giant | 1 | item(s) | 228 | 480 | 32 | 41 | 3 | 23 | 10.00 | — | — | — | 110 | 60 | 5.40 | 1440 | — | — | 0 | |
| Roast beef sandwich, regular | 1 | item(s) | 157 | 350 | 21 | 34 | 2 | 16 | 6.00 | — | — | — | 85 | 60 | 3.60 | 950 | — | — | 0 | |
| Roast chicken deluxe sandwich, light | 1 | item(s) | 194 | 260 | 23 | 33 | 3 | 5 | 1.00 | 5.00 | — | — | 40 | 100 | 2.70 | 1010 | — | — | 2 | |
| **Burger King** | | | | | | | | | | | | | | | | | | | | |
| BK Broiler chicken sandwich | 1 | item(s) | 258 | 550 | 30 | 52 | 3 | 25 | 5.00 | — | — | — | 105 | 60 | 3.60 | 1110 | — | — | 6 | |
| Croissan'wich w/sausage, egg, & cheese | 1 | item(s) | 157 | 520 | 19 | 24 | 1 | 39 | 14.00 | — | — | 1.93 | 210 | 300 | 4.50 | 1090 | — | — | 0 | |
| Fish Fillet sandwich | 1 | item(s) | 185 | 520 | 18 | 44 | 2 | 30 | 8.00 | — | — | 1.12 | 55 | 150 | 2.70 | 840 | — | — | 1 | |
| French fries, medium, salted | 1 | serving(s) | 117 | 360 | 4 | 46 | 4 | 18 | 5.00 | — | — | 4.50 | 0 | 20 | 0.72 | 640 | — | — | 9 | |
| Onion rings, medium | 1 | serving(s) | 91 | 320 | 4 | 40 | 3 | 16 | 4.00 | — | — | 3.50 | 0 | 97 | 0.00 | 460 | — | — | 0 | |
| Whopper | 1 | item(s) | 291 | 710 | 31 | 52 | 4 | 43 | 13.00 | — | — | 1 | 85 | 150 | 6.30 | 980 | — | — | 9 | |
| Whopper w/cheese | 1 | item(s) | 316 | 800 | 36 | 53 | 4 | 50 | 18.00 | — | — | 2 | 110 | 250 | 6.30 | 1420 | — | — | 9 | |
| **Chick-Fil-A** | | | | | | | | | | | | | | | | | | | | |
| Chargrilled chicken garden salad | 1 | item(s) | 275 | 180 | 22 | 9 | 3 | 6 | 3.00 | — | — | 0 | 70 | 150 | 0.72 | 660 | — | — | 30 | |
| Chargrilled deluxe chicken sandwich | 1 | item(s) | 195 | 290 | 27 | 31 | 2 | 7 | 1.50 | — | — | 0 | 70 | 80 | 1.80 | 990 | — | — | 5 | |
| Chicken biscuit w/cheese | 1 | item(s) | 151 | 450 | 19 | 43 | 5 | 23 | 7.00 | — | — | 2.85 | 45 | 150 | 2.70 | 1430 | — | — | 0 | |
| Chicken salad sandwich | 1 | item(s) | 153 | 350 | 20 | 32 | 1 | 15 | 3.00 | — | — | 0 | 65 | 150 | 1.80 | 880 | — | — | 0 | |
| Chick-n-Strips | 4 | item(s) | 127 | 290 | 29 | 14 | 2 | 13 | 2.50 | — | — | 0 | 65 | 20 | 0.36 | 730 | — | — | 0 | |
| Coleslaw | 1 | item(s) | 105 | 210 | 1 | 14 | 2 | 17 | 2.50 | — | — | 0 | 20 | 40 | 0.36 | 180 | — | — | 27 | |
| **Dairy Queen** | | | | | | | | | | | | | | | | | | | | |
| Banana split | 1 | item(s) | 369 | 510 | 8 | 96 | 3 | 12 | 8.00 | 3.00 | 0.50 | — | 30 | 250 | 1.80 | 180 | — | — | 15 | |
| Chocolate chip cookie dough blizzard, small | 1 | item(s) | 319 | 720 | 12 | 105 | 0 | 28 | 14.00 | — | — | 2.50 | 50 | 350 | 2.70 | 370 | — | — | 1 | |
| Chocolate malt, small | 1 | item(s) | 418 | 650 | 15 | 111 | 0 | 16 | 10.00 | — | — | 0.50 | 55 | 450 | 1.80 | 370 | — | — | 2 | |
| Vanilla soft serve | ½ | cup(s) | 94 | 140 | 3 | 22 | 0 | 5 | 3.00 | — | — | 0 | 15 | 150 | 0.72 | 70 | — | — | 0 | |
| **Domino's** | | | | | | | | | | | | | | | | | | | | |
| **Classic hand-tossed pizza** | | | | | | | | | | | | | | | | | | | | |
| America's favorite feast, 12" | 2 | slice(s) | 205 | 508 | 22 | 57 | 4 | 22 | 9.20 | — | — | — | 49 | 202 | 3.70 | 1221 | — | — | 1 | |
| Pepperoni feast, extra pepperoni & cheese, 12" | 2 | slice(s) | 196 | 534 | 24 | 56 | 3 | 25 | 10.92 | — | — | — | 57 | 279 | 3.36 | 1349 | — | — | <1 | |
| Vegi feast, 12" | 2 | slice(s) | 203 | 439 | 19 | 57 | 4 | 16 | 7.09 | — | — | — | 34 | 279 | 3.44 | 987 | — | — | 1 | |

| Food | Amt | Unit | Wt (g) | Energy (kcal) | Prot (g) | Carb (g) | Fiber (g) | Fat (g) | Sat. Fat (g) | Chol (mg) | Calc (mg) | Iron (mg) | Sodm (mg) |
|---|---|---|---|---|---|---|---|---|---|---|---|---|---|
| **Thin crust pizza** | | | | | | | | | | | | | |
| Extravaganzza, 12" | ¼ | item(s) | 159 | 425 | 20 | 34 | 3 | 24 | 9.41 | 53 | 245 | 1.95 | 1408 |
| Pepperoni, extra pepperoni & cheese, 12" | ¼ | item(s) | 159 | 420 | 20 | 32 | 2 | 24 | 10.46 | 54 | 316 | 1.34 | 1362 |
| Vegi, 12" | ¼ | item(s) | 159 | 338 | 16 | 34 | 3 | 17 | 7.08 | 34 | 317 | 1.42 | 1047 |
| **Ultimate deep dish pizza** | | | | | | | | | | | | | |
| America's favorite, 12" | 2 | slice(s) | 235 | 617 | 26 | 59 | 4 | 33 | 12.88 | 58 | 334 | 4.43 | 1573 |
| Pepperoni, extra pepperoni & cheese, 12" | 2 | slice(s) | 235 | 629 | 26 | 57 | 4 | 34 | 13.57 | 61 | 332 | 4.25 | 1650 |
| Vegi, 12" | 2 | slice(s) | 235 | 547 | 22 | 59 | 4 | 26 | 10.19 | 41 | 333 | 4.33 | 1334 |
| **In-n-Out Burger** | | | | | | | | | | | | | |
| Cheeseburger w/mustard & ketchup | 1 | item(s) | 268 | 400 | 22 | 41 | 3 | 18 | 9.00 | 55 | 200 | 3.60 | 1080 |
| Chocolate shake | 1 | item(s) | 425 | 690 | 9 | 83 | 0 | 36 | 24.00 | 95 | 300 | 0.72 | 350 |
| Double-Double cheeseburger w/mustard & ketchup | 1 | item(s) | 328 | 590 | 37 | 42 | 3 | 32 | 17.00 | 115 | 350 | 5.40 | 1510 |
| French fries | 1 | item(s) | 125 | 400 | 7 | 54 | 2 | 18 | 5.00 | 0 | 20 | 1.80 | 245 |
| Hamburger w/mustard & ketchup | 1 | item(s) | 243 | 310 | 16 | 41 | 3 | 10 | 4.00 | 35 | 40 | 3.60 | 720 |
| **Jack in the Box** | | | | | | | | | | | | | |
| Chicken club salad | 1 | item(s) | 535 | 310 | 28 | 15 | 5 | 16 | 6.00 | 65 | 300 | 3.60 | 890 |
| Hamburger | 1 | item(s) | 104 | 250 | 12 | 30 | 3 | 9 | 3.50 | 30 | 100 | 3.60 | 610 |
| Jack's Spicy Chicken sandwich | 1 | item(s) | 253 | 580 | 24 | 53 | 3 | 31 | 6.00 | 60 | 150 | 1.80 | 950 |
| Jumbo Jack hamburger w/cheese | 1 | item(s) | 294 | 690 | 26 | 60 | 3 | 38 | 16.00 | 75 | 250 | 4.50 | 1360 |
| Sourdough Jack | 1 | item(s) | 244 | 700 | 30 | 36 | 3 | 49 | 16.00 | 80 | 200 | 4.50 | 1220 |
| **Jamba Juice** | | | | | | | | | | | | | |
| Banana berry smoothie | 24 | fluid ounce(s) | 719 | 470 | 5 | 112 | 5 | 2 | 0.50 | 5 | 200 | 1.08 | 85 |
| Chocolate mood smoothie | 24 | fluid ounce(s) | 612 | 690 | 16 | 142 | 2 | 8 | 4.50 | 25 | 500 | 1.08 | 280 |
| Jamba powerboost smoothie | 24 | fluid ounce(s) | 730 | 440 | 6 | 103 | 7 | 2 | 0.00 | 0 | 1100 | 1.44 | 40 |
| Orange juice, freshly squeezed | 16 | fluid ounce(s) | 496 | 220 | 3 | 52 | 1 | 1 | 0.00 | 0 | 60 | 1.08 | 0 |
| Protein berry pizzaz smoothie | 24 | fluid ounce(s) | 710 | 440 | 20 | 92 | 6 | 2 | 0.00 | 0 | 1100 | 2.62 | 240 |
| **Kentucky Fried Chicken (KFC)** | | | | | | | | | | | | | |
| Extra Crispy chicken, breast | 1 | item(s) | 162 | 470 | 34 | 19 | 0 | 28 | 8.00 | 135 | 19 | 1.44 | 1230 |
| Hot & spicy chicken, whole wing | 1 | item(s) | 55 | 180 | 11 | 9 | 0 | 11 | 3.00 | 60 | 10 | 0.72 | 420 |
| Original Recipe chicken, drumstick | 1 | item(s) | 59 | 140 | 14 | 4 | 0 | 8 | 2.00 | 75 | 10 | 0.70 | 440 |
| **Long John Silver's** | | | | | | | | | | | | | |
| Baked cod | 1 | serving(s) | 101 | 120 | 22 | 1 | 0 | 5 | 1.00 | 90 | 20 | 0.72 | 240 |
| Batter dipped fish sandwich | 1 | item(s) | 177 | 440 | 17 | 48 | 3 | 20 | 5.00 | 35 | 60 | 3.60 | 1120 |
| Clam chowder | 1 | item(s) | 227 | 220 | 9 | 23 | 0 | 10 | 4.00 | 25 | 150 | 0.72 | 810 |
| Crunchy shrimp basket | 21 | item(s) | 114 | 340 | 12 | 32 | 2 | 19 | 5.00 | 105 | 500 | 1.80 | 720 |
| **McDonald's** | | | | | | | | | | | | | |
| Big Mac hamburger | 1 | item(s) | 216 | 590 | 24 | 47 | 3 | 34 | 11.00 | 85 | 300 | 4.50 | 1090 |
| Cheeseburger | 1 | item(s) | 121 | 330 | 15 | 36 | 2 | 14 | 6.00 | 45 | 250 | 2.70 | 830 |
| Chicken McNuggets | 4 | item(s) | 72 | 210 | 10 | 12 | 1 | 13 | 2.50 | 35 | 20 | 0.72 | 460 |
| Egg McMuffin | 1 | item(s) | 138 | 300 | 18 | 29 | 2 | 12 | 4.50 | 235 | 300 | 2.70 | 830 |
| Filet-o-fish sandwich | 1 | item(s) | 156 | 470 | 15 | 45 | 1 | 18 | 5.00 | 50 | 200 | 1.80 | 890 |
| French fries, small | 1 | serving(s) | 68 | 210 | 3 | 26 | 2 | 10 | 1.50 | 15 | 10 | 0.36 | 135 |
| Fruit n' yogurt parfait | 1 | item(s) | 338 | 380 | 10 | 76 | 2 | 5 | 2.00 | 5 | 300 | 1.80 | 240 |
| Hash browns | 1 | item(s) | 53 | 130 | 1 | 14 | 1 | 8 | 1.50 | 0 | 10 | 0.36 | 330 |
| Honey sauce | 1 | item(s) | 14 | 45 | 0 | 12 | 0 | 0 | 0.00 | 0 | 10 | 0.18 | 0 |
| McSalad Shaker garden salad | 1 | item(s) | 149 | 100 | 7 | 4 | 2 | 0 | 3.00 | 75 | 150 | 1.08 | 120 |
| McSalad Shaker grilled chicken caesar salad | 1 | item(s) | 163 | 100 | 17 | 3 | 1 | 3 | 1.50 | 40 | 100 | 1.08 | 240 |
| Newman's Own creamy Caesar salad dressing | 1 | item(s) | 59 | 190 | 2 | 4 | 0 | 18 | 3.50 | 20 | 60 | 0.18 | 500 |
| Plain hotcakes w/syrup & margarine | 3 | item(s) | 228 | 600 | 9 | 104 | 0 | 17 | 3.00 | 0 | 100 | 4.50 | 770 |
| Quarter Pounder hamburger | 1 | item(s) | 172 | 430 | 23 | 37 | 2 | 21 | 8.00 | 70 | 200 | 4.50 | 840 |
| Quarter Pounder hamburger w/cheese | 1 | item(s) | 200 | 530 | 28 | 38 | 2 | 30 | 13.00 | 95 | 350 | 4.50 | 1310 |
| Sausage McMuffin w/egg | 1 | item(s) | 164 | 450 | 20 | 29 | 2 | 28 | 10.00 | 255 | 300 | 2.70 | 930 |
| Vanilla milkshake | 8 | fluid ounce(s) | 227 | 254 | 9 | 40 | 0 | 7 | 4.28 | 27 | 331 | 0.23 | 215 |
| **Pizza Hut** | | | | | | | | | | | | | |
| Pepperoni Lovers stuffed crust pizza | 1 | slice(s) | 171 | 480 | 23 | 44 | 3 | 23 | 11.00 | 65 | 300 | 2.70 | 1300 |
| Pepperoni Lovers thin 'n crispy pizza | 1 | slice(s) | 94 | 270 | 13 | 22 | 2 | 13 | 7.00 | 40 | 200 | 1.44 | 700 |
| Personal Pan supreme pizza | 1 | slice(s) | 73 | 170 | 8 | 19 | 1 | 8 | 3.00 | 15 | 80 | 1.86 | 400 |
| Veggie Lovers stuffed crust pizza | 1 | slice(s) | 181 | 370 | 17 | 45 | 3 | 17 | 7.00 | 35 | 250 | 2.70 | 980 |
| Veggie Lovers thin 'n crispy pizza | 1 | slice(s) | 110 | 190 | 8 | 23 | 2 | 8 | 3.00 | 15 | 150 | 1.44 | 480 |

| Food Description | Qty | Measure | Wt (g) | Ener (cal) | Prot (g) | Carb (g) | Dietary Fiber (g) | Fat (g) | Fat Breakdown (g) Sat | Mono | Poly | Trans | Chol (mg) | Calc (mg) | Iron (mg) | Sodi (mg) | Vit E (mg) | Folate (mcg) | Vit C (mg) | Selenium (mcg) |
|---|---|---|---|---|---|---|---|---|---|---|---|---|---|---|---|---|---|---|---|---|
| **Starbucks** | | | | | | | | | | | | | | | | | | | | |
| Cappuccino, tall | 12 | fluid ounce(s) | 360 | 120 | 7 | 10 | 0 | 6 | 4.00 | — | — | — | 25 | 250 | 0.00 | 95 | — | — | 1 | — |
| Cinnamon spice mocha, tall nonfat w/o whipped cream | 12 | fluid ounce(s) | 360 | 170 | 11 | 32 | 0 | 0 | 0.50 | 0.00 | 0.00 | 0 | 5 | 300 | 0.72 | 150 | — | — | 0 | — |
| Frappuccino, tall chocolate | 12 | fluid ounce(s) | 360 | 290 | 13 | 52 | 1 | 5 | 1.00 | — | — | — | 3 | 400 | 1.80 | 300 | — | — | 5 | — |
| Latte, tall w/nonfat milk | 12 | fluid ounce(s) | 360 | 123 | 12 | 17 | 0 | 1 | 0.40 | 0.16 | 0.02 | 0 | 6 | 420 | 0.18 | 174 | — | 18 | 4 | — |
| Latte, tall w/whole milk | 12 | fluid ounce(s) | 360 | 212 | 11 | 17 | 0 | 11 | 6.90 | 3.24 | 0.42 | 0 | 46 | 400 | 0.18 | 165 | — | 17 | 3 | — |
| Macchiato, tall caramel w/whole milk | 12 | fluid ounce(s) | 360 | 190 | 6 | 27 | 0 | 7 | 4.00 | — | — | — | 25 | 200 | 0.36 | 105 | — | — | 1 | — |
| Tazo chai black tea, tall nonfat | 12 | fluid ounce(s) | 360 | 170 | 6 | 37 | 0 | 0 | 0.00 | 0.00 | 0.00 | 0 | 5 | 200 | 0.36 | 95 | — | — | 0 | — |
| **Subway** | | | | | | | | | | | | | | | | | | | | |
| Chocolate chip cookie | 1 | item(s) | 48 | 209 | 3 | 29 | 1 | 10 | 3.50 | — | — | 1.07 | 12 | 0 | 1.00 | 135 | — | — | 0 | — |
| Classic Italian B.M.T. sandwich, 6", white bread | 1 | item(s) | 250 | 453 | 21 | 40 | 3 | 24 | 8.00 | — | — | 0 | 56 | 100 | 2.70 | 1740 | — | — | 24 | — |
| Meatball sandwich, 6", white bread | 1 | item(s) | 284 | 501 | 23 | 46 | 4 | 25 | 10.00 | — | — | 0.75 | 56 | 100 | 3.60 | 1350 | — | — | 24 | — |
| Roast beef sandwich, 6", white bread | 1 | item(s) | 220 | 264 | 18 | 39 | 3 | 5 | 1.00 | — | — | 0 | 20 | 40 | 3.60 | 840 | — | — | 24 | — |
| Roasted chicken breast sandwich, 6", white bread | 1 | item(s) | 234 | 311 | 25 | 40 | 3 | 6 | 1.50 | — | — | 0 | 48 | 60 | 3.60 | 880 | — | — | 24 | — |
| Tuna sandwich, 6", white bread | 1 | item(s) | 252 | 419 | 18 | 39 | 3 | 21 | 5.00 | — | — | 0 | 42 | 100 | 2.70 | 1180 | — | — | 24 | — |
| Turkey breast sandwich, 6", white bread | 1 | item(s) | 220 | 254 | 16 | 39 | 3 | 4 | 1.00 | — | — | 0 | 15 | 40 | 2.70 | 1000 | — | — | 24 | — |
| **Taco Bell** | | | | | | | | | | | | | | | | | | | | |
| 7-layer burrito | 1 | item(s) | 283 | 530 | 18 | 67 | 10 | 22 | 8.00 | — | — | 3 | 25 | 300 | 3.59 | 1360 | — | — | 5 | — |
| Beef burrito supreme | 1 | item(s) | 248 | 440 | 18 | 51 | 7 | 18 | 8.00 | — | — | 2 | 40 | 200 | 2.70 | 1330 | — | — | 9 | — |
| Grilled chicken burrito | 1 | item(s) | 198 | 390 | 19 | 49 | 3 | 13 | 4.00 | — | — | 0 | 40 | 151 | 1.44 | 1240 | — | — | 2 | — |
| Taco | 1 | item(s) | 78 | 170 | 8 | 13 | 3 | 10 | 4.00 | — | — | 0.50 | 25 | 60 | 1.08 | 350 | — | — | 2 | — |
| Veggie fajita wrap supreme | 1 | item(s) | 255 | 470 | 11 | 55 | 3 | 22 | 7.00 | — | — | — | 30 | 150 | 1.44 | 990 | — | — | 6 | — |
| **CONVENIENCE MEALS** | | | | | | | | | | | | | | | | | | | | |
| **Budget Gourmet** | | | | | | | | | | | | | | | | | | | | |
| Cheese manicotti w/meat sauce | 1 | item(s) | 284 | 420 | 18 | 38 | 4 | 22 | 11.00 | 6.00 | 1.34 | — | 85 | 300 | 2.70 | 810 | — | 31 | 0 | — |
| Chicken w/fettuccine | 1 | item(s) | 284 | 380 | 20 | 33 | 3 | 19 | 10.00 | — | — | — | 85 | 100 | 2.70 | 810 | — | — | 0 | — |
| Light beef stroganoff | 1 | item(s) | 248 | 290 | 20 | 32 | 3 | 7 | 4.00 | — | — | — | 35 | 40 | 1.80 | 580 | — | 19 | 2 | — |
| Light sirloin of beef in herb sauce | 1 | item(s) | 269 | 260 | 19 | 30 | 5 | 7 | 4.00 | 2.30 | 0.31 | — | 30 | 40 | 1.80 | 850 | — | 38 | 6 | — |
| Light vegetable lasagna | 1 | item(s) | 298 | 290 | 15 | 36 | 5 | 9 | 1.79 | 0.89 | 0.60 | — | 15 | 283 | 3.03 | 780 | — | 75 | 59 | — |
| **Healthy Choice** | | | | | | | | | | | | | | | | | | | | |
| Chicken enchilada suprema meal | 1 | item(s) | 320 | 360 | 13 | 59 | 8 | 7 | 3.00 | 2.00 | 2.00 | — | 30 | 40 | 1.44 | 580 | — | — | 4 | — |
| Lemon pepper fish meal | 1 | item(s) | 303 | 280 | 11 | 49 | 5 | 5 | 2.00 | 1.00 | 2.00 | — | 30 | 40 | 0.36 | 580 | — | — | 30 | — |
| Traditional salisbury steak meal | 1 | item(s) | 354 | 360 | 23 | 45 | 5 | 9 | 3.50 | 4.00 | 1.00 | — | 45 | 80 | 2.70 | 580 | — | — | 21 | — |
| Traditional turkey breasts meal | 1 | item(s) | 298 | 330 | 21 | 50 | 4 | 5 | 2.00 | 1.50 | 1.50 | — | 35 | 40 | 1.44 | 600 | — | — | 0 | — |
| Zucchini lasagna | 1 | item(s) | 383 | 280 | 13 | 47 | 5 | 4 | 2.50 | — | — | — | 10 | 200 | 1.80 | 310 | — | — | 0 | — |
| **Stouffers** | | | | | | | | | | | | | | | | | | | | |
| Cheese enchiladas with Mexican rice | 1 | serving(s) | 276 | 370 | 12 | 48 | 5 | 14 | 5.00 | — | — | — | 25 | 200 | 1.44 | 890 | — | — | 12 | — |
| Chicken pot pie | 1 | item(s) | 284 | 740 | 23 | 56 | 4 | 47 | 18.00 | 12.41 | 10.48 | — | 65 | 150 | 2.70 | 1170 | — | — | 0 | — |
| Homestyle beef pot roast & potatoes | 1 | item(s) | 252 | 270 | 16 | 25 | 3 | 12 | 4.50 | — | — | — | 35 | 20 | 1.80 | 820 | — | — | 6 | — |
| Homestyle roast turkey breast w/stuffing & mashed potatoes | 1 | item(s) | 273 | 300 | 16 | 34 | 2 | 11 | 3.00 | — | — | — | 35 | 40 | 0.72 | 1190 | — | — | 0 | — |
| Lean Cuisine Everyday Favorites chicken chow mein w/rice | 1 | item(s) | 255 | 210 | 12 | 33 | 2 | 3 | 1.00 | 1.00 | 0.50 | 0 | 30 | 20 | 0.36 | 620 | — | — | 0 | — |
| Lean Cuisine Everyday Favorites lasagna w/meat sauce | 1 | item(s) | 291 | 300 | 19 | 41 | 3 | 8 | 4.00 | 2.00 | 0.50 | 0 | 30 | 200 | 1.08 | 650 | — | — | 5 | — |
| **Weight Watchers** | | | | | | | | | | | | | | | | | | | | |
| Smart Ones chicken enchiladas suiza entree | 1 | serving(s) | 255 | 270 | 15 | 33 | 2 | 9 | 3.50 | — | — | — | 50 | 250 | 1.08 | 660 | — | — | 4 | — |
| Smart Ones garden lasagna entree | 1 | item(s) | 312 | 270 | 14 | 36 | 5 | 7 | 3.50 | — | — | — | 30 | 350 | 1.80 | 610 | — | — | 6 | — |
| Smart Ones pepperoni pizza | 1 | item(s) | 158 | 390 | 23 | 46 | 4 | 12 | 4.00 | — | — | — | 45 | 450 | 1.80 | 650 | — | — | 5 | — |
| Smart Ones spicy penne pasta & ricotta | 1 | item(s) | 289 | 280 | 11 | 45 | 4 | 6 | 2.00 | — | — | — | 5 | 150 | 2.70 | 400 | — | — | 6 | — |
| Smart Ones spicy Szechuan style vegetables & chicken | 1 | item(s) | 255 | 220 | 11 | 39 | 3 | 2 | 0.50 | — | — | — | 10 | 150 | 1.80 | 730 | — | — | 2 | — |

# Glossary

## A

**Action stage** Stage of change in the transtheoretical model in which the individual is actively changing a negative behavior or adopting a new, healthy behavior.

**Activities of daily living** Everyday behaviors that people normally do to function in life (cross the street, carry groceries, lift objects, do laundry, sweep floors).

**Acupuncture** Chinese medical system that requires body piercing with fine needles during therapy to relieve pain and treat ailments and diseases.

**Addiction** Compulsive and uncontrollable behavior(s) or use of substance(s).

**Adenosine triphosphate (ATP)** A high-energy chemical compound that the body uses for immediate energy.

**Adequate Intake (AI)** The recommended amount of a nutrient intake when sufficient evidence is not available to calculate the EAR and subsequent RDA.

**Adipose tissue** Fat cells in the body.

**Aerobic** Describes exercise that requires oxygen to produce the necessary energy (ATP) to carry out the activity.

**Agility** The ability to quickly and efficiently change body position and direction.

**AIDS (acquired immunodeficiency syndrome)** Any of a number of diseases that arise when the body's immune system is compromised by HIV; the final stage of HIV infection.

**Air displacement** Technique to assess body composition by calculating the body volume from the air replaced by an individual sitting inside a small chamber.

**Alcohol** (ethyl alcohol) A depressant drug that affects the brain and slows down central nervous system activity; has strong addictive properties.

**Alcoholism** Disease in which an individual loses control over drinking alcoholic beverages.

**Altruism** Unselfish concern for the welfare of others.

**Alveoli** Air sacs in the lungs where gas exchange (oxygen and carbon dioxide) takes place.

**Alveoli** Air sacs in the lungs where oxygen is taken up and carbon dioxide (produced by the body) is released from the blood.

**Amenorrhea** Cessation of regular menstrual flow.

**Amino acids** Chemical compounds that contain nitrogen, carbon, hydrogen, and oxygen; the basic building blocks the body uses to build different types of protein.

**Amotivational syndrome** A condition characterized by loss of motivation, dullness, apathy, and no interest in the future.

**Amphetamines** A class of powerful central nervous system stimulants.

**Anabolic steroids** Synthetic versions of the male sex hormone testosterone, which promotes muscle development and hypertrophy.

**Anaerobic** Describes exercise that does not require oxygen to produce the necessary energy (ATP) to carry out the activity.

**Anaerobic threshold** The highest percentage of the $VO_{2max}$ at which an individual can exercise (maximal steady state) for an extended time without accumulating significant amounts of lactic acid (accumulation of lactic acid forces an individual to slow down the exercise intensity or stop altogether).

**Android obesity** Obesity pattern seen in individuals who tend to store fat in the trunk or abdominal area.

**Angina pectoris** Chest pain associated with coronary heart disease.

**Angiogenesis** Formation of blood vessels (capillaries).

**Angioplasty** A procedure in which a balloon-tipped catheter is inserted, then inflated, to widen the inner lumen of the artery.

**Anorexia nervosa** An eating disorder characterized by self-imposed starvation to lose and maintain very low body weight.

**Anthropometric measurement** Techniques to measure body girths at different sites.

**Antibodies** Substances produced by the white blood cells in response to an invading agent.

**Anticoagulant** Any substance that inhibits blood clotting.

**Antioxidants** Compounds such as vitamins C and E, beta-carotene, and selenium that prevent oxygen from combining with other substances in the body to form harmful compounds.

**Aquaphobic** Having a fear of water.

**Arrhythmias** Irregular heart rhythms.

**Arterial-venous oxygen difference (a-vO₂diff)** The amount of oxygen removed from the blood as determined by the difference in oxygen content between arterial and venous blood.

**Atherosclerosis** Fatty/cholesterol deposits in the walls of the arteries leading to formation of plaque.

**Atrophy** Decrease in the size of a cell.

**Autogenic training** A stress management technique using a form of self-suggestion, wherein an individual is able to place himself or herself in an autohypnotic state by repeating and concentrating on feelings of heaviness and warmth in the extremities.

**Ayurveda** Hindu system of medicine based on herbs, diet, massage, meditation, and yoga to help the body boost its own natural healing.

## B

**Balance** The ability to maintain the body in proper equilibrium.

**Ballistic (dynamic) stretching** Exercises done with jerky, rapid, bouncy movements or slow, short, and sustained movements.

**Basal metabolic rate (BMR)** The lowest level of oxygen consumption necessary to sustain life.

**Behavior modification** The process of permanently changing negative behaviors to positive behaviors that will lead to better health and well-being.

**Benign** Noncancerous.

**Binge-eating disorder** An eating disorder characterized by uncontrollable episodes of eating excessive amounts of food within a relatively short time.

**Bioelectrical impedance** Technique to assess body composition by running a weak electrical current through the body.

**Biofeedback** A stress management technique in which a person learns to influence physiologic responses that are not typically under voluntary control or responses that typically are regulated but for which regulation has broken down as a result of injury, trauma, or illness.

**Blood lipids (fat)** Cholesterol and triglycerides.

**Blood pressure** A measure of the force exerted against the walls of the vessels by the blood flowing through them.

**Bod Pod** Commercial name of the equipment used to assess body composition through the air displacement technique.

**Body composition** The fat and non-fat components of the human body; important in assessing recommended body weight.

**Body mass index (BMI)** Technique to determine thinness and excessive fatness that incorporates height and weight to estimate critical fat values at which the risk for disease increases.

**Bone integrity** A component of physiologic fitness used to determine risk for osteoporosis based on bone mineral density.

**Bradycardia** Slower heart rate than normal.

**Breathing exercises** A stress management technique wherein the individual concentrates on "breathing away" the tension and inhaling fresh air to the entire body.

**Bulimia nervosa** An eating disorder characterized by a pattern of binge eating and purging in an attempt to lose weight and maintain low body weight.

## C

**Calorie** The amount of heat necessary to raise the temperature of 1 gram of water 1 degree centigrade; used to measure the energy value of food and cost (energy expenditure) of physical activity.

**Cancer** Group of diseases characterized by uncontrolled growth and spread of abnormal cells.

**Capillaries** Smallest blood vessels carrying oxygenated blood to the tissues in the body.

**Carbohydrate loading** Increasing intake of carbohydrates during heavy aerobic training or prior to aerobic endurance events that last longer than 90 minutes.

**Carbohydrates** A classification of a dietary nutrient containing carbon, hydrogen, and oxygen; the major source of energy for the human body.

**Carcinogens** Substances that contribute to the formation of cancers.

**Carcinoma in situ** Encapsulated malignant tumor that has not spread.

**Cardiac output** Amount of blood pumped by the heart in one minute.

**Cardiomyopathy** A disease affecting the heart muscle.

**Cardiorespiratory endurance** The ability of the lungs, heart, and blood vessels to deliver adequate amounts of oxygen to the cells to meet the demands of prolonged physical activity.

**Cardiorespiratory endurance** The ability of the lungs, heart, and blood vessels to deliver adequate amounts of oxygen to the cells to meet the demands of prolonged physical activity.

**Cardiorespiratory training zone** Recommended training intensity range, in terms of exercise heart rate, to obtain adequate cardiorespiratory endurance development.

**Cardiovascular diseases** The array of conditions that affect the heart and the blood vessels.

**Carotenoids** Pigment substances in plants that are often precursors to vitamin A. More than 600 carotenoids are found in nature, about 50 of which are precursors to vitamin A, the most potent one being beta-carotene.

**Catecholamines** "Fight-or-flight" hormones, including epinephrine and norepinephrine.

**Cellulite** Term frequently used in reference to fat deposits that "bulge out"; these deposits are nothing but enlarged fat cells from excessive accumulation of body fat.

**Chiropractics** Health care system that proposes that many diseases and ailments are related to misalignments of the vertebrae and emphasizes the manipulation of the spinal column.

**Chlamydia** A sexually transmitted disease, caused by a bacterial infection, that can cause significant damage to the reproductive system.

**Cholesterol** A waxy substance, technically a steroid alcohol, found only in animal fats and oil; used in making cell membranes, as a building block for some hormones, in the fatty sheath around nerve fibers, and other necessary substances.

**Chronic diseases** Illnesses that develop as a result of an unhealthy lifestyle and last a long time.

**Chronological age** Calendar age.

**Chylomicrons** Triglyceride transporting molecules.

**Circuit training** Alternating exercises by performing them in a sequence of three to six or more.

**Cirrhosis** A disease characterized by scarring of the liver.

**Cocaine** 2-beta-carbomethoxy-3-beta-benzoxytropane, the primary psychoactive ingredient derived from coca plant leaves.

**Cold turkey** Eliminating a negative behavior all at once.

**Complementary and alternative medicine (CAM)** A group of diverse medical and health care systems, practices, and products that are not presently considered to be part of conventional medicine; also called unconventional, nonallopathic, or integrative medicine.

**Complex carbohydrates** Carbohydrates formed by three or more simple sugar molecules linked together; also referred to as polysaccharides.

**Concentric** Describes shortening of a muscle during muscle contraction.

**Contemplation stage** Stage of change in the transtheoretical model in which the individual is considering changing behavior within the next 6 months.

**Contraindicated exercises** Exercises that are not recommended because they may cause injury to a person.

**Controlled ballistic stretching** Exercises done with slow, short, gentle, and sustained movements.

**Conventional Western medicine** Traditional medical practice based on methods that are tested through rigorous scientific trials; also called allopathic medicine.

**Cool-down** Tapering off an exercise session slowly.

**Coordination** The integration of the nervous and muscular systems to produce correct, graceful, and harmonious body movements.

**Core strength training** A program designed to strengthen the abdominal, hip, and spinal muscles (the core of the body).

**Coronary heart disease (CHD)** Condition in which the arteries that supply the heart muscle with oxygen and nutrients are narrowed by fatty deposits, such as cholesterol and triglycerides.

**C-reactive protein (CRP)** A protein whose blood levels increase with inflammation, at times hidden deep in the body; elevation of this protein is an indicator of potential cardiovascular events.

**Creatine** An organic compound derived from meat, fish, and amino acids that combines with inorganic phosphate to form creatine phosphate.

**Creatine phosphate (CP)** A high-energy compound that the cells use to resynthesize ATP during all-out activities of very short duration.

**Cross-training** A combination of aerobic activities that contribute to overall fitness.

**Cruciferous vegetables** Plants that produce cross-shaped leaves (cauliflower, broccoli, cabbage, Brussels sprouts, kohlrabi), which seem to have a protective effect against cancer.

## D

**Daily Values (DVs)** Reference values for nutrients and food components used in food labels.

**Dentist** Practitioner who specializes in diseases of the teeth, gums, and oral cavity.

**Deoxyribonucleic acid (DNA)** Genetic substance of which genes are made; molecule that contains cell's genetic code.

**Diabetes mellitus** A disease in which the body doesn't produce or utilize insulin properly.

**Diastolic blood pressure** Pressure exerted by blood against walls of arteries during relaxation phase (diastole) of the heart; lower of the two numbers in blood pressure readings.

**Dietary fiber** A complex carbohydrate in plant foods that is not digested but is essential to digestion.

**Dietary Reference Intakes (DRI)** A general term that describes four types of nutrient standards that establish adequate amounts and maximum safe nutrient intakes in the diet: Estimated Average Requirements (EARs), Recommended Dietary Allowances (RDAs), Adequate Intakes (AIs), and Tolerable Upper Intake Levels (ULs).

**Disaccharides** Simple carbohydrates formed by two monosaccharide units linked together, one of which is glucose. The major disaccharides are sucrose, lactose, and maltose.

**Distress** Negative stress: Unpleasant or harmful stress under which health and performance begin to deteriorate.

**Dopamine** A neurotransmitter that affects emotional, mental, and motor functions.

**Dual energy X-ray absorptiometry (DEXA)** Method to assess body composition that uses very low dose beams of X-ray energy to measure total body fat mass, fat distribution pattern, and bone density.

**Dynamic constant external resistance (DCER)** See *fixed resistance*.

**Dynamic training** Strength-training method referring to a muscle contraction with movement.

**Dysmenorrhea** Painful menstruation.

## E

**Eccentric** Describes lengthening of a muscle during muscle contraction.

**Ecosystem** A community of organisms interacting with each other in an environment.

**Elastic elongation** Temporary lengthening of soft tissue.

**Electrocardiogram (ECG or EKG)** A recording of the electrical activity of the heart.

**Electrolytes** Substances that become ions in solution and are critical for proper muscle and neuron activation (include sodium, potassium, chloride, calcium, magnesium, phosphate, and bicarbonate among others).

**Emotional eating** The consumption of large quantities of food to suppress negative emotions.

**Emotional wellness** The ability to understand your own feelings, accept your limitations, and achieve emotional stability.

**Endorphins** Morphine-like substances released from the pituitary gland (in the brain) during prolonged aerobic exercise; thought to induce feelings of euphoria and natural well-being.

**Energy-balancing equation** A principle holding that as long as caloric input equals caloric output, the person will not gain or lose weight. If caloric intake exceeds output, the person gains weight; when output exceeds input, the person loses weight.

**Environmental wellness** The capability to live in a clean and safe environment that is not detrimental to health.

**Enzymes** Catalysts that facilitate chemical reactions in the body.

**Essential fat** Minimal amount of body fat needed for normal physiologic functions; constitutes about 3 percent of total weight in men and 12 percent in women.

**Estimated Average Requirement (EAR)** The amount of a nutrient that meets the dietary needs of half the people.

**Estimated energy requirement (EER)** The average dietary energy (caloric) intake that is predicted to maintain energy balance in a healthy adult of defined age, gender, weight, height, and level of physical activity, consistent with good health.

**Estrogen** Female sex hormone essential for bone formation and conservation of bone density.

**Eustress** Positive stress: Health and performance continue to improve, even as stress increases.

**Exercise** A type of physical activity that requires planned, structured, and repetitive bodily movement with the intent of improving or maintaining one or more components of physical fitness.

**Exercise intolerance** Inability to function during exercise because of excessive fatigue or extreme feelings of discomfort.

**Explanatory style** The way people perceive the events in their lives, from an optimistic or a pessimistic perspective.

## F

**Fast-twitch fibers** Muscle fibers with greater anaerobic potential and fast speed of contraction.

**Fats** A classification of nutrients containing carbon, hydrogen, some oxygen, and sometimes other chemical elements.

**Ferritin** Iron stored in the body.

**Fight or flight** Physiologic response of the body to stress that prepares the individual to take action by stimulating the body's vital defense systems.

**Fighting spirit** Determination; the open expression of emotions, whether negative or positive.

**FITT** An acronym used to describe the four cardiorespiratory exercise prescription variables: *f*requency, *i*ntensity, *t*ype (mode), and *t*ime (duration).

**Fixed resistance** Type of exercise in which a constant resistance is moved through a joint's full range of motion (dumbbells, barbells, machines using a constant resistance).

**Flexibility** The achievable range of motion at a joint or group of joints without causing injury.

**Folate** One of the B vitamins.

**Fortified foods** Foods that have been modified by the addition or increase of nutrients that either were not present or were present in insignificant amounts with the intent of preventing nutrient deficiencies.

**Free weights** Barbells and dumbbells.

**Frequency** Number of times per week a person engages in exercise.

**Functional capacity** The ability to perform the ordinary and unusual demands of daily living without limitations and excessive fatigue or injury.

**Functional foods** Foods or food ingredients containing physiologically active substances that provide specific health benefits beyond those supplied by basic nutrition.

**Functional independence** Ability to carry out activities of daily living without assistance from other individuals.

## G

**General adaptation syndrome (GAS)** A theoretical model that explains the body's adaptation to sustained stress which includes three stages: alarm reaction, resistance, and exhaustion/recovery.

**Genetically modified foods (GM foods)** Foods whose basic genetic material (DNA) is manipulated by inserting genes with desirable traits from one plant, animal, or microorganism into another one either to introduce new traits or to enhance existing ones.

**Genital herpes** A sexually transmitted disease caused by a viral infection of the herpes simplex virus types I and II. The virus can attack different areas of the body but typically causes blisters on the genitals.

**Genital warts** A sexually transmitted disease caused by a viral infection.

**Girth measurements** Technique to assess body composition by measuring circumferences at specific body sites.

**Glucose intolerance** A condition characterized by slightly elevated blood glucose levels.

**Glycemic index** A measure that is used to rate the plasma glucose response of carbohydrate-containing foods with the response produced by the same amount of carbohydrate from a standard source, usually glucose or white bread.

**Glycogen** Form in which glucose is stored in the body.

**Goals** The ultimate aims toward which effort is directed.

**Gonorrhea** A sexually transmitted disease caused by a bacterial infection.

**Gynoid obesity** Obesity pattern seen in people who store fat primarily around the hips and thighs.

## H

**Hatha yoga** A form of yoga that incorporates specific sequences of static-stretching postures to help induce the relaxation response.

**Health** A state of complete well-being—not just the absence of disease or infirmity.

**Health fitness standards** The lowest fitness requirements for maintaining good health, decreasing the risk for chronic diseases, and lowering the incidence of muscular-skeletal injuries.

**Health promotion** The science and art of enabling people to increase control over their lifestyles to move toward a state of wellness.

**Health-related fitness** Fitness programs that are prescribed to improve the individual's overall health.

**Healthy life expectancy (HLE)** Number of years a person is expected to live in good health; this number is obtained by subtracting ill-health years from the overall life expectancy.

**Heart rate reserve (HRR)** The difference between maximal heart rate and resting heart rate.

**Heat cramps** Muscle spasms caused by heat-induced changes in electrolyte balance in muscle cells.

**Heat exhaustion** Heat-related fatigue.

**Heat stroke** Emergency situation resulting from the body being subjected to high atmospheric temperatures.

**Hemoglobin** Iron-containing compound, found in red blood cells, that transports oxygen.

**Hemoglobin** Protein–iron compound in red blood cells that transports oxygen in the blood.

**Herbal medicine** Unconventional system that uses herbs to treat ailments and disease.

**Heroin** A potent drug that is a derivative of opium.

**High-density lipoproteins (HDLs)** Cholesterol-transporting molecules in the blood ("good" cholesterol) that help clear cholesterol from the blood.

**HIV (human immunodeficiency virus)** Virus that leads to acquired immunodeficiency syndrome (AIDS).

**Homeopathy** System of treatment based on the use of minute quantities of remedies that in large amounts produce effects similar to the disease being treated.

**Homeostasis** A natural state of equilibrium; the body attempts to maintain this equilibrium by constantly reacting to external forces that attempt to disrupt this fine balance.

**Homocysteine** An amino acid that, when allowed to accumulate in the blood, may lead to plaque formation and blockage of arteries.

**Human papillomavirus (HPV)** A group of viruses that can cause sexually transmitted diseases.

**Hydrostatic weighing** Underwater technique to assess body composition; considered the most accurate of the body composition assessment techniques.

**Hypertension** Chronically elevated blood pressure.

**Hypertrophy** An increase in the size of the cell, as in muscle hypertrophy.

**Hypokinetic diseases** "Hypo" denotes "lack of"; "kinetic" denotes "motion"; therefore, illnesses related to lack of physical activity.

**Hyponatremia** A low sodium concentration in the blood caused by overhydration with water.

**Hypotension** Low blood pressure.

**Hypothermia** A breakdown in the body's ability to generate heat; a drop in body temperature below 95°F.

**I**

**Imagery** Mental visualization of relaxing images and scenes to induce body relaxation in times of stress or as an aid in the treatment of certain medical conditions such as cancer, hypertension, asthma, chronic pain, and obesity.

**Immunity** The function that guards the body from invaders, both internal and external.

**Insulin** A hormone secreted by the pancreas; essential for proper metabolism of blood glucose (sugar) and maintenance of blood glucose level.

**Insulin resistance** Inability of the cells to respond appropriately to insulin.

**Intensity** In cardiorespiratory exercise, how hard a person has to exercise to improve or maintain fitness.

**Intensity** (for flexibility exercises) Degree of stretch when doing flexibility exercises.

**International unit (IU)** Measure of nutrients in foods.

**Interval training** A system of exercise in which a short period of intense effort is followed by a specified recovery period according to a prescribed ratio; for instance, a 1:3 work-to-recovery ratio.

**Isokinetic training** Strength-training method in which the speed of the muscle contraction is kept constant because the equipment (machine) provides an accommodating resistance to match the user's force (maximal) through the range of motion.

**Isometric training** Strength-training method referring to a muscle contraction that produces little or no movement, such as pushing or pulling against an immovable object.

**L**

**Lactic acid** End product of anaerobic glycolysis (metabolism).

**Lactovegetarians** Vegetarians who eat foods from the milk group.

**Lapse** (v.) To slip or fall back temporarily into unhealthy behavior(s); (n.) short-term failure to maintain healthy behaviors.

**Lean body mass** Body weight without body fat.

**Learning theories** Behavioral modification perspective stating that most behaviors are learned and maintained under complex schedules of reinforcement and anticipated outcomes.

**Life expectancy** Number of years a person is expected to live based on the person's birth year.

**Life expectancy** How many years a person is expected to live.

**Life Experiences Survey** A questionnaire used to assess sources of stress in life.

**Lipoproteins** Lipids covered by proteins, these transport fats in the blood. Types are LDL, HDL, and VLDL.

**Locus of control** A concept examining the extent to which a person believes he or she can influence the external environment.

**Low-density lipoproteins (LDLs)** Cholesterol-transporting molecules in the blood ("bad" cholesterol) that tend to increase blood cholesterol.

**Lymphocytes** Immune system cells responsible for waging war against disease or infection.

## M

**Magnetic therapy** Unconventional treatment that relies on magnetic energy to promote healing.

**Maintenance stage** Stage of change in the transtheoretical model in which the individual maintains behavioral change for up to 5 years.

**Malignant** Cancerous.

**Mammogram** Low-dose X-rays of the breasts used as a screening technique for the early detection of breast cancer.

**Marijuana** A psychoactive drug prepared from a mixture of crushed leaves, flowers, small branches, stems, and seeds from the hemp plant *cannabis sativa.*

**Massage therapy** The rubbing or kneading of body parts to treat ailments.

**Maximal heart rate (MHR)** Highest heart rate for a person, related primarily to age.

**Maximal oxygen uptake (VO$_{2max}$)** Maximum amount of oxygen the body is able to utilize per minute of physical activity, commonly expressed in mL/kg/min; the best indicator of cardiorespiratory or aerobic fitness.

**MDA** A hallucinogenic drug that is structurally similar to amphetamines.

**MDMA** A synthetic hallucinogen drug with a chemical structure that closely resembles MDA and methamphetamine; also known as Ecstasy.

**Meditation** A stress management technique used to gain control over one's attention by clearing the mind and blocking out the stressor(s) responsible for the increased tension.

**Mediterranean diet** Typical diet of people around the Mediterranean region, focusing on olive oil, red wine, grains, legumes, vegetables, and fruits, with limited amounts of meat, fish, milk, and cheese.

**Megadoses** For most vitamins, 10 times the RDA or more; for vitamins A and D, 5 and 2 times the RDA, respectively.

**Melanoma** The most virulent, rapidly spreading form of skin cancer.

**Mental wellness** A state in which your mind is engaged in lively interaction with the world around you.

**MET** Short for metabolic equivalent, the rate of energy expenditure at rest; 1 MET is the equivalent of a VO$_2$ of 3.5 mL/kg/min.

**Metabolic fitness** A component of physiologic fitness that denotes reduction in the risk for diabetes and cardiovascular disease through a moderate-intensity exercise program in spite of little or no improvement in cardiorespiratory fitness.

**Metabolic profile** A measurement of plasma insulin, glucose, lipid, and lipoprotein levels to assess risk for diabetes and cardiovascular disease.

**Metabolic syndrome** An array of metabolic abnormalities that contribute to the development of atherosclerosis triggered by insulin resistance. These conditions include low HDL-cholesterol, high triglycerides, high blood pressure, and an increased blood-clotting mechanism.

**Metabolism** All energy and material transformations that occur within living cells; necessary to sustain life.

**Metastasis** The movement of cells from one part of the body to another.

**Methamphetamine** A potent form of amphetamine.

**Minerals** Inorganic nutrients essential for normal body functions; found in the body and in food.

**Mitochondria** Structures within the cells where energy transformations take place.

**Mode** Form or type of exercise.

**Moderate physical activity** Activity that uses 150 calories of energy per day, or 1,000 calories per week.

**Monogamous** Describes a sexual relationship in which two people have sexual relations with only each other.

**Monosaccharides** The simplest carbohydrates (sugars), formed by five- or six-carbon skeletons. The three most common monosaccharides are glucose, fructose, and galactose.

**Morbidity** A condition related to or caused by illness or disease.

**Morphologic fitness** A component of physiologic fitness used in reference to body composition factors such as percent body fat, body fat distribution, and body circumference.

**Motivation** The desire and will to do something.

**Motor neurons** Nerves connecting the central nervous system to the muscle.

**Motor unit** The combination of a motor neuron and the muscle fibers that neuron innervates.

**Muscular endurance** The ability of a muscle to exert submaximal force repeatedly over time.

**Muscular strength** The ability of a muscle to exert maximum force against resistance (for example, 1 repetition maximum [or 1 RM] on the bench press exercise).

**Myocardial infarction** Heart attack; damage to or death of an area of the heart muscle as a result of an obstructed artery to that area.

**Myocardium** Heart muscle.

## N

**Naturopathic medicine** Unconventional system of medicine that relies exclusively on natural remedies to treat disease and ailments.

**Negative resistance** The lowering or eccentric phase of a repetition during a strength-training exercise.

**Neustress** Neutral stress; stress that is neither harmful nor helpful.

**Nicotine** Addictive compound found in tobacco leaves.

**Nitrosamines** Potentially cancer-causing compounds formed when nitrites and nitrates, which prevent the growth of harmful bacteria in processed meats, combine with other chemicals in the stomach.

**Nonmelanoma skin cancer** Cancer that spreads or grows at the original site but does not metastasize to other regions of the body.

**Nonresponders** Individuals who exhibit small or no improvements in fitness as compared with others who undergo the same training program.

**Nurse** Health-care practitioner who assists in the diagnosis and treatment of health problems and provides many services to patients in a variety of settings.

**Nutrient density** A measure of the amount of nutrients and calories in various foods.

**Nutrients** Substances found in food that provide energy, regulate metabolism, and help with growth and repair of body tissues.

**Nutrition** Science that studies the relationship of foods to optimal health and performance.

## O

**Obesity** An excessive accumulation of body fat, usually at least 30 percent above recommended body weight.

**Objectives** Steps required to reach a goal.

**Occupational wellness** The ability to perform your job skillfully and effectively under conditions that provide personal and team satisfaction and adequately reward each individual.

**Oligomenorrhea** Irregular menstrual cycles.

**Omega-3 fatty acids** Polyunsaturated fatty acids found primarily in cold-water seafood, flaxseed, and flaxseed oil; thought to lower blood cholesterol and triglycerides.

**Omega-6 fatty acids** Polyunsaturated fatty acids found primarily in corn and sunflower oils and most oils in processed foods.

**Oncogenes** Genes that initiate cell division.

**One repetition maximum (1 RM)** The maximum amount of resistance an individual is able to lift in a single effort.

**Ophthalmologist** Medical specialist concerned with diseases of the eye and prescription of corrective lenses.

**Opportunistic infections** Infections that arise in the absence of a healthy immune system, which would fight them off in healthy people.

**Optometrist** Health care practitioner who specializes in the prescription and adaptation of lenses.

**Oral surgeon** A dentist who specializes in surgical procedures of the oral-facial complex.

**Orthodontist** A dentist who specializes in the correction and prevention of teeth irregularities

**Osteopath** A medical practitioner with specialized training in musculoskeletal problems who uses diagnostic and therapeutic methods of conventional medicine in addition to manipulative measures.

**Osteoporosis** A condition of softening, deterioration, or loss of bone mineral density that leads to disability, bone fractures, and even death from medical complications.

**Overload principle** Training concept that the demands placed on a system (cardiorespiratory or muscular) must be increased systematically and progressively over time to cause physiologic adaptation (development or improvement).

**Overtraining** An emotional, behavioral, and physical condition marked by increased fatigue, decreased performance, persistent muscle soreness, mood disturbances, and feelings of "staleness" or "burnout" as a result of excessive physical training.

**Overweight** An excess amount of weight against a given standard, such as height or recommended percent body fat.

**Ovolactovegetarians** Vegetarians who include eggs and milk products in their diet.

**Ovovegetarians** Vegetarians who allow eggs in their diet.

**Oxygen free radicals** Substances formed during metabolism that attack and damage proteins and lipids, in particular the cell membrane and DNA, leading to diseases such as heart disease, cancer, and emphysema.

**Oxygen uptake ($VO_2$)** The amount of oxygen the human body uses.

## P

**Pedometer** An electronic device that senses body motion and counts footsteps. Some pedometers also record distance, calories burned, speeds, "aerobic steps," and time spent being physically active.

**Pelvic inflammatory disease (PID)** An overall designation referring to the effects of other STIs, primarily chlamydia and gonorrhea.

**Percent body fat** Proportional amount of fat in the body based on the person's total weight; includes both essential fat and storage fat; also termed "fat mass".

**Periodization** A training approach that divides the season into cycles using a systematic variation in intensity and volume of training to enhance fitness and performance.

**Peripheral vascular disease** Narrowing of the peripheral blood vessels.

**Peristalsis** Involuntary muscle contractions of intestinal walls that facilitate excretion of wastes.

**Personal trainer** A health/fitness professional who evaluates, motivates, educates, and trains clients to help them meet individualized, healthy, lifestyle goals.

**Physical activity** Bodily movement produced by skeletal muscles; requires expenditure of energy and produces progressive health benefits. Examples include walking, taking the stairs, dancing, gardening, yard work, house cleaning, snow shoveling, washing the car, and all forms of structured exercise.

**Physical fitness** The ability to meet the ordinary as well as the unusual demands of daily life safely and effectively without being overly fatigued and still have energy left for leisure and recreational activities.

**Physical fitness standards** A fitness level that allows a person to sustain moderate to-vigorous physical activity without undue fatigue and the ability to closely maintain this level throughout life.

**Physical wellness** Good physical fitness and confidence in your personal ability to take care of health problems.

**Physician assistant** Health-care practitioner trained to treat most standard cases of care.

**Physiologic fitness** A term used primarily in the field of medicine to mean biological systems affected by physical activity and the role of activity in preventing disease.

**Physiologic age** The biological and functional capacity of the body as it should be in relation to the person's maximal potential at any given age in the lifespan.

**Phytonutrients** Compounds found in fruits and vegetables that block formation of cancerous tumors and disrupt the progress of cancer.

**Pilates** A training program that uses exercises designed to help strengthen the body's core by developing pelvic stability and abdominal control; exercises are coupled with focused breathing patterns.

**Plastic elongation** Permanent lengthening of soft tissue.

**Plyometric exercise** Explosive jump training, incorporating speed and strength training to enhance explosiveness.

**Positive resistance** The lifting, pushing, or concentric phase of a repetition during a strength-training exercise.

**Power** The ability to produce maximum force in the shortest time.

**Prayer** Sincere and humble communication with a higher power.

**Precontemplation stage** Stage of change in the transtheoretical model in which an individual is unwilling to change behavior.

**Preparation stage** Stage of change in the transtheoretical model in which the individual is getting ready to make a change within the next month.

**Primary care physician** A medical practitioner who provides routine treatment of ailments; typically, the patient's first contact for health care.

**Principle of individuality** Training concept holding that genetics plays a major role in individual responses to exercise training and that these differences must be considered when designing exercise programs for different people.

**Probiotics** Healthy bacteria (abundant in yogurt) that help break down foods and prevent disease-causing organisms from settling in the intestines.

**Problem-solving model** Behavioral modification model proposing that many behaviors are the result of making decisions as the individual seeks to solve the problem behavior.

**Processes of change** Actions that help you achieve change in behavior.

**Progressive muscle relaxation** A stress management technique that involves sequential contraction and relaxation of muscle groups throughout the body.

**Progressive resistance training** A gradual increase of resistance over a period of time.

**Proprioceptive neuromuscular facilitation (PNF)** Mode of stretching that uses reflexes and neuromuscular principles to relax the muscles being stretched.

**Proteins** A classification of nutrients consisting of complex organic compounds containing nitrogen and formed by combinations of amino acids; the main substances used in the body to build and repair tissues.

## Q

**Quackery/fraud** The conscious promotion of unproven claims for profit.

## R

**Range of motion** Entire arc of movement of a given joint.

**Rate of perceived exertion (RPE)** A perception scale to monitor or interpret the intensity of aerobic exercise.

**Reaction time** The time required to initiate a response to a given stimulus.

**Recommended body weight** Body weight at which there seems to be no harm to human health; healthy weight.

**Recommended Dietary Allowance (RDA)** The daily amount of a nutrient (statistically determined from the EARs) that is considered adequate to meet the known nutrient needs of almost 98 percent of all healthy people in the United States.

**Recovery time** Amount of time the body takes to return to resting levels after exercise.

**Registered dietitian (RD)** A person with a college degree in dietetics who meets all certification and continuing education requirements of the American Dietetic Association or Dietitians of Canada.

**Relapse** (v.) To slip or fall back into unhealthy behavior(s) over a longer time; (n.) longer-term failure to maintain healthy behaviors.

**Relapse prevention model** Behavioral modification model based on the principle that high-risk situations can be anticipated through the development of strategies to prevent lapses and relapses.

**Repetitions** Number of times a given resistance is performed.

**Resistance** Amount of weight lifted.

**Responders** Individuals who exhibit improvements in fitness as a result of exercise training.

**Resting heart rate (RHR)** Heart rate after a person has been sitting quietly for 15–20 minutes.

**Resting metabolic rate (RMR)** The energy requirement to maintain the body's vital processes in the resting state.

**Resting metabolism** Amount of energy (expressed in milliliters of oxygen per minute or total calories per day) an individual requires during resting conditions to sustain proper body function.

**Reverse cholesterol transport** A process in which HDL molecules attract cholesterol and carry it to the liver, where it is changed to bile and eventually excreted in the stool.

**Ribonucleic acid (RNA)** Genetic material that guides the formation of cell proteins.

**RICE** An acronym used to describe the standard treatment procedure for acute sports injuries: *r*est, *i*ce (cold application), *c*ompression, and *e*levation.

**Risk factors** Lifestyle and genetic variables that may lead to disease.

## S

**Sarcopenia** Age-related loss of lean body mass, strength, and function.

**Sedentary** Description of a person who is relatively inactive and whose lifestyle is characterized by a lot of sitting.

**Sedentary Death Syndrome (SeDS)** Cause of deaths attributed to a lack of regular physical activity.

**Self-efficacy** One's belief in the ability to perform a given task.

**Self-esteem** A sense of positive self-regard and self-respect.

**Semivegetarians** Vegetarians who include milk products, eggs, and fish and poultry in the diet.

**Set** A fixed number of repetitions; one set of bench presses might be 10 repetitions.

**Setpoint** Weight control theory that the body has an established weight and strongly attempts to maintain that weight.

**Sexually transmitted infections (STIs)** Communicable diseases spread through sexual contact.

**Shin splints** Injury to the lower leg characterized by pain and irritation in the shin region of the leg.

**Side stitch** A sharp pain in the side of the abdomen.

**Simple carbohydrates** Formed by simple or double sugar units with little nutritive value; divided into monosaccharides and disaccharides.

**Skill-related fitness** Fitness components important for success in skillful activities and athletic events; encompasses agility, balance, coordination, power, reaction time, and speed.

**Skinfold thickness** Technique to assess body composition by measuring a double thickness of skin at specific body sites.

**Slow-sustained stretching** Exercises in which the muscles are lengthened gradually through a joint's complete range of motion.

**Slow-twitch fibers** Muscle fibers with greater aerobic potential and slow speed of contraction.

**SMART** An acronym used in reference to specific, measurable, attainable, realistic, and time-specific goals.

**Social cognitive theory** Behavioral modification model holding that behavior change is influenced by the environment, self-efficacy, and characteristics of the behavior itself.

**Social wellness** The ability to relate well to others, both within and outside the family unit.

**Specific adaptation to imposed demand (SAID) training** Training principle stating that, for improvements to occur in a specific activity, the exercises performed during a strength-training program should resemble as closely as possible the movement patterns encountered in that particular activity.

**Specificity of training** Principle that training must be done with the specific muscle the person is attempting to improve.

**Speed** The ability to rapidly propel the body or a part of the body from one point to another.

**Sphygmomanometer** Inflatable bladder contained within a cuff and a mercury gravity manometer (or aneroid manometer) from which blood pressure is read.

**Spiritual wellness** The sense that life is meaningful, that life has purpose, and that some power brings all humanity together; the ethics, values, and morals that guide you and give meaning and direction to life.

**Spontaneous remission** Inexplicable recovery from incurable disease.

**Spot reducing** Fallacious theory proposing that exercising a specific body part will result in significant fat reduction in that area.

**Step aerobics** A form of exercise that combines stepping up and down from a bench accompanied by arm movements.

**Sterols** Derived fats, of which cholesterol is the best-known example.

**Storage fat** Body fat in excess of essential fat; stored in adipose tissue.

**Strength training** A program designed to improve muscular strength and/or endurance through a series of progressive resistance (weight) training exercises that overload the muscle system and cause physiologic development.

**Stress** The mental, emotional, and physiologic response of the body to any situation that is new, threatening, frightening, or exciting.

**Stress electrocardiogram** An exercise test during which the workload is increased gradually until the individual reaches maximal fatigue, with blood pressure and 12-lead electrocardiographic monitoring throughout the test.

**Stressor** Stress-causing event.

**Stretching** Moving the joints beyond the accustomed range of motion.

**Stroke** Condition in which a blood vessel that feeds the brain ruptures or is clogged, leading to blood flow disruption to the brain.

**Stroke volume** Amount of blood pumped by the heart in one beat.

**Structured interview** Assessment tool used to determine behavioral patterns that define Type A and B personalities.

**Subcutaneous fat** Deposits of fat directly under the skin.

**Subluxation** Partial dislocation of a joint.

**Substrates** Substances acted upon by an enzyme (examples: carbohydrates, fats).

**Sun protection factor (SPF)** Degree of protection offered by ingredients in sunscreen lotion; at least SPF 15 is recommended.

**Supplements** Tablets, pills, capsules, liquids, or powders that contain vitamins, minerals, antioxidants, amino acids, herbs, or fiber that individuals take to increase their intake of these nutrients.

**Suppressor genes** Genes that deactivate the process of cell division.

**Synergistic action** The effect of mixing two or more drugs, which can be much greater than the sum of two or more drugs acting by themselves.

**Synergy** A reaction in which the result is greater than the sum of its two parts.

**Syphilis** A sexually transmitted disease caused by a bacterial infection.

**Systolic blood pressure** Pressure exerted by blood against walls of arteries during forceful contraction (systole) of the heart.

**Systolic blood pressure** Pressure exerted by blood against walls of arteries during forceful contraction (systole) of the heart; higher of the two numbers in blood pressure readings.

## T

**Tachycardia** Faster-than-normal heart rate.

**Tar** Chemical compound that forms during the burning of tobacco leaves.

**Techniques of change** Methods or procedures used during each process of change.

**Telomerase** An enzyme that allows cells to reproduce indefinitely.

**Telomeres** A strand of molecules at both ends of a chromosome.

**Termination/adoption stage** Stage of change in the transtheoretical model in which the individual has eliminated an undesirable behavior or maintained a positive behavior for more than 5 years.

**Thermogenic response** Amount of energy required to digest food.

**Trans fatty acid** Solidified fat formed by adding hydrogen to monounsaturated and polyunsaturated fats to increase shelf life.

**Transtheoretical model** Behavioral modification model proposing that change is accomplished through a series of progressive stages in keeping with a person's readiness to change.

**Triglycerides** Fats formed by glycerol and three fatty acids; also called free fatty acids.

**Type 1 diabetes** Insulin-dependent diabetes mellitus (IDDM), a condition in which the pancreas produces little or no insulin, also known as juvenile diabetes.

**Type 2 diabetes** Non-insulin-dependent diabetes mellitus (NIDDM), a condition in which insulin is not processed properly; also known as adult-onset diabetes.

**Type A** Behavior pattern characteristic of a hard-driving, overambitious, aggressive, at times hostile, and overly competitive person.

**Type B** Behavior pattern characteristic of a calm, casual, relaxed, and easygoing individual.

**Type C** Behavior pattern of individuals who are just as highly stressed as the Type A but do not seem to be at higher risk for disease than the Type B.

## U

**Ultraviolet A (UVA) rays** Light rays provided by sun lamps and tanning parlors known to damage skin and promote skin cancers.

**Ultraviolet B (UVB) rays** Portion of sunlight that causes sunburn and encourages skin cancers.

**Underweight** Extremely low body weight.

**Upper Intake Level (UL)** The highest level of nutrient intake that seems safe for most healthy people, beyond which exists an increased risk of adverse effects.

## V

**Variable resistance** Training using special machines equipped with mechanical devices that provide differing amounts of resistance through the range of motion.

**Vegans** Vegetarians who eat no animal products at all.

**Vegetarians** Individuals whose diet is of vegetable or plant origin.

**Very low calorie diet** A diet that allows an energy intake (consumption) of only 800 calories or less per day.

**Very-low-density lipoproteins (VLDLs)** Triglyceride-, cholesterol-, and phospholipid-transporting molecules in the blood that tend to increase blood cholesterol.

**Vigorous activity** Any exercise that requires an MET level equal to or greater than 6 METs (21 mL/kg/min). 1 MET is the energy expenditure at rest, 3.5 mL/kg/min, and METs are defined as multiples of this resting metabolic rate (examples of activities that require a 6-MET level include aerobics, walking uphill at 3.5 mph, cycling at 10 to 12 mph, playing doubles in tennis, and vigorous strength training).

**Vigorous exercise** Cardiorespiratory exercise that requires an intensity level of approximately 70 percent of capacity.

**Vitamins** Organic nutrients essential for normal metabolism, growth, and development of the body.

**Volume (in strength training)** The sum of all the repetitions performed multiplied by the resistances used during a strength-training session.

**Volume (of training)** The total amount of training performed in a given work period (day, week, month, or season).

## W

**Waist circumference (WC)** A waist girth measurement to assess potential risk for disease based on intra-abdominal fat content.

**Warm-up** Starting a workout slowly.

**Water** The most important classification of essential body nutrients, involved in almost every vital body process.

**Weight-regulating mechanism (WRM)** A feature of the hypothalamus of the brain that controls how much the body should weigh.

**Wellness** The constant and deliberate effort to stay healthy and achieve the highest potential for well-being. It encompasses seven dimensions—physical, emotional, mental, social, environmental, occupational, and spiritual—and integrates them all into a quality life.

**Workload** Load (or intensity) placed on the body during physical activity.

## Y

**Yoga** A school of thought in the Hindu religion that seeks to help the individual attain a higher level of spirituality and peace of mind.

# Answers to Assess Your Knowledge

| 1 | 2 | 3 | 4 | 5 | 6 | 7 | 8 | 9 | 10 | 11 | 12 | 13 | 14 | 15 |
|---|---|---|---|---|---|---|---|---|---|---|---|---|---|---|
| 1. c | 1. a | 1. b | 1. e | 1. b | 1. a | 1. c | 1. b | 1. d | 1. a | 1. e | 1. b | 1. e | 1. c | 1. e |
| 2. e | 2. a | 2. e | 2. b | 2. c | 2. d | 2. d | 2. e | 2. a | 2. c | 2. b | 2. a | 2. a | 2. b | 2. c |
| 3. d | 3. e | 3. c | 3. d | 3. e | 3. c | 3. a | 3. a | 3. b | 3. c | 3. a | 3. a | 3. c | 3. e | 3. b |
| 4. a | 4. d | 4. d | 4. a | 4. a | 4. c | 4. b | 4. a | 4. e | 4. e | 4. e | 4. e | 4. d | 4. e | 4. d |
| 5. e | 5. c | 5. d | 5. b | 5. b | 5. c | 5. d | 5. b | 5. d | 5. e | 5. e | 5. e | 5. d | 5. d | 5. e |
| 6. d | 6. d | 6. a | 6. e | 6. e | 6. e | 6. d | 6. e | 6. b | 6. e | 6. e | 6. e | 6. d | 6. a | 6. a |
| 7. c | 7. a | 7. a | 7. b | 7. a | 7. b | 7. c | 7. c | 7. a | 7. a | 7. e | 7. b | 7. d | 7. a | 7. e |
| 8. b | 8. b | 8. c | 8. b | 8. c | 8. d | 8. c | 8. b | 8. e | 8. a | 8. e | 8. e | 8. e | 8. d | 8. c |
| 9. a | 9. e | 9. a | 9. e | 9. d | 9. c | 9. e | 9. e | 9. a | 9. b | 9. e | 9. b | 9. e | 9. e | 9. e |
| 10. b | 10. e | 10. e | 10. e | 10. e | 10. c | 10. e | 10. d | 10. e | 10. c | 10. a | 10. e | 10. e | 10. c | 10. a |

# Index

# HEALTH-RELATED COMPONENTS OF PHYSICAL FITNESS

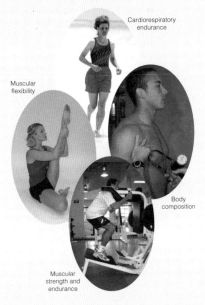

Cardiorespiratory endurance

Muscular flexibility

Body composition

Muscular strength and endurance

**Cardiorespiratory endurance** The ability of the lungs, heart, and blood vessels to deliver adequate amounts of oxygen to the cells to meet the demands of prolonged physical activity.

**Body composition** The fat and non-fat components of the human body; important in assessing recommended body weight.

**Muscular strength** The ability of a muscle to exert maximum force against resistance (for example, 1 repetition maximum [or 1 RM] on the bench press exercise).

**Muscular endurance** The ability of a muscle to exert submaximal force repeatedly over time.

**Flexibility** The achievable range of motion at a joint or group of joints without causing injury.

## HEALTHY LIFESTYLE HABITS

Research indicates that adhering to the following 12 lifestyle habits will significantly improve health and extend life.

| | I PLAN TO | I DID IT |
|---|---|---|
| 1. Participate in a lifetime physical activity program. | ☐ | ☐ |
| 2. Do not smoke cigarettes. | ☐ | ☐ |
| 3. Eat right. | ☐ | ☐ |
| 4. Avoid snacking. | ☐ | ☐ |
| 5. Maintain recommended body weight through adequate nutrition and exercise. | ☐ | ☐ |
| 6. Get enough rest. | ☐ | ☐ |
| 7. Lower your stress levels. | ☐ | ☐ |
| 8. Be wary of alcohol. | ☐ | ☐ |
| 9. Surround yourself with healthy friendships. | ☐ | ☐ |
| 10. Be informed about the environment. | ☐ | ☐ |
| 11. Increase education. | ☐ | ☐ |
| 12. Take personal safety measures. | ☐ | ☐ |

## ESTIMATED NUMBER OF STEPS TO WALK OR JOG A MILE BASED ON GENDER, HEIGHT, AND PACE

| | Pace (min/mile) | | | | |
|---|---|---|---|---|---|
| | Walking | | Jogging | | |
| Height | 20 | 15 | 12 | 10 | 8 |
| **Women** | | | | | |
| 5'0" | 2,371 | 2,054 | 1,997 | 1,710 | 1,423 |
| 5'2" | 2,343 | 2,026 | 1,970 | 1,683 | 1,396 |
| 5'4" | 2,315 | 1,998 | 1,943 | 1,656 | 1,369 |
| 5'6" | 2,286 | 1,969 | 1,916 | 1,629 | 1,342 |
| 5'8" | 2,258 | 1,941 | 1,889 | 1,602 | 1,315 |
| 5'10" | 2,230 | 1,913 | 1,862 | 1,575 | 1,288 |
| 6'0" | 2,202 | 1,885 | 1,835 | 1,548 | 1,261 |
| 6'2" | 2,174 | 1,857 | 1,808 | 1,521 | 1,234 |
| **Men** | | | | | |
| 5'2" | 2,310 | 1,993 | 1,970 | 1,683 | 1,396 |
| 5'4" | 2,282 | 1,965 | 1,943 | 1,656 | 1,369 |
| 5'6" | 2,253 | 1,937 | 1,916 | 1,629 | 1,342 |
| 5'8" | 2,225 | 1,908 | 1,889 | 1,602 | 1,315 |
| 5'10" | 2,197 | 1,880 | 1,862 | 1,575 | 1,288 |
| 6'0" | 2,169 | 1,852 | 1,835 | 1,548 | 1,261 |
| 6'2" | 2,141 | 1,824 | 1,808 | 1,521 | 1,234 |
| 6'4" | 2,112 | 1,795 | 1,781 | 1,494 | 1,207 |

Prediction Equations (pace in min/mile and height in inches):
Walking
Women: Steps/mile = 1,949 + [(63.4 × pace) − (14.1 × height)]
Men: Steps/mile = 1,916 + [(63.4 × pace) − (14.1 × height)]
Running
Women and Men: Steps/mile = 1,084 + [(143.6 × pace) − (13.5 × height)]
***Source:*** Werner W. K. Hoeger et al., "One-mile step count at walking and running speeds." *ACSM's Health & Fitness Journal,* Vol 12(1):14–19, 2008.

## STAGES OF CHANGE: MODEL OF PROGRESSION AND RELAPSE

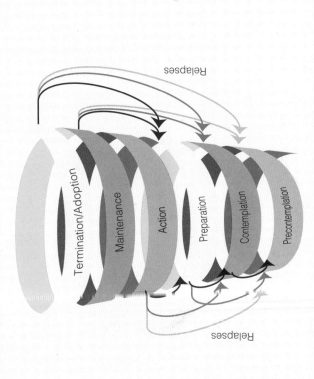

Relapses

Termination/Adoption

Maintenance

Action

Preparation

Contemplation

Precontemplation

Relapses

## STEPS FOR SUCCESSFUL BEHAVIOR MODIFICATION

| I PLAN TO | I DID IT | |
|---|---|---|
| ☐ | ☐ | 1. Acknowledge that you have a problem. |
| ☐ | ☐ | 2. Describe the behavior to change (increase physical activity, stop overeating, quit smoking). |
| ☐ | ☐ | 3. List advantages and disadvantages of changing the specified behavior. |
| ☐ | ☐ | 4. Decide positively that you will change. |
| ☐ | ☐ | 5. Identify your stage of change. |
| ☐ | ☐ | 6. Set a realistic goal (SMART goal), completion date, and sign a behavioral contract. |
| ☐ | ☐ | 7. Define your behavioral change plan: List processes of change, techniques of change, and objectives that will help you reach your goal. |
| ☐ | ☐ | 8. Implement the behavior change plan. |
| ☐ | ☐ | 9. Monitor your progress toward the desired goal. |
| ☐ | ☐ | 10. Periodically evaluate and reassess your goal. |
| ☐ | ☐ | 11. Reward yourself when you achieve your goal. |
| ☐ | ☐ | 12. Maintain the successful change for good. |

**TRY IT**

In your Online Journal or class notebook, record your answers to the following questions:

Have you consciously attempted to incorporate a healthy behavior into or eliminate a negative behavior from your lifestyle? If so, what steps did you follow, and what helped you achieve your goal?

## THE AMERICAN DIET: CURRENT AND RECOMMENDED CARBOHYDRATE, FAT, AND PROTEIN INTAKE EXPRESSED AS A PERCENTAGE OF TOTAL CALORIES

| | Current Percentage | Recommended Percentage* |
|---|---|---|
| Carbohydrates: | 50% | 45–65% |
| Simple | 26% | Less than **25%** |
| Complex | 24% | 20–40% |
| Fat: | 34% | 20–30%** |
| Monounsaturated: | 11% | Up to 20% |
| Polyunsaturated: | 10% | Up to 10% |
| Saturated: | 13% | Less than 7% |
| Protein: | 16% | 10–35% |

*Adapted from the 2002 recommended guidelines by the National Academy of Sciences.
**Up to 35% is allowed for individuals with metabolic syndrome who may need additional fat in the diet.

## COMPUTATION FOR FAT CONTENT IN FOOD

**Nutrition Facts**

Serving Size 1 cup (240 ml)
Servings Per Container 4

**Amount Per Serving**

**Calories** 120          Calories from Fat 45

| | % Daily Value* |
|---|---|
| **Total Fat** 5g | 8% |
| Saturated Fat 3g | 15% |
| **Cholesterol** 20mg | 7% |
| **Sodium** 120mg | 5% |
| **Total Carbohydrate** 12g | 4% |
| Dietary Fiber 0g | 0% |
| Sugars 12g | |
| **Protein** 8g | |

| | | | |
|---|---|---|---|
| Vitamin A | 10% | Vitamin C | 4% |
| Calcium | 30% | Iron | 0% |

* Percent Daily Values are based on a 2,000 calorie diet. Your daily values may be higher or lower depending on your calorie needs:

| | | Calories | 2,000 | 2,500 |
|---|---|---|---|---|
| Total Fat | Less than | | 65g | 80g |
| Sat Fat | Less than | | 20g | 25g |
| Cholesterol | Less than | | 300mg | 300mg |
| Sodium | Less than | | 2,400mg | 2,400mg |
| Total Carbohydrate | | | 300g | 375g |
| Fiber | | | 25g | 30g |

Calories per gram:
Fat 9 • Carbohydrate 4 • Protein 4

Percent fat calories = (grams of fat × 9) ÷ calories per serving × 100

5 grams of fat × 9 calories per grams of fat = 45 calories from fat

45 calories from fat ÷ 120 calories per serving × 100 = 38% fat

## GOOD SOURCES OF VITAMIN D

| Food | Amount | IU* |
|---|---|---|
| Multivitamins (most brands) | daily dose | 400 |
| Salmon | 3.5 oz | 360 |
| Mackerel | 3.5 oz | 345 |
| Sardines (oil/drained) | 3.5 oz | 250 |
| Shrimp | 3.5 oz | 200 |
| Orange juice (D-fortified) | 8 oz | 100 |
| Milk (any type/D-fortified) | 8 oz | 100 |
| Margarine (D-fortified) | 1 tbsp | 60 |
| Yogurt (D-fortified) | 6–8 oz | 60 |
| Cereal (D-fortified) | ¾–1 c | 40 |
| Egg | 1 | 20 |

*IU = international units

# CALORIC AND FAT CONTENT OF SELECTED FAST FOODS

| Burgers | Calories | Total Fat (grams) | Saturated Fat (grams) | Percent Fat Calories |
|---|---|---|---|---|
| McDonald's Big Mac | 590 | 34 | 11 | 52 |
| McDonald's Big N' Tasty with Cheese | 590 | 37 | 12 | 56 |
| McDonald's Quarter Pounder with Cheese | 530 | 30 | 13 | 51 |
| Burger King Whopper | 760 | 46 | 15 | 54 |
| Burger King Bacon Double Cheeseburger | 580 | 34 | 18 | 53 |
| Burger King BK Smokehouse Cheddar Griller | 720 | 48 | 19 | 60 |
| Burger King Whopper with Cheese | 850 | 53 | 22 | 56 |
| Burger King Double Whopper | 1,060 | 69 | 27 | 59 |
| Burger King Double Whopper with Cheese | 1,150 | 76 | 33 | 59 |
| Wendy's Baconator | 830 | 51 | 22 | 55 |

Continued on back

# SELECTING NUTRITIOUS FOODS

Do you regularly follow the habits below?

**To select nutritious foods:**

☐ I PLAN TO  ☐ I DID IT

☐ ☐ 1. Given the choice between whole foods and refined, processed foods, choose the former (apples rather than apple pie, potatoes rather than potato chips). No nutrients have been refined out of the whole foods, and they contain less fat, salt, and sugar.

☐ ☐ 2. Choose the leaner cuts of meat. Select fish or poultry often, beef seldom. Ask for broiled, not fried, to control your fat intake.

☐ ☐ 3. Use both raw and cooked vegetables and fruits. Raw foods offer more fiber and vitamins, such as folate and thiamin, that are destroyed by cooking. Cooking foods frees other vitamins and minerals for absorption.

☐ ☐ 4. Include milk, milk products, or other calcium sources for the calcium you need. Use low-fat or non-fat items to reduce fat and calories.

Continued on back

# CALORIC AND FAT CONTENT OF SELECTED FAST FOODS

| Mexican | Calories | Total Fat (grams) | Saturated Fat (grams) | Percent Fat Calories |
|---|---|---|---|---|
| Taco Bell Crunchy Taco | 170 | 10 | 4 | 53 |
| Taco Bell Taco Supreme | 220 | 14 | 6 | 57 |
| Taco Bell Soft Chicken Taco | 190 | 7 | 3 | 33 |
| Taco Bell Bean Burrito | 370 | 12 | 4 | 29 |
| Taco Bell Fiesta Steak Burrito | 370 | 12 | 4 | 29 |
| Taco Bell Grilled Steak Soft Taco | 290 | 17 | 4 | 53 |
| Taco Bell Double Decker Taco | 340 | 14 | 5 | 37 |
| **French Fries** | | | | |
| Wendy's, biggie (5½ oz) | 440 | 19 | 7 | 39 |
| McDonald's, large (6 oz) | 540 | 26 | 9 | 43 |
| Burger King, large (5½ oz) | 500 | 25 | 13 | 45 |

# SELECTING NUTRITIOUS FOODS

**When choosing from a vending machine:**

☐ ☐ 13. Choose cracker sandwiches over chips and pork rinds (virtually pure fat). Choose peanuts, pretzels, and popcorn over cookies and candy.

☐ ☐ 14. Choose milk and juices over cola beverages.

**TRY IT**

Based on what you have learned, list strategies you can use to increase food variety, enhance the nutritive value of your diet, and decrease fat and caloric content in your meals.

Adapted from W. W. K. Hoeger, L. W. Turner, & B. Q. Hafen. Wellness: Guidelines for a Healthy Lifestyle (Wadsworth Thomson Learning, 2007).

Continued on back

5. Learn to use margarine, butter, and oils sparingly. A little gives flavor, a lot overloads you with fat, calories, and increases disease risk.

6. Vary your choices. Eat broccoli today, carrots tomorrow, and corn the next day. Eat Chinese today, Italian tomorrow, and broiled fish with brown rice and steamed vegetables the third day.

7. Load your plate with vegetables and unrefined starchy foods. A small portion of meat or cheese is all you need for protein.

8. When choosing breads and cereals, choose the whole-grain varieties.

**To select nutritious fast foods:**

9. Choose the broiled sandwich with lettuce, tomatoes, and other goodies—and hold the mayo—rather than the fish or chicken patties coated with breadcrumbs and cooked in fat.

10. Select a salad—and use more plain vegetables than those mixed with oily or mayonnaise-based dressings.

11. Order chili with more beans than meat. Choose a soft bean burrito over tacos with fried shells.

12. Drink low-fat milk rather than a cola beverage.

| Sandwiches | Calories | Total Fat (grams) | Saturated Fat (grams) | Percent Fat Calories |
|---|---|---|---|---|
| Arby's Regular Roast Beef | 350 | 16 | 6 | 41 |
| Arby's Super Roast Beef | 470 | 23 | 7 | 44 |
| Arby's Roast Chicken Club | 520 | 28 | 7 | 48 |
| Arby's Market Fresh Roast Beef & Swiss | 810 | 42 | 13 | 47 |
| McDonald's Crispy Chicken | 430 | 21 | 8 | 43 |
| McDonald's Filet-O-Fish | 470 | 26 | 5 | 50 |
| McDonald's Chicken McGrill | 400 | 17 | 3 | 38 |
| Wendy's Chicken Club | 470 | 19 | 4 | 36 |
| Wendy's Breast Fillet | 430 | 16 | 3 | 34 |
| Wendy's Grilled Chicken | 300 | 7 | 2 | 21 |
| Burger King Specialty Chicken | 560 | 28 | 6 | 45 |
| Subway Veggie Delight* | 226 | 3 | 1 | 12 |
| Subway Turkey Breast | 281 | 5 | 2 | 16 |
| Subway Sweet Onion Chicken Teriyaki | 374 | 5 | 2 | 12 |
| Subway Steak & Cheese | 390 | 14 | 5 | 32 |
| Subway Cold Cut Trio | 440 | 21 | 7 | 43 |
| Subway Tuna | 450 | 22 | 6 | 44 |

| Shakes | Calories | Total Fat (grams) | Saturated Fat (grams) | Percent Fat Calories |
|---|---|---|---|---|
| Wendy's Frosty, medium (16 oz) | 440 | 11 | 7 | 23 |
| McDonald's McFlurry, small (12 oz) | 610 | 22 | 14 | 32 |
| Burger King, Old Fashioned Ice Cream Shake, medium (22 oz) | 760 | 41 | 29 | 49 |

| Hash Browns | | | | |
|---|---|---|---|---|
| McDonald's Hash Browns (2 oz) | 130 | 8 | 4 | 55 |
| Burger King, Hash Browns, small (2½ oz) | 230 | 15 | 9 | 59 |

**TRY IT**

Using the above information, record in your Online Journal or class notebook ways you can restructure fast-food consumption to decrease caloric value and fat and saturated fat content in your diet.

*6-inch sandwich with no mayo
**Source:** Adapted from Restaurant Confidential by Michael F. Jacobson and Jayne Hurley (Workman, 2002), by permission of Center for Science in the Public Interest.

## "SUPER" FOODS

The following "super" foods that fight disease and promote health should be included often in the diet. Are you eating these foods regularly?

I PLAN TO | I DID IT

☐ ☐ Avocados
☐ ☐ Bananas
☐ ☐ Beans
☐ ☐ Beets
☐ ☐ Blueberries
☐ ☐ Broccoli
☐ ☐ Butternut squash
☐ ☐ Carrots
☐ ☐ Grapes
☐ ☐ Kale
☐ ☐ Kiwifruit
☐ ☐ Flaxseeds
☐ ☐ Nuts (Brazil, walnuts)
☐ ☐ Salmon (wild)
☐ ☐ Soy
☐ ☐ Oats and oatmeal
☐ ☐ Olives and olive oil
☐ ☐ Onions
☐ ☐ Oranges

☐ ☐ Peppers
☐ ☐ Strawberries
☐ ☐ Spinach
☐ ☐ Tea (green, black, red)
☐ ☐ Tomatoes
☐ ☐ Yogurt

**TRY IT**

Using the above list, make a list of which super foods you can add to your diet and when you can eat them (snacks/meals). List meals that you can add these foods to.

## DISEASE RISK ACCORDING TO BODY MASS INDEX (BMI)

| BMI | Disease Risk | Classification |
|---|---|---|
| <18.5 | Increased | Underweight |
| 18.5–21.99 | Low | Acceptable |
| 22.0–24.99 | Very Low | Acceptable |
| 25.0–29.99 | Increased | Overweight |
| 30.0–34.99 | High | Obesity I |
| 35.0–39.99 | Very High | Obesity II |
| ≥40.00 | Extremely High | Obesity III |

## GUIDELINES FOR A HEALTHY DIET

I PLAN TO | I DID IT

☐ ☐ Base your diet on a large variety of foods.
☐ ☐ Consume ample amounts of green, yellow, and orange fruits and vegetables.
☐ ☐ Eat foods high in complex carbohydrates, including at least three 1-ounce servings of whole-grain foods per day.
☐ ☐ Obtain most of your vitamins and minerals from food sources.
☐ ☐ Eat foods rich in vitamin D.
☐ ☐ Maintain adequate daily calcium intake and consider a bone supplement with vitamin $D_3$.
☐ ☐ Consume protein in moderation.
☐ ☐ Limit daily fat, trans fat, and saturated fat intake.
☐ ☐ Limit cholesterol consumption to less than 300 mg per day.
☐ ☐ Limit sodium intake to 2,400 mg per day.
☐ ☐ Limit sugar intake.
☐ ☐ If you drink alcohol, do so in moderation (one daily drink for women and two for men).
☐ ☐ Consider taking a daily multivitamin (preferably one that includes vitamin $D_3$).
☐ ☐ Eat cold water fish at least two times per week.

**TRY IT**

Carefully analyze the above guidelines and note the areas where you can improve your diet. Work on one guideline each week until you are able to adhere to all of the above guidelines.

## TIPS FOR LIFETIME WEIGHT MANAGEMENT

Maintenance of recommended body composition is one of the most significant health issues of the 21st century. If you are committed to lifetime weight management, the following strategies will help:

I PLAN TO | I DID IT

☐ ☐ Accumulate 60 to 90 minutes of physical activity daily.
☐ ☐ Exercise at a vigorous aerobic pace for a minimum of 20 minutes three times per week.
☐ ☐ Strength train two to three times per week.
☐ ☐ Use common sense and moderation in your daily diet.
☐ ☐ Manage daily caloric intake by keeping in mind long-term benefits (recommended body weight) instead of instant gratification (overeating).
☐ ☐ "Junior-size" instead of "super-size."
☐ ☐ Regularly monitor body weight, body composition, body mass index, and waist circumference.
☐ ☐ Do not allow increases in body weight (percent fat) to accumulate; deal immediately with the problem through moderate reductions in caloric intake and maintenance of physical activity and exercise habits.

**TRY IT**

In your Online Journal or your class notebook, note which of these tips you are already using and which ones you can incorporate into your daily habits right away.

# PHYSICAL ACTIVITY GUIDELINES FOR WEIGHT MANAGEMENT

The following physical activity guidelines are recommended to effectively manage body weight:

**I PLAN TO** / **I DID IT**

☐ ☐ 30 minutes of physical activity on most days of the week if you do not have difficulty maintaining body weight (more minutes and/or higher intensity if you choose to reach a high level of physical fitness).

☐ ☐ 60 minutes of daily activity if you want to prevent weight gain.

☐ ☐ Between 60 and 90 minutes each day if you are trying to lose weight or attempting to keep weight off following extensive weight loss (30 pounds of weight loss or more). Be sure to include some high-intensity/low-impact activities at least twice a week in your program.

## TRY IT

In your Behavior Change Planner Progress Tracker, Online Journal, or class notebook, record how many minutes of daily physical activity you accumulate on a regular basis and record your thoughts on how effectively your activity has helped you manage your body weight. Is there one thing you could do today to increase your physical activity?

## CARDIORESPIRATORY EXERCISE PRESCRIPTION

Intensity of Exercise

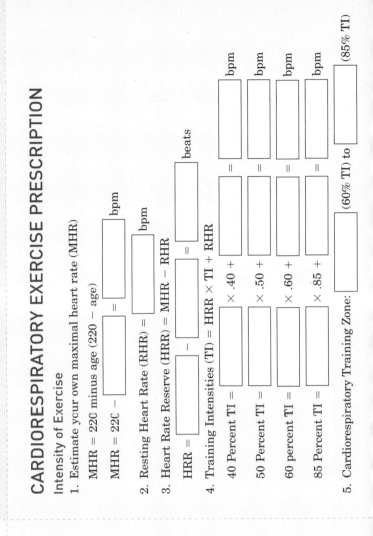

1. Estimate your own maximal heart rate (MHR)

   MHR = 220 minus age (220 − age)

   MHR = 220 − [ ] = [ ] bpm

2. Resting Heart Rate (RHR) = [ ] bpm

3. Heart Rate Reserve (HRR) = MHR − RHR

   HRR = [ ] − [ ] = [ ] beats

4. Training Intensities (TI) = HRR × TI + RHR

   40 Percent TI = [ ] × .40 + [ ] = [ ] bpm

   50 Percent TI = [ ] × .50 + [ ] = [ ] bpm

   60 percent TI = [ ] × .60 + [ ] = [ ] bpm

   85 Percent TI = [ ] × .85 + [ ] = [ ] bpm

5. Cardiorespiratory Training Zone: [ ] (60% TI) to [ ] (85% TI)

## CARDIORESPIRATORY EXERCISE PRESCRIPTION GUIDELINES

**Activity:** Aerobic (examples: walking, jogging, cycling, swimming, aerobics, racquetball, soccer, stair climbing)

**Intensity:** 40/50%–85% of heart rate reserve

**Duration:** 20–60 minutes of continuous aerobic activity

**Frequency:** 3 to 5 days per week

*Source:* American College of Sports Medicine, *ACSM's Guidelines for Exercise Testing and Prescription* (Philadelphia: Lippincott Williams & Wilkins, 2006).

## STRENGTH-TRAINING GUIDELINES

**Mode:** 8 to 10 dynamic strength-training exercises involving the body's major muscle groups

**Resistance:** 8 to 12 repetitions per set to complete or near-complete fatigue. A range of 3 to 20 repetitions to complete or near-complete fatigue, however, may also be used and appears to be just as effective. The number of repetitions is optional; you may use 3 to 6, 8 to 12, 12 to 15, or 16 to 20 repetitions.

**Sets:** A minimum of 1 set

**Frequency:** 2 to 3 days per week on nonconsecutive days

Adapted from American College of Sports Medicine, *Guidelines for Exercise Testing and Prescription* (Baltimore: Lippincott Williams & Wilkins, 2006).

# HEALTHY STRENGTH TRAINING

| I PLAN TO | I DID IT | |
|---|---|---|
| ❏ | ❏ | Make a progressive resistance strength-training program a priority in your weekly schedule. |
| ❏ | ❏ | Strength-train at least once a week; even better, twice a week. |
| ❏ | ❏ | Find a facility where you feel comfortable training and where you can get good professional guidance. |
| ❏ | ❏ | Learn the proper technique for each exercise. |
| ❏ | ❏ | Train with a friend or group of friends. |
| ❏ | ❏ | Consume a pre-exercise snack consisting of a combination of carbohydrates and some protein about 30 to 60 minutes before each strength-training session. |
| ❏ | ❏ | Use a minimum of 8 to 10 exercises that involve all major muscle groups of your body. |
| ❏ | ❏ | Perform at least one set of each exercise to near muscular fatigue. |
| ❏ | ❏ | To enhance protein synthesis, consume one post-exercise snack with a 4-to-l gram ratio of carbohydrates to protein immediately following strength training; and a second snack one hour thereafter. |
| ❏ | ❏ | Allow at least 48 hours between strength-training sessions that involve the same muscle groups. |

**TRY IT**
Attend the school's fitness or recreation center and have an instructor or fitness trainer help you design a progressive resistance strength-training program. Train twice a week for the next 4 weeks. Thereafter, evaluate the results and write down your feelings about the program.

# TIPS TO PREVENT LOW-BACK PAIN

| I PLAN TO | I DID IT | |
|---|---|---|
| ❏ | ❏ | Be physically active. |
| ❏ | ❏ | Stretch often using spinal exercises through a functional range of motion. |
| ❏ | ❏ | Regularly strengthen the core of the body using sets of 10 to 12 repetitions to near fatigue with isometric contractions when applicable. |
| ❏ | ❏ | Lift heavy objects by bending at the knees and carry them close to the body. |
| ❏ | ❏ | Avoid sitting (over 50 minutes) or standing in one position for lengthy periods of time. |
| ❏ | ❏ | Maintain correct posture. |
| ❏ | ❏ | Sleep on your back with a pillow under the knees or on your side with the knees drawn up and a small pillow between the knees. |
| ❏ | ❏ | Try out different mattresses of firm consistency before selecting a mattress. |
| ❏ | ❏ | Warm up properly using mild stretches before engaging in physical activity. |
| ❏ | ❏ | Practice adequate stress management techniques. |

**TRY IT**
In your class notebook, record how many of the above actions are a regular part of your healthy low-back program. If you are not using all of them, what is necessary to incorporate these behaviors into your lifestyle?

# GUIDELINES FOR FLEXIBILITY DEVELOPMENT

| | |
|---|---|
| **Mode:** | Slow-sustained, slow-controlled ballistic, slow-controlled proprioceptive neuromuscular facilitation stretching to include all major muscle groups |
| **Intensity:** | Stretch to tightness at the end of the range of motion |
| **Repetitions:** | Repeat each exercise 2 to 4 times and hold the final stretched position for 15 to 30 seconds |
| **Frequency:** | Minimal, 2 or 3 days per week |
| | Ideal, 5 to 7 days per week |

***Source:*** Adapted from American College of Sports Medicine, *ACSM's Guidelines for Exercise Testing and Prescription* (Baltimore: Williams & Wilkins, 2006).

# CONTRAINDICATIONS TO EXERCISE DURING PREGNANCY

Stop exercise and seek medical advice if you experience any of the following symptoms:

- Unusual pain or discomfort, especially in the chest or abdominal area
- Cramping, primarily in the pelvic or lower back areas
- Muscle weakness, excessive fatigue, or shortness of breath
- Abnormally high heart rate or a pounding (palpitations) heart rate
- Decreased fetal movement
- Insufficient weight gain
- Amniotic fluid leakage
- Nausea, dizziness, or headaches
- Persistent uterine contractions
- Vaginal bleeding or rupture of the membranes
- Swelling of ankles, calves, hands, or face

## STRESSORS IN THE LIVES OF COLLEGE STUDENTS

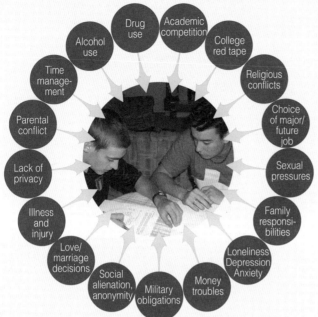

Drug use · Academic competition · College red tape · Alcohol use · Time management · Religious conflicts · Parental conflict · Choice of major/ future job · Lack of privacy · Sexual pressures · Illness and injury · Family responsibilities · Love/ marriage decisions · Loneliness Depression Anxiety · Social alienation, anonymity · Military obligations · Money troubles

Adapted from W. W. K. Hoeger, L. W. Turner, and B. Q. Hafen. *Wellness Guidelines for a Healthy Lifestyle.* Wadsworth/Thomson Learning, 2007.

## COMMON SYMPTOMS OF STRESS

Check those symptoms you experience regularly.

- ❑ Headaches
- ❑ Muscular aches (mainly in neck, shoulders, and back)
- ❑ Grinding teeth
- ❑ Nervous tic, finger tapping, toe tapping
- ❑ Increased sweating
- ❑ Increase in or loss of appetite
- ❑ Insomnia
- ❑ Nightmares
- ❑ Fatigue
- ❑ Dry mouth
- ❑ Stuttering
- ❑ High blood pressure
- ❑ Tightness or pain in the chest
- ❑ Impotence
- ❑ Hives
- ❑ Dizziness
- ❑ Depression
- ❑ Irritation
- ❑ Anger

- ❑ Hostility
- ❑ Fear, panic, anxiety
- ❑ Stomach pain, flutters
- ❑ Nausea
- ❑ Cold, clammy hands
- ❑ Poor concentration
- ❑ Pacing
- ❑ Restlessness
- ❑ Rapid heart rate
- ❑ Low-grade infection
- ❑ Loss of sex drive
- ❑ Rash or acne

### TRY IT

If you regularly experience some of the above symptoms, use your Online Journal or class notebook to keep a log of when these symptoms occur and under what circumstances. You may find out that a pattern emerges when experiencing distress in life.

## TIPS TO MANAGE ANGER

| I PLAN TO | I DID IT | |
|---|---|---|
| ❑ | ❑ | Commit to change and gain control over the behavior. |
| ❑ | ❑ | Remind yourself that chronic anger leads to illness and disease and may eventually kill you. |
| ❑ | ❑ | Recognize when feelings of anger are developing and ask yourself the following questions: |
| | | • Is the matter really that important? |
| | | • Is the anger justified? |
| | | • Can I change the situation without getting angry? |
| | | • Is it worth risking my health over it? |
| | | • How will I feel about the situation in a few hours? |
| ❑ | ❑ | Tell yourself, "Stop, my health is worth it" every time you start to feel anger. |
| ❑ | ❑ | Prepare for a positive response: Ask for an explanation or clarification of the situation, walk away and evaluate the situation, exercise, or use appropriate stress management techniques (breathing, meditation, imagery) before you become angry and hostile. |
| ❑ | ❑ | Manage anger at once; do not let it build up. |
| ❑ | ❑ | Never attack anyone verbally or physically. |

*Continued on back*

## CHOLESTEROL GUIDELINES

| | Amount | Rating |
|---|---|---|
| Total cholesterol | <200 mg/dL | Desirable |
| | 200–239 mg/dL | Borderline high |
| | ≥240 mg/dL | High risk |
| LDL cholesterol | <100 mg/dL | Optimal |
| | 100–129 mg/dL | Near or above optimal |
| | 130–159 mg/dL | Borderline high |
| | 160–189 mg/dL | High |
| | ≥190 mg/dL | Very high |
| HDL cholesterol | <40 mg/dL | Low (high risk) |
| | ≥60 mg/dL | High (low risk) |

From National Cholesterol Education Program.

## TRIGLYCERIDES GUIDELINES

| Amount | Rating |
|---|---|
| <150 mg/dL | Desirable |
| 150–199 mg/dL | Borderline high |
| 200–499 mg/dL | High |
| ≥500 mg/dL | Very high |

***Source:*** National Heart, Lung and Blood Institute.

## BLOOD GLUCOSE GUIDELINES

| Amount | Rating |
|---|---|
| ≤100 mg/dL | Normal |
| 101–125 mg/dL | Pre-diabetes |
| ≥126 mg/dL | Diabetes* |

*Confirmed by two tests on different days.

- ❑ | ❑   Keep a journal and ponder the situations that cause you to be angry.
- ❑ | ❑   Seek professional help if you are unable to overcome anger by yourself: You are worth it.

**TRY IT**

If you and others feel that anger is disrupting your health and relationships, the above management strategies are critical to help restore a sense of well-being in your life. In your Online Journal or class notebook, list all of the strategies on a separate sheet of paper, study them each morning, and then evaluate yourself every night for the next week. If you gain control over the behavior, continue with the exercise until it becomes a healthy behavior. If you still struggle, professional help is recommended. "You are worth it."

## BLOOD PRESSURE GUIDELINES (mm Hg)

| Rating | Systolic | Diastolic |
|---|---|---|
| Normal | <120 | <80 |
| Prehypertension | 121–139 | 81–89 |
| Stage 1 hypertension | 140–159 | 90–99 |
| Stage 2 hypertension | ≥160 | ≥100 |

*Source:* National High Blood Pressure Education Program.

## DIAGNOSIS OF METABOLIC SYNDROME

| Components | Men | Women |
|---|---|---|
| Waist circumference | >40 inches | >35 inches |
| Blood pressure | >130/85 mm Hg | >130/85 mm Hg |
| Fasting blood glucose | >110 mg/dL | >110 mg/dL |
| Fasting HDL cholesterol | <40 mg/dL | <50 mg/dL |
| Fasting triglycerides | >150 mg/dL | >150 mg/dL |

Note: Metabolic syndrome is identified by the presence of at least three of the above components.

## SIGNS OF HEART ATTACK AND STROKE

Any or all of the following signs may occur during a heart attack or a stroke. If you experience any of these and they last longer than a few minutes, call 911 and seek medical attention immediately. Failure to do so may cause irreparable damage and even result in death.

### Warning Signs of a Heart Attack

- Chest pain, discomfort, pressure, or squeezing that lasts for several minutes. These feelings may go away and return later.
- Pain or discomfort in the shoulders, neck, or arms or between the shoulder blades
- Chest discomfort with shortness of breath, lightheadedness, cold sweats, nausea and/or vomiting, a feeling of indigestion, sudden fatigue or weakness, fainting, or sense of impending doom

### Warning Signs of Stroke

- Sudden weakness or numbness of the face, arm, or leg—particularly on one side of the body
- Sudden severe headache
- Sudden confusion, dizziness, or difficulty with speech and understanding
- Sudden difficulty walking; loss of balance or coordination
- Sudden visual difficulty

## 2006 AMERICAN HEART ASSOCIATION DIET AND LIFESTYLE RECOMMENDATIONS FOR CARDIOVASCULAR DISEASE RISK REDUCTION

| I PLAN TO | I DID IT | |
|---|---|---|
| ☐ | ☐ | Balance caloric intake and physical activity to achieve or maintain a healthy body weight. |
| ☐ | ☐ | Consume a diet rich in vegetables and fruits. |
| ☐ | ☐ | Consume whole-grain, high-fiber foods. |
| ☐ | ☐ | Consume fish, especially oily fish, at least twice a week. |
| ☐ | ☐ | Limit your intake of saturated fat to less than 7 percent and trans fat to less than 1 percent of total daily caloric intake. |
| ☐ | ☐ | Limit cholesterol intake to less than 300 mg per day. |
| ☐ | ☐ | Minimize your intake of beverages and foods with added sugars. |
| ☐ | ☐ | Choose and prepare foods with little or no salt. |
| ☐ | ☐ | If you consume alcohol, do so in moderation. |
| ☐ | ☐ | When you eat food that is prepared outside of the home, follow the above recommendations. |
| ☐ | ☐ | Avoid use of and exposure to tobacco products. |

### TRY IT

In your Online Journal or class notebook, record which of the above recommendations you fall short on and propose at least one thing you could do to improve.

# AMERICAN HEART ASSOCIATION DIET AND LIFESTYLE GOALS FOR CARDIOVASCULAR DISEASE RISK REDUCTION

| I PLAN TO | I DID IT | |
|---|---|---|
| ☐ | ☐ | Consume an overall healthy diet. |
| ☐ | ☐ | Aim for a healthy body weight. |
| ☐ | ☐ | Aim for recommended levels of LDL cholesterol, HDL cholesterol, and triglycerides. |
| ☐ | ☐ | Aim for a normal blood pressure. |
| ☐ | ☐ | Aim for normal blood glucose levels |
| ☐ | ☐ | Be physically active. |
| ☐ | ☐ | Avoid use of and exposure to tobacco products. |

## TRY IT

To significantly offset the risk of cardiovascular disease, you need to aim for all of the above goals. You are now aware of the necessary lifestyle and dietary guidelines to do so. In your Online Journal or class notebook, outline the lifestyle changes that are required for you to meet the above goals.

# TIPS FOR A HEALTHY CANCER-FIGHTING DIET

Increase intake of phytonutrients, fiber, cruciferous vegetables, and more antioxidants by

| I PLAN TO | I DID IT | |
|---|---|---|
| ☐ | ☐ | Eating a predominantly vegetarian diet |
| ☐ | ☐ | Eating more fruits and vegetables every day (six to eight servings per day maximize anticancer benefits) |
| ☐ | ☐ | Increasing the consumption of broccoli, cauliflower, kale, turnips, cabbage, kohlrabi, Brussels sprouts, hot chili peppers, red and green peppers, carrots, sweet potatoes, winter squash, spinach, garlic, onions, strawberries, tomatoes, pineapple, and citrus fruits in your regular diet |
| ☐ | ☐ | Eating vegetables raw or quickly cooked by steaming or stir-frying |
| ☐ | ☐ | Substituting tea and fruit and vegetable juices for coffee and soda |
| ☐ | ☐ | Eating whole-grain breads |
| ☐ | ☐ | Including calcium in the diet (or from a supplement) |
| ☐ | ☐ | Including soy products in the diet |

*Continued on back*

# LIFESTYLE FACTORS THAT DECREASE CANCER RISK

Do you have these healthy lifestyle factors working in your favor?

| I PLAN TO | I DID IT | Factor | Function |
|---|---|---|---|
| ☐ | ☐ | Physical activity | Controls body weight, may influence hormone levels, strengthens the immune system. |
| ☐ | ☐ | Fiber | Contains anti-cancer substances, increases stool movement, blunts insulin secretion. |
| ☐ | ☐ | Fruits and vegetables | Contain phytonutrients and vitamins that thwart cancer. |
| ☐ | ☐ | Recommended weight | Helps control hormones that promote cancer. |
| ☐ | ☐ | Healthy grilling | Prevents formation of heterocyclic amines (HCAs) and polycyclic aromatic hydrocarbons (PAHs), both carcinogenic substances. |
| ☐ | ☐ | Tea | Contains polyphenols that neutralize free radicals, including epigallocatechin gallate (EGCG), which protects cells and the DNA from damage believed to cause cancer. |

*Continued on back*

# SIX-STEP SMOKING CESSATION APPROACH

The following six-step plan is a guide to help you quit smoking. The total program should be completed in 4 weeks or less. Steps One through Four should take no longer than 2 weeks. A maximum of 2 additional weeks are allowed for the rest of the program.

| | I PLAN TO | I DID IT | |
|---|---|---|---|
| Step One | ☐ | ☐ | Decide positively that you want to quit. Now prepare a list of the reasons why you smoke and why you want to quit. |
| Step Two | ☐ | ☐ | Initiate a personal diet and exercise program. Exercise and decreased body weight cause a greater awareness of healthy living and increase motivation for giving up cigarettes. |
| Step Three | ☐ | ☐ | Decide on the approach you will use to stop smoking. You may quit cold turkey or gradually decrease the number of cigarettes smoked daily. Many people have found that quitting cold turkey is the easiest way to do it. Although it may not work the first time, after several attempts, all of a sudden smokers are able to overcome the habit without too much difficulty. Tapering off cigarettes can be done in several ways. You may start by eliminating cigarettes that you do not necessarily need, you can switch to a brand lower in |

*Continued on back*

| | | |
|---|---|---|
| ❑ | ❑ | Using whole-wheat flour instead of refined white flour in baking |
| ❑ | ❑ | Using brown (unpolished) rice instead of white (polished) rice |

Decrease daily fat intake to 20 percent of total caloric intake by

| | | |
|---|---|---|
| ❑ | ❑ | Limiting consumption of beef, poultry, or fish to no more than 3 to 6 ounces (about the size of a deck of cards) once or twice a week |
| ❑ | ❑ | Trimming all visible fat from meat and removing skin from poultry prior to cooking |
| ❑ | ❑ | Decreasing the amount of fat and oils used in cooking |
| ❑ | ❑ | Substituting low-fat for high-fat dairy products |
| ❑ | ❑ | Using salad dressings sparingly |
| ❑ | ❑ | Using only half to three-quarters of the amount of fat required in baking recipes |
| ❑ | ❑ | Limiting fat intake to mostly monounsaturated (olive oil, canola oil, nuts, and seeds) and omega-3 fats (fish, flaxseed, and flaxseed oil) |
| ❑ | ❑ | Eating fish once or twice a week |
| ❑ | ❑ | Including flaxseed oil in the diet |

**TRY IT**

Make a copy of these "Cancer-Fighting Diet" tips and each week incorporate into your lifestyle two additional dietary behaviors from the above list.

---

**Step Four** nicotine or tar every couple of days, you can smoke less of each cigarette, or you can simply decrease the total number of cigarettes smoked each day. Set the target date for quitting. Choose a special date to add a little extra incentive: An upcoming birthday, anniversary, vacation, graduation, family reunion—all are examples of good dates to free yourself from smoking.

**Step Five** Stock up on low-calorie foods—carrots, broccoli, cauliflower, celery, popcorn (butter- and salt-free), fruits, sunflower seeds (in the shell), sugarless gum, and plenty of water. Keep such food handy on the day you stop and the first few days following cessation. Use it whenever you want a cigarette.

**Step Six** This is the day that you will quit smoking. On this day and the first few days thereafter, do not keep cigarettes handy. Stay away from friends and events that trigger your desire to smoke. Drink large amounts of water and fruit juices and eat low-calorie foods. Replace the old behavior with new behavior. You will need to replace smoking time with new positive substitutes that will make smoking difficult or impossible. When you desire a cigarette, take a few deep breaths and then occupy yourself by doing a number of things such as talking to someone else, washing your hands, brushing your teeth, eating a healthy snack, chewing on a straw, doing dishes, playing sports, going for a walk or bike ride, going swimming, and so on.

| | | |
|---|---|---|
| ❑ | ❑ | Step Four |
| ❑ | ❑ | Step Five |
| ❑ | ❑ | Step Six |

---

| | | | |
|---|---|---|---|
| ❑ | ❑ | Spices | Provide phytonutrients and strengthen the immune system. |
| ❑ | ❑ | Vitamin D | Disrupts abnormal cell growth. |
| ❑ | ❑ | Monounsaturated fat | May contribute to cancer cell destruction. |

**TRY IT**

In your Online Journal or class notebook, note ways you can incorporate all of these factors into your everyday lifestyle.